26 Update in Intensive Care and Emergency Medicine

Edited by J.-L. Vincent

Springer-Verlag Berlin Heidelberg GmbH

J. L. Rombeau   J. Takala   (Eds.)

Gut Dysfunction in Critical Illness

With 80 Figures and 29 Tables

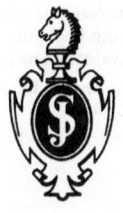

Springer

Series Editor

Prof. Jean-Louis Vincent
Clinical Director, Department of Intensive Care
Erasme University Hospital
Route de Lennik 808, B-1070 Brussels, Belgium

Volume Editors

Prof. J. L. Rombeau
Pennsylvania University Hospital
Department of Surgery
3400 Spruce Street, PA 19104 Philadelphia, USA

Prof. J. Takala
Kuopio University Hospital
Department of Intensive Care
Critical Care Research Program
FIN-70211 Kuopio, Finland

ISBN 978-3-642-80226-3   ISBN 978-3-642-80224-9 (eBook)
DOI 10.1007/978-3-642-80224-9

Library of Congress Cataloging-in-Publication Data applied for

Die Deutsche Bibliothek – CIP-Einheitsaufnahme
Gut dysfunction in critically illness : with 29 tables / J. L. Rombeau ; J. Takala (ed.). – Berlin ;
Heidelberg ; New York ; Barcelona ; Budapest ; Hong Kong ; London ; Milan ; Paris ; Santa
Clara ; Singapore ; Tokyo : Springer, 1996
   (Update in intensive care and emergency medicine ; 26)
NE: Rombeau, J. L. [Hrsg.]; GT

Typesetting and printing: Zechnersche Buchdruckerei, Speyer
Bookbinding: J. Schäffer, Grünstadt
SPIN: 10527313   19/3133-5 4 3 2 1 0 – Printed on acid-free paper

Table of Contents

List of Contributors

Bahrami S.
Ludwig Boltzmann Institute
for Experimental and Clinical
Traumatology,
Donaueschingenstrasse 13,
1200 Vienna, Austria

Cabie A.
Dept of Infectious Diseases,
Hôpital Bichat-Claude Bernard,
46 Rue Henri Huchard,
75018 Paris, France

Carlet J.
Dept of Intensive Care,
Hôpital Saint Joseph,
Rue Pierre Larousse 7,
75674 Paris Cedex 14, France

Cerra F. B.
Dept of Surgery,
University of Minnesota Hospital,
420 Delaware Street SE, Minneapolis
MN 55455, USA

Chagnon J. L.
Dept of Anesthesiology, Valenciennes
Hospital, Avenue Desandroins,
59322 Valenciennes Cédex, France

Cholley B.
Dept of Anesthesiology,
Lariboisière Hospital,
2 rue Ambroise Paré,
75010 Paris, France

Erlandsen S. L.
Dept of Cell Biology and
Neuroanatomy,
University of Minnesota,
420 Delaware Street SE,
Minneapolis MN 55455-0374, USA

Evans T. W.
Dept of Critical Care,
National Heart & Lung Institute,
Royal Brompton Hospital,
Sydney Street, London SW3 6NP,
United Kingdom

Faehnrich J.
Dept of Anesthesiology,
Duke University Medical Center
POBox 3094, Durham NC 27710, USA

Fink M. P.
Dept of Surgery, Beth Israel Hospital,
330 Brookline Avenue,
Boston MA 02215, USA

Frankel H. L.
Dept of Surgery, Hospital
of the University of Pennsylvania,
3400 Spruce Street,
Philadelphia PA 19104, USA

Fürst P.
Institute for Biological Chemistry
and Nutrition,
University of Hohenheim,
Garbenstrasse 30, 70593 Stuttgart,
Germany

Georgieff M.
Universitätsklinik für Anästhesiologie,
Klinikum der Universität,
Steinhovelstrasse 9,
89075 Ulm, Germany

Goris R. J. A.
Dept of Surgery,
University Hospital Nijmegen,
G. Grooteplein 14,
6500 HB Nijmegen,
The Netherlands

Groeneveld A. B. J.
Medical Intensive Care Unit,
Free University Hospital,
De Boelelaan 1117,
1081 HV Amsterdam, The Netherlands

Haglund U.
Dept of Surgery, University Hospital,
751 85 Uppsala, Sweden

Jansen M. M. J.
Dept of Surgery,
University Hospital Nijmegen,
G. Grooteplein 14,
6500 HB Nijmegen, The Netherlands

Kubes P.
Dept of Medical Physiology,
University of Calgary,
3330 Hospital Drive, Calgari Alberta
T2N 4N1, Canada

Marshall J. C.
Dept of General and Critical Care
Surgery, Toronto General Hospital,
200 Elizabeth Street, Eaton North,
9-234, Toronto ONT M5G 2C4, Canada

McVay L. D.
Dept of Microbiology, University of
Pennsylvania School of Medicine,
1033 Blockley Hall,
Philadelphia PA 19104-6021, USA

Moore E. E.
Dept of Surgery, University of
Colorado Health Sciences Center,
Denver CO, USA

Moore F. A.
Dept of Surgery,
University of Texas Medical School,
6431 Fannin, MSB 4.264,
Houston TX 77030, USA

Mythen M.
Dept of Anesthesiology and Critical
Care, Duke University Medical Center
PO Box 3094, Durham NC 27710,
USA

Nevière R.
Dept of Anesthesiology,
Calmette Hospital,
Bld du Prof. Leclercq,
59037 Lille Cedex, France

Nieuwenhuijzen, G. A. P.
Dept of Surgery,
University Hospital Nijmegen,
G. Grooteplein 14,
6500 HB Nijmegen, The Netherlands

Payen D.
Dept of Anesthesiology,
Lariboisière Hospital,
2 rue Ambroise Paré,
75010 Paris, France

Radermacher P.
Universitätsklinik für Anästhesiologie,
Klinikum der Universität,
Steinhovelstrasse 9, 89075 Ulm,
Germany

Redl H.
Ludwig Boltzmann Institute for
Experimental and Clinical
Traumatology,
Donaueschingenstrasse 13,
1200 Vienna, Austria

Rombeau J. L.
Dept of Surgery,
University of Pennsylvania Hospital,
3400 Spruce Street,
Philadelphia PA 19104, USA

Schlag G.
Ludwig Boltzmann Institute
for Experimental and Clinical
Traumatology,
Donaueschingenstrasse 13,
1200 Vienna, Austria

Schumacker P. T.
Dept of Pulmonary and Critical Care
Medicine, The University of Chicago,
5841 South Maryland Avenue,
Chicago IL 60637, USA

Sinclair D. G
Dept of Critical Care,
National Heart & Lung Institute,
Royal Brompton Hospital,
Sydney Street, London SW3 6NP,
United Kingdom

Singer M.
Dept of Intensive Care Medicine,
Bloomsbury Institute of Intensive Care
Medicine, Rayne Institute Building,
University Street, London WC1E 6JJ,
United Kingdom

Soeters P. B.
Dept of Surgery,
University Hospital Maastricht,
P. Debyelaan 25,
6202 AZ Maastricht,
The Netherlands

Stoutenbeek C. P.
Dept of Intensive Care,
Academic Medical Center,
Meibergdreef 9,
1105 AZ Amsterdam,
The Netherlands

Takala J.
Dept of Intensive Care,
Kuopio University Hospital,
70211 Kuopio, Finland

Tamion F.
Dept of Intensive Care,
Centre Hospitalier Universitaire,
76000 Rouen, France

Vallet B.
Dept of Anesthesiology,
Claude Huriez Hospital,
Place de Verdun,
59037, Lille Cedex, France

van der Hulst R. R. W. J.
Dept of Surgery,
University Hospital Maastricht,
P. Debyelaan 25,
6202 AZ Maastricht,
The Netherlands

van Saene H. K. F.
Dept of Intensive Care,
Academic Medical Center,
Meibergdreef 9, 1105 AZ Amsterdam,
The Netherlands

Vincent J. L.
Dept of Intensive Care,
Erasme University Hospital,
Route de Lennik 808, 1070 Brussels,
Belgium

von Meyenfeldt M. F.
Dept of Surgery,
University Hospital Maastricht,
P. Debyelaan 25,
6202 AZ Maastricht, The Netherlands

Wells C. L.
Dept of Laboratory Medicine,
Pathology and Surgery,
University of Minnesota,
420 Delaware Street
SE, Minneapolis MN 55455-0374, USA

Zhang H.
Dept of Intensive Care,
Erasme University Hospital,
Route de Lennik 808,
1070 Brussels, Belgium

Ziegler T. R.
Dept of Endocrinology and
Metabolism, Emory University
1365 Clifton Road,
Atlanta GA 30322, USA

Common Abbreviations

ADP	Adenosine diphosphate
ARDS	Acute respiratory distress syndrome
ATI	Abdominal trauma index
ATP	Adenosine triphosphate
BPI	Bactericidal permeability increasing protein
BT	Bacterial translocation
cAMP	Cyclic adenosine monophosphate
CPB	Cardiopulmonary bypass
DNA	Desoxyribonucleic acid
DO_2	Oxygen delivery/supply
EGF	Epidermal growth factor
EN	Enteral nutrition
GALT	Gut-associated lymphoid tissue
GF	Growth factors
GH	Growth hormone
GI	Gastrointestinal
Glu	Glutamine
GM-CSF	Granulocyte macrophage colony stimulating factor
GSH	Glutathione
I/R	Ischemia/reperfusion
ICG	Indocyanine green
ICU	Intensive care unit
IFN-γ	Interferon gamma
IGF	Insulin-like growth factor
IL	Interleukin
iNOS	Inducible nitric oxide synthase
ISS	Injury severity score
LBP	Lipopolysaccharide binding protein
LPS	Lipopolysaccharide

MALT	Mucosal-associated lymphoid tissue
MCP	Monocyte-chemoattractant protein
MLN	Mesenteric lymph nodes
MODS	Multiple organ dysfunction syndrome
MOF	Multiple organ failure
mRNA	Messenger ribonucleic acid
NO	Nitric oxide
O_2ER	Oxygen extraction
ODC	Ornithine decarboxylase
OFR	Oxygen free radical
PAF	Platelet activating factor
PDH	Pyruvate dehydrogenase
pHi	Gastric intramucosal pH
PMN	Polymorphonuclear leukocyte
TPN	Total parenteral nutrition/feeding
ROM	Reactive oxygen metabolites
SBF	Splanchnic blood flow
SBS	Short bowel syndrome
SCFA	Short chain fatty acids
SDD	Selective digestive decontamination
SIRS	Systemic inflammatory response syndrome
SNAP	S-nitroso-N-acetylpenicillamine
TGF	Transforming growth factor
TNF	Tumor necrosis factor
VO_2	Oxygen consumption/uptake

Gastrointestinal Structure and Function

Pathophysiology of Gut Dysfunction in Shock and Sepsis

U. Haglund

Introduction

It is generally assumed that gut dysfunction occurs early in shock, sepsis and following trauma, and that gut dysfunction may influence the further development into multiple organ failure (MOF) [1]. The concept that gut dysfunction and mucosal injury of the gut is an unfavorable prognostic sign in surgical critical illness is fairly widely accepted [2, 3]. However, there is much more controversy as to whether there is a causal relationship between mucosal injury and development of MOF, and if so by which mechanisms this relation is excerpted.

This chapter is concentrated on the mechanisms by which gut dysfunction occurs in shock conditions.

Intestinal Blood Flow

The intestines have a relative overperfusion as related to the needs of the tissue [4]. This is partly due to the fact that blood flow to the intestines in addition to providing oxygen (O_2) to the tissue and transporting metabolites from the tissue also is a vehicle for absorbed nutritions. Intestinal blood flow is through the portal system an important provider of O_2 to the liver.

The regulation of the intestinal blood flow is complex [5]. The vascular smooth muscle cells have an intrinsic control, autoregulating blood flow over a wide pressure range. In addition, local metabolites, nervous influence, peptide hormones, and various circulating vasoactive substances cooperate in the control of intestinal blood flow [4, 5]. Hemorrhage decreases intestinal blood flow [6]. This is not only due to reduced cardiac output. Especially following hemorrhage and cardiac tamponade, there is a disproportionate reduction of intestinal blood flow. There is evidence that the renin-angiotensin system is very important for the intestinal vascular control during hemorrhage and cardiac tamponade [7]. In sepsis, blood flow is reduced in proportion to changes in cardiac output, and the renin-angiotensin system seems to exert little or no influence [8].

The intestinal vascular bed can compensate for the reduced blood flow by increased O_2 extraction (O_2ER). Consequently, the intestinal blood flow can be reduced to about 50% of control without any significant effect on the local intestinal oxygen consumption (VO_2) [9]. As a consequence of the increased intestinal O_2ER, the intestinal venous blood contains very little O_2 in this situation. Low oxygen delivery (DO_2) with the portal blood flow cannot be compensated fully by increased hepatic arterial blood flow and, hence, flow-dependent hepatic hypoxia is a likely consequence. This has also been demonstrated to be the consequence in experimental peritonitis [10].

The small intestine is best regarded as several independent vascular circuits coupled in parallel [11]. The mucosal circuit is of especial interest during critical illness. The vascular arrangement in the mucosa is peculiar. The villus layer has a countercurrent exchange situation between the centrally located arterial vessels and the subepithelial network of small veins and capillaries. The arterial vessel does not branch until it reaches the tip of the villus. The distance between these two sets of vessels with mainly opposite direction of flow is small enough to allow diffusion equilibrium for easily diffusible substances [12]. In this context, the possibility for diffusion of O_2 from the arterial to the venous side at the base of the villi is of considerable interest. Such short-circuiting of O_2 has been demonstrated experimentally [12]. It has, further more, been demonstrated that the O_2 concentration at the tip of the villi is very low also in normal situations [13] and it becomes close to zero in hypotension. The normally low oxygenation of the tips of the villi explains how the addition of fairly low amounts of O_2 by intralumenal perfusion of oxygenated saline can protect from hypoxic injury [12, 14]. Reduced blood flow, prolonging the time available for obtaining a diffusion equilibrium of O_2 will further exaggerate the hypoxic situation. As a consequence, the tip of the villi might become anoxic despite an almost normal volume of blood flowing through the tissue [12, 14].

Intramucosal pH

The superficial mucosa is the part of the intestinal vascular bed which most rapidly demonstrate dysfunction and morphologic signs of injury. The oxygenation of the superficial part of the intestinal mucosa can be monitored by tonometry as described by Fiddian-Green and co-workers [15, 16]. This technique, which will be described in more details elsewhere in this volume, has provided means for more detailed analyses of the pathophysiology of gut dysfunction in shock.

Using the tonometric technique for monitoring intramucosal pH (pHi) it was demonstrated that reduced pHi was rapidly seen following hemorrhage [17], endotoxemia [18], bacteriemic sepsis [19], and peritonitis [20]. Experiments performed on pigs revealed a simultaneous shift, qualitatively to a very similar degree, when pHi was followed in the stomach, the small intestine and in the sigmoid colon during hemorrhage and bacteriemic sepsis. In hemorrhagic shock, pHi became only slightly abnormal after 1 h of blood pressure at 80 mmHg, but significantly reduced after 1 h at 45 mmHg at which situation arterial pH was not abnormal [17]. In bacteriemic sepsis, pHi decreased before arterial blood pressure or arterial pH indicated critical illness [20]. In septic conditions, pHi decreased despite maintained or even increased O_2 metabolism [18, 20]. Interestingly, in a recent series of experiments, intestinal mucosal permeability increased and pHi decreased in the animals made septic by continuous endotoxin infusion, while non-septic animals with partial occlusion of the superior mesenteric artery – graded to give an equal reduction of intestinal blood flow – had an unchanged permeability [20]. It could be concluded that there is something in addition to intestinal ischemia that causes reduced pHi and increased permeability in sepsis.

In recent experiments in our laboratory, it was demonstrated that intramucosal pH of the small intestine decreased rapidly following induction of fecal peritonitis [19, 22, 23]. This occurred despite maintained DO_2 and despite an approximately 70% increase in VO_2 (Fig. 1) [10, 19]. It was hypothesized that recruitment to the tissue and activation there of circulating white blood cells was of importance for the increased splanchnic tissue O_2 in sepsis. Therefore, experiments were repeated using a monoclonal antibody against the CD11/CD18 complex to prevent adherence of white blood cells to the vascular endothelium. It could be concluded from those experiments that circulating white blood cells probably do not contribute significantly to the increased splanchnic consumption during sepsis [24]. There is still an open question whether activated resident white blood cells and macrophages are of importance.

There are several recent findings indicating that O_2 metabolism might be disturbed during sepsis [25]. Recent data from our laboratory have indicated that

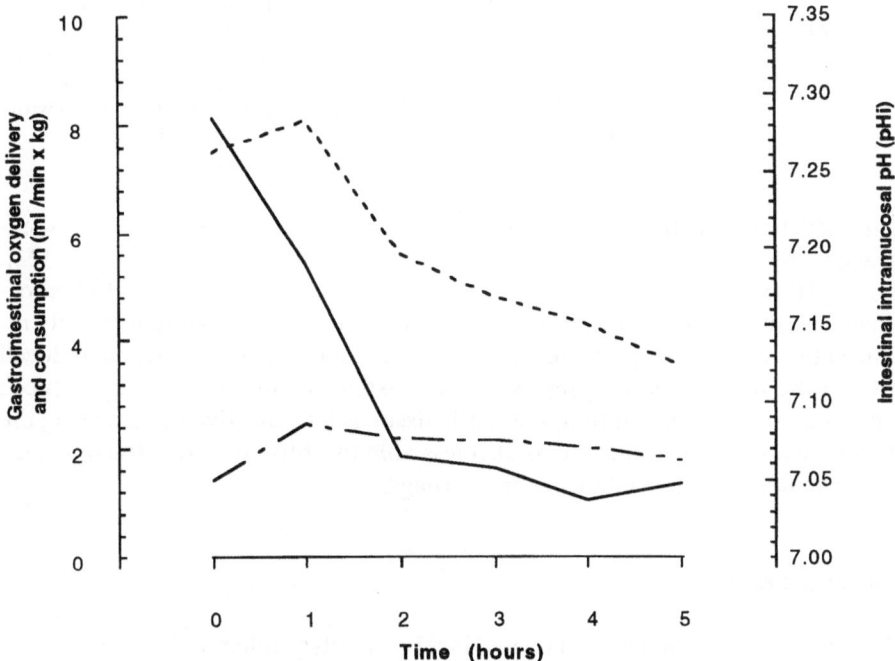

Fig. 1. Intestinal DO_2 (upper interrupted line), pHi obtained by a tonometer (solid line), and intestinal VO_2 (lower interrupted line) during fecal peritonitis. Note the sharp decrease of pH, despite elevated DO_2 and VO_2 maintained at least at 60% of baseline. (Adapted from [19]).

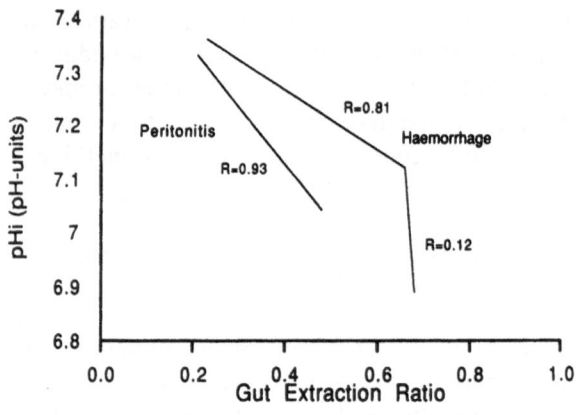

Fig. 2. Association between gut pHi and O_2ER of the gut. Note the increased extraction in hemorrhage which seems to reach a cut off at approximately 2/3. More pronounced ischemia does not provoke higher O_2ER by the small intestine. (From [23] with permission).

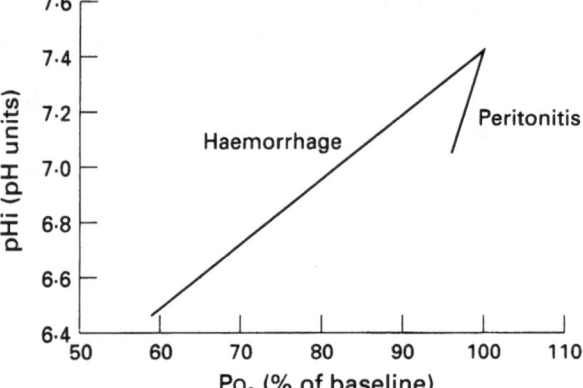

Fig. 3. Association between pH and pO_2 of the superficial gut mucosa. The difference in R. values (0.06 vs 0.63) is statistically significant ($p < 0.002$). (From [22] with permission).

the reduction in pHi in sepsis occurs despite a much less increase in the O_2 extraction by the tissue compared to the situation in hemorrhage (Fig. 2) [22]. Also, pHi falls in sepsis despite a maintained local pO_2 (Fig. 3) [23]. In hemorrhage, on the contrary, the reduction in pHi is associated with a significantly reduced tissue pO_2. It is concluded from the series of experiments that the reduced pHi of the intestine during sepsis to some extent might be caused by reduced DO_2 (blood flow). In addition, the septic tissue is less effective in increasing the O_2 extraction ratio, and it seems also less able to utilise the O_2 extracted compared to normal tissue following hemorrhage.

Mucosal Injury

Shock, intestinal ischemia and related insults rapidly produce a characteristic injury to the intestinal mucosa [26, 27]. The pathogenesis of the intestinal mucosal injury is briefly outlined in Table 1. This injury has been characterized by Chiu and coworkers (1970) using a grading system from 0 (normal mucosa) to 5 (de-

Table 1. Mechanisms causing mucosal injury of the gut during critical illness

1. Ischemic components of injury
   - Decreased oxygen delivery
   - - Reduce blood flow to the organ
   - - Uneven distribution of blood flow (oxygen) within the organ
   - Increased oxygen demand
   - Decreased oxygen extraction
   - Decreased oxygen utilization
2. Reperfusion component
   - Increased generation of oxygen derived free radicals

struction of the mucosa) [28]. The grading system suggested by these authors has more or less generally been adhered to in subsequent reports, probably because this system is logically based on the pathogenesis of mucosal injury. The Chiu grading system is based on the appearance in the light microscope. Experimental data has demonstrated that the grade of injury is indirectly related to the amount of blood flow to the intestine and directly proportional to the duration of the ischemia [28]. The initial form of tissue injury following reduced DO_2 is characterized by lifting of the epithelial cells at the tips of the villi. In more severe grades of mucosal injury, the villus core structure is injured. It is characteristic for this type of tissue injury that deeper mucosal structures than the villus layer is never affected during ischemia induced by circulatory shock states [29]. This type of mucosal injury has most frequently been studied in animal experiments. The *post mortem* autolysis induces a very similar change. However, it is demonstrated, studying biopsies taken at surgery, that also patients in shock develop the same injury [29]. We do not know, on the other hand, how severe the hemodynamic situation has to be or how long it has to be impaired to induce injury, nor do we know in which frequency critically ill patients do develop intestinal mucosal injury.

In a situation with mechanical occlusion of the intestinal blood flow, the deeper layers of the intestine will demonstrate microscopic signs of injury, ultimately transmural infarction which may be evident after 8–16 h [30]. It takes about 20 min for light microscopic mucosal changes to be apparent in the light microscope following total occlusion of intestinal blood flow [31]. Changes are detectable much earlier in the electron microscope [32]. Following shock and sepsis, it takes 1–2 h to develop injury detectable in the light microscope.

There is abundant experimental evidence to support that even supply of minor amounts of O_2 by intraluminal perfusion prevents the developments of the mucosal injury following shock conditions [14, 33, 34]. The low normal tissue pO_2 at the tips of the villi explains how addition of such small amounts of O_2 may benefit [13]. Also following occlusion of the superior mesenteric artery, perfusion with O_2 containing solutions intraluminally can prevent mucosal injury and even intramucosal acidosis [34]. This strongly suggests the hypoxic nature of the mucosal injury.

The superficial mucosal injury confined to the villi may heal rapidly provided the hemodynamic situation is normalized. Superficial injury of the very tips seems to heal within 4 h, while deeper villous injury was not healed until 18 h after restoration of normal blood flow [35].

Reperfusion Injury

There is abundant experimental evidence that mucosal injury caused by ischemia may be exacerbated following ischemia at reperfusion [29, 34–39]. This reperfusion component of injury is dependent on a certain degree of proceeding ischemic injury. On the other hand, as is illustrated also in other organs like the kidney, a severe ischemic injury will make exacerbation at reperfusion undetectable [31, 40]. The background for the development of the reperfusion component is an increased generation of O_2 free radicals [36, 38, 39]. The basic mechanism for generation of O_2 free radicals at reperfusion is probably the xanthine oxidase pathway as originally proposed by Granger and co-workers [36]. Xanthine dehydrogenase is abundantly available in the intestinal mucosa. It is converted by a proteolytic process during ischemia to xanthine oxidase [41, 42]. Hypoxanthine becomes converted to xanthine and urea upon reperfusion when O_2 is available in high amounts. This process is catalysed by xanthine oxidase, and as a consequence superoxide anion is created. This O_2 derived radical might cause microcirculatory disturbance and further tissue injury by injury to endothelial cells. In addition, radicals might be formed in various chain reactions and more aggressive radicals than superoxide anion will result. Another consequence of radical formation is activation of leukocytes which in turn generate more O_2 free radicals. The end-process will be significantly disturbed tissue microcirculation and exacerbation of tissue injury [43]. The reperfusion component of intestinal ischemic injury is very interesting from a theoretical stand point but there is no support for the concept that reperfusion of the intestine plays an important role in critical illness. Increased generation of O_2 free radicals, probably caused by other mechanisms in addition to reperfusion, may during the course of severe disease be very important for subcellular events, such as those responsible for increased intestinal mucosal permeability, and for triggering macrophages and polymorphonuclear leukocytes (PMNs) in the septic response.

Importance of Gut Dysfunction

Reduced pHi is considered the initial indicator of tissue dysfunction in critical illness. The first functional variable demonstrated to deteriorate during shock is the barrier function and especially the mucosal permeability for solutes like inulin, manitol and Cr^{51}-EDTA [21, 44]. It has been hypothesized that this increased mucosal permeability to some extent might reflect a possibility for increased translocation of bacteria and endotoxin. This latter phenomenon has been repeatedly demonstrated in small experimental animals [45], but data from larger animals and especially clinical data are less convincing [46, 47].

The recently most often discussed dysfunction caused by hypoxia, and during certain circumstances exacerbated at reperfusion, may cause translocation of bacteria and endotoxin. Increased intestinal mucosal permeability has been demonstrated by several groups experimentally and clinically. However, there is conflicting data as whether the increased intestinal mucosal permeability is related to septic complications and the development of MOF in severely injured patients or not [48, 49]. Release of cardiotoxic substances and other toxic substances has been described as a consequence of intestinal mucosal injury although their clinical importance is not yet well defined [50–53]. Recently, the importance of intestinal component of the immune system has been emphasized. Ischemia is likely to cause significant changes in that system [54]. In addition, release of mediators from the intestine, influencing the activity of total body immune system, has also been described during ischemia and shock conditions [55, 56].

Conclusion

There is a considerable evidence indicating that the gut frequently becomes hypoxic during critical illness. A hypoxic gut becomes acidotic, and increased permeability and signs of morphologic mucosal injury develop rapidly. These changes are generally regarded as serious prognostic signs although the exact mechanism by which the dysfunctioning gut promotes the further development of irreversible shock and multiple organ failure remains to be defined.

References

1. Marston A, Bulkley GB, Fiddian-Green RG, Haglund UH (eds) (1989) Splanchnic ischemia and multiple organ failure, Edward Arnold, London
2. Gutierrez G, Palizas F, Doglio G, et al (1992) Gastric intramucosal pH as a therapeutic index of tissue oxygenation in critically ill patients. Lancet 339:195–199
3. Maynard N, Bihari D, Beale R, et al (1993) Assessment of splanchnic oxygenation by gastric tonometry in patients with acute circulatory failure. JAMA 270:1203–1210
4. Lundgren O (1989) Physiology of the intestinal circulation. In: Marston A, Bulkley GB, Fiddian-Green RG, Haglund U (eds), Splanchnic ischemia and multiple organ failure, Edward Arnold, London, pp 29–40
5. Folkow B (1971) Regulation of the peripheral circulation. Br Heart J 33 (Suppl):27–31
6. Haglund U, Lundgren O (1972) The effects of vasoconstrictor fibre stimulation on the consecutive vascular sections of the small intestine of the cat during prolonged regional hypotension. Acta Physiol Scand 85:547–558
7. Bailey RW, Bulkley GB, Hamilton SR, et al (1987) Protection of the small intestine from nonocclusive mesenteric ischemic injury due to cardiogenic shock. Am J Surg 153:108–116
8. Arvidsson D, Lindgren S, Almqvist P, et al (1990) Role of the renin-angiotensin system in liver blood flow reduction produced by positive end-expiratory pressure ventilation. Acta Chir Scand 156:353–358
9. Bulkley GB, Kvietys PR, Parks DA, et al (1985) Relationship of blood flow and oxygen consumption to ischemic injury in the canine small intestine. Gastroenterology 89:852–857
10. Arvidsson D, Rasmussen I, Almqvist P, et al (1991) Splanchnic oxygen consumption in septic and hemorrhagic shock. Surgery 2:190–197

11. Folkow B (1967) Regional adjustments of intestinal blood flow. Gastroenterology 2: 423–432
12. Lundgren O, Haglund U (1978) The pathophysiology of the intestinal countercurrent exchanger. Life Sciences 23: 1411–1422
13. Bohlen HG (1980) Intestinal tissue PO_2 and microvascular responses during glucose exposure. Am J Physiol 238 (Heart Circ Physiol 7): H164–H171
14. Falk A, Redfors S, Myrvold HE, et al (1985) Small intestinal mucosal lesions in feline septic shock: A study on the pathogenesis. Circ Shock 17: 327–337
15. Grum CM, Fiddian-Green RG, Pittenger GL, et al (1984) Adequacy of tissue oxygenation in intact dog intestine. J Appl Physiol 56: 1065–1069
16. Fiddian-Green RG (1989) Studies in splanchnic ischemia and multiple organ failure. In: Marston A, Bulkley GB, Fiddian-Green RG, Haglund U (eds) Splanchnic ischemia and multiple organ failure, Edward Arnold, London, pp 347–363
17. Montgomery A, Hartmann M, Jönsson K, et al (1989) Intramucosal pH measurement with tonometers for detecting gastrointestinal ischemia in porcine hemorrhagic shock. Circ Shock 29: 319–327
18. Fink MP, Cohn SM, Lee PC, et al (1989) Effect of lipopolysaccharide on intestinal intramucosal hydrogen ion concentration in pigs. Evidence of gut ischemia in a normodynamic model of septic shock. Crit Care Med 17: 641–646
19. Rasmussen I, Haglund U (1992) Early gut ischemia in experimental fecal peritonitis. Circ Shock 38: 22–28
20. Montgomery A, Almqvist P, Arvidsson D, et al (1990) Early detection of gastrointestinal mucosal ischemia in porcine E. coli sepsis. Acta Chir Scand 146: 613–620
21. Fink MP, Cohn SM, Lee PC, et al (1991) Maintenance of superior mesenteric arterial perfusion prevents increased intestinal mucosal permeability in endotoxic pigs. Surgery 110: 154–161
22. Antonsson JB, Haglund UH (1995) Gut intramucosal pH and intraluminal PO_2 in a porcine model of peritonitis or haemorrhage. Gut 37: 791–797
23. Antonsson JB, Engström L, Rasmussen I, et al (1995) Changes in gut intramucosal pH and gut oxygen extraction ratio in a porcine model of peritonitis and hemorrhage. Crit Care Med 23: 1872–1881
24. Wollert S, Rasmussen I, Lundberg C, et al (1993) Inhibition of CD18-dependent adherence of polymorphonuclear leukocytes does not affect liver oxygen consumption in fecal peritonitis in pigs. Circ Shock 41: 230–238
25. Gutierrez G, Lund N, Bryan-Brown CW (1989) Cellular oxygen utilization during multiple organ failure. Crit Care Med 5: 271–287
26. Haglund U (1991) Hypoxic damage of the gut in shock. In: Schalg G, Redl H, Siegel JH, Traber DL (eds) Shock sepsis and organ failure. Springer-Verlag, Berlin, pp 314–321
27. Wollert S, Antonsson J, Gerdin B, et al (1995) Intestinal mucosal injury during porcine faecal peritonitis. Eur J Surg 161: 741–750
28. Chiu Dd-J, McArdle AH, Brown R, et al (1970) Intestinal mucosal lesion in low-flow states. I. A Morphological, hemodynamic and metabolic reappraisal. Arch Surg 101: 478–483
29. Haglund U, Hultén L, Lundgren O, et al (1975) Mucosal lesions in the human small intestine in shock. Gut 16: 979–984
30. Haglund U, Bulkley GB, Granger DN (1987) On the pathophysiology of intestinal ischemic injury. Acta Chir Scand 153: 321–324
31. Park PO, Haglund U, Bulkley GV, et al (1990) The sequence of development of intestinal tissue injury following strangulation ischemia and reperfusion. Surgery 107: 574–580
32. Brown RA, Chiu C-J, Scott HJ, et al (1970) Ultrastructural changes in the canine ileal mucosal cell after mesenteric arterial occlusion. Arch Surg 101: 290–297
33. Shute K (1976) Effect of intraluminal oxygen on experimental ischaemia of the intestine. Gut 17: 1001–1006
34. Haglund U (1993) Therapeutic potential of intraluminal oxygenation. Crit Care Med 21: S69–S71
35. Park PO, Haglund U (1992) Regeneration of small bowel mucosa after intestinal ischemia. Crit Care Med 20: 135–139

36. Granger DN, Rutili G, McCord JM (1981) Superoxide radicals in feline intestinal ischemia. Gastroenterology 81:22-29
37. Parks DA, Bulkley GB, Granger DN, et al (1982) Ischemic injury in the cat small intestine: Role of superoxide radicals. Gastroenterology 82:9-15
38. Schoenberg MH, Poch B, Younes M, et al (1991) Involvement of neutrophils in post-ischaemic damage to the small intestine. Gut 32:905-912
39. Morris JB, Haglund UH, Bulkley GB, et al (1986) Direct demonstration of oxygen free radical generation from a living, intact organ (the feline intestine). Surg Forum 37:123-125
40. Hoshino T, Maley WR, Bulkley GB, et al (1988) Arbation of free radical-mediated reperfusion injury for the salvage of kidneys taken from non-heartbeating donors. Transplantation 45:284-289
41. Parks DA, Williams TK, Beckman JS (1988) Conversion of xanthine dehydrogenase to oxidase in ischemic rat intestine: A reevaluation. Am J Physiol (Gastrointest Liver Physiol 17) 254:G768-G774
42. Bulkely GB (1994) Reactive oxygen metabolites and reperfusion injury: Aberrant triggering of reticuloendothelial function. Lancet 344:934-936
43. Granger DN (1988) Role of xanthine oxidase and granulocytes in ischemia-reperfusion injury. Am J Physiol 255 (Heart Circ Physiol 24):H1269-H1275
44. Schlichting E, Grotmol T, Kähler H, et al (1995) Alterations in mucosal morphology and permeability, but no bacterial or endotoxin translocation take place after intestinal ischemia and early reperfusion in pigs. Shock 3:116-124
45. Deitch E (1992) Multiple organ failure. Ann Surg 216:117-134
46. Moore FA, Moore EE, Poggetti R, et al (1991) Gut bacterial translocation via the portal vein: A clinical perspective with major torso trauma. J Trauma 31:629-638
47. Brathwaite CEM, Ross SE, Nagele R, et al (1993) Bacterial translocation occurs in humans after traumatic injury: Evidence using immunofluorescence. J Trauma 34:586-590
48. Pape HC, Dwenger A, Regel G, et al (1994) Increased gut permeability after multiple trauma. Br J Surg 81:850-852
49. Roumen RMH, Hendriks T, Wevers A, et al (1993) Intestinal permeability after severe trauma and hemorrhagic shock is increased without relation to septic complications. Arch Surg 128:453-457
50. Haglund U, Lundgren O (1973) Cardiovascular effects of blood borne material release from the cat small intestine during simulated shock conditions. Acta Physiol Scand 89:558-570
51. Haglund U, Myrvold H, Lundgren O (1978) Cardiac and pulmonary function in regional intestinal shock. Arch Surg 113:963-969
52. Hallström S, Doidl B, Müller U, et al (1991) A cardiodepressant factor isolated from blood blocks Ca^{2+} current in cardiomyocytes. Am J Physiol 260 (Heart Circ Physiol 29) 260: H869-H876
53. Parrillo JE, Burch C, Shelhamer JH, et al (1985) A circulating myocardial depressant substance in humans with septic shock. Septic shock patients with a reduced ejection fraction have a circulating factor that depresses in vitro myocardial cell performance. J Clin Invest 76:1539-1553
54. Österberg J, Johnsson C, Gannedahl G, et al (1996) Alterations in mucosal immune cell distribution in septic rats. Shock (in press) (Abst)
55. Deitch EA, Dazhong X, Franko L, et al (1994) Evidence favoring the role of the gut as a cytokine-generating organ in rats subjected to hemorrhagic shock. Shock 1:141-146
56. Moore EE, Moore FA, Franciose RJ, et al (1994) The postischemic gut serves as a priming bed for circulating neutrophils that provoke multiple organ failure. J Trauma 37:881-887

Intestinal Mucosal Hyperpermeability in Critical Illness

M. P. Fink

Introduction

The gut serves not only as a physiologic portal for the entry of water and nutrients into the body, but also as a barrier limiting the systemic absorption of intraluminal microbes and/or microbial products. The intestinal epithelium *per se* represents a critical barrier against systemic absorption of intralumenal microbes and microbial products. The ability of the intestinal epithelium to selectively permit the absorption of nutrients, electrolytes, and water, but restrict the passage from the lumen of larger, potentially toxic hydrophilic compounds is thought to be mediated by the tight junctions ("zonula occludens") surrounding each cell in the epithelial sheet [1]. Under normal circumstances, tight junctions exclude passive movement of hydrophilic noncharged compounds with a molecular radius > 11.5 Å [1]. Substances that are therefore prevented from paracellular transepithelial movement include the amphipathic compound, lipopolysaccharide (LPS) [2], as well as a variety of other bacteria-derived proinflammatory hydrophilic compounds, such as formyl-methionyl-leucyl-phenylalanine (FMLP) [3] and peptidoglycan-polysaccharides [4], which are present in high concentration within the lumen of the distal small intestine and colon.

Epithelial permeability to hydrophilic solutes is not constant, but is dynamically regulated under both physiologic and pathophysiologic conditions [1]. Thus, intestinal epithelial permeability can be modulated by a number of factors, including changes in intracellular cAMP concentration [5], insulin [6], insulin-like growth factors [7], activators of protein kinase C [8], and cytokines [9, 10].

Modulation of Intestinal Epithelial Permeability under Pathophysiologic Conditions

Mucosal Hypoxia

Certain pathophysiologic processes can reduce oxygen delivery (DO_2) to the mucosa below a critical value (DO_{2crit}) such that oxygen consumption (VO_2) becomes supply-dependent [11]. Supply-dependency of VO_2 can occur as a result of tissue hypoperfusion, arterial hypoxemia, or anemia. Hypermetabolism, secondary to sepsis and other critical illnesses, necessitates a higher VO_2, thereby increasing DO_{2crit} [12]. Alone or in combination, these factors may limit intracellular PO_2 to levels inadequate to support normal mitochondrial respiration.

There are two important consequences of impaired mitochondrial respiration due to intracellular hypoxia. First, the cell attempts to preserve adequate levels of adenosine triphosphate (ATP) by increasing the rate of anaerobic glycolysis. In contrast to oxidative phosphorylation, substrate level phosphorylation of adenosine diphosphate (ADP) during glycolysis leads to the net production of protons; in other words, intracellular acidosis is an inevitable consequence of enhanced anaerobic metabolism [13]. Second, if mitochondrial respiration is sufficiently limited, then intracellular levels of ATP will be depleted. As will be discussed below, both intracellular acidosis and ATP depletion can lead to increases in intestinal epithelial permeability.

Oxidant Stress

Oxidants have been implicated in a variety of causes of intestinal barrier dysfunction. In experimental animals, intestinal ischemia followed by reperfusion leads to mucosal hyperpermeability and biochemical evidence of oxidant stress [14, 15]. During the reperfusion phase, spin trapping techniques have been used to demonstrate the formation of free radicals [16].

There are two main sources of reactive oxygen metabolites (ROMs) in intestinal ischemia/reperfusion:
1) the reaction catalyzed by xanthine oxidase, and
2) the reaction catalyzed by NADPH oxidase in neutrophils sequestered in the intestinal microvasculature.

Agents which scavenge ROMs or inhibit xanthine oxidase have been shown to ameliorate derangements in intestinal barrier function following intestinal ischemia/reperfusion [17]. These strategies also have been shown to have salutary effects on barrier function in animals subjected to hemorrhage [18] or systemic inflammation [19–21].

The mechanisms whereby oxidants impair barrier function are not well understood. In various *in vitro* models, however, oxidants, such as hydrogen peroxide (H_2O_2) or superoxide radical ($O_2^{-\bullet}$) have been shown to increase the permeability of epithelial [22] or endothelial [23] monolayers. Oxidants also disrupt the cytoskeleton (by promoting excessive actin polymerization) [23, 24]. ROMs can lead to ATP depletion [25–27]. As will be discussed below, ATP depletion is another potential factor contributing to epithelial barrier dysfunction. The mechanisms responsible for oxidant-mediated ATP depletion probably include inhibition of glyceraldehyde-3-phosphate dehydrogenase (in the glycolytic pathway) and inhibition of mitochondrial phosphorylation of ADP [28].

Mucosal Acidosis

As already noted, acidosis is a consequence of increased substrate level phosphorylation of ADP during glycolysis in hypoxic cells. In sepsis, tissue acidosis can occur even in the absence of hypoperfusion or hypoxia [29, 30]. Sepsis downregulates the activity of pyruvate dehydrogenase (PDH), the enzyme complex catalyzing the first irreversible step in the mitochondrial oxidative pathway [31]. The shift of PDH to its inactive form in sepsis fosters increased flux through the glycolytic pathway without a commensurate increase in mitochondrial oxidative phosphorylation. Glycolytic flux also may be increased in sepsis as a result of increased availability of glucose transporters on the surface of cells [32]. Using both *in vivo* and *in vitro* model systems, our group has investigated the effects of acidosis on intestinal epithelial permeability. When pigs are subjected to either systemic endotoxemia or partial mechanical occlusion of the mesenteric artery [33], there is a strong direct correlation between the degree of ileal mucosal acidosis and the degree of ileal mucosal hyperpermeability induced by these perturbations (Fig. 1). This finding suggests that the adverse effects of endotoxemia or ischemia on intestinal epithelial permeability might be related to the resultant derangements in tissue pH rather than simply the changes in tissue oxygenation *per se*. This notion is further supported by the observation that ileal epithelial permeability is increased in pigs when mucosal acidosis is induced in the absence of tissue hypoxia by acutely elevating arterial carbon dioxide (CO_2) tension (Fig. 2).

In other studies, we have employed cultured Caco-2$_{BBe}$ cells growing on permeable supports in bicameral chambers as a reductionist model of the intestinal epithelium. Caco-2 cells reproduce many of the features of normal absorptive small intestinal epithelium [34]. The use of an *in vitro* model system, such as Caco-2 monolayers, permits much more control over experimental conditions than is possible in studies using experimental animals. *In vitro* models using cultured cells, however, inevitably represent an oversimplification of the complex *in vivo* environment. Moreover, immortalized cell lines, like Caco-2, may not accurately mimic all the characteristics of normal enterocytes. Using the Caco-2 model system, we have shown that acidosis increases permeability *in vitro* (unpublished observations).

The mechanism(s) whereby acidosis promotes epithelial hyperpermeability are unknown. It has been established, however, that acidosis can promote the formation of oxidants. A number of studies have shown that acidosis promotes lipid peroxidation [35–39], a finding which we have confirmed in the Caco-2$_{BBe}$ system (unpublished observations). Acidosis promotes mobilization of free iron from intracellular stores [40, 41], and evidence has been presented supporting the view that oxidant stress under conditions of acidosis depends, at least in part, on iron delocalization [41]. Recent findings [42] suggest that another mechanism whereby acidosis enhances oxidant-mediated damage is inhibition of two key enzymes: glutathione reductase which is required to regenerate reduced glutathione (GSH), and glutathione peroxidase which uses GSH to convert H_2O_2 to water.

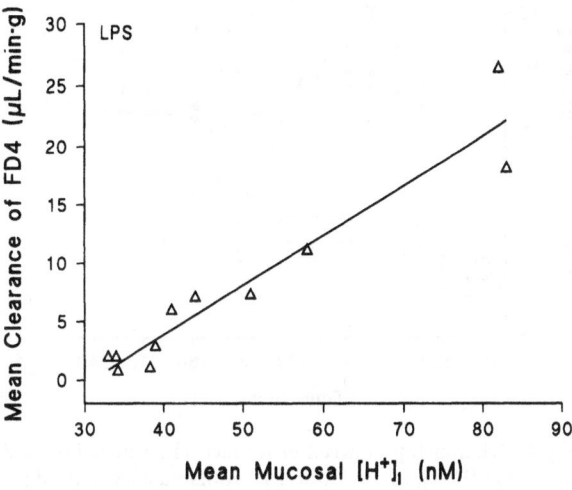

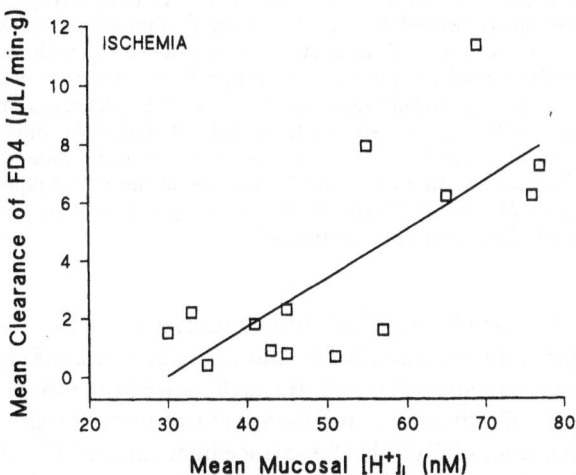

Fig. 1. Relationship between ileal mucosal permeability and ileal mucosal hydrogen ion concentration $[H^+]_i$ in anesthetized pigs subjected to mesenteric ischemia induced by infusion of LPS (upper panel) or partial mechanical occlusion of the superior mesenteric artery (lower panel). Mucosal permeability was assessed by measuring the plasma-to-lumen clearance of fluorescein isothiocyanate dextran with an average molecular mass of 4000 Daltons (FD4). Each point represents the mean values for $[H^+]_i$ (x-axis) and FD4 clearance (y-axis) obtained in a single animal over a 4-h period of observation. Over a broad range of responses to LPS, mean $[H^+]_i$ and mean FD4 clearance were strongly and linearly correlated ($R^2 = 0.93$; $p < 0.0001$). Similary, when mesenteric ischemia was induced by partial mechanical occlusion of the superior mesenteric artery, mean $[H^+]_i$ and mean FD4 clearance were linearly correlated ($R^2 = 0.58$, $p < 0.002$). (From [33] with permission)

Another way the acidosis might alter epithelial permeability is by increasing intracellular calcium concentration ($[Ca^{2+}]_i$) [43]. Possible mechanisms for the tendency of low gastric intramucosal pH (pHi) to increase $[Ca^{2+}]_i$ in epithelial

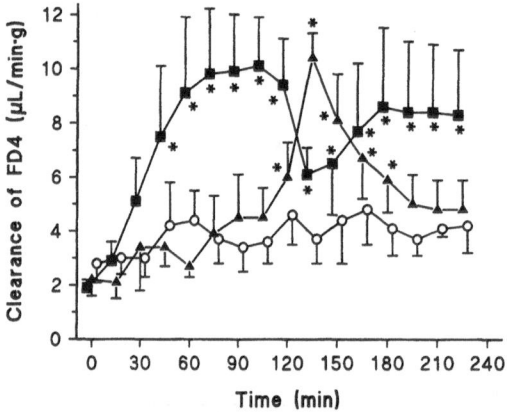

Fig. 2. Relationship between ileal mucosal permeability and ileal mucosal hydrogen ion concentration $[H+]_i$ in mechanically ventilated anesthetized pigs breathing a normal gas mixture (open circles), a hypoxic gas mixture (solid squares), or a hypercapnic gas mixture (solid triangles). After a period of stabilization during which time all animals were ventilated with a normal gas mixture, ventilation with the hypoxic or hypercapnic gas mixtures was started at $T = 0$ min and continued throught $T = 120$ min. At the end of the 120 min experimental period, ventilation with a normal gas mixture was resumed for an additional 120 min period of observation. In the normal gas mixture, the fractional oxygen concentration was 0.5 and the fractional carbon dioxide concentration was < 0.01. In the hypoxic gas mixture, the fractional oxygen concentration was ~ 0.1 and the fractional carbon dioxide concentration was < 0.01. In the hypercapnic gas mixture, the fractional oxygen concentration was 0.5 and the fractional carbon dioxide concentration was 0.25. Values are means ± SE. * points which are significantly different ($p < 0.05$) than the baseline value within group (one-way analysis of variance and Dunnett's test). (From [33] with permission)

cells include increased mitochondrial Ca^{2+}-H^+ exchange, modulation of Ca^{2+} flux into the smooth ER, and activation of a pH-dependent plasma membrane Ca^{2+} channel [43]. The effects of ionized calcium on epithelial integrity are complex. On the one hand, formation of normal tight junctions depends upon the presence of Ca^{2+} in the extracellular milieu [44]. On the other hand, elevations in *intracellular* $[Ca^{2+}]$ loosen tight junctions and increase epithelial permeability [45–48].

Although alterations in epithelial permeability to hydrophilic solutes are generally thought to represent changes in the size of the water-filled paracellular "pore," recent findings from our laboratory call this idea into question. In our studies using monolayers of Caco-2_{BBe} cells to study acidosis-induced epithelial hyperpermeability, we employed fluorescence confocal microscopy to visualize a fluorescent probe, fluorescein-labelled dextran with an average molecular weight of 4000 Da (FD4). Using this technique, we showed that FD4 is localized to the apical surface of cells incubated under physiological (i.e. normal pH) conditions (unpublished observations). The apical localization of FD4 probably represents uptake of the probe via endocytotic fluid-phase pinocytosis. In similar studies, Hidalgo et. al. [49] have demonstrated that presentation of horseradish peroxidase to the apical surface of polarized Caco-2 monolayers at 37 °C results in fluid-phase pinocytosis of this macromolecule into numerous multivesicular bodies that are clustered just beneath the terminal web.

In contrast to the normal apical uptake of FD4, Caco-2$_{BBe}$ cells that have been exposed to an acidic milieu for 24 h take up large quantities of FD4 and the fluorescent probe is present in both the apical and basolateral regions of the enterocytes (unpublished observations). This finding suggests that acidosis-induced hyperpermeability might be caused, at least in part, by an increase in the transcellular movement of hydrophilic macromolecules across the intestinal epithelial monolayer. Transcellular transport of the hydrophilic probe could occur as a result of either accelerated endocytotic fluid-phase pinocytosis or simple diffusion through compromised plasma membranes. However, since pinocytosis is an energy requiring process, and monolayer ATP levels are significantly reduced after incubation at low pH, it is unlikely that this mechanism is increased under acidotic conditions. Furthermore, studies have demonstrated that cytoplasmic acidification below pH 6.8 inhibits the endocytotic uptake of fluid-phase markers, as well as overall intracellular vesicular trafficing [50].

In order to further investigate the mechanism of acidosis-induced hyperpermeability, we assessed the temperature dependency of the flux of another fluorescent probe, fluorescein sulfonic acid (FS) across Caco-2$_{BBe}$ monolayers incubated under normal or acidic conditions. Incubation of monolayers at 4 °C significantly reduces permeability to FS under both control (pH$_0$ 7.40) and acidic (pH$_0$ 5.43) conditions. However, the cold-induced decrease in permeability is significantly greater for monolayers incubated at pH 5.43 as compared to pH 7.40. The apparent activation energy for permeation by FS across Caco-2$_{BBe}$ monolayers maintained at pH 7.40 is about 8 kcal/mole. This value agrees well with the calculated activation energy (8.2 kcal/mole) for permeation of monolayers by another hydrophilic solute of similar size, namely the chemotactic peptide N-formylmethionyl-leucyl-phenylalanine [51]. Activation energies in this range are consistent with permeation via a paracellular pathway [51–53]. In contrast, the apparent activation energy for permeation by FS across Caco-2$_{BBe}$ monolayers maintained at pH 5.43 is about 15 kcal/mole, which suggests contribution from a transcellular pathway [53]. The increase in enthalpy for FS permeation across the Caco-2$_{BBe}$ monolayers is consistent with diffusion of a hydrophilic molecule through a lipid barrier (i.e. compromised plasma membranes). The observed decrease in FS permeability under acidotic conditions at 4 °C compared to 37 °C is probably related to a temperature-induced decrease in plasma membrane fluidity.

ATP Depletion

As noted above, ATP depletion is a consequence of impaired mitochondrial function due to intracellular hypoxia. ATP depletion also can be caused by oxidant stress, leading to inhibition of glyceraldehyde-3-phosphate dehydrogenase (in the glycolytic pathway) and inhibition of mitochondrial phosphorylation of ADP [28]. Acidosis, in a form of positive feed-back, also can promote ATP depletion [54], perhaps by inhibiting the rate-limiting phosphofructokinase step in glycolysis [55, 56] or via other poorly understood mechanisms [54].

In order to investigate the role of ATP depletion as a factor leading to intestinal hyperpermeability, we recently studied the effects of chronic hypoxia or glycolytic inhibition with 2-deoxyglucose (2-DOG) in glucose-free buffer on Caco-2_{BBe} monolayers [57]. In both scenarios, we found that relatively minor reductions (<30%) in ATP content were sufficient to increase the permeability of Caco-2_{BBe} monolayers. The mechanism appears to involve derangements in the actin-based cytoskeleton, since laser confocal micrographs using rhodamine-phalloidin to stain polymerized (F) actin demonstrated perijunctional condensation of actin filaments after prolonged 2-DOG exposure.

In these studies, we observed that Caco-2_{BBe} monolayers are much more sensitive to glycolytic inhibition than hypoxia [57]. Whereas hypoxia is associated with the development of lactic acidosis, ATP depletion caused by glycolytic inhibition does not lead to a decrease in intracellular pH. Apparently, hypoxia-induced acidosis, provided that the decrease in intracellular pH is relatively minor, helps Caco-2_{BBe} cells defend against ATP depletion [57]. Similar protective effects of mild acidosis have been observed in other systems [58–60]. Thus, depending upon the degree of pH change, acidosis can either protect against or promote epithelial barrier dysfunction.

Nitric Oxide

Nitric oxide (NO) is an important regulator and/or effector of many phenomena in the cardiovascular, nervous, and immune systems [61]. It is becoming increasingly apparent that NO also plays a versatile role in the physiology and pathophysiology of the gastrointestinal (GI) tract [62]. A large variety of cell types in the gut are potential sources of NO. These cell types include myenteric neurons [63–66], vascular endothelial cells [66, 67], and interstitial cells of Cajal [68]. Inflammatory cells in the submucosa, including mast cells [69], macrophages [70, 71], and polymorphonuclear leukocytes [72, 73], are capable of producing NO. Luminal bacteria represent another potential source of NO in the GI tract [74].

Enterocytes also appear to be capable of producing NO, at least under certain conditions. Tepperman et al. [75], however, have documented upregulation of inducible nitric oxide synthase (iNOS) activity in enterocytes harvested from the colons of rats injected 4 h earlier with LPS. Prior administration of an anti-neutrophil antiserum prevents LPS-induced leukosequestration in the colonic mucosa, but has no effect on measured levels of iNOS activity, supporting the view that infiltrating neutrophils are not the source of the iNOS activity in enterocytic preparations from endotoxic rats. Grisham et al. [76] have demonstrated that exposure of cultured IEC-18 (rat intestinal epithelial) cells to LPS, interleukin-1 (IL-1), or tumor necrosis factor α (TNF-α) plus interferon gamma (IFN-γ) increases the production nitrite plus nitrate (markers of NO production). Dignass et al. [77] showed that incubation of cultures of another rat enterocytic cell line (IEC-6) with a number of different cytokines (e.g. IL-2, TNF-α) results in modest increases in the production of nitrogen oxides. Recently, our group [10] has shown that incubation of Caco-2$_{BBe}$ cells with the proinflammatory cytokine, IFN-γ, increases the release of markers of increased NO production (nitrite and nitrate anions) into the media. Even more recently, we have shown that incubation of Caco-2$_{BBe}$ cells with INF-γ upregulates expression of iNOS messenger ribonucleic acid (mRNA) (unpublished observations).

NO appears to be capable of modulating intestinal epithelial permeability. Depending upon the experimental system employed, NO can either diminish or increase intestinal permeability to various water-soluble molecules. Low (i.e. physiologic) concentrations of NO tend to preserve mucosal function under both normal conditions [78] and in certain pathological states, such as ischemia/reperfusion injury [79, 80] or endotoxemia [81, 82]. Nevertheless, overproduction of NO can damage the integrity of the intestinal mucosal barrier. For example, Lopez-Belmonte et al. [83] showed that close arterial infusion of NO donors, SNP or S-nitroso-N-acetylpenicillamine (SNAP), causes gastric mucosal damage in the rat when infused at high concentrations. Similarly, Tepperman et al. [75] reported that NO donors, such as SNP or SNAP, decrease the *ex vivo* viability of freshly harvested rat colonic epithelial cells [75]. Tepperman et al. [75, 84] also showed that *in vivo* administration of LPS decreases the viability of gut epithelial cells via a NO-dependent mechanism. Recently, our group [85] demonstrated that NO$^\bullet$ donors (SNP or SNAP) as well as authentic NO gas are capable of increasing the permeability of Caco-2$_{BBe}$ monolayers to a variety of hydrophilic macromolecules. The deleterious effect of NO on barrier function appears to be mediated through derangements in intracellular ATP production and cytoskeletal organization [85].

Cytokines

Recent studies performed using cultured enterocytic monolayers suggest that certain proinflammatory cytokines, namely IFN-γ and IL-4, are capable of increasing the permeability of model epithelia [9, 86, 87]. The mechanism(s) whereby cytokines, such as IFN-γ, induces intestinal epithelial hyperpermeability has not been determined. It is known, however, that IFN-γ, acting either alone or in combination with other cytokines, is capable of triggering increased production of NO by a number of different cell types [88–91]. Thus, it seems plausible that cytokine-induced intestinal epithelial hyperpermeability is mediated through induction iNOS leading excess NO production. In support of this view are recent data published by our group [10] showing that: 1) incubation of Caco-2$_{BBe}$ (enterocytic) cells with IFN-γ increases the release of NO oxidation products (nitrite and nitrate) into culture supernatants (Fig. 3); 2) Caco-2$_{BBe}$ monolayers can be rendered hyperpermeable by incubation in media containing IFN-γ (Fig. 4); and 3) co-incubation of Caco-2$_{BBe}$ monolayers with INF-γ and various NOS inhibitors significantly blunts the development of hyperpermeability (Fig. 4).

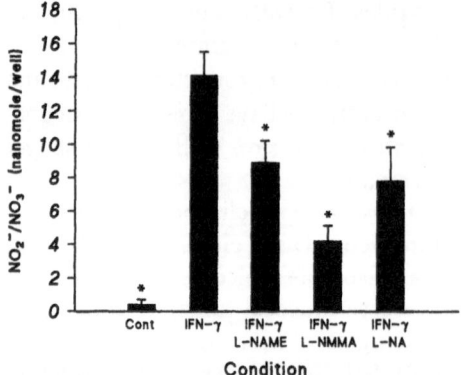

Fig. 3. Accumulation of nitrite (NO_2^-) and nitrate (NO_3^-) products of nitric oxide (NO) oxidation, supernatants of cultured Caco-2$_{BBe}$ intestinal epithelial monolayers incubated with the cytokine, interferon- γ (IFN-γ), for 7 days. IFN-γ was present in the incubation medium at a concentration of 1000 U/mL. In some cases, various inhibitors of NO biosynthesis were added as well. These inhibitors included: N^G-nitro-L-arginine methyl ester (L-NAME; 5 mM), N^G-monomethyl-L-arginine (L-NMMA; 5 mM), and N^G-nitro-L-arginine (L-NA, 1 mM). Means ± SE. * $p < 0.05$ for comparisons with monolayers incubated with IFN-γ alone. (From [10] with permission)

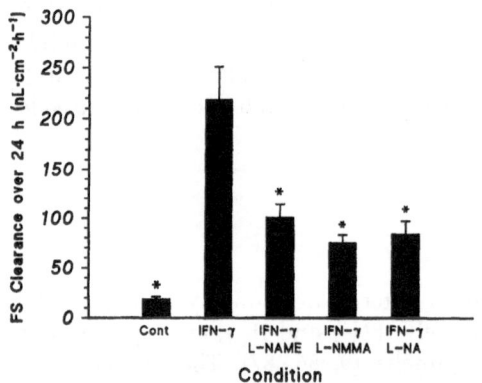

Fig. 4. Effects of incubation with the cytokine, interferon-γ (IFN-γ), for 7 days in the presence or absence of various inhibitors of NO synthesis on the permeability of Caco-2$_{BBe}$ monolayers to the fluorescent probe, fluorescein sulfonic acid (FS). Permeability is expressed as the apical-to-basolateral clearance of the probe over the final 24 h of incubation. The following nitric oxide synthesis inhibitors were employed: N^G-nitro-L-arginine methyl ester (L-NAME; 5 mM), N^G-monomethyl-L-arginine (L-NMMA; 5 mM), and N^G-nitro-L-arginine (L-NA, 1 mM). Means ± SE. * $p < 0.01$ for comparisons with monolayers incubated with IFN-γ alone. (From [10] with permission)

Conclusion

One important component of the intestinal barrier is the epithelium itself. Under normal circumstances, tight junctions between adjacent enterocytes enable the epithelium to manifest selectively permeability, such that the absorption of water and nutrients is permitted, but larger, potentially toxic or pro-inflammatory substances are excluded from the subepithelial compartment. In critical illness, a number of factors may play a role in causing increases in intestinal epithelial permeability. Some possible mechanisms leading to epithelial hyperpermeability in critical illness are suggested by studies performed *in vivo* using various animal models and *in vitro* using cultured enterocytic monolayers as a model of the intestinal epithelium. Factors contributing to the development of hyperpermeability in critically ill patients may include mucosal hypoxia, oxidant stress, mucosal acidosis, toxic effects of nitric oxide, and deleterious effects of certain cytokines.

Acknowledgement: This work was supported by a grant (2 R01 GM37631-11) from the National Institutes of Health.

References

1. Madara JL (1989) Loosening tight junctions: Lessons from the intestine. J Clin Invest 83: 1089-1094
2. van Deventer SJM, tenCate JW, Tytgat GNJ (1988) Intestinal endotoxemia: Clinical significance. Gastroenterology 94:823-831
3. Chadwick VS, Mellor DM, Myers DB, et al (1988) Production of peptides inducing chemotaxis and lysozomal enzyme release in human neutrophils by intestinal bacteria *in vitro* and *in vivo*. Scand J Gastroenterol 23:121-128
4. Lichtman SN, Okoruwa EE, Keku J, et al (1992) Degradation of endogenous bacterial cell wall polymers by the muralytic enzyme mutanolysin prevents hepatobiliary injury in genetically susceptible rats with experimental intestinal bacterial overgrowth. J Clin Invest 90: 1313-1322
5. Duffey ME, Hainau B, Ho S, et al (1981) Regulation of epithelial tight junction permeability by cyclic AMP. Nature 294:451-453
6. McRoberts JA, Aranda R, Riley N, et al (1990) Insulin regulates the paracellular permeability of cultured intestinal epithelial cell monolayers. J Clin Invest 85:1127-1134
7. McRoberts JA, Riley NE (1992) Regulation of T84 cell monolayer permeability by insulin-like growth factors. Am J Physiol 262:C207-C213
8. Stenson WF, Easom RA, Riehl TE, et al (1993) Regulation of paracellular permeability in Caco-2 cell monolayers by protein kinase C. Am J Physiol 265:G995 (Abst)
9. Adams RB, Planchon SM, Roche JK (1993) IFN-γ modulation of epithelial barrier function: Time course, reversibility, and site of cytokine binding. J Immunol 150:2356-2363
10. Unno N, Menconi MJ, Smith M, et al (1995) Nitric oxide mediates interferon-gamma-induced hyperpermeability in cultured human intestinal epithelial monolayers. Crit Care Med 23:1170-1176
11. Hochachka PW (1987) Metabolic suppression and oxygen availability. Can J Zool 66:152-158
12. Heard SO, Baum TD, Wang H, et al (1991) Systemic and mesenteric O_2 metabolism in endotoxic pigs: Effect of graded hemorrhage. Circ Shock 35:44-52
13. Mommsen TP, Hochachka PW (1983) Protons and anaerobiasis. Science 219:1391-1397
14. Granger DN, Rutili G, McCord JM (1981) Superoxide radicals in feline intestinal ischemia. Gastroenterology 81:22-29
15. Granger DN (1988) Role of xanthine oxidase and granulocytes in ischemia-reperfusion injury. Am J Physiol 255:H1269-H1275
16. Nilsson UA, Lundgren O, Haglind E, et al (1989) Radical production during *in vivo* intestinal ischemia and reperfusion in the cat. Am J Physiol 257:G409-G414
17. Otamiri T (1989) Oxygen radicals, lipid peroxidation, and neutrophil infiltration after small-intestinal ischemia and reperfusion. Surgery 105:593-597

18. Deitch EA, Bridges W, Baker J, et al (1988) Hemorrhagic shock-induced bacterial transloca-
    tion is reduced by xanthine oxidase inhibition or inactivation. Surgery 104:191–198
19. Deitch EA, Specian RD, Berg RD (1991) Endotoxin-induced bacterial translocation and mu-
    cosal permeability: Role of xanthine oxidase, complement activation, and macrophage pro-
    ducts. Crit Care Med 19:785–791
20. Mainous MR, Xu D, Deitch EA (1993) Role of xanthine oxidase and prostaglandins in in-
    flammatory-induced bacterial translocation. Circ Shock 40:99–104
21. Deitch EA, Ma L, Ma JW, et al (1989) Inhibition of endotoxin-induced bacterial transloca-
    tion in mice. J Clin Invest 84:36–42
22. Welsh MJ, Shasby DM, Husted RM (1985) Oxidants increase paracellular permeability in a
    cultured epithelial cell line. J Clin Invest 76:1155–1168
23. Hinshaw DB, Burger JM, Beals TF, et al (1991) Actin polymerization in cellular oxidant in-
    jury. Arch Biochem Biophys 288:311–316
24. Hinshaw DB, Burger JM, Miller MT, et al (1993) ATP depletion induces an increase in the
    assembly of a labile pool of polymerized actin in endothelial cells. Am J Physiol 264:
    C1171–C1179
25. Wilson J, Winter M, Shasby DM (1990) Oxidants, ATP depletion, and endothelial permeabi-
    lity to macromolecules. Blood 76:2578–2582
26. Hinshaw DB, Burger JM, Armstrong BC, et al (1989) Mechanism of endothelial cell shape
    change in oxidant injury. J Surg Res 46:339–349
27. Hinshaw DB, Burger JM (1990) Protective effect of glutamine on endothelial cell ATP in oxi-
    dant injury. J Surg Res 49:222–227
28. Hyslop PA, Hinshaw DB, Halsey WA Jr, et al (1988) Mechanism of oxidant-mediated cell
    injury: The glycolytic and mitochondrial pathways of ADP phosphorylation are major in-
    tracellular targets inactivated by hydrogen peroxide. J Biol Chem 253:1665–1675
29. Hotchkiss RS, Karl IE (1992) Reevaluation of the role of cellular hypoxia and bioenergetic
    failure in sepsis. J Am Med Assoc 267:1503–1509
30. Vandermeer TJ, Wang H, Fink MP (1995) Endotoxemia causes ileal mucosal acidosis in the
    absence of mucosal hypoxia in a normodynamic porcine model of septic shock. Crit Care
    Med 23:1217–1226
31. Vary TC, Siegel JH, Nakatani T, et al (1986) Effect of sepsis on activity of pyruvate dehydro-
    genase complex in skeletal muscle and liver. Am J Physiol 250:E634–E640
32. Zeller WP, The SM, Sweet M, et al (1991) Altered glucose transporter mRNA abundance in a
    rat model of endotoxic shock. Biochem Biophys Res Commun 176:535–540
33. Salzman AL, Wang H, Wollert PS, et al (1994) Endotoxin-induced ileal mucosal hyperper-
    meability in pigs: Role of tissue acidosis. Am J Physiol 266:G633–G646
34. Pinto M, Robine-Leon S, Appay MD, et al (1983) Enterocyte-like differentiation and pola-
    rization of the human colon carcinoma cell line Caco-2 in culture. Biol Cell 47:323–330
35. Bralet J, Bouvier C, Schrieber L, et al (1991) Effect of acidosis on lipid peroxidation in brain
    slices. Brain Res 539:175–177
36. Rehncrona S, Hauge HN, Siesjo BK (1989) Enhancement of iron-catalyzed free radical
    formation by acidosis in brain homogenates: Differences in effect by lactic acid and CO_2.
    J Cereb Blood Flow Metab 9:65–70
37. Siesjo BK, Bendek G, Koide T, et al (1985) Influence of acidosis on lipid peroxidation in
    brain tissues *in vitro*. J Cereb Blood Flow Metab 5:253–258
38. Cancela JM, Bralet J, Beley A (1994) Effects of iron-induced lipid peroxidation and of acido-
    sis on choline uptake by synaptosomes. Neurochem Res 19:833–837
39. Musleh W, Bruce A, Malfroy B, et al (1994) Effects of EUK-8, a synthetic catalytic superoxide
    scavenger, on hypoxia- and acidosis-induced damage in hippocampal slices. Neuropharm
    33:929–934
40. Bralet J, Schreiber L, Bouvier C (1992) Effect of acidosis and anoxia on iron delocalization
    from brain homogenates. Biochem Pharmacol 43:979–983
41. Oubidar M, Boquillon M, Marie C, et al (1994) Ischemia-induced brain iron delocalization:
    Effect of iron chelators. Free Rad Biol Med 16:861–867
42. Rodeheaver DP, Schnellman RG (1993) Extracellular acidosis ameliorates metabolic-inhibi-
    tor-induced and potentiates oxidant-induced cell death in renal proximal tubules. J Phar-
    macol Exp Ther 265:1355–1360

43. Burns KD, Homma T, Breyer MD, et al (1991) Cytosolic acidification stimulates a calcium influx that activates Na$^+$-H$^+$ exchange in LLC-PKX1 cells. Am J Physiol 261:F617–F625
44. Martinez-Palomo A, Meza I, Beaty G, et al (1980) Experimental modulation of occluding junctions in a cultured transporting epithelium. J Cell Biol 87:746–754
45. Lowe PJ, Miyai K, Steinbach JH, et al (1988) Hormonal regulation of hepatocyte tight junctional permeability. Am J Physiol 255:G454–G461
46. Kan KS, Coleman R (1988) The calcium ionophore A23187 increases the tight-junctional permeability in rat liver. Biochem J 256:1039–1041
47. Fleming I, Gray GA, Stoclet JC (1993) Influence of endothelium on induction of the L-arginine-nitric oxide pathway in rat aortas. Am J Physiol 264:H1200–H1207
48. Peterson MW, Gruenhaupt D (1990) A23187 increases permeability of MDCK monolayers independent of phospholipase activation. Am J Physiol 259:C69–C76
49. Hidalgo IJ, Raub TJ, Borchardt RT (1989) Characterization of human colonic carcinoma cell line (Caco-2) as a model system of intestinal epithelial permeability. Gastroenterology 96:736–749
50. Shibuya I, Douglas WW (1992) Calcium channels in rat melanotrophs are permeable to manganese, cobalt, cadmium, and lanthanum, but not to nickel: Evidence provided by fluorescence changes in fura-2-loaded cells. Endocrinology 131:1936–1941
51. Riehl TE, Stenson WF (1994) Mechanisms of transit of lipid mediators of inflammation and bacterial peptides across intestinal epithelia. Am J Physiol 267:G687–G695
52. van Os CH, de Jong MD, Slegers JFG (1974) Dimensions of polar pathways through rabbit gallbladder epithelium. J Membrane Biol 15:363–382
53. Hingson DJ, Diamond JM (1972) Comparison of non-electrolyte permeability patterns in several epithelia. J Membrane Biol 10:93–135
54. Suleymanlar G, Zhou HZ, McCormack M, et al (1992) Mechanism of impaired energy metabolism during acidosis: Role of oxidative metabolism. Am J Physiol 262:H1818–H1822
55. Carpenter JF, Hand SC (1986) Reversible dissociation and inactivation of phosphofructokinase in ischemic rat heart. Am J Physiol 250:R512–R518
56. Trivedi B, Danforth WH (1966) Effect of pH on the kinetics of frog muscle phosphofructokinase. J Biol Chem 241:4110–4114
57. Unno N, Menconi MJ, Salzman AL, et al (1996) Hyperpermeability and ATP depletion induced by chronic hypoxia or glycolytic inhibition in Caco-2$_{BBe}$ monolayers. Am J Physiol (in press)
58. Gores GJ, Nieminen AL, Wray BE, et al (1989) Intracellular pH during "chemical hypoxia" in cultured rat hepatocytes: Protection by intracellular acidosis against the onset of cell death. J Clin Invest 83:386–396
59. Rouslin W, Erickson JL, Soaro J (1986) Effects of oligomycin and acidosis on rates of ATP depletion in ischemic heart muscle. Am J Physiol 250:H503–H508
60. Fish EM, Molitoris B (1994) Extracellular acidosis minimizes actin cytoskeletal alterations during ATP depletion. Am J Physiol 267:F566–F572
61. Nathan C (1992) Nitric oxide as a secretory product of mammalian cells. FASEB J 6:3051–3064
62. Stark ME, Szurszewski JH (1992) Role of nitric oxide in gastrointestinal and hepatic function and disease. Gastroenterology 103:1928–1949
63. Bredt DS, Snyder SH (1990) Localization of nitric oxide synthase indicating a neural role for nitric oxide. Nature 347:768–770
64. Llewellyn-Smith IJ, Song Z-M, Costa M, et al (1992) Ultrastructural localization of nitric oxide synthase immunoreactivity in guinea-pig enteric neurons. Brain Res 577:337–342
65. Ward SM, Xue C, Shuttleworth CW, et al (1992) NADPH diaphorase and nitric oxide synthase colocalization in enteric neurons of canine proximal colon. Am J Physiol 263:G277–G284
66. Nichols K, Staines W, Krantis A (1993) Nitric oxide synthase distribution in the rat intestine: A histochemical analysis. Gastroenterology 105:1651–1661
67. Pique JM, Whittle BJR, Esplugues JV (1989) The vasodilator role of endogenous nitric oxide in the rat gastric microcirculation. Eur J Pharmacol 174:293–296
68. Publicover NG, Hammond EM, Sanders KM (1993) Amplification of nitric oxide signaling by interstitial cells isolated from canine colon. Proc Natl Acad Sci 90:2087–2091

69. Hogaboam CM, Befus AD, Wallace JL (1993) Modulation of rat mast cell reactivity by IL-1β: Divergent effects on nitric oxide and platelet activating factor release. J Immunol 151: 1367–1374
70. Granger DL, Hibbs JB, Perfect JR, et al (1990) Metabolic fate of L-arginine in relation to microbiostatic capability of murine macrophages. J Clin Invest 85:264–273
71. Stuehr DJ, Nathan CF (1989) Nitric oxide: A macrophage product responsible for cytostasis and respiratory inhibition in tumor target cells. J Exp Med 169:1543–1555
72. Grisham MB, Ware K, Gilleland HE Jr, et al (1992) Neutrophil-mediated nitrosamine formation: Role of nitric oxide in rats. Gastroenterology 103:1260–1266
73. Malzwista SE, Montgomery RR, van Blaricom G (1992) Evidence for reactive nitrogen intermediates in killing of staphylococci by human neutrophil cytoplasts. A new microbicidal pathway for polymorphonuclear leukocytes. J Clin Invest 90:631–635
74. Goretski J, Zafiriou OC, Hollocher TC (1990) Steady-state nitric oxide concentrations during denitrification. J Biol Chem 265:11 535–11 538
75. Tepperman BL, Brown JF, Korolkiewicz R, et al (1994) Nitric oxide synthase activity, viability and cyclic GMP levels in rat colonic epithelial cells: Effect of endotoxin challenge. J Pharmacol Exp Ther 271:1477–1482
76. Grisham MB (1993) Nitric oxide production by intestinal epithelial cells. Gastroenterology 104:A710 (Abst)
77. Dignass A, Podolsky D, Rachmilewitz D (1994) Nitric oxide generation by intestinal epithelial cells is stimulated by cytokines and bacterial endotoxin. Gastroenterology 106:A673 (Abst)
78. Kubes P (1992) Nitric oxide modulates epithelial permeability in the feline small intestine. Am J Physiol 262:G1138–G1142
79. Payne D, Kubes P (1993) Nitric oxide donors reduce the rise in reperfusion-induced intestinal mucosal permeability. Am J Physiol 265:G189–G195
80. Kubes P (1993) Ischemia-reperfusion in the feline small intestine: A role for nitric oxide. Am J Physiol 264:G143–G149
81. Boughton-Smith NK, Hutcheson IR, Deakin AM, et al (1990) Protective effect of S-nitroso-N-acetyl-penicillamine in endotoxin-induced acute intestinal damage in the rat. Eur J Pharmacol 191:485–488
82. Hutcheson IR, Whittle BJ, Boughton-Smith NK (1990) Role of nitric oxide in maintaining vascular integrity in endotoxin-induced intestinal damage in the rat. Br J Pharmacol 101: 815–820
83. Lopez-Belmonte J, Whittle BJ, Moncada S (1993) The actions of nitric oxide donors in the prevention or induction of injury to the rat gastric mucosa. Br J Pharmacol 108:73–78
84. Tepperman BL, Brown JF, Whittle BJR (1993) Nitric oxide synthase induction and intestinal cell viability in rats. Am J Physiol 265:G214–G218
85. Salzman AL, Menconi MJ, Unno N, et al (1995) Nitric oxide dilates tight junctions and depletes ATP in cultured Caco-2BBe intestinal epithelial monolayers. Am J Physiol 268: G361–G373
86. Madara JL, Stafford J (1989) Interferon-γ directly affects barrier function of cultured intestinal epithelial monolayers. J Clin Invest 83:724–727
87. Colgan SP, Resnick MB, Parkos CA, et al (1994) IL-4 directly modulates function of a model human intestinal epithelium. J Immunol 153:2122–2129
88. Williams G, Brown T, Becker L, et al (1994) Cytokine-induce expression of nitric oxide synthase in C2C12 skeletal muscle myocytes. Am J Physiol 267:R1021–R1025
89. Koide M, Kawahara Y, Tsuda T, et al (1994) Expression of nitric oxide synthase by cytokines in vascular smooth muscle cells. Hypertension 23:145–148
90. Markewitz BA, Michael JR, Kohan DE (1993) Cytokine-induced expression of a nitric oxide synthase in rat renal tubule cells. J Clin Invest 91:2138–2143
91. Vodovotz Y, Kwon NS, Pospischill M, et al (1994) Inactivation of nitric oxide synthase after prolonged incubation of mouse macrophages with IFN-γ and bacterial lipopolysaccharide. J Immunol 152:4110–4118

Molecular Mechanisms of Intestinal Injury, Repair, and Growth

T. R. Ziegler

Introduction

Severe catabolic illness is associated with markedly altered structure and function of intestinal mucosal cells [1, 2]. For example, burn injury, major trauma, infection, shock, and lack of enteral feeding are all associated with atrophy of the intestinal mucosa, increased gut permeability, diminished intestinal barrier and gut immune function, and apparent gut-origin sepsis in animal models [1–3]. Bowel ischemia may increase enterocyte sloughing and result in frank mucosal ulcerations or erosions [1–3]. Local and systemic cytokines appear to mediate, at least in part, intestinal tissue damage during mucosal inflammation and injury [4–11]. Intestinal cell injury may also be caused by mucosal production of oxygen free radicals, with concomitant depletion of systemic and local antioxidant defenses [12, 13].

Putative mediators of intestinal injury have been extensively studied; however, the mechanisms which regulate intestinal growth, regeneration and repair during catabolic stress remain poorly understood, especially at the molecular level. Enteral feeding is one element known to increase gut mucosal regeneration in models of critical illness [14, 15]. Animal studies also demonstrate potent gut-trophic effects with recombinant peptide growth factor (GF) administration in various catabolic states [16, 17]. The interactions between exogenous nutrients and peptide GF on intestinal growth are beginning to be examined in clinical models, with promising results. However, underlying molecular mechanisms operative during gut atrophy and in the gut-trophic effects of nutrients and GF are generally unknown. The possible interactions between mediators of intestinal damage and factors which facilitate intestinal repair are also poorly understood.

This chapter will focus primarily on some of the putative molecular mechanisms involved in intestinal damage during catabolic states and in nutrient and GF-induced intestinal growth and repair.

Mediators of Intestinal Injury During Catabolic States

Intestinal Cytokine Production

Recent studies have documented increased production of cytokines at the messenger ribonucleic acid (mRNA) and protein level in gut mucosal cells during inflammation and other states of mucosal damage [4–11]. In addition, movement of endotoxin and microorganisms across the gut mucosal barrier ("translocation") may activate the reticuloendothelial system to increase plasma cytokine levels, with secondary elaboration of classical catabolic stress hormones such as glucocorticoids and catecholamines [1–3]. The proinflammatory effects of some cytokines are probably important local effectors of intestinal cell damage in catabolic states. Cytokines such as interleukins (IL), tumor necrosis factor (TNF) and monocyte-chemoattractant protein-1 (MCP-1) may variously activate B- and T-lymphocytes and polymorphonuclear leukocytes, induce immune cell chemotaxis, upregulate endothelial adhesion molecules, modulate lipid mediators including prostaglandin and platelet activating factor (PAF), and contribute to shock and tissue injury during sepsis, among other important functions [4–11].

Significantly increased mRNA levels of IL-1, IL-6 and IL-8 were present in activated macrophages obtained from colonic mucosa of patients with active inflammation compared to non-inflamed areas of colonic mucosa or healthy control tissue [4]. IL-1β and transforming GF-β (TGF-β) mRNA levels were greater from small intestinal and colonic mucosa of patients with Crohn's disease compared to normal intestine, where low levels were detected [5]. These and other molecular studies indicate that inflammation of both the small and large intestinal mucosa is associated with increased local cytokine production in humans [4–11]. Mononuclear cells (MNC) which infiltrate the mucosal lamina propria are believed to be the major source of mucosal cytokines during injury [4–6]. However, in situ hybridization techniques have been used to localize cellular mRNA expression in the gut epithelial cells themselves. Classical cytokines including IL-1 [5], IL-8 [6], TNF [7], MCP-1 [9] are all able to be produced in gut epithelium. Production of cytokines by gut-associated MNC and by intestinal epithelial cells themselves may each individually contribute to multiple organ failure and the overall hemodynamic, immune and protein-catabolic effects of critical illness [1–3].

Nitric oxide (NO) can be made by gut epithelial cells, and rat IEC-6 intestinal epithelial cell lines produce both the calcium-dependent constitutive and the lipopolysaccharide (LPS)-inducible NO synthase (iNOS) [11]. NO production was significantly induced in IEC-6 cells by cytokines (IL-1, -2, -8, interferon (IFN), TNF) and by GF, including epidermal GF (EGF), TGF-α, and basic fibroblast GF (bFGF) [11]. Thus, stimulation of NO production by cytokines and some GF may regulate gut mucosal integrity through NO-induced effects on local blood vessel dilation. In addition to alterations in local vasoactive substances, bowel ischemia related to cardiovascular failure, emboli, and fluid or blood loss may increase enterocyte sloughing and/or result in frank gut mucosal ulcerations or erosions [1–3].

Oxidant-mediated Tissue Damage

Catabolic states are associated with increased production of oxygen free radical (OFR) species which play important roles in arachidonic acid metabolism, phagocyte action and cytokine generation. Increased tissue levels of OFRs are thought to mediate cellular injury and organ dysfunction during catabolic states and critical illness by damage to DNA, proteins and cell membrane lipids [12, 13]. The body has an elaborate antioxidant system which serves to inhibit tissue damage due to excess production of OFRs, via their conversion to stable molecular products. The antioxidant system also includes non-enzymatic antioxidant nutrients such as vitamins A, C, E, beta carotene, cysteine, taurine and glutathione (GSH) [18, 19]. In addition, a number of enzymes, including glutathione peroxidase, superoxide dismutase and catalase, function as antioxidants by metabolizing OFRs and thus preventing their accumulation in tissues and plasma [13, 18, 19]. The function of these key antioxidant enzymes is dependent upon nutrient trace elements including selenium, copper, zinc and manganese [18, 19].

GSH is a tripeptide composed of cysteine, glutamate and glycine and is considered the body's central antioxidant [18]. In addition, GSH plays key roles in cellular proliferation and metabolism, tissue repair, immune function, leukotriene and prostaglandin metabolism, immune function and host defense[18, 19]. GSH protects against lipid peroxidation by several mechanisms, including

1) reducing oxidized forms of vitamin C back to the functional, reduced form;
2) utilization as a hydrogen donor by glutathione peroxidase to quench toxic peroxides; and
3) function through the enzyme glutathione S-transferase to detoxify reactive aldehydes generated via lipid peroxidation [12, 13, 18, 19].

Numerous studies demonstrate that depletion of GSH and other antioxidant nutrient defenses, including vitamins E and C, selenium and zinc, commonly occurs during malnutrition, liver dysfunction, sepsis, burns, trauma, chemotherapy, and other catabolic states associated with OFR-mediated cell damage [12, 13, 20–23]. Studies in ICU patients document marked reductions in plasma and muscle concentrations of GSH, with associated increased levels of malondialdehyde, a marker of lipid membrane peroxidation [24, 25].

Of interest, GSH has been shown to be critical for intestinal growth and function [26, 27]. Sources of GSH in the gut lumen include the diet, transport in bile, desquamated gut epithelial cells and direct efflux from mucosal cells into the lumen [26, 27]. Although data are limited, it is likely that intestinal cell GSH depletion contributes to loss of intestinal mucosal cell integrity and function during various catabolic states. Cysteine is normally the rate-limiting amino acid for GSH production; however, a series of animal studies indicate that provision of intravenous or enteral glutamine (Gln) is able to maintain or upregulate tissue and blood levels of GSH during catabolic states [20–23, 28, 29]. Parenteral nutrition enriched in L-Gln prevented hepatic damage induced by chemotherapy [20], endotoxin administration [21] or acetaminophen toxicity [22] in rats, and im-

Table 1. Some factors which contribute to intestinal cell damage during critical illness

- Reduced splanchnic blood flow and frank cell ischemia
- Effects of cytokines (endocrine, autocrine/paracrine delivery)
- Injury mediated by oxygen free radicals
- Depletion of antioxidant capacity, including diminished availability of nutrient antioxidants (GSH, Gln, zinc, selenium, vitamins A, C, and E)
- Lack of enteral feeding with impaired mucosal structure and function
- Insufficient supply of exogenous gut-trophic nutrients (Gln, SCFA, others)
- Diminished ability of gut cells to utilize trophic nutrients (reduced Gln uptake)
- Cellular resistance to hormonal growth factor action (GH-IGF-I action pathway)
- Other mechanisms

GHS: glutathione, Gln: glutamine, SCFA: short chain fatty acids, GH: growth hormone, IGF: insulin-like growth factor

proved survival in all of these models. Enteral Gln administration preserves small bowel mucosa GSH levels during intestinal ischemia/reperfusion injury in rats and reduces indices of intestinal damage [23]. Gln-enriched enteral diets also coordinately increased hepatic Gln uptake and hepatic GSH release in a rat model of inflammatory stress [28]. Enteral diets enriched in L-Gln also increased intestinal GSH levels and diminished gut mucosal injury in an animal model of chronic radiation enteropathy [29]. The exact mechanisms by which intravenous or enteral Gln upregulates GSH production in tissues such as the gut is unknown. However, cytokine administration in animals diminishes plasma and tissue GSH levels [18, 19]. Further, sepsis and cytokine administration reduce intestinal uptake and utilization of Gln [30]. Thus, an inability of the gut to utilize Gln for cellular production of GSH may contribute to intestinal injury during sepsis and other catabolic states [30]. Factors which may contribute to intestinal cell damage during critical illness are shown in Table 1.

Intestinal Atrophy and Growth during Altered Nutrition

The mammalian intestinal mucosa is one of the most rapidly replicating tissues in the body [31]. The small intestinal enteric epithelium is completely replaced in 2–3 days in rodents and presumably almost as rapidly in man [31]. The crypt regions of the colonic and small intestinal mucosa are the sites of intestinal cell differentiation and proliferation. In small bowel, stem cells located in the crypt region differentiate into enterocytes, enteroendocrine cells, and mucous-secreting goblet cells. These specialized cells move along the intestinal villus and are eventually extruded into the gut lumen [31, 32]. In contrast, Paneth cells, whose function remains unclear, move downward into the crypt base region [32, 33]. The overall small bowel mucosal thickness is determined by two major factors: the villus cell lifespan and the crypt cell division rate [31–33].

Increased intestinal cell proliferation (hypertrophy and hyperplasia) may occur in remnant bowel after resection (intestinal adaptation); during recovery after physical or chemical mucosal injury, with adrenergic or cholinergic nervous stimulation, or in response to a number of hormones and specific nutrients. In contrast, decreased cell proliferation occurs in defunctionalized bowel segments, with ionizing irradiation, mucosal ischemia or inflammation, with folate, zinc, or vitamin B12 deficiency, after hypophysectomy, and with fasting or parenteral nutrition (PN) administration [2, 31]. Despite knowledge of the physiology of epithelial cell renewal and factors which may affect it, the molecular mechanisms responsible for intestinal cell atrophy and growth remain unclear.

Fasting/Refeeding and Route of Nutrient Delivery

During total starvation or severe protein-calorie malnutrition, the enteric mucosal and muscular layers atrophy to a disproportionate degree compared to the changes in total body mass and weight of other tissues [31, 34, 35]. Protein restriction alone is also associated with gut mucosal cell atrophy [36]. Malnutrition is also associated with altered or diminished intestinal cell digestive/absorptive capacity [31, 37, 38] and with impaired gut barrier function [2]. In rats, fasting markedly reduced small intestinal brush border mRNA content of ornithine decarboxylase (ODC; the rate-limiting enzyme in the synthesis of polyamines); ODC mRNA was restored with enteral refeeding [33]. Local polyamine production in tissues is believed to be critical for cellular growth, but polyamines are apparently available to gut cells through their presence in some foods [31].

Fasting has been shown to significantly reduce specific activity and mRNA levels of certain digestive enzymes in the small bowel mucosa [33, 37]. In contrast, mRNA levels of lactase were increased in small intestinal mucosa of fasted rats [33]. In rabbits, a 72-h fast significantly reduced transport capacity for Gln and arginine in small bowel brush border membrane vesicles, due to a decreased number of functional amino acid transporter proteins per mg mucosal protein [38]. Several rat small intestinal amino acid and peptide transporters have recently been cloned using reverse transcriptase polymerase chain reaction (RT-PCR) technology [39]. mRNA levels for two of the peptide transporters, termed rPepT 1 and rpt-1, were found to be evenly distributed along the longitudinal axis of the rat small intestine. However, these mRNAs, as well as the mRNA for the high affinity glutamate transporter EAAC1, were markedly upregulated in the distal 1/3 of the small intestine when high protein enteral diets were given after a period of low protein feeding [39]. This molecular study suggests that the distal small intestine (ileum), in contrast to the more proximal duodenal-jejunal segments, plays an important role in adaptive amino acid absorption in response to changes in dietary protein.

The route of feeding also influences intestinal cell proliferation [31, 37, 40]. Parenteral nutrition (PN) is commonly administered during critical illness when the intestinal tract is dysfunctional due to ileus, intra-abdominal infection, bleeding and the like. How-ever, both PN and provision of elemental or semi-elemental enteral diets are associated with mucosal atrophy in rodents [2, 37, 40] and in man [41–43]. This occurs despite provision of adequate micronutrients,

Table 2. Possible mechanisms of intestinal growth related to luminal nutrition

- Enhanced blood flow with oxygen, nutrient and growth factor delivery to basolateral mucosal cell membranes
- Increased gut neuronal activity and peristalsis
- Effects of salivary, gastric, mucosal and pancreatic-biliary secretions (eg delivery of growth factors)
- Direct delivery of nutrients to mucosal cells via the lumen
- Provision of antioxidant nutrients present in food
- Delivery of specific compounds such as glutamine, polyamines and fiber which enhance cell growth
- Mucosal generation of growth factors for endocrine, paracrine and/or autocrine action
- Increased sloughing of enterocytes at villus tip, with subsequent stimulation of crypt region

calories, fats and amino acids, presumably because these modalities provide inadequate gut-trophic nutrients or do not stimulate factors important in mucosal cell renewal. The atrophic effects of PN are rapidly reversed when complex enteral diets are given [31, 35, 37, 40, 42]. Luminal nutrients increase pancreatic-biliary secretions, gut neuronal activity, peristalsis, and splanchnic blood flow [31]. Enteral nutrition (EN) in rats increases mucosal production of insulin-like GF-I (IGF-I) after fasting [35, 44] and during intestinal adaptation after bowel resection [17], as outlined in more detail below. In addition, food contains compounds such as polyamines and dietary fibers which may exert specific trophic effects on the bowel [15, 31, 45]. The potential mechanisms by which enteral nutrients facilitate gut growth are listed in Table 2.

Gut-trophic Effects of Specific Nutrients

PN is limiting in specific nutrients and compounds which appear to be important for gut growth and regeneration [2, 15, 23]. These include Gln, short-chain fatty acids (SCFA), dietary fibers, polyamines and possibly other nutrients such as arginine. The available data strongly suggests that Gln becomes conditionally essential during critical illness (see chapter by van der Hulst et al. in this volume) [15, 46]. Gln is utilized intensively by small bowel and colonic mucosal cells during critical illness probably as a major fuel source or for other functions [15, 46–48]. The benefits of Gln supplementation of parenteral and enteral diets in intestinal health have become increasingly apparent. Although most data are derived from rat studies, recent human studies show that PN supplemented with glutamine dipeptides enhances D-xylose absorption, an index of small bowel absorptive capacity, in critically ill patients [49]. Gln-enriched enteral diets were recently shown to increase splanchnic blood flow in the rat [50]. This effect may theoretically be important in mucosal growth and function by facilitating growth factor and nutrient delivery to the gut.

A number of animal studies suggest an important role for Gln supplementation in states of gut mucosal injury, inflammation and also in intestinal adaptation (reviewed in [15, 46–48]). When supplemented to otherwise complete enteral or parenteral diets, Gln attenuated intestinal and pancreatic atrophy associated with PN and elemental EN; decreases hepatic steatosis; attenuated gut mucosal damage, and reduces bacteremia and mortality after chemotherapy, irradiation or following sepsis or endotoxemia; enhances intestinal adaptation after massive small bowel resection; and improves gut immune function [15, 46–48]. Gln feeding increases systemic, hepatic and intestinal GSH concentrations [20–23] which may play a key role in protecting intestinal tissues from oxidant-mediated injury during or following sepsis, endotoxemia and blood loss [19, 26]. Of interest, sepsis inhibits intestinal Gln utilization *in vitro* in rat and human small bowel mucosa [30]. In addition, ICU patients have increased Gln content in duodenal mucosa, suggesting that Gln utilization by the small bowel mucosa is impaired in human critical illness [51].

Both water soluble and insoluble fibers elicit stimulatory effects on small and large bowel mucosal growth and cell proliferation in normal rats [52, 53]. In a model of massive small bowel resection, the addition of pectin, a water soluble fiber, to an elemental diet enhanced mucosal adaptation, as indicated by mucosal weight, DNA content, mucosal thickness and disaccharidase activity [53]. Fermentable fibers (such as pectins and gums) and other unabsorbed carbohydrates may either resist digestion or escape absorption in the upper-intestinal tract. Anaerobic bacteria may metabolize these to SCFA (acetate, propionate and butyrate), hydrogen gas, carbon dioxide, methane and water. The SCFA are readily absorbed by the colonic mucosa and utilized for energy [54–57]. Thus, some of the carbohydrate calories that would have otherwise been lost because of upper-intestinal tract malabsorption, can be salvaged by this process [56]. Furthermore, animal data indicates that the SCFA enhance sodium and water absorption [15, 54], reduced mucosal atrophy associated with PN after extensive bowel resection [55], and exert trophic effects both on the small intestine and in the colon [57]. The possible role of dietary fibers in production of gut mucosal GF is under investigation. Specific micronutrients including folate, vitamin B12 and especially zinc are also critical for intestinal growth [31]. For example, zinc depletion is associated with diarrhea [58] and significantly reduced gut adaptation and regrowth following bowel resection [59]. This atrophic response can be reversed by zinc repletion, presumably due to the important role of zinc in cell proliferation processes (see below) [58, 59].

Specific Hormones and Intestinal Growth

The intestinal mucosa is known to synthesize a number of peptide hormones which may function as important GF for this tissue [17, 31, 35, 60, 61]. A complete review of the metabolic and growth-promoting effects of intestinal hormones is beyond the scope of this chapter, but is covered in depth in an additional chapter in this volume. Numerous animal studies suggest a possible role for exogenous administration of IGF-I, growth hormone (GH), epidermal GF (EGF), neurotensin, TGF-α, insulin and possibly other hormones in enhancing intestinal adaptation and rehabilitation. To date, very little human data on exogenous administration of GF and intestinal growth or function is available. This section will briefly highlight some of the important observations related to administration of EGF, GH, IGF-I and insulin in terms of gut anabolism.

EGF Administration

EGF is a known mitogen for intestinal mucosal cells, and is secreted by the salivary glands and by specialized enteroendocrine cells lining the upper small intestinal mucosa [62, 63]. As with several other hormones (most notably IGF-I), EGF may exert actions in an endocrine fashion (via transport in the blood to distant sites of action) or via autocrine/paracrine modes of action (via actions on adjacent cells or on the cell secreting the peptide itself) [61]. Numerous studies demonstrate gut-trophic effects of EGF administration in catabolic animal models. For example, EGF administration attenuated the atrophic effects of malnutrition in rat small bowel [62]. *In vivo* studies in rabbits documented EGF-stimulated jejunal absorption of water, sodium, chloride and glucose, suggesting a role for EGF in the control of intestinal nutrient transport [63]. Systemic and luminal EGF appears to be able to regulate activity and/or production of mucosal brush border digestive enzymes in association with maintenance of gut cell proliferation [64, 65]. Intraperitoneal EGF infusion increased wound breaking strength of healing wounds in stomach, ileum and colon in pigs compared to untreated animals [66]. Additional studies in animals documented gut-trophic effects and decreased bacterial translocation with exogenous EGF administration after burn injury [67]. EGF therapy was also significantly decreased in PN-associated small bowel mucosal atrophy in unstressed rats [68].

GH Administration

GH and IGF-I, which is believed to mediate many of GH-induced anabolic effects, play critical roles in somatic growth, cell proliferation and cell differentiation in non-intestinal tissues [15]. Several lines of evidence support the concept that exogenous GH administration exerts trophic effects in the intestine. In animal studies, partial reversal of small intestinal atrophy and increased absorption of fluid, sodium, chloride, potassium and calcium occur with GH treatment in hypophysectomized rats [69, 70]. Growth and differentiation of fetal rat intestinal transplants were shown to be stimulated by GH administration [71]. GH administration increased strength and collagen deposition in rat colonic anastomoses [72], and increased ileal weight and ileal mucosal height after 75% small bowel resection [73]. In a rat model of experimental colitis, exogenous GH administration significantly decreased the level of colonic inflammation and mucosal damage, concomitant with enhanced colonic breaking strength [74]. Finally, GH transgenic mice exhibited significantly increased small bowel mucosal mass and villus height compared to pair-fed control mice [75, 76]. Data on specific intestinal effects of GH as a single trophic agent in humans are limited. However, in a recent study, adult patients receiving daily subcutaneous (s.c.) recombinant GH for 3 days prior to intestinal surgery demonstrated significantly increased ($\approx 35\%$) jejunal and ileal amino acid transport, as measured *in vitro* in brush border membrane vesicles [77]. These findings suggest that GH may facilitate intestinal nutrient absorption in man.

IGF-I Administration

Exogenous recombinant human IGF-I administration has marked trophic effects on the intestinal mucosa in a variety of rat models associated with altered mucosal growth, including experimental short bowel syndrome (SBS) [78–81], dexamethasone administration during PN [82], and after orthotopic jejunal transplantation [83]. Both recombinant native IGF-I or a modified form of IGF-I with little affinity to IGF binding proteins enhanced enteral nitrogen absorption in a rat model of SBS [84]. In a study of burn injured rats (50% body surface area), a 5-day infusion of IGF-I improved body weight, spleen weight and significantly increased proximal small bowel desoxyribonucleic acid (DNA) and protein content and distal small bowel DNA content vs burned controls [85]. In addition, IGF-I therapy reduced bacterial translocation to mesenteric lymph nodes from 89 to 30%, possibly due to enhanced anatomic and/or immune barrier function of the gut [85]. Finally, IGF-I-enriched formula increased small bowel cellularity in neonatal calves, in association with increased plasma IGF-I levels [86], while intra-ileal luminal IGF-I infusion stimulated ileal mucosal growth in one study of normal rats [87].

Insulin and other Hormonal Growth Factors

Insulin is a potent somatic GF, but anabolic effects of this peptide on the intestine have been little studied. Oral insulin administration was shown to induce trophic effects on ileal mucosa in growing pigs [88], and a stimulatory effect of s.c. insulin on DNA synthesis in suckling mouse colon was documented [89]. Keratinocyte growth factor (KGF) was recently found to be present along the crypt-villus axis in rat intestine and exogenous KGF administration induced proliferation of both hepatocytes and epithelial cells throughout the rat gastrointestinal tract [90]. Finally, numerous other hormones have trophic bowel effects in various models including neurotensin, bombesin, TGF-α and enteroglucagon [61].

Interactions between Nutrients and Hormones in Gut Anabolism

GH-IGF-I Axis and Nutrient Availability

It is well documented that nutritional status markedly effects the GH/IGF-I axis in man [91]. In humans and animal models, serum and tissue levels of IGF-I are reduced in proportion to the severity of malnutrition, and rise over time with refeeding. Available data in animals and humans suggest that both energy and protein intake are important for IGF-I production [91]. Animal studies demonstrated that mRNA levels for the GH receptor, a proximal mediator of GH-induced IGF-I production, is significantly reduced by fasting. Additional studies in rats suggest that protein restriction is associated with normal hepatic GH-receptor binding but a blunted hepatic IGF-I response at both the protein and mRNA level [91]. Taken together, the available data suggest that malnutrition (protein depletion) induces GH resistance at both receptor and post-receptor sites. It is possible that undernutrition deprives cells of essential nutrients required for IGF-I production [15].

Both the quantity and quality of food intake are known to regulate gastrointestinal hormones that are important in gut growth and repair, including somatotatin, gastrin, EGF and IGF-I [92]. Milk of various species is a nutrient source rich in a variety of gut-trophic GF including GH, IGF-I, insulin, prolactin and EGF [93]. These may interact with receptors in gut mucosa to stimulate regeneration and function of enterocytes or may be absorbed for systemic effects on the whole body [88, 93]. Thus the gut is a target tissue for IGF-I, a classical nutrient-stimulated GF which may be available to mucosal cells via the circulation (endocrine route), the gut lumen (via milk, saliva, pancreatic-biliary secretions) and mucosal cells themselves (autocrine/paracrine route) (Table 3).

In rats, a 3-day total fast markedly reduced jejunal IGF-I mRNA levels versus fed controls; with enteral *ad libitum* chow refeeding, gut IGF-I mRNA levels were rapidly normalized, concomitant with rapidly increased gut cellularity (Fig. 1) [35]. Similar observations in rat small intestine were observed by others with fasting and refeeding [44]. These findings suggest a role for gut mucosal IGF-I production in the anabolic response to enteral nutrient delivery following malnutrition [35, 44].

Table 3. Sources of nutrient-stimulated IGF-I for gut mucosal growth

- Circulation (interaction with basolateral region)
- Mucosal cells (autocrine/paracrine effects)
- Gut lumen (interaction with apical region)
- - pancreatic-biliary secretions
- - mucosal secretions/sloughed enterocytes
- - saliva
- - milk

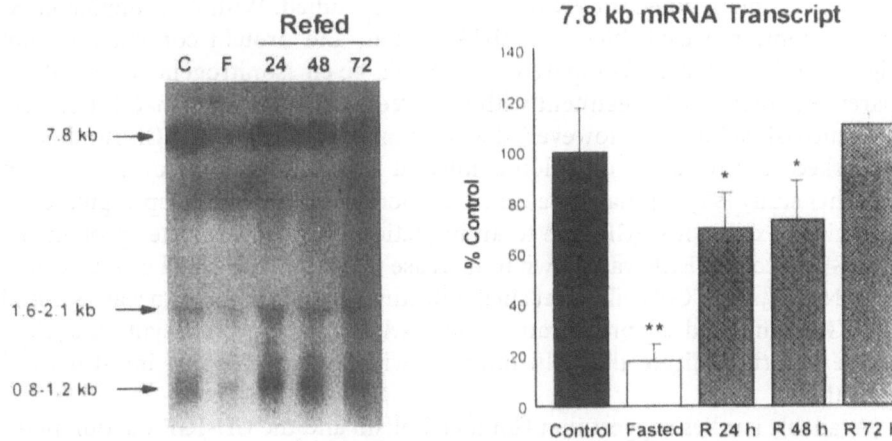

Fig. 1. Rat jejunal IGF-I mRNA expression with fasting and enteral refeeding. A Northern blot of jejunal RNA derived from control fed (C), 72-h fasted (F) and 24-h, 48-h, and 72-h refed conditions is shown on the left. Quantitative data for the 7.8 kb IGF-I transcript is shown on the right. * $p < 0.05$ vs 72-h refed; ** $p < 0.01$ vs all other groups. (From [35] with permission)

Effects of Specific Nutrients on the GH-IGF-I Axis

Deficiencies of a number of micronutrients downregulate IGF-I levels in plasma and IGF-I production in tissues and are associated with diminished tissue anabolism and repair. For example, zinc depletion is common in catabolic and hospitalized patients due to urinary, gastrointestinal and wound losses, coupled with insufficient intake. Zinc depletion inhibits gut adaptation and growth after partial small bowel resection [59]. In rats and lambs, zinc depletion is associated with significantly reduced plasma insulin, GH and IGF-I levels, and reduced hepatic mRNA levels for IGF-I; these changes are reversed with zinc repletion [94, 95].

Another example of nutrient-GF interactions is the reduction in rat plasma and tissue IGF-I concentrations and tissue IGF-I mRNA levels with potassium or magnesium depletion [96]. Finally, experimental thiamine deficiency in rats reduces IGF-I levels in plasma and tissues by 40%, while thiamine repletion enhanced the IGF-I response to GH administration in this model [97].

Interactions Between Dietary Gln and Growth Factors

Several studies suggest that the anabolic and tissue-specific trophic effects of dietary Gln are enhanced by exogenous EGF or GH therapy in a synergistic or additive fashion, suggesting that the metabolism of Gln and certain peptide GF are physiologically interactive. Both EGF and dietary Gln administration are each individually trophic to gut mucosa in experimental animals [15]. In one study [98], the effects of Gln-enriched PN with or without s.c. recombinant

EGF in rats maintained on PN for 4 days were studied. With Gln supplementation, colonic mucosal thickness, DNA content and protein content were not significantly increased compared to controls given isonitrogenous, isocaloric parenteral diets; EGF treatment with Gln-free feeding similarly had little effect on mucosal cellularity. However, the combination of Gln and EGF resulted in a marked additive effect on colonic mucosal DNA and protein content [98]. In an other study [99], jejunal glutamine transport was significantly up-regulated in rats given exogenous EGF, due to an induction of Gln transporter proteins by this GF. Recently, EGF was shown to increase Gln uptake by small intestine during PN [100]. In IEC-6 cells, a rat small intestinal crypt cell line, Gln was essential for EGF-stimulated cell proliferation and DNA, RNA and protein synthesis [101]. These reports indicate that Gln interacts with EGF to support intestinal cell growth.

Available studies suggest that Gln metabolism and the GH-IGF-I action pathways are interactive in humans. Enteral administration of L-Gln to healthy adults stimulates GH release [102]. Administration of recombinant GH to postoperative patients significantly attenuated the usual fall in muscle intracellular Gln concentrations [103]. In hypophysectomized rats, GH administration upregulates hepatic specific activity and mRNA for Gln synthetase, the rate-limiting enzyme involved in endogenous Gln synthesis [104]. In experimental short bowel syndrome in rats, the combination of Gln-enriched enteral diets and s.c. IGF-I administration synergistically increased ileal protein content, ileal wet weight and plasma IGF-I and Gln levels, compared to treatment with Gln or IGF-I alone [81].

In a series of studies, Byrne et al [105, 106] investigated the combined effects of intravenous or enteral Gln, parenteral GH, and a modified enteral diet in PN-dependent adult patients with gastrointestinal failure and SBS. Markedly improved intestinal absorption of protein, carbohydrate, calories, sodium and water occurred using the combined therapy in a subgroup of patients with SBS, suggesting that GH/Gln/diet treatment enhanced bowel function, possibly through increased mucosal surface area and/or alterations in gut blood flow or transit time [105]. A larger group of SBS patients was given the combined nutrient-GF therapy for 3 weeks, then were maintained on a Gln-supplemented modified diet (without GH) indefinitely. Therapy was associated with an 80% elimination or reduction in PN requirements after an average of one year of follow-up [106]. Further work is required to determine the molecular mechanisms and the nature of the synergistic effect of combined Gln and GH therapy in human intestinal function.

Dietary Proteins and Growth Factor Function in the Intestine

A recent study documented an important potential role of EN in preserving function of luminally-derived gut GF. Fasting human jejunal secretions destroyed the structure and bioactivity of EGF and TGF-α. In contrast, EGF (but not TGF-α) bioactivity was preserved when casein or protease inhibitors were combined with the jejunal secretions. Elemental EN solutions added in place of casein or enzyme inhibitors did not protect either GF from destruction by small intestinal juice [107]. In addition, diversion of rat pancreatic secretions to the mid-small intestine significantly increased EGF bioactivity in the lumen and enhanced gut growth in the proximal, enzyme-free, gut segment [107]. In a more recent study, Xian and colleagues [108] determined that degradation of IGF-I in the adult rat intestinal tract occurred very rapidly in ligated duodenal and ileal segments. However, IGF-I structural integrity and receptor binding activity were markedly preserved in the presence of casein, and to a lesser extent, bovine serum albumin and lactoferrin in the small intestine [108].

These studies suggest that intact complex dietary proteins may protect certain endogenous or exogenous GF from destruction in the lumen by intestinal or pancreatic enzymes. This may in turn allow the GF to optimally influence mucosal repair and regeneration. These data also provide one possible mechanism for the gut-trophic effects of oral diets containing intact complex proteins, as compared to the atrophic responses to enteral elementar diets. Consistent with this concept, elemental PN solutions given enterally do not alter jejunal IGF-I mRNA levels after fasting in rats [44], whereas refeeding with complex rat chow markedly increased jejunal IGF-I mRNA expression in this model [35].

Molecular Mechanisms of Growth, Adaptation and Repair in Intestinal Cells

Expression and Signaling of Growth Factors and their Receptors in Intestinal Cells

An explosion of new information has been published in recent years concerning GF receptors and signaling pathways, but these functional studies are primarily from non-intestinal cells and tissues. However, multiple putative GF and their specific receptors have been localized to intestinal cells at the mRNA level by Northern blotting and in situ hybridization methods, and at the protein level using immunohistochemistry, immunoblotting, radiolabeling and ligand binding techniques. Most publications focus on gut-trophic peptides, including neurotensin, bombesin, gastrin, enteroglucagon, glucagon-like peptide 1 (GLP-1), peptide YY, EGF, TGF-α, GH, IGF-I, and KGF [35, 44, 60, 61, 75, 90]. However, certain peptide hormones, including somatostatin [109] and TGF-β [110], clearly have negative regulatory effects on intestinal cell growth.

In human fetal intestine (15 to 20 weeks of gestation), TGF-α mRNA was detected from the stomach distally to the colon, but mRNA levels were much higher in duodenum and jejunum [111]. EGF mRNA was present throughout the fetal small bowel and colon in this study [111]. In rats, EGF and EGF-receptor gene expression was increased in the healing colonic anastomosis tissue compared to non-anastomotic tissue [112]. Of interest, both EGF and TGF-α binds to the EGF receptor; thus, expression and functions of these gut peptides are probably interactive [111–113]. This is evidenced by studies demonstrating EGF-induced upregulation of TGF-α mRNA in rat intestinal epithelial cells [113]. In human intestine, EGF-receptor immunoreactivity is present in fetal small bowel villi and crypts, and exogenous EGF markedly increased TGF-α gene expression in human jejunal explants [111]. Recently, EGF and TGF-α were shown to activate a common signaling pathway in IEC-6 gut epithelial cells [114]. In this study, both peptides increased cell thymidine incorporation, in association with markedly increased activity of the cytoplasmic mitogen-activated protein kinases (MAP kinases) p42 and p44 [114].

In brief, the MAP kinase signaling pathway for mitogens including EGF, TGF-α, insulin, GH, and IGF-I involves a cascade of phosphorylations which link cell surface events (triggered by ligand-receptor binding) and nuclear events mediated by downstream substrate activation [114–116]. Some of these downstream phosphorylated substrates include intracellular enzymes, such as S6 kinases, and also the immediate-early genes (eg *c-fos, c-jun and c-myc*). The immediate-early genes presumably encode transcription factor proteins which may stimulate secondary nuclear target genes involved in mediating metabolic effects of the ligand [115–117]. In gut cell lines (IEC-6 and HT-29 cells), EGF-enriched medium rapidly stimulates *c-fos, c-jun* and *jun-B* mRNA expression [118]. Transcription factor mRNA was similarly upregulated in residual ileum within several hours after small bowel resection in rats [119]. In the latter study, animals were unfed prior to tissue harvest; thus, immediate-early gene expression in the gut was independent of nutrient intake [119]. Nutrient-independent increases in proglucagon and ODC mRNA in residual intestine were observed in another study in experimental rat SBS [120]. Therefore, growth-related molecular events are stimulated by nutrient-induced and non-nutrient-induced pathways in gut cells during intestinal adaptation [35, 44, 45, 118, 119].

The hormonal signal for some gut-related peptides, including GLP-1, bombesin, and neurotensin, is transduced by a superfamily of specific cell surface, GTP binding, (G)-protein-coupled receptors which are single polypeptide chains with seven transmembrane domains [121]. Ligand binding to G-protein receptors trigger a series of events coupled to changes in membrane-bound enzymes, notably adenylyl cyclase, which catalyses cAMP formation from adenosine triphosphate (ATP) and ultimately leads to phosphorylation of substrate proteins critical for the biological responses of the ligand [121]. These molecular events contrast with signaling pathways of the two other major classes of gut peptide or cytokine receptors, namely the cytokine/hematopoietic receptor superfamily [115] and the insulin/IGF-I family of tyrosine kinase receptors [35, 44, 122, 123]. Of interest, the GH receptor and several cytokine receptors (eg IL-2, IL-3, IL-4, IL-6, among others) are also single transmembrane proteins, and are able to phosphorylate similar cytoplasmic protein tyrosine kinases, including members of the Janus kinase (JAK) family [115–117]. JAK 2 is apparently the prominent molecule in the JAK system, and is able to associate with and phosphorylate the GH receptor and several cytokine receptors [115–117]. JAK 2 also stimulates MAP kinases and other key transcription factors within the cell [116]. Thus, post-receptor action pathways for GH, a major somatic GF, several interleukins, and other cytokines have similar characteristics (Table 4). Studies on functional

Table 4. Some signaling mechanisms identified for selected intestinal growth factors

Peptide	Signal pathway
Neurotensin, bombesin, GLP-1, etc.	G-protein-coupled receptor adenylyl cyclase/cAMP system
EGF and TGF-α	EGF receptor (TK mediated), MAP kinases, immediate-early genes (eg *c-fos*, *c-jun*)
GH, cytokines	cytokine/hematopoietic receptor cytoplasmic TK, Janus kinase (JAK) family, STATS, MAP kinases, immediate-early genes
Insulin, IGF-I	Heterotetrameric TK receptors, insulin receptor substrate-1 (IRS-1), P-I-3-kinase, MAP kinases, immediate-early genes

GH: growth hormone, EGF: epidermal growth factor, IGF: insulin-like growth factor, MAP: mitogen activated protein

indices of the GH/cytokine receptor superfamily in gut tissue have not yet been published; however, these may be interactive during intestinal cell damage and regeneration.

Expression of GH-IGF-I Action Pathway Genes in the Intestine

Following small intestinal or colonic resection in animal models (rat, pig, dog), the remnant bowel undergoes an adaptive response involving structural and functional changes which eventually lead to enhanced nutrient absorption. This dynamic process includes both intestinal cell hyperplasia and hypertrophy, and is termed intestinal adaptation [31]. Small intestinal resection results in increased villus height and microvillus surface area, increased crypt depth, enhanced mucosal cell mitotic activity and cell migration along the crypt-villus axis, increased mucosal and submucosal protein and DNA content, dilation and lengthening of the intestinal remnant, and increased gut muscle wall circumference [16, 31]. The acceleration in cell growth is associated with increased digestive enzyme capacity and absorptive surface area, which eventually lead to improved nutrient absorptive capacity. The degree of small bowel adaptive changes are directly proportional to the extent of bowel resection, and is greater in distal (eg ileal) versus proximal (eg duodenal) small bowel segments [31]. Data on intestinal adaptation in humans are limited, and no systematic studies of intestinal adaptation have been reported in man. The underlying molecular mechanisms which underlie intestinal adaptation in SBS have been little studied to date.

The insulin and IGF-I receptors are major heterotetrameric transmembrane tyrosine kinases localized in non-intestinal [122, 123] and intestinal cells of several different species including rat, pig, rabbit and man [35, 44, 124–127]. The IGF–I and insulin receptors share structural and functional homology [122].

IGF-I, insulin, and IGF-II all bind to the IGF-I receptor in descending order of affinity. Both receptors interact with and phosphorylate insulin-receptor-substrate-1 (IRS-1) in the cytoplasm of the cell [122]. IRS-1 serves as docking protein for SH2-containing proteins, and mediates distal signaling systems within cells that are being increasingly defined [122].

As discussed above, several lines of evidence support the concept that the intestine is a major target tissue for GH, IGF-I and possibly insulin. In rat intestine, cellular localization of both IGF-I receptors [124-127] and GH receptors [128] is predominant in the crypt region, strongly suggesting that GH and IGF-I are involved in intestinal cell renewal and/or differentiation. However, both IGF-I and insulin receptors appear to be expressed in multiple cell types in the intestine, including cells of the muscularis and lamina propria in addition to the epithelium [127]. Epithelial cell IGF-I and insulin receptors are present on both the basolateral and apical brush border membranes [127]. The mRNA for the IGF-I receptor in the rat is located throughout the intestine in an increasing proximal to distal gradient, with the highest receptor mRNA abundance in the colon (Ziegler TR et al, unpublished observations).

In humans, recent studies demonstrated specific, high-affinity IGF-I binding sites [129, 130] and GH receptor (GH-R) mRNA [131, 132] in the intestinal mucosa. GH-R mRNA was identified throughout the human small intestinal and colonic mucosa and submucosa, but was most abundant in the intestinal crypt cells [131, 132]. As in animal models, crypt cell localization of GH-R suggests a potential role for GH in human intestinal cell proliferation and/or differentiation, and supports the concept that exogenous GH may have important effects in human small intestine and colon. Expression of both GH-R and IGF-I-R is regulated by nutrients in tissues [25, 91], but no data are available on nutrient regulation of GH-R or IGF-I-R in human intestine.

In the human fetal intestine, IGF-I mRNA was localized to mesenchymal cells and the lamina propria of stomach and small intestine [133], suggesting that mesenchymal cell-derived IGF-I exerts paracrine or autocrine effects in the human intestine. IGF-I mRNA is also found throughout all regions of the gastrointestinal tract in adult rats; levels fall after hypophysectomy or fasting and rose with GH treatment or refeeding [16, 35, 44]. These studies suggest a role for GH and IGF-I in regulating bowel growth via the GH and/or IGF-I receptor pathway. IGF-II is another potential modulator of intestinal growth, and both IGF-II mRNA and IGF-II receptors have been identified in rat intestinal tissues [16]. However, IGF-II is not GH-responsive and the potential role of this peptide in gut growth is much less clear than for IGF-I.

IGF-I and IGF-II may be bound to the six known IGF-binding proteins (BPs) (IGF-BP 1-6) which circulate in plasma and are synthesized in multiple animal tissues, including the gut [17, 44, 80, 81]. The various IGF-BPs appear to modulate IGF availability (eg by binding or sequestration), action (by unknown mechanisms), and/or cellular transport (eg by influencing movement of IGFs across cell membranes) [91, 92]. However, the actual physiological functions of IGF-BPs in tissues and plasma remain unclear. We and others have shown that IGF-BP-3 and IGF-BP-4 mRNA are both abundantly expressed in rat intestinal tissues [44, 80, 81, 84]. Multiple IGF-BPs have now been identified in human fetal intestine [134, 135], and also in rat intestinal cells [136–138]. Immunohisto-chemical analysis has revealed IGF-BPs-1, 2 and 3 to be abundantly localized in the epithelial lining of the stomach and ileum of human second trimester fetuses [134]. Of interest, these IGF-BPs were expressed in a coordinate fashion in intes-tine, and localized primarily in the columnar cells lining the villi, compared to much weaker IGF-BP staining in the crypt region [134]. In marked contrast, re-cent *in situ* hybridization studies demonstrate that IGF-BP-4, 5 and 6 mRNA expression in human fetal intestine is localized primarily in the crypt cell region, suggesting a role for these IGF-BPs in gut cell division and differentiation [135]. Thus, in human intestine, IGF-BPs exhibit differential cellular localization, sug-gesting distinct functional roles which may directly or indirectly regulate local IGF-I action and/or alter intestinal responses to exogenous GH. Overall, little is known about the regulation and role of human intestinal IGF-I and IGF-BPs, and no studies have determined the effect of exogenous GH or specific nutrients on these components of the GH-IGF-I action pathway.

Expression of IGF System Genes with Intestinal Adaptation

As noted above, GH, insulin and especially IGF-I administration have been shown to exert potent gut-trophic effects in various models. In several non-intes-tinal tissues in rats, fasting for 48 h significantly increased IGF-I binding and IGF-I receptor mRNA levels [123]. We performed studies investigating the ef-fects of enteral nutrient availability on jejunal insulin and IGF-I receptor protein and steady-state mRNA levels, and on IGF-I mRNA levels, using a 3-day fast as a model of intestinal atrophy, and enteral refeeding as a model of rapid intestinal cell proliferation [35]. Fasting for 72 h induced jejunal atrophy, lowered plasma IGF-I concentrations, and markedly decreased full-thickness jejunal IGF-I mRNA abundance (Fig. 1, lane 2). These changes were reversed by enteral refeed-ing for 24 to 72 h (Fig. 1, lanes 3, 4 and 5). IGF-I-R number and receptor mRNA expression changed little with fasting, but increased significantly following re-feeding (Fig. 2). These changes were markedly discoordinate from changes in in-sulin receptor expression, which exhibited a marked increase with fasting and significant downregulation with refeeding.

These data suggests that
1) the capacity for IGF-I action, via the small intestinal population of IGF-I re-ceptors, is maintained during fasting-induced intestinal atrophy; and
2) a critical component of the gut IGF-I action pathway is upregulated at a time when plasma IGF-I and local jejunal IGF-I mRNA are also increased, strong-ly suggesting a role for IGF-I in the gut-trophic response to enteral refeeding in rats.

A similar study confirmed these findings and demonstrated that fasting in rats reduces jejunal expression of IGF-BP-3, and this alteration is unaffected by en-teral refeeding [44].

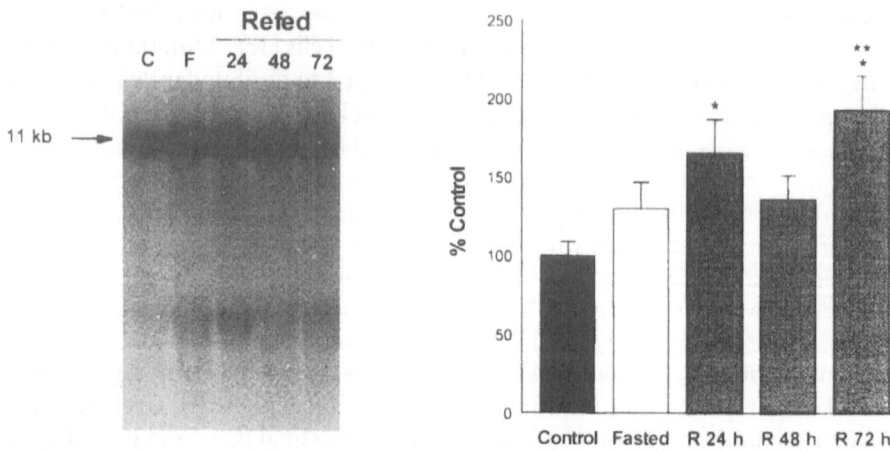

Fig. 2. IGF-I receptor mRNA expression in jejunum during fasting and refeeding. A Northern blot demonstrating the 11.0 kb rat IGF-I-R transcript from control (C), 72-h fasted (F) and 24-h, 48-h and 72-h refed conditions is shown on the left. Quantitative data from multiple experiments are shown on the right. * $p < 0.01$ vs control; ** $p < 0.05$ vs fasted. (From [35] with permission)

In a study of IGF-I system mRNAs during intestinal adaptation in adult rats, we demonstrated a significant increase in ileal IGF-I mRNA expression ($\approx 250\%$ of transected controls), concomitant with increased ileal weight, DNA and protein content (Fig. 3) [80]. Following resection and 7 days of s.c. IGF-I infusion, ileal DNA content and mass was enhanced further, and ileal IGF-I mRNA levels remained significantly elevated compared to levels in control rats ($\approx 200\%$ of transected animals) (Fig. 3). These changes occurred concomitant with significantly increased plasma IGF-I during IGF-I infusion. Ileal IGF-I-R mRNA expression was maintained near control levels with resection or IGF-I infusion. Further, increased intestinal cell proliferation after resection and/or IGF-I infusion was associated with significantly increased ileal IGF-BP-4 mRNA expression (250–300% of control) [80].

Similar enhancement of IGF-I and IGF-BP-4 during ileal adaptation was documented in rats subjected to 80% small bowel resection, then given isocaloric, isonitrogenous enteral diets without supplemental Gln or IGF-I infusion [81]. Both Gln and IGF-I individually increased adaptive cell hyperplasia in residual ileum. Resection alone (resection + standard diet + vehicle infusion) significantly increased ileal IGF-I mRNA levels. Of interest, IGF-I infusion after resection further increased IGF-I mRNA. Ileal IGF-BP-4 increased slightly with resection, but was markedly increased with resection + IGF-I [81]. In contrast, IGF-BP-3 expression was unaltered under these conditions. Dietary Gln had no effect on expression of any of these gut mRNAs and did not have additive or synergistic effects on intestinal cell proliferation, as assessed by DNA content. Interestingly, combined Gln and IGF-I treatment synergistically increased plasma levels of IGF-I and Gln, as well as ileal wet weight and protein content. These findings

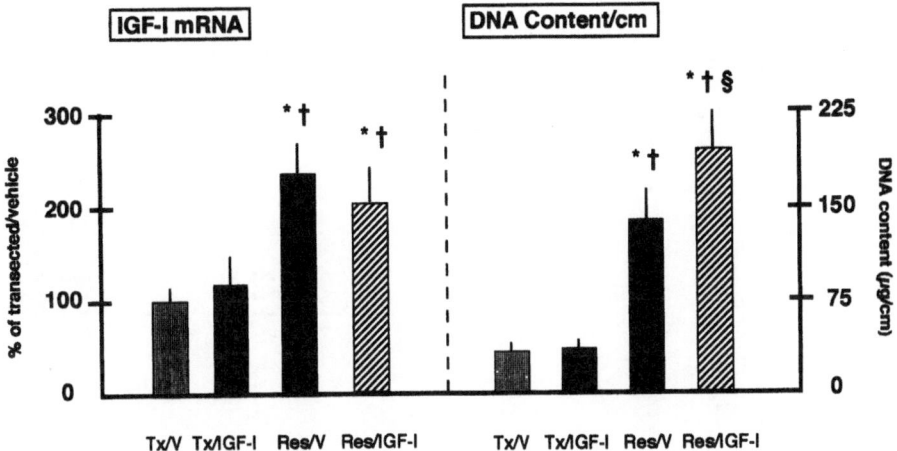

Fig. 3. Coordinate IGF-I mRNA expression (left) and DNA content/cm (right) in ileum of rats following 80% small bowel resection ± IGF-I infusion and gastrostomy feeding for 7 days. Tx/V = transected/vehicle infused; Tx/IGF-I = transected/IGF-I infused; Res/V = resected/ vehicle infused; Res/IGF-I = resected/IGF-I infused. * p < 0.01 vs Tx/V; † p<0.01 vs Tx/IGF-I; $ p<0.01 vs Res/V

suggest that the Gln and IGF-I actions are metabolically interactive, and that gut-trophic effects of Gln are not mediated by local expression of IGF-I in ileum [81].

In a rat model of 60% small bowel and partial colonic resection, colonic IGF-I and IGF-BP-4 mRNA expression were significantly increased compared to expression in transected animals (Fig. 4) [17]. IGF-I administration in this model of SBS markedly increased colonic cellularity and significantly increased water absorption (80% above control). This improvement gut absorptive function occurred in association with a sustained increase in colonic IGF-I mRNA expression (Fig. 4). Colonic IGF-I-R mRNA levels fell moderately with resection ± IGF-I infusion (NS), while IGF-BP-3 mRNA expression was discoordinate from that of IGF-BP-4 [17].

Finally, in a rat model of partial small bowel-colonic resection combined with jejunal orthotopic transplantation, 10 days of IGF-I infusion significantly increased glucose absorption (25%) and water absorption (15%) across the transplanted jejunal isograft, compared to absorption in control rats receiving saline [83]. IGF-I infusion significantly increased IGF-BP-3 mRNA, isograft crypt cell production rate, villus height, and crypt depth in both transplanted and control animals. IGF-BP-4 or IGF-I-R mRNA expression was unaltered in this model. Increased cell proliferation in the isografts was associated with significantly increased isograft expression of IGF-I mRNA, with or without IGF-I infusion (275–375% of control) [83]. IGF-I infusion also markedly reduced bacterial translocation to mesenteric lymph nodes in this model [83].

Taken together, these animal data demonstrate that IGF-I, IGF-I-R and IGF-BP-3 and 4 are measurable throughout the rat intestine, and that IGF-I adminis-

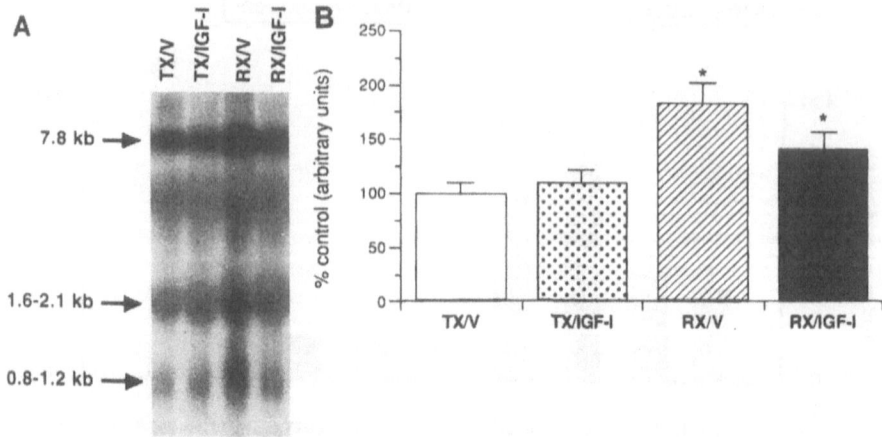

Fig. 4. Colonic IGF-I mRNA expression after partial small bowel-colonic resection in rats ± IGF-I infusion and gastrostomy feeding for 7 days. A Northern blot of colonic total RNA derived from transected/vehicle infused (Tx/V); transected/IGF-I infused (Tx/IGF-I); resected/ vehicle infused (Res/V); and resected/IGF-I infused (Res/IGF-I) is shown on the left. Quantitative data for the 7.8 kb IGF-I mRNA transcript is shown on the right. * p<0.01 versus Tx/V. (From [17] with permission)

tration improves intestinal structure and functional capacity. The data suggest that intestinal IGF-I synthesis is involved in gut-trophic responses, including the effects of enteral refeeding, intestinal adaptation in SBS, and also during IGF-I administration (when plasma IGF-I levels are elevated). Maintained or increased intestinal IGF-I-R and IGF-BP-4 mRNA levels during these states of accelerated gut growth further suggest a role for the GH-IGF-I pathway in mediating these responses. In our rat studies, mRNA levels for IGF-BP-3 were generally discoordinate from those of IGF-BP-4 [17, 80, 81, 84], suggesting differential functional roles for these intestinal IGF-BP species during intestinal growth [136–138].

Interactions between Growth Factors in Intestinal Cells

Several sets of observations indicate that certain peptide GF are interactive in gut cell growth pathways. For example, in IEC-6 cells, EGF induced cell growth and *c-fos*, *c-jun* and *jun-B* production [109]. The trophic effects of EGF were markedly attenuated with somatostatin pre-treatment of these rat crypt-derived cells [109]. Somatostatin is a peptide made in gut cells, the brain and other tissues, and is well known to inhibit pituitary GH and pancreatic insulin secretion. Thus, increased local intestinal or systemic production of this hormone may negatively influence gut growth *in vivo*. In another rat intestinal epithelial cell line, IEC-18 cells, IGF-I and EGF synergistically enhanced cell proliferation [139]. It was also determined that EGF acted as a critical competence factor which primed the cells for subsequent IGF-I-induced trophic effects [110]. In a molecular regulation study, EGF and IGF-I each individually stimulated DNA synthesis in IEC-6 cells, but in combination, cell DNA production was increased synergistically [140]. Both hormones increased IEC-6 cell mRNA levels of immediate-early genes. IGF-1 treatment diminished IGF-I-R mRNA in the cells; however, addition of EGF to the media significantly attenuated this effect. IGF-BP-2 appears to be inhibitory for cell growth in IEC-6 cells. Addition of either IGF-I and EGF to the cell culture system reduced IGF-BP-2 mRNA expression, but when the hormones were combined, inhibition of IGF-BP-2 gene expression was additive [140]. Thus, the effects of EGF on the IGF-I-R and on levels of IGF-BP-2 mRNA in these gut crypt cells may enhance IGF-I responsiveness and contribute to synergistic growth-related effects [140].

Conclusion

This chapter has summarized some of the molecular mechanisms of intestinal cell injury, repair, and growth *in vivo* and in cell culture models. Further knowledge in this area will have potentially beneficial implications for patients with critical illness, which is associated with intestinal damage, and also in conditions when intestinal rehabilitation is possible. Intestinal cell damage during critical illness may occur due to alterations in splanchnic blood flow with cellular ischemia, effects of cytokines, such as interleukins and TNF, and injury mediated by oxygen free radicals, depletion of antioxidant capacity and diminished availability of nutrient antioxidants. Further, lack of enteral feeding, with secondarily impaired mucosal structure and function, insufficient supply of exogenous gut-trophic nutrients, and diminished ability of gut cells to utilize trophic nutrients probably contributes to gut injury in ICU patients. Specific nutrients such as Gln and SCFA are gut-trophic in animals and probably in humans, but clinical data are still limited.

Exogenous administration of certain growth factors (eg GH, IGF-I, EGF) exerts potent gut-trophic effects in animal models. General nutritional status and specific nutrients (eg zinc, potassium, magnesium) have a major regulatory effect on the GH-IGF-I axis, with malnutrition decreasing and nutritional repletion increasing IGF-I synthesis in tissues. Gln-enriched feeding also enhances the effects of gut-trophic hormones (GH, IGF-I, EGF) in animal models, but little human data are available. Growth factor peptides are expressed in a cell and/or site-specific manner along the intestinal crypt-villus axis. Signaling mechanisms are being identified for selected growth factors in intestinal cells, and these appear to be similar as those in non-intestinal tissues. Certain growth factors are interactive and synergistic in intestinal cell growth and signaling pathways. Finally, IGF-I system mRNAs and other growth-related genes (EGF, *c-fos*) are activated during intestinal adaptation, nutrient-induced gut cell growth and with intestinal healing after cell damage. Taken together, it appears that interactions between specific nutrients and peptide growth factors are critical for optimal intestinal structure and function. The role these various factors play in the ICU patients will need to be determined by randomized controlled trials.

References

1. Carrico CJ, Meakins JL, Marshall JC, Fry D, Maier RV (1986) Multiple organ failure syndrome. Arch Surg 121:196-208
2. Wilmore DW, Smith RJ, O'Dwyer ST, Jacobs DO, Ziegler TR, Wang XD (1988) The gut: A central organ after surgical stress. Surgery 104:917-923
3. Ziegler TR, Smith RJ, O'Dwyer ST, Demling RH, Wilmore DW (1988) Increased intestinal permeability associated with infection in burn patients. Arch Surg 123:1313-1319
4. Isaacs KL, Sartor RB, Haskill S (1992) Cytokine messenger RNA profiles in inflammatory bowel disease mucosa detected by polymerase chain reaction amplification. Gastroenterology 103:1587-1595
5. McCabe RP, Secrist H, Botney M, Egan M, Peters MG (1993) Cytokine mRNA expression in intestine from normal and inflammatory bowel disease patients. Clin Immun Immunopath 66:52-58
6. Mazzucchelli L, Hauser C, Zgraggen K, et al (1994) Expression of interleukin-8 gene in inflammatory bowel disease is related to the histological grade of active inflammation. Am J Path 144:997-1007
7. Huang L, Tan X, Crawford SE, Hsueh W (1994) Platelet-activating factor and endotoxin induce tumour necrosis factor gene expression in rat intestine and liver. Immunology 83:65-69
8. Reinecker H-C, Loh EY, Ringler DJ, Mehta A, Rombeau JL, MacDermott RP (1995) Monocyte-chemoattractant protein 1 gene expression in intestinal epithelial cells and inflammatory bowel disease. Gastroenterology 108:40-50
9. Radema SA, Tytgat GNJ, van Deventer SJH (1995) *In situ* detection of interleukin-1β and interleukin 8 in biopsy specimens from patients with ulcerative colitis. In: Mestecky J et al (eds) Advances in Mucosal Immunology. Plenum Press, New York, pp 1297-1299
10. Panja A, Siden E, Mayer L (1995) Synthesis and regulation of accessory/proinflammatory cytokine by intestinal epithelial cells. Clin Exp Immunol 100:298-305
11. Dignass AU, Podolsky DK, Rachmilewitz D (1995) NO_x generation by cultured small intestinal epithelial cells. Dig Dis Sci 40:1859-1865
12. Bray TM, Taylor CG (1994) Enhancement of tissue glutathione for antioxidant and immune functions in malnutrition. Biochem Pharmacol 47:2113-2123
13. Robinson MK, Rounds JD, Hong RW, Jacobs DO, Wilmore DW (1992) Glutathione deficiency increases organ dysfunction after hemorrhagic shock. Surgery 112:140-149
14. Saito H, Trocki O, Alexander JW (1987) The effect of nutrient administration on the nutritional state, catabolic hormone secretion, and gut mucosal integrity after burn injury. J Parent Enteral Nutr 11:1-7
15. Ziegler TR (1995) New developments in specialized nutrition support. In: Bion JF, Burchardi H, Dellinger RP, Dobb GJ (eds) Current Topics in Intensive Care. WB Saunders Co, London, pp 144-174
16. Vanderhoof JA (1993) Regulatory peptides and intestinal growth. Gastroenterology 104: 1205-1208
17. Mantell MP, Ziegler TR, Roth BA, et al (1995) Resection-induced colonic adaptation is augmented by IGF-I and associated with upregulation of colonic IGF-I mRNA. Am J Physiol 269:G974-G980
18. Meister A (1991) Glutathione deficiency produced by inhibition of its synthesis, and its reversal: Applications in research and therapy. Pharmacol Ther 51:155-194
19. Bray TM, Taylor CG (1994) Enhancement of tissue glutathione for antioxidant and immune functions in malnutrition. Biochem Pharmacol 47:2113-2123
20. Hong RW, Helton WS, Rounds JD, Wilmore DW (1990) Glutamine-supplemented TPN preserves hepatic glutathione and improves survival following chemotherapy. Surg Forum 41:9-11
21. Hong RW, Robinson MK, Rounds JD, Wilmore DW (1991) Glutamine protects the liver following corynebacterium parvum/endotoxin-induced hepatic necrosis. Surg Forum 42:1-3
22. Hong RW, Rounds JD, Helton WS, Wilmore DW (1992) Glutamine preserves liver glutathione after lethal hepatic injury. Ann Surg 215:114-119

23. Harward TRS, Coe D, Souba WW, Klingman N, Seeger JM (1994) Glutamine preserves gut glutathione levels during intestinal ischemia/reperfusion. J Surg Res 56:351-355
24. Goode HF, Cowley HC, Walker BE, Howdle PD, Webster NR (1995) Decreased antioxidant status and increased lipid peroxidation in patients with septic shock and secondary organ dysfunction. Crit Care Med 23:646-651
25. Hammarqvist F, Luo J, Andersson K, Wernerman J (1995) Glutathione and amino acid concentrations in ICU patients. J Parent Enteral Nutr 19 (suppl 1):19S (Abst)
26. Martensson J, Jain A, Meister A (1990) Glutathione is required for intestinal function. Proc Natl Acad Sci USA 87:1715-1719
27. Hagan TM, Jones DP (1987) Transepithelial transport of glutathione in vascularly perfused small intestine of rat. Am J Physiol 252:G607-G613
28. Welbourne TC, King AB, Horton K (1993) Enteral glutamine supports hepatic glutathione efflux during inflammation. J Nutr Biochem 4:236-242
29. Jensen JC, Schaefer R, Nwokedi E, et al (1994) Prevention of chronic radiation enteropathy by dietary glutamine. Ann Surg Oncol 1:157-163
30. Salloum RM, Copeland EM, Souba WW (1991) Brush border transport of glutamine and other substrates during sepsis and endotoxemia. Ann Surg 213:401-410
31. Johnson LR (1988) Regulation of gastrointestinal mucosal growth. Physiol Rev 68:456-502
32. Gordon JI (1989) Intestinal epithelial cell differentiation: New insights from chimeric and transgenic mice. J Cell Biol 108:1187-1194
33. Hodin RA, Chamberlain SM, Meng S (1995) Pattern of rat intestinal brush border enzyme gene expression changes with epithelial growth state. Am J Physiol 269:C385-C391
34. Steiner M, Bourges HR, Freedman LS, Gray SJ (1968) Effect of starvation on the tissue composition of the small intestine in the rat. Am J Physiol 215:75-77
35. Ziegler TR, Almahfouz A, Pedrini MT, Smith RJ (1995) A comparison of rat small intestinal insulin and IGF-I receptors during fasting and refeeding. Endocrinology 136:5148-5154
36. Prosper J, Murray RL, Kern F (1968) Protein starvation and the small intestine. Gastroenterology 55:223-228
37. Levine GM, Deren JJ, Steiger E, Zinno R (1974) Role of oral intake in maintenance of gut mass and disaccharide activity. Gastroenterology 67:975-982
38. Sarac TP, Souba WW, Miller JH, et al (1994) Starvation induces differential small bowel luminal amino acid transport. Surgery 116:679-686
39. Erickson RH, Gum JR, Lindstrom MM, McKean D, Kim YS (1995) Regional expression and dietary regulation of rat small intestinal peptide and amino acid transporter mRNAs. Biochem Biophys Res Com 216:249-257
40. Ford WDA, Boelhouwer RU, King W, deVries JE, Ross JS, Malt RA (1984) Total parenteral nutrition inhibits intestinal adaptive hyperplasia in young rats: Reversal by feeding. Surgery 112:527-533
41. Buchman AL, Moukarzel AA, Bhuta S, et al (1995) Parenteral nutrition is associated with intestinal morphologic and functional changes in humans. J Parent Enteral Nutr 19:453-460
42. Pironi L, Paganelli GM, Miglioli M, et al (1994) Morphologic and cytoproliferative patterns of duodenal mucosa in two patients after long-term total parenteral nutrition: Changes with oral refeeding and relation to intestinal resection. J Parent Enteral Nutr 18:351-354
43. Cummins A, Chu G, Faust L, et al (1995) Malabsorption and villous atrophy in patients receiving enteral feeding. J Parent Enteral Nutr 19:193-198
44. Winesett DE, Ulshen MH, Hoyt EC, Mohapatra NK, Fuller CR, Lund PK (1995) Regulation and localisation of the insulin-like growth factor system in small bowel during altered nutrient status. Am J Physiol 268:G631-G640
45. Wang JY, McCormack SA, Viar MJ, Johnson LR (1991) Stimulation of proximal small intestinal mucosal growth by luminal polyamines. Am J Physiol 261:G504-G511
46. Souba WW (1993) Intestinal glutamine metabolism and nutrition. J Nutr Biochem 4:2-9
47. Ziegler TR, Gatzen C, Wilmore DW (1994) Strategies for attenuating protein-catabolic responses in the critically ill. Annu Rev Med 45:459-480

48. Stehle P, Furst P (1995) Glutamine and the gut. In: Cynober L, Furst P, Lawin P (eds) Pharmacological Nutrition-Immune Nutrition. W. Zuckschwerdt Verlag, Munich, pp 105–115
49. Tremel H, Kienle B, Weilemann LS, Stehle P, Furst P (1994) Glutamine dipeptide supplemented TPN maintains intestinal function in the critically ill. Gastroenterology 107: 1595–1601
50. Houdijk APJ, Van Leeuwen PAM, Boermeester MA, et al (1994) Glutamine-enriched enteral diet increases splanchnic blood flow in the rat. Am J Physiol 267:G1035–G1040
51. Ahlman B, Ljungqvist O, Perrson B, Bindslev L, Wernerman J (l995) Intestinal amino acid content in critically ill patients. J Parent Enteral Nutr 19:272–278
52. Sigleo S, Jackson MJ, Vahouny GV (1984) Effects of dietary fiber constituents on intestinal morphology and nutrient transport. Am J Physiol 246:G34–G39
53. Koruda MJ, Rolandelli RH, Settle RG, Saul SH, Rombeau JL (1986) The effect of a pectin-supplemented elemental diet on intestinal adaptation to massive bowel resection. J Parent Enteral Nutr 10:343–350
54. Roediger WEW, Rae DA (1982) Trophic effect of short chain fatty acids on mucosal handling of ions by the defunctioned colon. Br J Surg 69:23–25
55. Koruda MJ, Rolandelli RH, Settle RG, Zimmaro DM, Rombeau JL (1988) Effect of parenteral nutrition supplemented with short-chain fatty acids on adaptation to massive small bowel resection. Gastroenterology 95:715–720
56. McNeil NI (1984) The contribution of the large intestine to energy supplies in man. Am J Clin Nutr 39:338–342
57. Rombeau JL, Kripke SA (1990) Metabolic and intestinal effects of short-chain fatty acids. J Parent Enteral Nutr 14 (Suppl):S181–S185
58. Prasad AS (1983) Zinc deficiency in human subjects. Prog Clin Biol Res 129:1–33
59. Tamada H, Nezu R, Matsuo M, Takagi Y, Okada A, Imamura I (1992) Zinc-deficient diet impairs adaptive changes in the remaining intestine after massive small bowel resection in the rat. Br J Surg 79:959–963
60. Besterman HS, Adrian TE, Mallinson CN, et al (1982) Gut hormone release after intestinal resection. Gut 23:854–861
61. Taylor RG, Fuller BP (1994) Humoral regulation of intestinal adaptation. Ballière's Clin Endocrinol Metab 8:165–183
62. Majumdar APN (1984) Postnatal undernutrition: Effect of epidermal growth factor on growth and function of the gastrointestinal tract in rats. J Ped Gastroenterol Nutr 3: 618–625
63. Opleta-Madsen K, Hardin J, Gall DG (1991) Epidermal growth factor upregulates intestinal electrolyte and nutrient transport. Am J Physiol 260:G807–G814
64. Goodlad RA, Raja KB, Peters TJ, Wright NA (1991) Effects of urogastrone-epidermal growth factor on intestinal brush border enzymes and mitotic activity. Gut 32:994–998
65. Ulshen MH, Lyn-Cook LE, Raasch RH (1986) Effects of intraluminal epidermal growth factor on mucosal proliferation in the small intestine of adult rats. Gastroenterology 91: 1134–1140
66. Kingsnorth AN, Vowles R, Nash JR (1990) Epidermal growth factor increases tensile stength in intestinal wounds in pigs. Br J Surg 77:409–412
67. Zapata-Sirvent RL, Hansbrough JF, Wolf P, et al (1993) Epidermal growth factor limits structural alterations in gastrointestinal tissues and decreases bacterial translocation in burned mice. Surgery 113:564–573
68. Goodlad RA, Lee CY, Wright NA (1992) Cell proliferation in the small intestine and colon of intravenously fed rats: Effects of urogastrone-epidermal growth factor. Cell Prolif 25: 393–404
69. Mainoya JR (1975) Effects of bovine growth hormone, human placental lactogen and ovine prolactin on intestinal fluid and ion transport in the rat. Endocrinology 96:1165–1170
70. Mainoya JR (1982) Influence of bovine growth hormone on water and NaCl absorption by the rat proximal jejunum and distal ileum. Comp Biochem Physiol 71A:477–479
71. Cooke PS, Yonemura CU, Russell SM, Nicoll CS (1986) Growth and differentiation of fetal rat intestine explants: Dependence on insulin and growth hormone. Biol Neonate 49: 211–218

72. Christensen H, Oxlund H, Laurberg S (1991) Postoperative biosynthetic human growth hormone increases the strength and collagen deposition of experimental colonic anastomoses. Int J Colorectal Dis 6:133–138.

73. Shulman DI, Hu CS, Duckett G, et al (1992) Effects of short-term growth hormone therapy in rats undergoing 75% small intestinal resection. J Pediatr Gastroenterol Nutr 14:3–11

74. Christensen H, Flyvbjerg A, Orskov H, et al (1993) Effect of growth hormone on the inflammatory activity of experimental colitis in rats. Scand J Gastroenterology 28:503–511

75. Ulshen MH, Dowling RH, Fuller CR, Zimmerman E, Lund PK (1993) Enhanced growth of small bowel in transgenic mice overexpressing bovine growth hormone. Gastroenterology 104:973–980

76. Bird AR, Croom WJ, Black BL, Fan YK, Daniel LR (1994) Somatotropin transgenic mice have reduced jejunal active glucose transport rates. J Nutr 124:2189–2196

77. Inoue Y, Copeland EM, Souba WW (1994) Growth hormone enhances amino acid uptake by the human small intestine. Ann Surg 219:715–724

78. Lemmey AB, Martin AA, Read LC, Tomas FM, Owens PC, Ballard FJ (1991) IGF-I and the truncated analogue des-(1-3)-IGF I enhance growth in rats after gut resection. Am J Physiol 260:E213–E219

79. Vanderhoof JA, McCusker RH, Clark R, et al (1992) Truncated and native insulin-like growth factor I enhance mucosal adaptation after jejunoileal resection. Gastroenterology 102:1949–1956

80. Mantell MP, Ziegler TR, Smith RJ, Rombeau JL (1993) Regulation of the intestinal insulin-like growth factor-I (IGF-I) action pathway after massive small bowel resection and IGF-I administration. Surg Forum 44:1–4

81. Ziegler TR, Mantell MP, Rombeau JL, Smith RJ (1994) Effects of glutamine and IGF-I administration on intestinal growth and the IGF pathway after partial small bowel resection. J Parent Enteral Nutr 18 (Suppl 1):20S (Abst)

82. Yang H, Grahn M, Schalch DS, Ney DM (1994) Anabolic effects of IGF-I coinfused with total parenteral nutrition in dexamethasone-treated rats. Am J Physiol 266:E690–E698

83. Zhang W, Frankel WL, Adamson WT, et al (1995) Insulin-like growth factor I (IGF-I) improves mucosal structure and function in transplanted rat small intestine. Transplantation 59:755–761

84. Lemmey AB, Ballard FJ, Martin AA, Tomas FM, Howarth GS, Read LC (1994) Treatment with IGF-I peptides improves function of the remnant gut following small bowel resection in rats. Growth Factors 10:243–252

85. Huang KF, Chung DH, Herndon DN (1993) Insulin-like growth factor I reduces gut atrophy and bacterial translocation after severe burn injury. Arch Surg 128:47–54

86. Baumrucker CR, Hadsell DL, Blum JW (1994) Effects of dietary insulin-like growth factor-I on growth and insulin-like growth factor receptors in neonatal calf intestine. J Anim Sci 72:428–433

87. Olanrewaju H, Patel L, Seidel ER (1992) Trophic action of local intraileal infusion of insulin-like growth factor-I: Polyamine dependence. Am J Physiol 263:E282–E286

88. Schulman R (1990) Oral insulin increases small intestinal mass and disaccharidase activity in newborn miniature pig. Ped Res 28:171–175

89. Menard D, Dagenais P (1993) Stimulatory effect of insulin on DNA synthesis in suckling mouse colon. Biol Neonate 63:310–315

90. Housley RM, Morris CF, Boyle W, et al (1994) Keratinocyte growth factor induces proliferation of hepatocytes and epithelial cells throughout the rat gastrointestinal tract. J Clin Invest 94:1764–1777

91. Thissen JP, Ketelslegers JM, Underwood LE (1994) Nutritional regulation of the insulin-like growth factors. Endocrine Rev 15:80–101

92. Lund P (1993) Nutritional control of genes encoding gastrointestinal peptides. In: Berdanier CD, Hargrove JL (eds): Nutrition and Gene Expression. CRC Press, Boca Raton, FL, pp 91–116

93. Donovan SM, Hintz RL, Wilson DM, Rosenfeld RG (1991) Insulin-like growth factors I and II and their binding proteins in rat milk. Pediatr Res 29:50–55

94. Droke EA, Spears JW, Armstrong JD, Kegley EB, Simpson RB (1993) Dietary zinc affects serum concentrations of insulin and insulin-like growth factor-I in growing lambs. J Nutr 123:13-19
95. Ninh NX, Thissen JP, Maiter D, Adam E, Mulumba N, Ketelslegers JM (1995) Reduced liver insulin-like growth factor-I gene expression in young zinc-deprived rats is associated with a decrease in liver growth hormone (GH) receptors and serum GH-binding protein. J Endocrinol 144:449-456
96. Dorup I (1994) Magnesium and potassium deficiency: Its diagnosis, occurrence and treatment in diuretic therapy and its consequences for growth, protein synthesis and growth factors. Acta Physiol Scand 52:1-55
97. Molina PE, Fan J, Lang CH, Abumrad NN (1994) Thiamine deficiency modulation of the IGF system response to growth hormone. Clin Nutr 14 (suppl 2):18 (Abst)
98. Jacobs DO, Evans DA, Mealy K, O'Dwyer S, Smith RJ, Wilmore DW (1988) Combined effects of glutamine and epidermal growth factor (EGF) on the rat intestine. Surgery 108:358-364
99. Salloum RM, Stevens BR, Schultz GS, Souba WW (1993) Regulation of small intestinal glutamine transport by epidermal growth factor. Surgery 113:552-559
100. Wang JY, Zhang LH, Song WL (1996) Epidermal growth factor regulates intestinal glutamine uptake during total parenteral nutrition. Clin Nutr 15:21-23
101. Ko TC, Beauchamp RD, Townsend CM, Thompson JC (1993) Glutamine is essential for epidermal growth factor-stimulated intestinal cell proliferation. Surgery 114:147-154
102. Welbourne TC (1995) Increased plasma bicarbonate and growth hormone after an oral glutamine load. Am J Clin Nutr 61:1058-1061
103. Hammarqvist F, Stromberg C, Decken von der A, et al (1992) Biosynthetic human growth hormone preserves both muscle protein synthesis and the decrease in muscle free glutamine, and improves whole-body nitrogen economy after operation. Ann Surg 216:184-191
104. Nolan EM, Masters JN, Dunn A (1990) Growth hormone regulation of hepatic glutamine synthetase mRNA levels in rats. Mol Cell Endocrinol 69:101-110
105. Byrne TA, Morrissey TB, Nattakom TV, Ziegler TR, Wilmore DW (1995) Growth hormone, glutamine and a modified diet enhance nutrient absorption in patients with the severe short bowel syndrome. J Parent Enteral Nutr 19:296-302
106. Byrne TA, Persinger RL, Young LS, Ziegler TR, Wilmore DW (1995) A new treatment for patients with the short bowel syndrome: Growth hormone, glutamine and a modified diet. Ann Surg 222:243-255
107. Playford RJ, Woodman AC, Clark P, et al (1993) Effect of luminal growth factor preservation on intestinal growth. Lancet 341:843-848
108. Xian CJ, Shoubridge CA, Read LC (1995) Degradation of IGF-I in the adult gastrointestinal tract is limited by a specific antiserum or the dietary protein casein. J Endocrinol 146:215-225
109. Hodin RA, Saldinger P, Meng S (1995) Small bowel adaptation: Counterregulatory effects of epidermal growth factor and somatostatin on the program of early gene expression. Surgery 118:206-211
110. Ko TC, Beauchamp D, Townsend CM, Thompson EA (1994) Transforming growth factor-β inhibits rat intestinal cell growth by regulating cell cycle specific gene expression. Am J Surg 167:14-20
111. Miettinen PJ (1993) Transforming growth factor-alpha and epidermal growth factor expression in human fetal gastrointestinal tract. Pediatr Res 33:481-486
112. Brasken P, Renvall S, Sandberg M (1991) Expression of epidermal growth factor and epidermal growth factor receptor genes in healing colonic anastomosis in rats. Eur J Surg 157:607-611
113. Suemori A, Ciacci C, Podolsky DK (1991) Regulation of transforming growth factor expression in rat intestinal epithelial cell lines. J Clin Invest 87:2214-2221
114. Oliver BL, Shaafi RI, Hajjar JJ (1995) Transforming growth factor-alpha and epidermal growth factor activate mitogen-activated protein kinase and its substrates in intestinal epithelial cells. Proc Soc Exp Med Biol 210:162-170

115. Horseman ND, Yu-Lee LY (1994) Transcriptional regulation by the helix bundle peptide hormones: Growth hormone, prolactin, and hematopoietic cytokines. Endo Rev 15: 627–648

116. Carter-Su C, Argetsinger LS, Campbell GS, Wang X, Ihle J, Witthuhn B (1994) The identification of JAK 2 tyrosine kinase as a signaling molecule for growth hormone. Proc Soc Exp Med Biol 206:210–215

117. Rotwein P, Gronowski AM, Thomas MJ (1994) Rapid nuclear actions of growth hormone. Horm Res 42:170–175

118. Hodin RA, Meng S, Nguyen D (1994) Immediate-early gene expression in EGF-stimulated intestinal epithelial cells. J Surg Res 56:500–504

119. Sacks AI, Warwick GJ, Barnard JA (1995) Early proliferative events following intestinal resection in the rat. J Pediatr Gastroenterol Nutr 21:158–164

120. Rountree DB, Ulshen MH, Selub S, et al (1992) Nutrient-independent increases in proglucagon and ornithine decarboxylase mRNAs after jejunoileal resection. Gastroenterology 103:462–468

121. Laburthe M, Couvineau A, Amiranoff B, Voisin T (1994) Receptors for gut regulatory peptides. Ballière's Clin Endocrinol Metab 8:77–110

122. Pedrini MF, Giorgino F, Smith RJ (1994) cDNA cloning of the rat IGF-I receptor: Structural analysis of the rat and human IGF-I and insulin receptors reveals differences in alternative splicing and receptor-specific domain conservation. Biochem Biophys Res Comm 202:1038–1046

123. Lowe WL, Adamo M, Werner H, Roberts CT, LeRoith D (1989) Regulation by fasting of rat insulin-like growth factor I and its receptor: Effects on gene expression and binding. J Clin Invest 84:619–626

124. LaBurthe M, Rouyer-Fessard C, Gammeltoft S (1988) Receptors for insulin-like growth factors I and II in rat gastrointestinal epithelium. Am J Physiol 254:G457–G462

125. Heinz-Erian P, Kessler U, Funk B, Gais P, Kiess W (1991) Identification and in situ localization of the insulin-like growth factor-II/mannose-6-phosphate (IGF-II/M6P) receptor in the rat gastrointestinal tract:Comparison with the IGF-I receptor. Endocrinology 129: 1769–1778

126. Ryan J, Costigan DC (1993) Determination of the histological distribution of insulin-like growth factor I receptors in the rat gut. Gut 34:1693-1697

127. MacDonald RS, Park JHY, Thornton WH (1993) Insulin, IGF-I, and IGF-II receptors in rat small intestine following massive small bowel resection: Analysis by binding, flow cytometry and immunohistochemistry. Dig Dis Sci 38:1658–1669

128. Lobie PE, Breipohl W, Waters MJ (1990) Growth hormone receptor expression in the rat gastrointestinal tract. Endocrinology 126:299–306

129. Rouyer-Fessard C, Gammeltoft S, LaBurthe M (1990) Expression of two types of receptor for insulin-like growth factors in human colonic epithelium. Gastroenterology 98: 703–707

130. Singh P, Rubin N (1993) Insulin-like growth factors and binding proteins in colon cancer. Gastroenterology 105:1218–1237

131. Delehaye-Zervas MC, Mertani H, Martini JF, Nihoul-Fekete C, Morel G, Postel-Vinay MC (1994) Expression of the growth hormone receptor gene in human digestive tissues. J Clin Endocrinol Metab 78:1473–1480

132. Nagano M, Chastre E, Choquet A, Bara J, Gespach C, Kelly PA (1995) Expression of prolactin and growth hormone receptor and their isoforms in the gastrointestinal tract. Am J Physiol 68:G431–G442

133. Han VK, D'Ercole AJ, Lund PK (1987) Cellular localization of somatomedin (insulin-like growth factor) messenger RNA in the human fetus. Science 236:193–197

134. Hill DJ, Clemmons DR (1992) Similar distribution of insulin-like growth factor binding proteins-1, -2, -3 in human fetal tissues. Growth Factors 6:315–326

135. Delhanty PJD, Hill DJ, Shimasaki S, Han VKM (1993) Insulin-like growth factor binding protein -4, -5 and -6 mRNAs in the human fetus: Localization to sites of growth and differentiation. Growth Regulation 3:8–11

136. Yang H, Ney DM, Peterson CA, Lo HC, Adamo ML (1995) Hepatic and jejunal responses to IGF-I and GH in rats maintained with total parenteral nutrition are associated with differential responses of IGF-I and IGF-BP-5 gene expression. Proceedings of the 77th Clinical Congress of the Endocrine Society, Washington, D.C. 173 (Abst)
137. Albiston AL, Taylor RG, Herington AC, Beveridge DJ, Fuller PJ (1992) Divergent ileal IGF-I and IGF-BP-3 gene expression after small bowel resection: A novel mechanism to amplify IGF action? Mol Cell Endocrinol 83:R17–R20
138. Singh P, Dai B, Dhruva B, Widen SG (1994) Episomal expression of sense and antisense insulin-like growth factor (IGF)-binding protein-4 complementary DNA alters the mitogenic response of a human colon cancer cell line (HT-29) by mechanisms that are independent of and dependent upon IGF-I. Cancer Res 54:6563–6570
139. Duncan MD, Korman LY, Bass BL (1994) Epidermal growth factor primes intestinal epithelial cells for proliferative effect of insulin-like growth factor-I. Dig Dis Sci 39:2197–2201
140. Simmons JG, Hoyt EC, Westwick JK, Brenner DA, Pucilowska JB, Lund PK (1995) Insulin-like growth factor-I and epidermal growth factor interact to regulate growth and gene expression in EC-6 intestinal epithelial cells. Mol Endo 9:1157–1165

Regulation of Gut Perfusion

B. Cholley and D. Payen

Introduction

Today, multiple organ failure (MOF) is still a common cause of death in ICU despite the efforts to prevent this ultimate evolution of critical illness. Among the different mechanisms involved in the complex pathophysiology of MOF, injury to the gut may play a key role [1–3]. The gut mucosa constitutes a barrier protecting the internal milieu from the intraluminal content. Since any insult to the barrier results in increased permeability to large molecules [4, 5], it has been hypothesized that bacteria or bacterial products such as endotoxin, could be "translocated" into the blood stream, subsequently promoting systemic inflammatory responses and development of MOF [2, 6–8].

Prior to the availability of monitoring tools to estimate gut perfusion, the digestive tract was generally not considered at risk of indirect injury during severe systemic disorders. With the emergence of gastric tonometry, splanchnic hypoxia and subsequent mucosal acidosis have been detected in critically ill patients and shown to correlate with poor outcome [9–12]. Moreover, there is experimental evidence that hypoxia (especially in the splanchnic territory and in the lungs) may trigger a cascade of pro-inflammatory cytokines and amplify the systemic inflammatory response [13]. Therefore, maintaining adequate gut perfusion during resuscitation of critical illness has to be one of the priorities of all resuscitation strategies [14].

The goal of the present chapter is to review the different mechanisms involved in the regulation of gut perfusion during physiological and pathological circumstances.

Main Features of Intestinal Vascular Anatomy

There is a great variability in the patterns of blood supply to the gut, but the three main visceral arteries (celiac trunk, superior and inferior mesenteric arteries) corresponding to the three distinct embryological areas of the gastrointestinal (GI) tract, are constant. In most cases, the upper part of the gut (stomach and duodenum) receives its blood from the celiac trunk, the entire small intestine and two thirds of the colon are supplied by the superior mesenteric artery (Fig. 1), while the left colon and rectum depend on the inferior mesenteric artery.

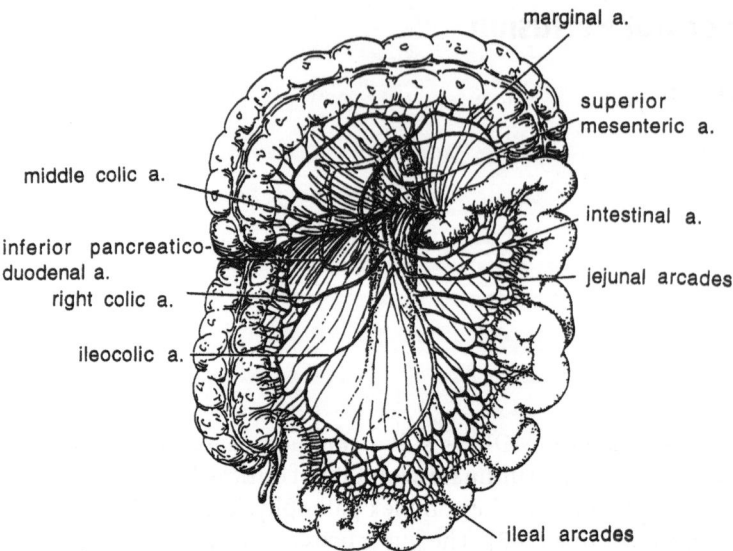

marginal a.

superior
mesenteric a.

middle colic a.

intestinal a.

inferior pancreatico-
duodenal a.

jejunal arcades

right colic a.

ileocolic a.

ileal arcades

Fig. 1. Main branches of the superior mesenteric artery (a.). Note that the "arcades" system is well developed at the level of the small intestine but not in the large bowel. (Adapted from [17])

In-between the main arteries and the microvessels are the "intermediate" vessels, characterized at the level of the small bowel by their many anastomoses realizing the arcade system (Fig. 1). This arrangement prevents any damage to result from obstruction of a single vessel. In the colon however, the anastomoses are much less developed with critical areas of anastomotic supply such as the junction between the superior and inferior mesenteric territories.

The intramural architecture of the microcirculation is similar in the small bowel and the colon [15]. An intermediate artery (ileal arcade, or one of the vasa recta in the colon) penetrates obliquely through the muscularis propria to enter the submucosa. In the submucosa, these rather large tortuous arteries are found around the whole circumference of the gut and anastomose freely to each other. They give origin to smaller vessels going to the mucosa and to recurrent branches going to the muscularis propria, which also receives blood from the serosal plexus. This dual blood supply may explain in part the resistance of the muscularis to ischemia.

Unlike the intramural pattern, the mucosal distribution of microvessels differs greatly between the large and small bowel. In the colon, branches of the submucosal plexus extend toward the base of the mucosa and then anastomose to realize a surface mucosal plexus. In the small bowel, a rich basal mucosal plexus is also present from which a single arteriole passes upwards through the middle of the villus to reach its tip. At this point, the vessel branches into several descending capillaries form an anastomotic network on the outer surface of the villus. This architecture is the basis of the countercurrent exchange system discussed below. Precapillary sphincters are present at the entrance to many ($\approx 75\%$) of the mucosal arterioles [16].

The alimentary veins follow closely the path of the arteries. They are remarkable in that they have no valves, so that changes in portal pressure are communicated directly to the gut wall [17]. The intestinal venous outflow drains in the portal vein and provides normally two thirds of the hepatic oxygen delivery (DO_2), one third only coming from the hepatic arterial inflow.

Intestinal Microcirculation: Countercurrent Exchanger of the Intestinal Villus

The anatomical disposition of the vessels in the intestinal villi implies opposite directions of blood flow in the central arteriole and in the subepithelial capillaries and venules resulting in a countercurrent exchanger (Fig. 2). The distance between the ascending and descending vessels is close to 20 µm, allowing diffusion of small molecules (like oxygen, water, or sodium) from one vessel to another according to the concentration gradient between the two sites [18, 19]. The intestinal countercurrent exchanger may act as a multiplier for actively transported solutes such as sodium, by maintaining a gradient between the intestinal lumen and the superficial capillaries. It may also induce hypoxia of the villous tip by allowing shunting of oxygen between arteriole and venous capillaries at the base of the villus [20, 21]. The only limiting factor to small molecule diffusion is the transit time of blood in these vessels. In the cat, under resting conditions (intestinal flow 20–40 mL/min/100 g), the transit time of blood between the base and the tip of the villus has been measured as 4–8 sec. It decreases to about 1 sec after maximal vasodilation and increases to 20–30 sec when intestinal blood flow is reduced to 5–10 mL/min/100 g [22]. During hypovolemic shock, the low perfusion pressure relaxes precapillary sphincters resulting in an increased number of perfused capillaries to try to maintain blood flow. A low pressure as well as an increased number of perfused capillaries are responsible for prolonging the mean transit time of blood through the villi and allow very poor DO_2 at the tip of the villus due to oxygen diffusion at its base. The villous apical hypoxia due to this countercurrent system is responsible for tissue damage during hypotension and is further aggravated by free radical exposure during reperfusion [23].

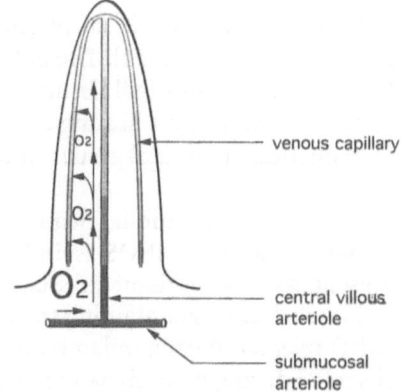

Fig. 2. Schematic representation of the intestinal villous countercurrent exchanger, where oxygen can diffuse away from the central arteriole towards the venous capillaries. This may lead to very low PaO_2 at the top of the villus, especially when the mean transit time of red blood cells increases

Control Mechanisms Acting on the Intestinal Circulation

Many different factors influence the smooth muscle tone of the splanchnic vessels, regulating intestinal blood volume and flow.

Sympathetic Nervous System

Sympathetic innervation is found in the mesentery (outside the gut itself) and in the gut wall as well, but not in the villi where the vessels lack smooth muscles. Experimentally, α-adrenergic stimulation increases intestinal resistance and reduces global splanchnic blood flow [24]. This reflects the high density of α-adrenergic receptors on the mesenteric vessels. The effects of α-adrenergic stimulation on blood flow partition between mucosa and muscularis are somewhat controversial. Some authors observed an increased blood flow towards the villi at the expense of the crypts [25], whereas others demonstrated a redistribution of blood flow from the mucosa towards the muscularis [26, 27]. On the other hand β$_2$-agonists do increase global mesenteric blood flow but also selectively vasodilate the mucosal microcirculation [14, 28]. The role of dopaminergic receptors in the mesenteric circulation remains unclear due to the lack of specific agonist. Indeed, even low-dose dopamine infusion stimulates α-receptors sufficiently to blunt the β$_2$- and dopaminergic vasodilator effects of the drug at the mucosa level [26]. Sympathetic activation of the splanchnic territory can be reflexly triggered by carotid baroreceptors activation [29] as well as chemoreceptors via increased arterial PCO_2, decreased PO_2, or decreased pH [30].

Parasympathetic Nervous System

The colon has some parasympathetic innervation provided by the pelvic nerves, but the small intestine apparently lacks parasympathetic vascular control [31].

Nitric Oxide (NO) Pathway

NO plays a central role in the physiology and the response to critical illness of the gastrointestinal tract [32]. The potential sources of NO in the gut include:
1) the intrinsic intestinal tissue;
2) resident and/or infiltrating cells as neutrophils and monocytes; and
3) reduction of luminal gastric nitrate.

Under resting conditions, two isoforms of NO synthase (bNOS and cNOS) are expressed, whereas iNOS is induced only when an inflammatory process is present. As in other tissues, the basal vasodilating tone is related to NO release by endothelial cells, maintaining the mucosal perfusion. The larger concentrations of NO released during inflammation may participate to the mucosal hyperemia observed during hyperdynamic sepsis.

In addition to its vascular effects, NO mediates the coordination of intestinal peristalsis and sphincters as a neurotransmitter of the non-adrenergic, non-cholinergic enteric nervous system.

Cyclooxygenase (COX) Pathway

Prostacyclin participates in the basal vasodilating tone, in parallel to NO, and is physiologically produced by a constitutive isoform of cyclooxygenase (COX I). In disease states such as portal hypertension or sepsis, an inducible form of the enzyme (COX II) is expressed and produces exagerate amounts of prostacyclin [33–35]. The NO secretion resulting from the expression of iNOS in the smooth muscle cells exerts an inhibitory effect on the production of prostacyclin by COX II [36].

Hormonal Control of the Intestinal Blood Flow

Several substances have been proposed to play a role in the splanchnic hemodynamics, especially the postprandial hyperemia. These include the cholecystokinine (CCK), gastrin, gastric inhibitory polypeptide (GIP), glucagon, neurotensin and secretin. However, none of them (alone or in association) was found to have a relaxing effect on intestinal arteriolar smooth muscle tone at physiologic concentrations [25]. The splanchnic circulation is very responsive to vasoconstrictive hormones like angiotensin II and vasopressin. The predominance of splanchnic vasoconstriction during hypovolemic shock is largely mediated by these two molecules [37].

Local Chemical Control of the Intestinal Circulation

The local chemical surrounding influences blood flow to tissues. When DO_2 is reduced, the number of perfused capillaries increases to facilitate oxygen extraction [38, 39]. Adenosine, low PO_2, high PCO_2, hyperosmolality, potassium ions, have all been proposed as potential mediators of postprandial hyperemia. Specifically to the intestine, the intraluminal chemical environment may influence perfusion, and substances like lipids, breakdown products of carbohydrates together with bile have been shown to participate in the reactive hyperemia [31].

Local Nervous Reflex Control

Described by Biber et al. [22] this control involves the mechanical stimulation of the villi by food and possibly secretion of vasoactive intestinal polypeptide (VIP) among the mediators responsible for postprandial vasodilation.

Physiological Variations in Splanchnic Perfusion

At Rest

The splanchnic circulation normally receives about 25% of the cardiac output and extracts only 15 to 20% of the oxygen available. Therefore the saturation of the portal blood entering the liver is quite high in comparison with venous blood from other territories. The resting blood flow per unit weight of the intestine is ten times higher than that of skeletal muscle and twice less than that of brain or heart. However, perfusion levels vary along the digestive tract, and there is a gradient in blood flow, expressed per unit weight of tissue, between the duodenum receiving up to 40 mL/min/100 g and the colon that receives roughly half of it. These values of resting blood flow can be doubled during ingestion of food or even increased by as much as one order of magnitude with vasodilators or during fulminant ulcerative colitis, mainly as the result of mucosal vasodilation.

Distribution of blood flow within the gut wall is important to consider, since muscularis and mucosa have very different behaviors related to their functional differences. For example, absorption and secretion are two metabolically demanding activities located in the mucosa. It is also possible that mucosal blood flow exceeds that required for oxygen and metabolites delivery in order to satisfy the needs of the absorption process. The partition of blood flow between mucosa-submucosa/muscularis at rest is approximately 75/25%, respectively. Few information exist regarding how this ratio is altered during critical illness or during treatment with vasoactive agents in humans.

Although less pronounced than in the kidney or the brain, the splanchnic circulation exhibits some degree of autoregulation [40]. In the liver, the hepatic arterial buffer response compensates for any decrease in portal blood flow (i.e. mesenteric blood flow) to maintain DO_2 [41]. In the intestine, the flow can be maintained fairly constant with variations in perfusion pressure from 80 to 160 mmHg. The precapillary arterioles are responsible for maintaining blood flow constant when perfusion pressure is reduced. This is accomplished by an increase in the number of capillaries perfused, resulting in increased intestinal blood volume and prolonged mean transit time of blood through the villi. The exact mechanism involved is not known and may involve the myogenic response of the precapillary sphincters to variations in perfusion pressure and/or the accumulation of vasoactive metabolites in the circumstances of low flow.

During Exercise

The splanchnic circulation contains 20–25% of the total blood volume, therefore any alteration in the splanchnic blood flow (SBF) or volume is expected to play a significant role in the cardiovascular response to stress. During exercise, blood is redistributed away from the splanchnic vascular bed and splanchnic blood flow can be reduced by 80% when maximum oxygen consumption (VO_2) is reached, compared to resting state [25]. SBF and blood volume are reduced as a consequence of sympathetically-mediated increase in mesenteric arterial resistance and reduction in portal venous bed capacitance [25, 42, 43]. However this reduction in DO_2 is counterbalanced by an increase in oxygen extraction ratio (O_2ER) and does not impair the metabolic rate of the splanchnic organs.

During Food Intake

Intestinal blood flow is considerably altered during the ingestion and digestion of food. The circulatory changes during anticipation and ingestion of food involve reflex sympathetic activation, whereas the vascular responses during digestion are mainly determined by the nature of the food taken, the concentration within the bowel lumen of the products of digestion, and the secondary effects of GI hormones [44]. In conscious dogs, the hemodynamic changes following food intake consist of two phases. The first one, occurring during anticipation of the meal and lasting until 3–10 min after ingestion, is characterized by an increase in heart rate, cardiac output and blood pressure resulting from sympathetic activation and lasting for up to 30 min. This initial increase in mesenteric resistance is abolished by sympathetic blockade. Then, digestion is followed by a two- or three-fold increase in mesenteric blood flow. The mechanisms accounting for this increase in flow are multiple and include effects of digestive hormones (CCK, secretin, ...) as well as direct mechanical effects of intestinal lumen distension. The visceral (especially the hepatic) autonomic nervous system also plays an important role in postprandial hemodynamic changes in humans, since the increase in portal blood flow (reflecting mesenteric outflow) is not detected any more following orthotopic liver transplantation [45]. The chemical specificity of the food (carbohydrates, lipids, or proteins) ingested also influences the splanchnic hyperemia [45, 46]. Bohlen demonstrated that glucose exposure was responsible for dilating mucosal microvessels independently of the glucose concentration. This mucosal hyperemia was at least in part secondary to a major decrease in mucosal tissue PO_2 [21, 47].

Pathological Variations in Splanchnic Perfusion

Effects of Intra-Thoracic and Intra-Abdominal Pressures

Mechanical ventilation with positive end-expiratory pressure (PEEP) increases the right atrial pressure which constitutes the back pressure opposing the venous return. As a consequence, venous pressure has to increase to maintain constant flow, resulting in passive distension of the veins and pooling of blood, notably in the splanchnic territory [48]. When PEEP increases, venous return drops and there is a proportional fall in cardiac and mesenteric blood flow [49]. However, the intra-abdominal location of the gut prevents large variations in splanchnic blood flow to result from positive pressure breathing. When direct intra-thoracic pressure is applied to mesenteric artery following esophageal reconstruction using an ileo-colic graft, deleterious effects of PEEP on graft blood flow is much more relevant [50, 51].

Hypovolemic and Cardiogenic Shock

During hypovolemic or cardiogenic shock, there is a generalized vasoconstriction, but in the splanchnic territory the increase in total peripheral resistance may be two- to five-fold greater than that calculated in the systemic circulation, reflecting a selective splanchnic vasospasm [52]. In an experimental model of circulatory shock using cardiac tamponade, a 50% reduction in cardiac output was accompanied by a 90% reduction in SBF [53]. Following moderate hemorrhagic hypovolemia in rats, Scalia et al. [54] observed an arteriolar vasoconstriction in the ileal mucosa that persisted despite volume restoration. In healthy humans, simulated hypovolemia was accompanied by a parallel decrease in cardiac output and splanchnic perfusion, but SBF remained low a long time after cardiac output had returned to baseline values [55]. This increase in mesenteric resistance is mediated by an increase in sym-pathetic tone and vasoconstrictive hormones, mainly angiotensin II and vasopressin [37]. In experimental animals undergoing cardiogenic or hypovolemic shock, this mesenteric vasoconstriction was responsible for ischemic mucosal damage [56, 57].

Septic Shock

Severe alterations in vascular properties occur during septic shock, attesting for the close interrelation between the vascular and immune systems. Vascular cells are a privileged target for cytokines (mainly tumor necrosis factor (TNF) and interleukin (IL)-1) responsible for their phenotypic immunomodulation. At the level of the endothelial cell, cytokines induce procoagulant and proinflammatory changes resulting in thrombosis, leukocyte adhesion, and hyperpermeability phenomena. At the level of the smooth muscle cell, cytokines induce the expression of iNOS and of COX II. These two enzymes can produce large amounts of NO and prostacyclin accounting for the septic vasoplegia.

The classical hemodynamic pattern of septic shock associating high cardiac output and low peripheral resistance may vary according to different factors. In the absence of fluid resuscitation, septic shock has much of the hemodynamic features of a hypovolemic or hemorrhagic shock, with low cardiac output, low mean arterial pressure and elevated systemic resistance [58].

The endocrine status, especially endogenous corticoids level, can also modify the vascular alterations during sepsis via a modulation of the expression of proinflammatory cytokines as well as that of iNOS [59]. Finally, the metabolic (glycemic) status may modulate the production of cytokines by the liver and influence the systemic hemodynamic response.

The vascular hyporeactivity leading to vasoplegia during sepsis has been experimentally demonstrated on large conductive vessels such as the aorta. However, some regional variations exist regarding the contractile response to norepinephrine after exposure to endotoxin or IL-1: in rabbits, this response was depressed at the level of aorta, pulmonary and carotid arteries, whereas it was preserved at the level of the renal and mesenteric arteries [60]. Splanchnic blood flow is low during unresuscitated septic shock [61, 62], but can be maintained or even increased during hyperdynamic shock following fluid resuscitation [5, 62, 63]. In humans with hyperdynamic sepsis, SBF was found to be elevated in comparison with normal volunteers or resuscitated trauma patients [64–66]. However, the increase in splanchnic VO_2 was proportionately larger than the increase in DO_2, suggesting that the gut mucosa might still be at risk of ischemic damage [65]. Furthermore, the microvascular alterations present during sepsis impair mucosal perfusion and hence, DO_2 to the metabolically most active portion of the gut [67, 68].

Experimentally, NO donors help maintaining flow and vascular integrity in the splanchnic territory, whereas NO inhibitors have opposite effects and increase the mortality rate in septic animals [61, 69, 70].

The beneficial effect of NO on splanchnic microcirculation results mainly from a network of actions:
1) maintenance of mucosal perfusion;
2) inhibition of neutrophil adhesion to mesenteric endothelial cells; and
3) inhibition of platelet aggregation and adhesion.

Conversely, excessive NO release can directly injure the mucosa, altering the mucosal barrier. At this high NO concentration, tight junctions are dilated and the barrier becomes hyperpermeable. Thus inhibition of NOS ameliorates the barrier dysfunction when iNOS yields "toxic" concentrations of NO. As for other tissues, it seems reasonable to maintain NO released by cNOS to protect the GI tract, but possibly to inhibit excessive NO production by iNOS, although the benefit of the administration of non-selective NO inhibitors is not established for the moment.

Conclusion

The splanchnic blood flow is subject to large physiological variations. It may double or more in order to face the metabolic demand associated with absorption of nutrients, and it may fall drastically as a consequence of blood volume and flow redistribution during exercise or hypovolemia. The multiple mechanisms regulating blood volume and flow in the splanchnic territory and their interrelations are not completely characterized. For the intensivist aware of the importance of protecting the intestinal barrier in critically ill patients, more information is needed regarding the effects of vasoactive drugs on gut mucosal perfusion, or the clinical usefulness of modulating NO or cyclooxygenase pathways during sepsis. Today, no specific therapeutic strategy has proven clear beneficial effect in terms of reducing the incidence of multiple organ failure and mortality.

References

1. Fiddian-Green R (1988) Splanchnic ischemia and multiple organ failure in the critically ill. Ann R Coll Surg 70:128–134
2. Landow L, Andersen L (1994) Splanchnic ischemia and its role in multiple organ failure. Acta Anaesthesiol Scand 38:626–639
3. Fink M (1993) Adequacy of gut oxygenation in endotoxemia and sepsis. Crit Care Med 21: S4–S8
4. Fink M, Antonsson J, Wang H, Rotschild H (1991) Increased intestinal permeability in endotoxic pigs. Mesenteric hypoperfusion as an etiologic factor. Arch Surg 126:211–218
5. Fink M, Kaups K, Wang H, Rotschild H (1991) Maintenance of superior mesenteric arterial perfusion prevents increased intestinal mucosal permeability in endotoxic pigs. Surgery 110:154–161
6. Border J, Hasset J, LaDuca J, et al (1987) The gut origin septic states in blunt multiple trauma (ISS=40) in the ICU. Ann Surg 206:427–448
7. Meakins J, Marshall J (1989) The gut as the "motor" of multiple system organ failure. In: Fiddian Green R (eds) Splanchnic ischemia and multiple organ failure. Mosby, St Louis Missouri, pp 339–348
8. Andersen L, Landow L, Baek L, Jansen E, Baker S (1993) Association between gastric intramucosal pH and splanchnic endotoxin, antibody to endotoxin, and tumor necrosis factor-α concentrations in patients undergoing cardiopulmonary bypass. Crit Care Med 21: 210–217
9. Doglio G, Pusajo J, Egurrola M, et al (1991) Gastric mucosal pH as a prognostic index of mortality in the critically ill patients. Crit Care Med 19:1037–1040
10. Guttierrez G, Palizas F, Doglio G, et al (1992) Gastric intramucosal pH as a therapeutic index of tissue oxygenation in critically ill patients. Lancet 339:195–199
11. Marik P (1993) Gastric intramucosal pH: A better predictor of multiorgan dysfunction syndrome and death than oxygen-derived variables in patients with sepsis. Chest 104: 225–229
12. Maynard N, Bihari D, Beale R, et al (1993) Assessment of splanchnic oxygenation by gastric tonometry in patients with acute circulatory failure. JAMA 270:1203–1248
13. Shreenivas R, Koga S, Karakurum M, et al. (1992) Hypoxia-mediated induction of endothelial cell interleukin-1α. J Clin Invest 90:2333–2339
14. Maynard N, Bihari D, Dalton R, Smithies M, Mason R (1995) Increasing splanchnic blood flow in the critically ill. Chest 108:1648–1654
15. Carr N (1989) Microscopic anatomy. In: Marston A, Bulkley G, Fiddian Green R, Haglund U (eds) Splanchnic ischemia and multiple organ failure. Mosby, St Louis, Missouri, pp 17–28
16. Gore R, Bohlen H (1977) Microvascular pressures in rat intestinal muscle and mucosal villi. Am J Physiol 233:H685–H693
17. Marston A, Pegington J (1989) Macroscopic anatomy. In: Marston A, Bulkley G, Fiddian Green R, Haglund U (eds) Splanchnic ischemia and multiple organ failure. Mosby, St Louis, Missouri, pp 3–16
18. Hallbeck D-A, Hulten L, Jodal M, Lindhagen J, Lundgreen O (1978) Evidence for the existence of a countercurrent exchanger in the small intestine in man. Gastroenterology 74: 683–690
19. Kampp M, Lundgreen O, Nilsson N (1968) Extravascular shunting of oxygen in the small intestine of the cat. Acta Physiol Scand 72:396–403
20. Kvietys P, Granger D (1982) Vasoactive agents and splanchnic oxygen uptake. Am J Physiol 243:G1–G9
21. Bohlen H (1980) Intestinal tissue PO_2 and microvascular responses during glucose exposure. Am J Physiol 238:H164–H171

22. Biber B, Lundgreen O, Stage L, Svanvik J (1973) An indicator-dilution method for studying intestinal hemodynamics in the cat. Acta Physiol Scand 87:433–447
23. Haglund U, Abe T, Ahren C, Braide I, Lundgreen O (1976) The intestinal mucosal lesions in shock: I. Studies on the pathogenesis. Eur Surg Res 8:435–447
24. Shepherd A, Pawlik W, Mailman D, Burks T, Jacobson E (1976) Effects of vasoconstrictors on intestinal vascular resistance and oxygen extraction. Am J Physiol 230:298–305
25. Donald D (1983) Splanchnic circulation. In: Geiger S (ed) Handbook of Physiology. William & Wilkins, Bethesda, Maryland, pp 219–240
26. Giraud G, MacCannel K (1984) Decreased nutrient blood flow during dopamine- and epinephrine-induced intestinal vasodilation. J Pharmacol Exp Ther 230:214–220
27. Segal J, Phang P, Walley K (1992) Low-dose dopamine hastens onset of gut ischemia in a porcine model of hemorragic shock. J Appl Physiol 73:1159–1164
28. Shepherd A, Riedel G, Maxwell L, Kiel J (1984) Selective vasodilators redistribute intestinal blood flow and depress oxygen uptake. Am J Physiol 247:G377–G384
29. Hadjiminas J, Öberg B (1968) Effects of carotid baroreceptor reflexes on venous tone of skeletal muscle and intestine in the cat. Acta Physiol Scand 72:518–532
30. Auden R, Donald D (1975) Reflex responses of the isolated *in situ* portal vein of the dog. J Surg Res 18:35–42
31. Lundgreen O (1989) Physiology of the intestinal circulation. In: Marston A, Bulkley G, Fiddian-Green R, Haglund U (eds) Splanchnic ischemia and multiple organ failure. Mosby, St Louis, Missouri, pp 29–40
32. Saltzman A (1995) Nitric oxide in the gut. New Horizons 3:33– 45
33. Wu Y, Burns R, Sitzman J (1993) Effects of nitric oxide and cyclooxygenase inhibition on splanchnic hemodynamics in portal hypertension. Hepatology 18:1416–1421
34. Maier A, Hla T, Maciag T (1990) Cyclooxygenase is an immediate-early gene induced by interleukin-1 in human endothelial cells. J Biol Chem 265:10805–10808
35. Ohkawa F, Ikeda U, Kawasaki K, Kusano E, Igarashi M, Shimada K (1994) Inhibitory effect of interleukin-6 on vascular smooth muscle contraction. Am J Physiol 266:H898–H902
36. Swierkosz T, Mitchell J, Wood E, Warner T, Thiermermann C, Vane J (1993) Co-release and interactions of nitric oxide and prostanoids *in vitro* and *in vivo* following exposure to bacteria and lipopolysaccharide. Endothelium 1:S45 (Abstr 175)
37. McNeil J, Stark R, Greenway C (1970) Intestinal vasoconstriction after hemorrhage: Roles of vasopressin and angiotensin. Am J Physiol 219:1342–1347
38. Shepherd A (1982) Role of capillary recruitment in the regulation of intestinal oxygenation. Am J Physiol 242:G435–G441
39. Shepherd A (1982) Local control of intestinal oxygenation and blood flow. Annu Rev Physiol 44:13–27
40. Granger D, Richardson P, Kvietys P, Mortillaro N (1980) Intestinal blood flow. Gastroenterology 78:837–863
41. Richardson P, Withrington P (1981) Liver blood flow. I. Intrinsic and nervous control of liver blood flow. Gastroenterology 81:159–173
42. Rowell L (1974) Human cardiovascular adjustments to exercise and thermal stress. Physiol Rev 54:75–159
43. Greenway C (1983) Role of splanchnic venous system in overall cardiovascular homeostasis. Federation Proc 42:1678–1684
44. Chou C (1983) Splanchnic and overall cardiovascular hemodynamics during eating and digestion. Federation Proc 42:1658–1661
45. Payen D, Fratacci M, Dupuy P, et al (1990) Portal and hepatic arterial blood flow measurements of human transplanted liver by implanted Doppler probes: Interest for early complications and nutrition. Surgery 107:417–427
46. Chou C, Kvietys P, Post J, Sit S (1978) Constituents of chyme responsible for postprandial intestinal hyperhemia. Am J Physiol 235:H677–H682
47. Bohlen H (1980) Intestinal mucosal oxygenation influences absorbtive hyperhemia. Am J Physiol 239:H489–H493
48. Manyari D, Wang Z, Cohen J, Tyberg J (1993) Assessment of the human splanchnic venous volume-pressure relation using radionuclide plethysmography. Circulation 87:1142–1151

49. Winso O, Biber B, Gustavson B, Milsom C, Niedman D (1986) Portal blood flow in man during positive end-expiratory pressure ventilation. Intensive Care Med 12:80–85
50. Jacob L, Boudaoud S, Rabary O, et al (1994) Decreased mesenteric blood flow supplying retrosternal esophageal ileocoloplastic grafts during positive pressure breathing. J Thorac Cardiovasc Surg 107:68–73
51. Jacob L, Rabary O, Boudaoud S, et al (1992) Usefulness of perioperative pulsed Doppler flowmetry in predicting postoperative local ischemic complication after ileocolic esophagoplasty. J Thorac Cardiovasc Surg 104:385–390
52. Vatner S (1974) Effects of hemorrhage on regional blood flow distribution in dogs and primates. J Clin Invest 54:225–235
53. Bulkley G, Kvietys P, Perry D, Granger D (1983) Effects of cardiac tamponade on colonic hemodynamics and oxygen uptake. Am J Physiol 244:G604–G612
54. Scalia S, Burton H, Van Wylen D, et al (1990) Persistent arteriolar constriction in microcirculation of the terminal ileum following moderate hemorrhagic hypovolemia and volume restoration. J Trauma 30:713–718
55. Edouard A, Degrémont A, Duranteau J, Pussard E, Berdeaux A, Samii K (1994) Heterogeneous vascular responses to simulated transient hypovolemia in man. Intensive Care Med 20:414–420
56. Bailey R, Bulkley G, Hamilton S, Morris J (1987) Protection of the small intestine from nonocclusive mesenteric ischemic injury due to cardiogenic shock. Am J Surg 153:108–116
57. Porter J, Sussman M, Bulkley G (1989) Splanchnic vasospasm in circulatory shock. In: Marston A, Bulkley G, Fiddian-Green R, Haglund U (eds) Splanchnic ischemia and multiple organ failure. Mosby, St Louis, Missouri, pp 73–88
58. Cholley B, Lang R, Berger D, Korcarz C, Payen D, Shroff S (1995) Alterations in systemic arterial mechanical properties during septic shock: Role of fluid resuscitation. Am J Physiol 269:H375–H384
59. Szabo C, Thiermermann C, Wu C, Peretti M, Vane J (1994) Attenuation of the induction of nitric oxide synthase by endogenous glucocorticoids accounts for endotoxin tolerance *in vivo*. Proc Natl Acad Sci USA 91:271–275
60. Robert R, Chapelain B, Neliat G (1993) Different effects of Interleukin-1 on reactivity of arterial vessels isolated from various vascular beds in the rabbit. Circulatory Shock 40:139–143
61. Pastor C, Losser M, Payen D (1995) Nitric oxyde donor prevents hepatic and systemic perfusion decrease induced by endotoxin in anesthetized rabbits. Hepatology 22:1547–1553
62. Vallet B, Lund N, Curtis S, Kelly D, Cain S (1994) Gut and muscle tissue PO_2 in endotoxemic dogs during shock and resuscitation. J Appl Physiol 76:793–800
63. Swan K, Barton R, Reynolds D (1971) Mesenteric hemodynamics during endotoxemia in the baboon. Gastroenterology 61:872–876
64. Dahn M, Lange P, Wilson R, Jacobs L, Mitchell R (1990) Hepatic blood flow and splanchnic oxygen consumption measurements in clinical sepsis. Surgery 107:295–301
65. Dahn M, Lange P, Lobdell K, Hans B, Jacobs L, Mitchell R (1987) Splanchnic and total body oxygen consumption differences in septic and injured patients. Surgery 101:69–80
66. Ruokonen E, Takala J, Kari A, Saxen H, Mertsola J, Hansen E (1993) Regional blood flow and oxygen transport in septic shock. Crit Care Med 21:1296–1303
67. Drazenovic R, Samsel R, Wylam M, Doerschuk C, Schumacker P (1992) Regulation of perfused capillary density in canine intestinal mucosa during endotoxemia. J Appl Physiol 72:259–265
68. Theuer C, Wilson M, Steeb G, Garrison R (1993) Microvascular vasoconstriction and mucosal hypoperfusion of the rat small intestine during bacteremia. Circulatory Shock 40:61–68
69. Hutchinson I, Whittle B, Boughton-Smith N (1990) Role of nitric oxide in maintaining vascular integrity in endotoxin-induced acute intestinal damage in the rat. Br J Pharmacol 101:815–820
70. Pastor C, Payen D (1994) Effect of modifying nitric oxide pathway on liver circulation in a rabbit endotoxin shock model. Shock 2:196–202

Regulation of Gut Oxygen Delivery, Cellular Oxygen Supply and Metabolic Activity

P. T. Schumacker

Introduction

Over the past three decades, a large number of studies have examined the physiological regulation of blood flow, oxygen supply (DO_2) and oxygen extraction (O_2ER) in the gut using a wide variety of different models and experimental approaches. More recently, with a growing recognition of the potential significance of gut dysfunction in critical illness, investigators have explored the behavior of the gut under pathophysiological conditions, in terms of its regulation of cellular O_2 supply and epithelial barrier function. In this review, we begin with a brief overview of the physiological regulation of intestinal blood flow and oxygen transport, and then proceed to examine the potential significance of these findings for the function of the gut during critical illness, and especially during sepsis.

In an anatomical sense, the wall of the small intestine consists of an outer layer of smooth muscle comprised of longitudinal and circular layers, a submucosal layer of connective tissue, and an inner mucosal layer comprised of crypts and intestinal villi. Branches of the mesenteric artery supplying the small intestine form a plexus at the surface of the mesenteric attachment, and vessels coursing through the smooth muscle layers form a plexus of microvessels within the submucosa and at the submucosa-muscularis interface [1]. Microvessels supplying the mucosal crypts and villi originate in this plexus, although venous return from the villi travel by a separate route. This arrangement facilitates the capability for developing collateral blood flow under conditions where a single vessel may become transiently obstructed due to mechanical distortion of the mesentery or gut wall. In a study of the intestinal microcirculation, Gore and Bohlen [2] measured the longitudinal distribution of vascular resistance using micropipettes, and estimated that mucosal capillary hydrostatic pressure was less than in the muscularis as a consequence of differences in the vascular resistance in vessels upstream from the capillary bed. In a classical paper, Folkow [3] described the gut microcirculation in terms of three parallel vascular networks supplying mucosa, muscularis, and the submucosa. Because the metabolic demands of the connective tissue in the submucosa are low, and because some early anatomical studies suggested that arteriovenous anastomoses may exist in stomach submucosa [4, 5], flow to the submucosa was regarded as "shunt flow". However, more recent studies have failed to identify arteriovenous anastomoses in the gut of humans [1] or of the dog [6]. A useful modification to Folkow's model was described by Shepherd et al. [7] who proposed that the mucosa and muscularis functioned as two "parallel" vascular beds, each with its own (relatively small) vascular resistance. These parallel vessels were supplied by a single upstream segment containing a "series" resistance influencing the overall flow to the gut wall (Fig. 1). Most of the vascular resistance in the gut resides in the series element, and vasoactive drugs or extrinsic neural stimulation [8] appear to exert the majority of their effect on the series element. In that model, factors that alter the series resistance have a major influence on the overall blood flow to the gut wall, while relative changes in the parallel resistances in mucosal and muscularis can alter the intramural distribution between those regions. That model is consistent with the measurements made by Gore and Bohlen [2], and is quite useful in interpreting experimental data involving changes in gut vascular resistance, O_2ER, and the distribution of blood flow between mucosa and muscularis. As discussed below, experimental interventions can affect the relative magnitudes of these regional resistances, thereby influencing the relationships among pressure, flow and O_2ER in the gut wall.

Important regional differences in the regulation of blood flow have been identified within mucosa and muscularis, and the responses within these regions to vasoactive drugs, hypoxia, extrinsic neural stimulation, metabolic stimulation, systemic hemorrhage and transient ischemia have been found to differ markedly. These differences probably relate to the fundamental structural and functional differences: mucosa has high metabolic demands arising from the active cell division and epithelial transport functions, while the oxygen demand (VO_2) in muscularis is relatively small [9]. In fact, muscularis is capable of sustaining contractions even in the absence of blood flow.

The regional differences in the factors contributing to the regulation of blood flow between mucosa and muscularis are manifested in the different responses to stimuli seen in these areas. For example, the reactive hyperemia seen after a transient cessation of blood flow is largely due to an increase in mucosal as compared with muscularis flow [10]. These differences in reactive hyperemia were further magnified when the metabolic activity of the mucosa was augmented by placing absorbable solutes in the intestinal lumen [11]. Stimulation of the perivascular nerve bundle leads to an increase in vascular resistance and a decrease

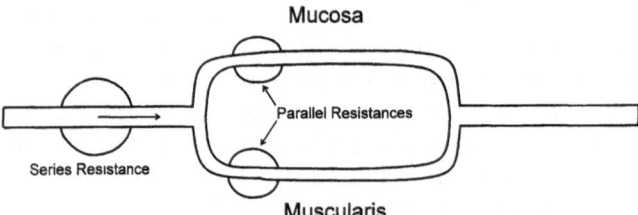

Fig. 1. Vascular model of blood flow regulation in the gut. Most of the resistance to blood flow occurs in the "series resistance". Although the "parallel" resistances represent a small fraction of the overall blood flow resistance, they determine the distribution of flow between mucosa and muscularis regions

in blood flow [8], which is followed by an eventual "autoregulatory escape" [12]. However, probably as a consequence of the higher metabolic rate in mucosa, the restoration of blood flow during sympathetic nerve stimulation is greater than in muscularis [13].

The local intestinal response to systemic hemorrhage provides and example of the competition for blood flow between mucosa and muscularis. In studies of isolated intestine segments that were perfused with blood from the femoral artery at systemic arterial pressure (i.e. autoperfused), progressive hemorrhage of the animal resulted in a progressive decrease in gut vascular resistance and a progressive decrease in gut blood flow and DO_2. When gut DO_2 reached a critical extraction of approximately 65%, gut VO_2 became DO_2-limited in that model [14]. In later experiments where an isolated gut segment was perfused with blood using an occlusive roller pump, it was possible to locally reduce gut blood flow while keeping the animal systemically normotensive, thereby separating the direct effects of hypoperfusion from the integrated response seen with the baroreflex response to systemic hemorrhage [15]. Interestingly, the local ability of the gut to increase O_2ER in response to a decrease in pump speed and DO_2 was significantly impaired when the animal was kept normotensive, averaging only 45%. By contrast, if the animal was progressively hemorrhaged to augment baroreflex vasoconstriction, local gut critical O_2ER averaged 69%, a value that was similar to the critical O_2ER seen in the autoperfused preparation. Further evidence was obtained in normovolemic animals where local gut flow was reduced below the critical delivery by lowering pump speed. While holding gut DO_2 constant at that point, subsequent hemorrhage of the animal caused an increase in local gut O_2 and O_2ER, demonstrating that the extraction ability could be restored by augmenting baroreflex vasoconstriction [15].

At the critical point, gut vascular resistance was significantly higher in the hemorrhaged compared with the normovolemic group, suggesting that the increased vasoconstrictor tone contributed to the improved ability to extract O_2. Attempts to block the increase in vascular resistance (and thus the improvement in O_2ER) during hemorrhage using the α blocker phenoxybenzamine were unsuccessful. Although α-blockade significantly attenuated the increase in vascular resistance produced by hemorrhage, it did not significantly impair the local gut O_2ER ability, which still reached 62% at the critical point. These observations may be interpreted using the vascular model proposed by Shepherd et al. [7]. Hemorrhage of the animal appears to have increased overall vascular resistance by augmenting both the "series" resistance and each of the "parallel" resistances in mucosa and muscularis. α-adrenergic blockade appeared to act primarily at the series element, lowering resistance without interfering with the appropriate partitioning of flow between mucosa and muscularis. The balance in resistances between these regions is the most likely determinant of the critical O_2ER ability, because the intrinsic metabolic rates in these regions differ, as do their capacities for augmenting VO_2. Because phenoxybenzamine did not appear to undermine the partitioning of blood flow between mucosa and muscularis, it did not affect the ability of the gut to adjust O_2ER in response to decreases in blood flow. Collectively, these findings support the work of Granger et al. [16–18] by demonstrating the important functional differences between "resistance" vessels and those responsible for regulating the "distribution" of blood flow.

Heterogeneity of Blood Flow in Gut Mucosa and Muscularis

Factors that alter the distribution of blood flow between muscularis and mucosa in the gut can significantly affect the ability of the tissue to maintain cellular DO_2. If the vascular tone regulating the flow distribution between these regions is lost, a "vascular steal" [7, 10, 19] by muscularis may deprive mucosa of sufficient DO_2, causing the onset of supply-limited metabolism even though overall extraction by the gut wall is low.

As is the case in many tissues, an optimal ability to utilize delivered O_2 in the mucosa exists when the microvascular regulation of capillary blood flow is precisely matched to the local O_2 demands of the surrounding cells. Under normal conditions, it is reasonable to propose that different cells or regions within mucosa may exhibit different metabolic activities and O_2 demands, by virtue of their different functional roles. For example, placing glucose and bile into the lumen of small intestine caused overall VO_2 to increase by 62% [20]; it is likely that more of this occurred in intestinal villous epithelium than in cells in the crypts. To the extent that some regions of the mucosa exhibit different metabolic demands than others, capillary blood flow would need to be distributed in accordance with demand in order to optimize utilization. Connolly et al. [21] recently measured the heterogeneity of blood flow within mucosa and muscularis in perfused segments of canine small intestine. Microspheres (15 μm) were used to label the distribution of flow, and the mucosa of the gut loop was divided into tissue aliquots averaging 600 μg for analysis. In that study, a significant degree of regional heterogeneity was present among aliquots, with some regions receiving five times the blood flow of others. A similar degree of heterogeneity was found within muscularis. It is not known whether this intrinsic heterogeneity is a reflection of the normal regulation of blood flow among regions of mucosa with differing O_2 demands, or whether it reflects an intrinsic limitation in the regulation of mucosal perfusion. In either case, the degree of heterogeneity did not change significantly when overall blood flow to the gut was decreased, nor did it change significantly when baroreflex vasoconstriction was increased by hemorrhaging the animal. However, systemic hemorrhage did cause an intramural redistribution of blood flow, resulting in a greater perfusion of mucosa at the expense of muscularis. Interestingly, under supply-limited conditions, the extent of this redistribution correlated with the improvement in gut O_2ER elicited by hemorrhaging the animal. Collectively, these findings demonstrate that significant heterogeneity of blood flow normally exists in gut mucosa and muscularis, and that changes in vasoconstrictor tone have a greater effect on the partitioning of flow between mucosa and muscularis than within each of those compartments.

Pathophysiology of Gut Oxygen Extraction in Sepsis

A large body of literature strongly supports the view that the tissues comprising the gut are especially sensitive to the effects of septicemia. In experimental models, administration of bacterial endotoxin causes a decrease in intestinal perfusion, decreases in gut mucosal pH, and increases in gut epithelial permeability to solutes in animal models [22, 23]. Within the gut wall, the mucosa has been identified as the primary target of injury during sepsis or endotoxemia, although the mechanisms responsible for this susceptibility are unclear. Increasingly, the gut is regarded as a "sentinel organ" in septic patients [24], and studies utilizing tonometric estimates of mucosal pH [25] indicate that such measurements may provide a reliable prognostic indicator in patients with critical illness [26, 27], especially when combined with measurements of arterial lactate [28]. In addition to being a target of injury in sepsis, the gut may also play an initiating role in the development of multiple organ injury by contributing to the onset of sepsis after hemorrhage [29], trauma [30] or burn injury [31]. In this regard, an increase in the permeability of the epithelial barrier or an attenuation of the antibacterial defenses within the mucosa may lead to an increase in translocation of bacteria or endotoxins following an injury to the gut mucosa [32]. These events could, in turn, initiate or accelerate the development of systemic sepsis. However, the factors that render the mucosa more susceptible to injury during sepsis are not known, and widely disparate views on the potential role of O_2 exist.

What role does O_2 transport play in the gut mucosal injury seen during sepsis? One line of evidence points toward cellular DO_2 as a central element in the sequence of events leading to gut mucosal dysfunction. In support of this notion is the observation that the local ability of the gut to adjust its O_2ER in response to changes in gut DO_2 is impaired in experimental models of sepsis [33, 34]. According to this theory, the O_2ER dysfunction is due to a defect in the regulation of the distribution of perfusion within the mucosa, leading to the existence of tissue regions with inadequate DO_2 adjacent to other regions that receive excess flow with respect to their metabolic needs. If sepsis or endotoxemia renders microvessels in the mucosa incapable of adjusting perfused capillary density [19] or alters the distribution of perfusion within and between mucosa and muscularis in response to changes in gut DO_2, cells in the more poorly perfused regions would be liable to sustain hypoxic cellular injury whenever systemic and/or gut DO_2 is transiently depressed.

In support of this line of reasoning, Drazenovic et al. [35] found evidence of impaired regulation of intestinal mucosal capillary recruitment in a canine model of endotoxemia. In that study, endotoxemia ablated the increase in perfused capillary density in more poorly perfused segments of small intestine that was observed in non-septic control animals. In a study of gut mucosa, Vallet et al. [36] found that lipopolysaccharide infusion caused an acute decrease in cardiac output and blood pressure, and that gut perfusion and gut VO_2 likewise decreased. Those changes were associated with a decrease in the mean tissue O_2 tension (PO_2) both in mucosa and muscularis. During fluid resuscitation, the tissue PO_2 within muscularis returned to baseline levels, but tissue PO_2 within mucosa remained near anoxic levels suggesting that mucosal perfusion did not recover to the same extent as muscularis. In a study of pump-perfused canine intestine in our laboratory, Connolly et al. [21] found that the redistribution of blood flow toward mucosa that normally occurs when systemic baroreflex vasoconstriction is activated was abolished during endotoxemia, although the degree of heterogeneity within each of those regions was not worsened. Collectively, these findings support the conclusion that the regulation of blood flow in mucosa is disrupted in experimental models of sepsis.

By what mechanisms can sepsis influence the regulation of blood flow so as to alter O_2ER capability of the intact tissue? One line of evidence implicates nitric oxide (NO) synthesis in the impaired vascular responsiveness seen in models of sepsis. Exposure to cytokines including interleukin-1 (IL-1) and tumor necrosis factor-α (TNF-α) is known to initiate a variety of responses in vascular myocytes, including the expression of the inducible form of NO synthase (iNOS) [37–42]. These changes are associated with a decrease in the responsiveness of intact vessels to vasoactive substances, although the specific responses differ among different animal species that have been studied. For example, *in vivo* administration of endotoxin significantly decreased contractile responses to phenylephrine, angiotensin II, serotonin and potassium chloride in isolated blood vessels from rats and rabbits *ex vivo* [43], but not from dogs [34]. The impaired responsiveness in rats and rabbits was improved by N^G-nitro-L-arginine, but not by indomethacin or endothelial denudation. Endothelium-dependent relaxation to acetylcholine was impaired in rats, rabbits [43] and dogs given endotoxin [44], while relaxation responses to sodium nitroprusside were unaffected. Some studies have suggested that the vascular dysfunction associated with sepsis may be mediated by excessive NO synthesis, and can be reversed by inhibitors of NOS [45, 46]. However, the hypothesis that the vascular defect during sepsis is due entirely to excessive NO synthesis appears too simplistic, in that the inhibition of NOS *in vivo* fails to completely restore systemic vascular resistance in the dog. More importantly, it fails to restore a normal O_2ER response in canine intestine segments during endotoxemia [34].

Thus, there is strong indirect evidence linking the existence of a defect in vascular control in gut mucosa with the existence of an impaired ability to regulate local DO_2. However, no direct evidence has been presented to link a failure of cellular DO_2 with the development of hypoxic cellular injury in the gut, or in other tissues, during sepsis. While there is little doubt that the ability of the gut to adjust local O_2ER is impaired in sepsis, it is not clear whether this contributes to the cause of the organ failure or whether it is merely an indicator of the presence of cellular injury that is caused by other factors.

Could the gut mucosal injury seen during sepsis be a manifestation of cellular "histotoxic" injury unrelated to DO_2? Some of the support for this theory comes from the weaknesses in the arguments favoring DO_2 as the explanation [47]. For example, moderate elevations in circulating lactate levels are often cited as evidence for tissue ischemia, yet hypoxia need not be present to explain a moderate increase in arterial lactate concentrations because increases in glycolytic flux or a partial inhibition of the pyruvate dehydrogenase complex could produce a similar increase [48]. Other studies have used non-invasive techniques such as near-infrared spectroscopy to evaluate the reduction state of cytochrome aa3 as an index of cellular DO_2. In this regard, Schaefer et al. [49] used near-infrared spectroscopy in rat small intestine during lethal endotoxemia. They found that resuscitated endotoxemic animals showed an increase in the reduction state of cytochrome aa3 while intestinal VO_2 was maintained. They interpreted this as evidence of a toxic cellular effect rather than a limitation of DO_2.

In another study [50], the same group found endotoxin dose-related increases in the reduction state of cytochrome aa3 in the intestine, but concluded that this did not reflect tissue hypoxia because
1) tissue HbO_2 levels were not reduced significantly;
2) the redox shift did not recover after restoration of gut blood flow; and
3) systemic VO_2 was not decreased.

While intriguing, these results do not provide a critical test of the hypothesis because the fraction of cells that are hypoxic at any given instant may be relatively small, and beyond the resolution ability of detection. For similar reasons, conclusions regarding the presence or absence of tissue hypoxia based on overall hemoglobin saturation may be inaccurate. Finally, a histotoxic effect of sepsis would presumably limit cellular VO_2 and ATP production even if tissue O_2 availability were normal, yet VO_2 and metabolic rates in sepsis tend to be elevated rather than depressed. A definitive answer to the question of whether tissue DO_2 is the cause of organ failure in the gut, or whether it is merely a marker of cellular injury, awaits an experimental approach that can accurately and simultaneously assess cellular DO_2 and cellular function in the intact tissue during sepsis.

Alternative Factors Contributing to Gut Mucosal Injury

What other factors might contribute to gut mucosal dysfunction? Ischemia-reperfusion injury may be an important etiologic factor in the cellular dysfunction that develops in gut mucosa during sepsis. Although the generation of reactive O_2 species is accelerated by ischemia and reperfusion, the activation of this process in the context of endotoxemia is not fully known. Conceivably, an ischemia/reperfusion (I/R) injury could develop as a consequence of microvascular dysfunction, which could produce a transient ischemia in hypoperfused regions of mucosa. The possibility of such an event occurring in gut mucosa is highlighted by the data of Vallet et al. [36] who found that mucosal perfusion failed to return after transient hypoperfusion in a model of endotoxemia. Other studies also provide supportive evidence for this theory. For example, Tokyay et al. [31] found that burn injury produced a transient gut vasoconstriction in pigs, which was followed by an increase in the translocation of bacteria and endotoxin, conceivably as a consequence of the transient ischemia. In rats, Xu et al. [51] found decreases in gut blood flow in a hyperdynamic model of endotoxemia, which was associated with increased mucosal permeability to ^{51}Cr-EDTA. These changes were prevented by allopurinol, an inhibitor of xanthine oxidase. Likewise, Vaughan et al. [52] found that allopurinol attenuated the increases in intestinal permeability in a model of I/R in rats. However, Fink et al. [23] concluded that the increases in gut mucosal permeability in a porcine model of endotoxemia were not solely due to the decrease in gut perfusion. In a later study [22], that group found that mucosal acidosis, even in the absence of tissue ischemia, may be an important factor contributing to the endotoxin-induced increases in mucosal permeability. Moreover, additional mucosal injury may result from the localization of neutrophils in the gut during I/R injury [53], which can alter both epithelial as well as endothelial permeability. At the systemic level, some studies suggest a beneficial effect of antioxidant therapy using N-acetylcysteine. For example, Bakker et al. [54] found that pretreatment with this drug led to a more rapid normalization of blood lactate levels in a canine model of endotoxemia. In a clinical study of N-acetylcysteine, Spies et al. [55] found limited evidence of a beneficial effect on VO_2 and gut mucosal pH. However, because this drug also reduces the release of TNF-α in response to sepsis, it is not known whether the beneficial effects related to the antioxidant activity or to other effects. In summary, the possibility that oxidant-mediated I/R injury may contribute to the gut mucosal injury during endotoxemia, but the role of transient ischemia in initiating this response, and the relative contributions of radical productions in mucosal cells as opposed to marginated leukocytes, is not fully clear.

Conclusion

Perfusion to the gut can be described as two parallel vascular beds comprised of mucosa and muscularis. Although the vascular resistance in these regions is small relative to the total gut vascular resistance, small changes in the ratio of these resistances can have a major influence on the partitioning of flow between mucosa and muscularis. Most of the vascular resistance in the gut is located in the blood vessels upstream from these beds, the so-called "series" resistance. Because the intrinsic metabolic rates differ between mucosa and muscularis, flow redistribution can play an important role in assuring the adequacy of oxygen supply, especially to mucosa. By contrast, relatively large changes in the series resistance vessels may have little effect on oxygen extraction ability, unless the distribution between mucosa and muscularis is also affected. In sepsis, cellular injury to mucosa may lead to an impairment in its barrier function. Although circumstantial evidence points to a role for impaired microvascular perfusion and oxygen transport as the cause of the cellular damage, the definitive cause of the mucosal dysfunction is not known. Other conceivable contributors include ischemia/reperfusion oxidant injury, or histotoxic cellular injury. Evidence for the latter of these is limited, but a definitive answer to this question will require further study.

Acknowledgement: This work was supported by NHLBI grants HL32646 and HL35440.

References

1. Lundgren O (1991) Microcirculation of the gastrointestinal tract and pancreas. In: Renkin EM, Michel CC (eds) Handbook of Physiology. The Microcirculation. Am Physiol Soc, pp 799–863
2. Gore RW, Bohlen HG (1977) Microvascular pressures in rat intestinal muscle and mucosal villi. Am J Physiol 233:H685–H693
3. Folkow B (1967) Regional adjustments of intestinal blood flow. Gastroenterology 52: 423–432
4. Barlow TE (1951) Arterio-venous anastomoses in the human stomach. J Anatomy 85:1–4
5. Vajda J, Raposa T, Herpai Z (1968) Structural bases of blood flow regulation in the small intestine. Acta Morphologica Acad Sci Hung 16:331–340
6. Schnitzlein HN (1957) Regulation of blood flow through the stomach of the rat. Anat Rec 127:735–753
7. Shepherd AP, Riedel GL, Maxwell LC, Kiel JW (1984) Selective vasodilators redistribute intestinal blood flow and depress oxygen uptake. Am J Physiol 247:G377–G384
8. Hultén L, Lindhagen J, Lundgren O (1977) Sympathetic nervous control of intramural blood flow in the feline and human intestines. Gastroenterology 72:41–48
9. Martin AW, Fuhrman FA (1955) The relationship between summated tissue respiration and metabolic rate in mouse and dog. Physiol Zool 28:18–34
10. Shepherd AP, Riedel GL (1984) Differences in reactive hyperemia between the intestinal mucosa and muscularis. Am J Physiol 247:G617–G622
11. Shepherd AP (1982) Metabolic control of intestinal oxygenation and blood flow. Fed Proc 41:2084–2089
12. Folkow B, Lewis DH, Lundgren O, Mellander S, Wallentin I (1964) The effect of graded vasoconstrictor fibre stimulation on the intestinal resistance and capacitance vessels. Acta Physiol Scand 61:445–457
13. Shepherd AP, Riedel GL (1988) Intramural distribution of intestinal blood flow during sympathetic stimulation. Am J Physiol 255:H1091–H1095
14. Nelson DP, King CE, Dodd SL, Schumacker PT, Cain SM (1987) Systemic and intestinal limits of O_2 extraction in the dog. J Appl Physiol 63:387–394
15. Samsel RW, Schumacker PT (1994) Systemic hemorrhage augments local O_2 extraction in canine intestine. J Appl Physiol 77:2291–2298
16. Granger DN, Kvietys PR, Perry MA (1982) Role of exchange vessels in the regulation of intestinal oxygenation. Am J Physiol 242:G570–G574
17. Granger HJ, Goodman AH, Granger DN (1976) Role of resistance and exchange vessels in local microvascular control of skeletal muscle oxygenation in the dog. Circ Res 38:379–385
18. Holm-Rutili L, Perry MA, Granger DN (1981) Autoregulation of gastric blood flow and oxygen uptake. Am J Physiol 241:G143–G149
19. Shepherd AP (1982) Local control of intestinal oxygenation and blood flow. Annu Rev Physiol 44:13–27
20. Shepherd AP, Riedel GL (1985) Laser-Doppler blood flowmetry of intestinal mucosal hyperemia induced by glucose and bile. Am J Physiol 248:G393–G397
21. Connolly HV, Maginniss LA, Schumacker PT (1995) Effects of blood flow and sympathetic tone on intestinal microvascular transit time heterogeneity. Am J Resp Critical Care Med 151:A325 (Abst)
22. Salzman AL, Wang H, Wollen PS, et al (1994) Endotoxin-induced ileal mucosal hyperpermeability in pigs: Role of tissue acidosis. Am J Physiol 266:G633–G646
23. Fink MP, Antonsson JB, Wang HL, Rothschild HR (1991) Increased intestinal permeability in endotoxic pigs. Mesenteric hypoperfusion as an etiologic factor. Arch Surg 126:211–218
24. Landow L, Andersen LW (1994) Splanchnic ischaemia and its role in multiple organ failure. Anaesth Scand 38:626–639
25. Clark CH, Gutierrez G (1992) Gastric intramucosal pH: A non-invasive method for the indirect measurement of tissue oxygenation. Am J Critical Care 1:53–60
26. Gutierrez G, Palizas F, Doglio G, et al (1992) Gastric intramucosal pH as a therapeutic index of tissue oxygenation in critically ill patients. Lancet 339:195–199

27. Gutierrez G, Clark C, Brown SD, Price K, Ortiz L, Nelson C (1994) Effect of dobutamine on oxygen consumption and gastric mucosal pH in septic patients. Am J Resp Crit Care Med 150:324–329
28. Friedman G, Berlot G, Kahn RJ, Vincent JL (1995) Combined measurements of blood lactate concentrations and gastric intramucosal pH in patients with severe sepsis. Crit Care Med 23:1184–1193
29. Zhi-Yong S, Dong YL, Wang XH (1992) Bacterial translocation and multiple system organ failure in bowel ischemia and reperfusion. J Trauma 32:148–153
30. Andersen LW, Landow L, Baek L, Jansen E, Baker S (1993) Association between gastric intramucosal pH and splanchnic endotoxin, antibody to endotoxin, and tumor necrosis factor-alpha concentrations in patients undergoing cardiopulmonary bypass. Crit Care Med 21:210–217
31. Tokyay R, Zeigler ST, Traber DL, et al (1993) Postburn gastrointestinal vasoconstriction increases bacterial and endotoxin translocation. J Appl Physiol 74:1521–1527
32. Baron P, Traber LD, Traber DL, et al (1994) Gut failure and translocation following burn and sepsis. J Surg Res 57:197–204
33. Nelson DP, Samsel RW, Wood LDH, Schumacker PT (1988) Pathological supply dependence of systemic and intestinal O_2 uptake during endotoxemia. J Appl Physiol 64: 2410–2419
34. Schumacker PT, Kazaglis J, Connolly HV, Samsel RW, O'Connor MF, Umans JG (1995) Systemic and gut O_2 extraction during endotoxemia: Role of nitric oxide synthesis. Am J Resp Critical Care Med 151:107–115
35. Drazenovic R, Samsel RW, Wylam ME, Doerschuk CM, Schumacker PT (1992) Regulation of perfused capillary density in canine intestinal mucosa during endotoxemia. J Appl Physiol 72:259–265
36. Vallet B, Lund N, Curtis SE, Kelly D, Cain SM (1994) Gut and muscle tissue PO_2 in endotoxemic dogs during shock and resuscitation. J Appl Physiol 76:793–800
37. Beasley D (1990) Interleukin-1 and endotoxin activate soluble guanylate cyclase in vascular smooth muscle. Am J Physiol 259:R38–R44
38. Beasley D, Cohen RA, Levinsky NG (1989) Interleukin-1 inhibits contraction of vascular smooth muscle. J Clin Invest 83:331–335
39. Beasley D, Cohen RA, Levinsky NG (1990) Endotoxin inhibits contraction of vascular smooth muscle *in vitro*. Am J Physiol 258:H1187–H1192
40. Fleming I, Julou-Schaeffer G, Gray GA, Parratt JR, Stoclet JC (1991) Evidence that an L-arginine/nitric oxide dependent elevation of tissue cyclic GMP content is involved in depression of vascular reactivity by endotoxin. Br J Pharm 103:1047–1052
41. Bigaud M, Julou-Schaeffer G, Parratt JR, Stoclet JC (1990) Endotoxin-induced impairment of vascular smooth muscle contractions elicited by different mechanisms. Eur J Pharm 190: 185–192
42. Nelson S, Steward RH, Traber LD, Traber DL (1991) Endotoxin-induced alterations in contractility of isolated blood vessels from sheep. Am J Physiol 260:H1790–H1794
43. Umans JG, Wylam ME, Samsel RW, Edwards J, Schumacker PT (1993) Effects of endotoxin in vivo on endothelial and smooth muscle function in rabbit and rat aorta. Am Rev Respir Dis 148:1638–1645
44. Wylam ME, Samsel RW, Umans JG, Mitchell RW, Leff AR, Schumacker PT (1990) Endotoxin impairs endothelium-dependent relaxation of canine arteries *in vitro*. Am Rev Respir Dis 142:1263–1267
45. Kilbourn RG, Gross SS, Jubran A, et al (1990) N^G-methyl-L-arginine inhibits tumor necrosis factor-induced hypotension: Implications for the involvement of nitric oxide. Proc Natl Acad Sci USA 87:3629–3632
46. Kilbourn RG, Jubran A, Gross SS, et al (1990) Reversal of endotoxin-mediated shock by N^G-methyl-L-arginine, an inhibitor of nitric oxide synthesis. Biochem Biophy Res Comm 172: 1132–1138
47. Cain SM (1992) Oxygen supply dependency in the critically ill – A continuing conundrum. Adv Exp Med Biol 317:35–45

48. Hotchkiss RS, Karl IE (1992) Reevaluation of the role of cellular hypoxia and bioenergetic failure in sepsis. JAMA 267:1503–1510
49. Schaefer CF, Biber B (1993) Effects of endotoxemia on the redox level of brain cytochrome a,a₃ in rats. Circ Shock 40:1–8
50. Schaefer CF, Lerner MR, Biber B (1991) Dose-related reduction of intestinal cytochrome a,a₃ induced by endotoxin in rats. Circ Shock 33:17–25
51. Xu D, Qi L, Guillory D, Cruz N, Berg R, Deitch EA (1993) Mechanisms of endotoxin-induced intestinal injury in a hyperdynamic model of sepsis. J Trauma 34:676–682
52. Vaughan WG, Horton JW, Walker PB (1992) Allopurinol prevents intestinal permeability changes after ischemia-reperfusion injury. J Pediatr Surg 27:968–972
53. Granger DN, Korthuis RJ (1995) Physiologic mechanisms of posischemic tissue injury. Annu Rev Physiol 57:311–332
54. Bakker J, Zhang H, Depierreux M, van Asbeck S, Vincent JL (1994) Effects of N-acetylcysteine in endotoxin shock. J Crit Care 9:236–243
55. Spies CD, Reinhart K, Witt I, et al (1994) Influence of N-acetylcysteine on indirect indicators of tissue oxygenation in septic shock patients: Results from a prospective, randomized, double-blind study. Crit Care Med 22:1738–1746

Immunology of the Gut

L. D. McVay

Introduction

The mucosal-associated lymphoid tissue (MALT) comprises all the lymphoid and mononuclear cells in the epithelia and lamina propria beneath the mucosal surface. MALT includes the upper respiratory tract and tonsils, the bronchial-associated lymphoid tissue (BALT), the salivary, lacrimal and lactating mammary glands, the gut-associated lymphoid tissue (GALT) and the uro-genital tract.

The immune system is an integral part of the mucosal-associated tissue. The immune compartment in the GALT, which includes the oral cavity, the small intestine and the colon, is a dynamic and highly complex group of specialized structures and cell types that function in areas of the body that are continuously exposed to environmental antigens. These unique structures include Peyer's patches, mesenteric lymph nodes and intestinal lamina propria, and contain complex populations of cells consisting of both effector and regulatory subsets of T lymphocytes, B lymphocytes, macrophages, mast cells and small numbers of dendritic cells, natural killer (NK) cells, neutrophils and eosinophils. Together with epithelial cells and enterocytes which maintain the integrity of the mucosal barrier, the gastrointestinal mucosal immune system maintains a delicate balance protecting the host against potential pathogens crossing mucosal barriers, and of providing immune tolerance against the plethora of food antigens and normal intestinal flora that interface with intestinal tissue. Understanding the role of the intestinal immune system in normal intestinal physiology will help to unravel the role of the immune system in gut dysfunction and critical illness.

Lymphocytes

In adults, the bone marrow is the major site of hematopoiesis and is the source of precursor lymphocytes. B cell precursors mature in the bone marrow while T cell precursors migrate to the thymus and differentiate there. These lymphocytes are "naive" (have not yet encountered cognate antigen). These cells traffic between the different secondary lymphoid tissues, which capture and accumulate antigen, such as the lymph node, Peyer's patch and spleen until they recognize their cognate antigens with their antigen receptors. The potency of the immune system lies in its capacity to generate billions of different antigen receptors on T cells and B cells from multiple gene segments that are assembled by somatic mutation [1]. The large array of antigen-recognition molecules expressed on the cell surface of lymphocytes comprises the T cell receptor (TCR) repertoire on T cells, and the immunoglobulin (Ig) receptor repertoire on B cells, and provides the basis for cellular (T cell) and humoral (B cell) immunity.

Once activated, T cells and B cells become effector and memory lymphocytes. One hallmark of many activated lymphocytes is that they selectively migrate back to the tissues in which they initially encountered antigen. This is particularly true for cells in the GALT; T and B cells that encounter antigen in mucosal-associated tissue tend to "home" back to the mucosal-associated tissue such as the GALT. Importantly, during inflammation, this specific homing or migratory behavior of lymphocytes is less selective and results in an influx of any activated leukocytes into intestinal tissue. The gut has been called a "sink-hole" for activated cells in the immune system and this may have some bearing on the development of inflammation and gut dysfunction, an important aspect of critical illness.

Immunoglobulin (Ig) is the Antigen Receptor for B Lymphocytes

All lymphocytes express a receptor on their cell surface that recognizes foreign antigen. The antigen receptor expressed on B lymphocytes is the immunoglobulin (Ig) receptor, or antibody receptor. A B cell which recognizes its cognate antigen with its antigen receptor undergoes molecular changes that allow it to secrete a soluble form of the receptor (or antibody) in the tissue or blood resulting in an antigen-specific antibody response.

Immunoglobulins

There are 5 classes of immunoglobulin, or antibody that provide humoral protection in normal health and disease. All immunoglobulin molecules have a basic structural unit of two heavy and two light chains and are held together by intra- and interchain disulfide bonds. The variable region of immunoglobulin confers the antigen-binding function. The constant region of each class of immunoglobulin is different and confers biologic functions specific for each class, shown in Table 1. Collectively, immunoglobulins provide host defense in three major ways 1) neutralization of the pathogen or its secreted products i.e. bacteria, bacterial toxin, virus particles; 2) opsonization; and 3) complement activation.

In the mucosa-associated immune system, IgA is the predominant class of immunoglobulin found. There are two forms or allotypes of IgA, IgA1 and IgA2, which can be distinguished by the amino acid sequence in the constant region of the molecule. IgA1 predominates in the serum and they are equally represented in normal mucosa. However, IgA2 production is associated with increased bacterial load [2].

Table 1. Function of different immunoglobulin isotypes

	Human immunoglobulin isotypes				
	IgD	IgM	IgG	IgE	IgA
Neutralization	−	+	−	−	+ +
Opsonization	−	−	+ + +	−	+
Activates complement system	−	+ + +	+ +	−	−
Mast cell sensitization	−	−	−	+ + +	−
Transport in epithelial cells	−	* −	* −	−	+ + +

* IgM and IgG molecules participate in transport in epithelial cells only when complexed to multivalent antigen/dIgA

IgA has several structural features that distinguish its function in the mucosal environment (Fig. 1). IgA, like IgM, has a unique constant region that allows it to react with a plasma cell-derived protein called J (joining) chain [3, 4], which is thought to aid in polymerization of IgM into pentamers and IgA into dimers. The capacity of these antibodies to polymerize is important since this increases the avidity or binding strength of the antibody for antigen. Dimeric IgA comprises ∼ 90% of all antibody in the gut with IgM and IgG comprising ∼ 10%. IgA can also exist as a monomer, primarily in the peripheral blood.

A novel mechanism of transport of IgA immune complexes has been defined in the intestine [5]. Mucosal IgA dimers can react with an epithelial cell-derived protein historically called secretory component (SC). Recently, SC was shown to be the poly Ig receptor [6]; it provides two important functions: 1) it acts as a transporter of IgA from the lamina propria into the lumen [5], and 2) it protects IgA dimers by preventing degradation by intestinal proteases (Fig. 2). Dimeric IgA (or a dimeric IgA complex) binds to the poly-Ig receptor at the baso-lateral end of the epithelial cell, is endocytosed and transported across the epithelial cell where it is released on the apical side of the epithelial cell into the lumen.

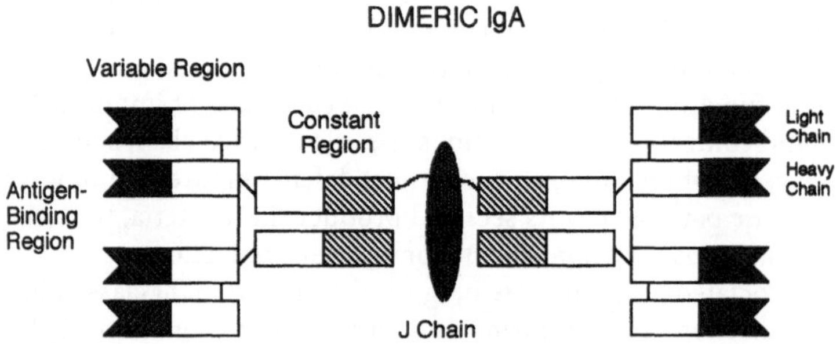

DIMERIC IgA

Fig. 1. Structure of dimeric IgA. IgA, like IgM, has a unique constant region that allows it to interact with a plasma-derived protein called J (joining) chain. This allows polymerization of IgA subunits into dimers, a biologically functional form of IgA in the GALT. (Adapted from [3, 4])

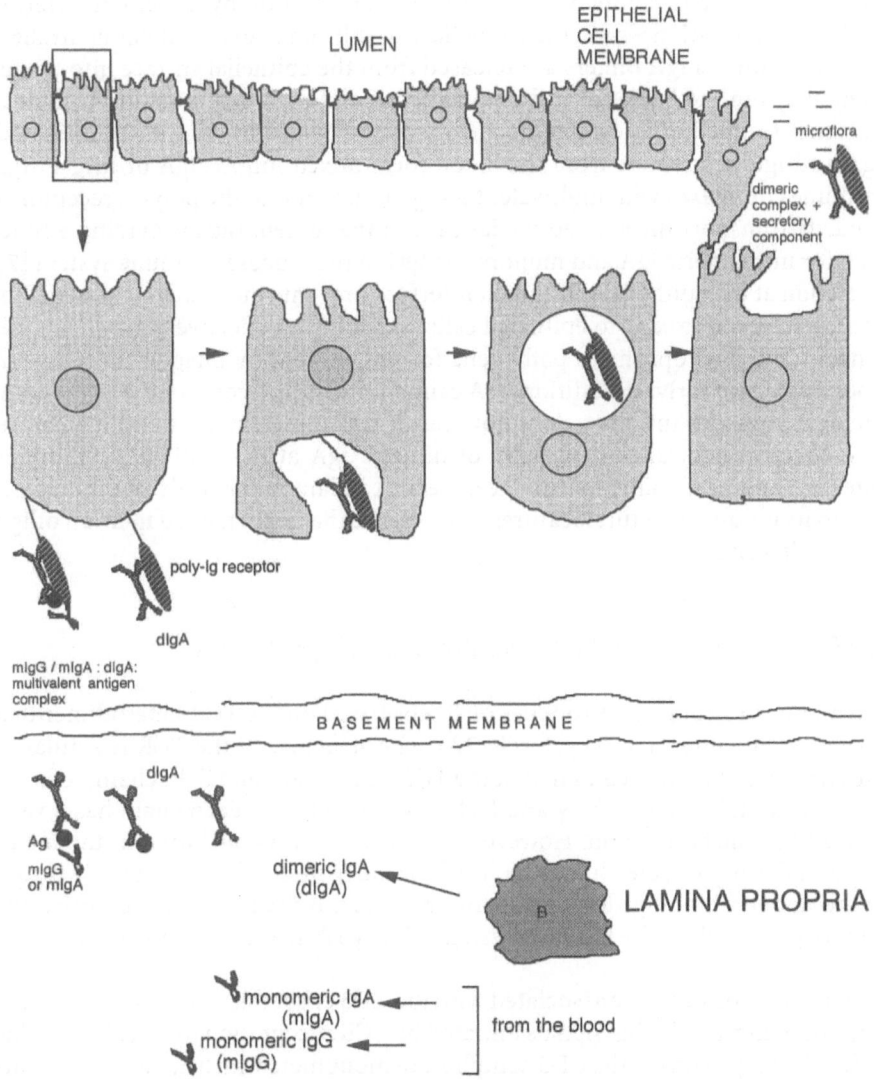

Fig. 2. Transcytosis of dimeric IgA across a single epithelial cell is mediated by the poly-Ig receptor. Plasma cells activated in Peyer's patch migrate to the lamina propria and secrete antigen-specific antibody (80–90% IgA, ~ 10% IgM or IgG) which binds antigen there, within the epithelial cell, or at the epithelial cell/mucosal interface. Monomeric IgA, IgG and IgM, while minor Igs in the lamina propria, can form complexes with multivalent antigen and dIgA. (Adapted from [5–8])

The transport of dIgA-SC-poly Ig across the epithelial cell can provide two functions (Fig. 2): 1) neutralization function *within* the epithelial cell. The epithelial cell lining is susceptible to infection by viral and other obligate intracellular parasites. Recent *in vitro* studies using Sendai virus have shown the capacity of dIgA-SC-poly Ig complex to neutralize viral infection by directly interfering with viral replication within the epithelial cell [6]; and 2) extracellular neutralization function. As IgA dimers are released from the epithelial surface into the lumen, they bind to bacterial and viral antigens and this "agglutination complex" becomes trapped in intestinal mucous, secreted by goblet cells, and eliminated. IgA and IgG monomers from the blood form mixed mIgA/dIgA or mIgG/dIgA immune complexes with multivalent antigen that bind to the poly-Ig receptor to mediate transport through epithelial cells to the lumen, thus providing a function for monomeric IgA and monomeric IgG in the mucosal immune system [7]. Secretion at the epithelial cell/lumen interface prevents the attachment of pathogenic bacteria or toxins to epithelial cells providing an effective neutralizing defense. While IgG opsonizes pathogens for engulfment by phagocytic cells, IgA does this very poorly. In addition, IgA cannot bind C3b, a component of the complement pathway and thus, does not recruit inflammatory cells and mediators. The effective neutralizing capacity of dimeric IgA at the epithelial cell/lumen interface and its inability to activate or recruit inflammatory cells and mediators due to its unique structural features, underscore the important adaptation of IgA in this vital site.

The T Cell Receptor (TCR) is the Antigen Receptor for T lymphocytes

T lymphocytes comprise two types of T cells based on the TCR heterodimer that is expressed, either $\alpha:\beta$ or $\gamma:\delta$ (Fig 3A). The structure of the TCR is similar to the structure of Ig molecules in that the TCR has a heavy and light chain, referred to as the α and β chains, or γ and δ chains, respectively. Each chain has a variable and a constant region. However, the TCR is always anchored in the membrane and is not secreted like Ig molecules. Like Ig molecules, the variable region is the antigen-binding domain of the molecule. $\alpha\beta$TCR+ cells comprise the majority of T cells in the immune system while $\gamma\delta$TCR+ cells comprise a minority.

Both types of TCRs are associated with the CD3 ensemble of molecules that are important in transducing signals initiated by TCR recognition [8, 9] (Fig 3B). The γ, δ, ϵ, ζ and η chains of the CD3 complex are monomers which are non-covalently associated with the TCR and with each other forming homodimers ($\zeta:\zeta$) and heterodimers ($\zeta:\eta$, $\epsilon:\delta$, $\epsilon:\delta$).

Fig. 3. **A** The T cell receptor (TCR) expressed on $\alpha\beta$ and $\gamma\delta$ T cells is a heterodimer. Each chain ▶ of the TCR heterodimer has a variable region and a constant region. The variable region is the antigen-binding portion of the TCR. **B** Components of the TCR-CD3 complex. The components of the CD3 complex (δ, ϵ, γ, η, ζ) are primarily involved in signal transduction, initiated by TCR recognition of an antigen complex. (Adapted from [9–13]). **C** $\alpha\beta$ TCR+ T cells recognize peptide antigen complexed with Class I or Class II molecules expressed on antigen-presenting cells. However, the biochemical and cell biologic pathways used to generate the peptides that will be presented by Class I and Class II molecules are distinct. (Adapted from [14, 15]). **D** The helper T cell and cytotoxic/killer T cell subsets are distinguished by expression of the co-receptors CD4 and CD8. (From [13] with permission)

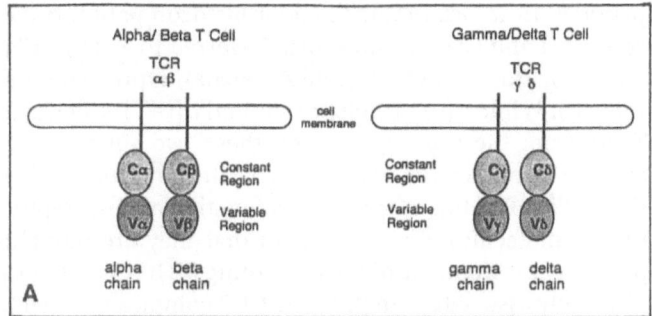

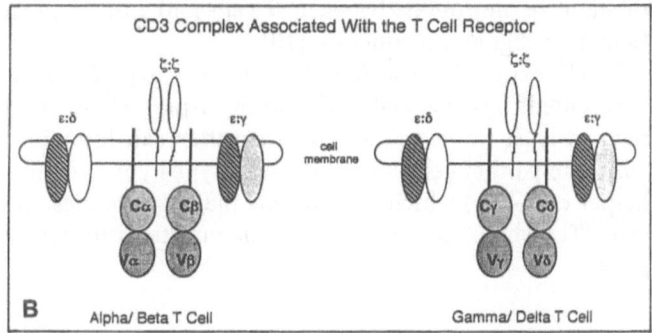

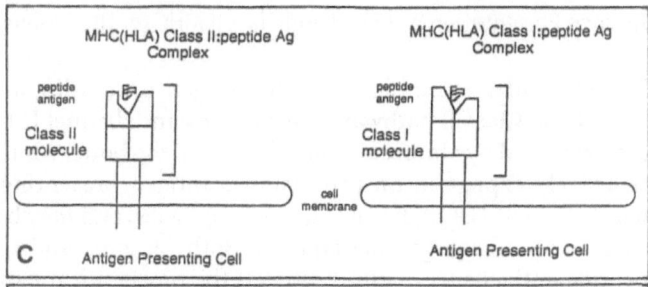

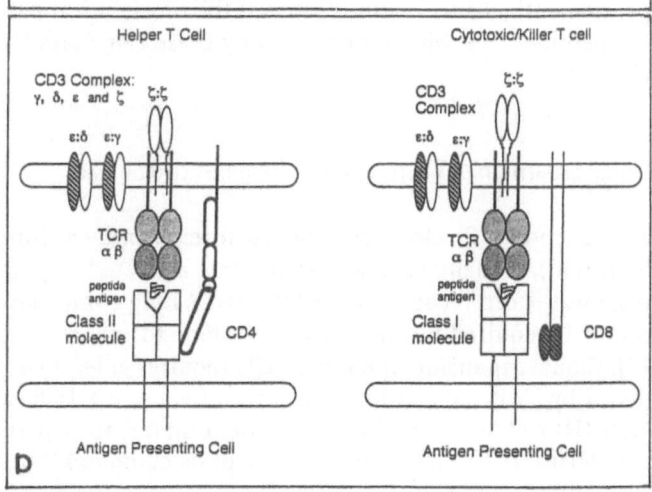

The hallmark of αβ T cells is their capacity to recognize foreign antigens, as peptides, in association with *major histocompatibility complex*, or MHC-encoded Class I and Class II molecules (referred to as HLA Class I and Class II in humans, for *Human Lymphocyte Antigens*), expressed on antigen-presenting cells (Fig 3C). While αβ + T helper cells and αβ + T killer/cytotoxic cells derive their TCRs from the same gene pool, these two subsets are phenotypically distinguished by expression of lineage-specific molecules called CD4 and CD8, respectively (Fig 3D) [10]. CD4 and CD8 function as co-receptors for MHC Class II and Class I molecules, respectively, in that they are thought to interact with non-polymorphic domains of the presenting MHC Class I or Class II molecule, and to physically associate with the TCR-CD3 complex in order to enhance adhesion of, or stabilize the contact between, T cells and antigen presenting cells and to participate in signal transduction [10].

T cells express a TCR that can recognize peptides from foreign proteins when "presented" by other cells called antigen-presenting cells (APCs). T lymphocytes have at least three major functions: they can function as 1) helper cells (Th) which help other cells mount delayed-type hypersensitivity (DTH) responses; 2) helper cells (Th) which help B cells make antibodies; and 3) killer or cytotoxic cells (Tc) which eliminate other cells infected with virus or intracellular pathogens.

Antigen Presentation by Class I and Class II MHC (or HLA) Molecules

The molecular events involved in antigen processing and presentation in the Class I and Class II pathways are complex and distinct [11, 12]. Class I molecules are expressed by almost all somatic cells in the body, while Class II molecules are selectively expressed on professional antigen presenting cells (APCs) such as dendritic cells (DCs), B cells and macrophages, and may be induced by cytokines such as interferon gamma (IFN-γ). Both Class I$^+$ and Class II$^+$ APCs present peptide antigens to T cells, however, the biochemical pathway used to generate the peptides that will be presented by Class I or Class II molecules are distinct [11, 12].

Clonal Expansion of T Lymphocytes Requires two Signals

The function of T cells is to recognize foreign antigens (discriminating 'self' from 'non-self'), clonally expand and become activated to participate in an immune response. T cell recognition of MHC(HLA):Ag complexes with their antigen receptor is required but not sufficient alone to mount an immune response [13, 14]. Clonal expansion of naive T cells requires at least two signals. Signal 1 is induced by TCR recognition of a ligand (where αβ TCR$^+$ CD4$^+$ cells recognize MHC(HLA) Class II: antigenic peptide complex, and αβ TCR$^+$ CD8$^+$ cells recognize MHC(HLA) Class I: antigenic peptide complex) (Fig. 4). The second signal, a co-stimulatory signal, is provided by one or more accessory molecules expressed on professional antigen-presenting cells (dendritic cell (DC), macrophage or B cell) and on T cells (Fig. 4). Co-stimulatory signals are neither antigen-specific nor MHC(HLA)-restricted; yet they have the capacity to induce maximal T lymphocyte proliferation, cytokine secretion and subsequent effector function (reviewed in [15]). In the absence of the engagement of the TCR by MHC(HLA): antigen complexes *or* in the absence of co-stimulation, the T cell becomes unresponsive or "anergized' (unable to secrete IL-2, but can proliferate in the presence of exogenous IL-2; and refractory to stimulation through the TCR/CD3 complex) [15].

Many co-stimulatory molecules can be expressed on APCs, but the most critical molecule to prevent anergy is B7; CD28 and CTLA-4 are the counter-receptors for B7 (reviewed in [15]). CD28 is the major counter-receptor for B7 on naive T cells, but on activated T cells, CTLA-4 binds B7 with a greater affinity than CD28, as depicted in Fig 4. While CD28 delivers a co-stimulatory signal, "signal 2", CTLA-4 does not provide a co-stimulatory signal but enhances that delivered by CD28 (reviewed in [15]). Recent studies suggest that CTLA-4 may provide a negative signal [16].

There are several pairs of co-stimulatory molecules on APC and counter-receptors on T cells (Fig. 5). T cell accessory receptors such as CD2 and CD28 can initiate antigen-independent T cell activation with the cell-surface integrin molecule LFA-3 (CD58), and B7, respectively. This has important implications in the immune system in the intestine since the major phenotype of T cells in the intes-

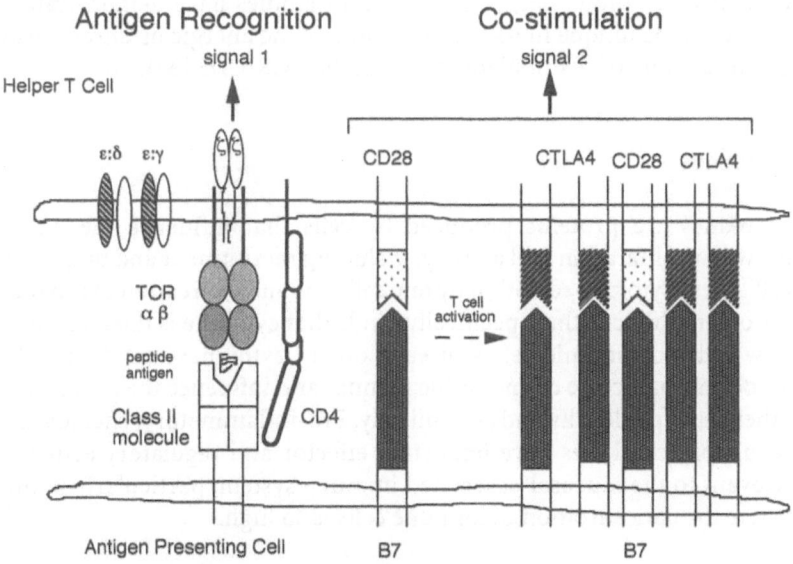

Fig. 4. Activation of T cells requires two signals. Signal 1 is mediated by ligation of antigen-recognition molecules (TCR/CD3/MHC). Signal 2 is mediated by a co-stimulatory signal provided by CD28 expression on the T cell and B7 expression on the antigen-presenting cell. Once activated, the expression of CTLA4, another co-stimulatory molecule, is upregulated and interacts with B7 molecules as well [16–91]

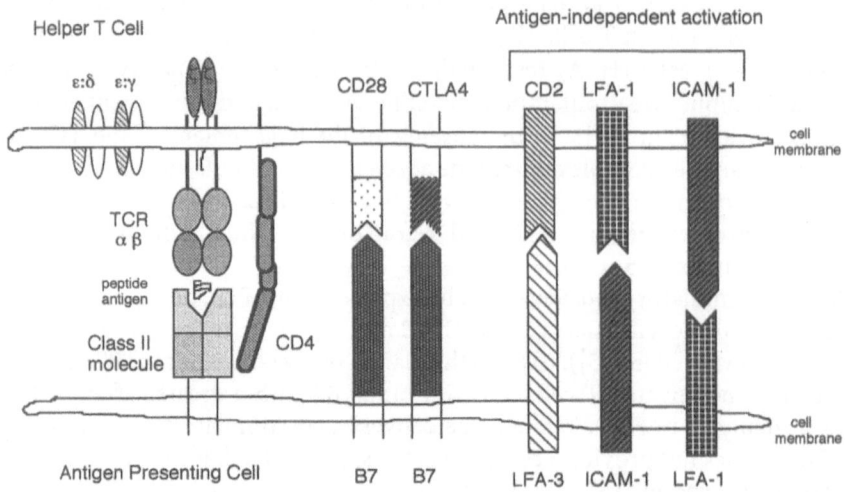

Fig. 5. Antigen-independent co-stimulation of T cells. Cell adhesion molecules such as CD2/LFA3, LFA-1/ICAM-1, ICAM-1/LFA-1 are expressed on T cells/APCs, respectively, and can induce T cell proliferation independent of antigen. (From [18] with permission)

tinal mucosa is characterized by unresponsiveness when stimulated through the TCR/CD3 complex, yet is susceptible to proliferation and cytokines production by anti-CD2 stimulation [17–19]. Recent studies have demonstrated that CD2 appears to be unique in its ability to reverse the anergic or unresponsive state of T cells unable to be stimulated through the TCR/CD3 [20].

Cytokines

Cytokines are proteins produced by cells that influence the differentiation, growth, proliferation and activity, including recruitment and migration, of other cell types. Cytokine secretion by one cell type and expression of a cytokine receptor on another cell that specifically binds that cytokine is the molecular basis for how cells "communicate" with each other. Cytokines may be regulated in an autocrine, paracrine or endocrine manner and influence the genetic programs of other cell types locally and systemically. Pro-inflammatory, chemoattractant and regulatory cytokines have important effector and regulatory activities that are relevant to the mucosal-associated immune system, particularly in the intestine where the concentration of immune cells is so high.

Cytokine Receptors

Cytokines interact with target cells expressing specific high affinity membrane-anchored receptors that function as signal transduction molecules to mediate cellular responses. Cytokine receptor + cells are continuously being identified on many cell types, including intestinal epithelial cells [21].

Functional Distinction Between CD4⁺ T Cell Subsets and Their Cytokine Profile

Functionally, CD4⁺ T cells were known to effect two functions as T "helper" cells: 1) to help delayed-type hypersensitivity (DTH) responses; and 2) to help B cell antibody responses. Murine studies by Mosmann and others analysed the cytokine patterns secreted by individual clones of CD4⁺ T cells. Two distinct patterns of cytokine production were found [22]: CD4⁺ T helper cells that participated in DTH/pro-inflammatory types of reactions were shown to secrete interleukin (IL)-2, lymphotoxin (LT) and IFN-γ and called CD4⁺ Th1 cells; CD4⁺ T helper cells that participated in helping B cell antibody responses were shown to secrete IL-4, IL-5, IL-6, IL-9, IL-10 and IL-13 and called CD4⁺ Th2 cells (Fig. 6) (reviewed in [23]). Another cell type and cytokine pattern, Th0, has also been described which includes both Th1 and Th2 cytokine profiles. Importantly, the different cytokines secreted by Th1 and Th2 cells have been shown to negatively regulate each other. For example, Th1-mediated DTH is inhibited by two Th2 cytokines, IL-4 and IL-10. Likewise, Th2-mediated help for B cell production is inhibited by IFN-γ, a potent Th1 cytokine (reviewed in [23]).

Th1-like and Th2-like patterns have been identified in human CD4⁺ T helper cell clones. In addition to CD4⁺ T cells, Th1- and Th2-like cytokine patterns have been identified in CD8⁺ killer/cytotoxic T cells (Tc). Analysis of CD8⁺ murine clones have demonstrated a Th1-like cytokine pattern while analysis of some human CD8⁺ clones were shown to secrete both IL-4 and IFN-γ (reviewed in [23]).

The relevancy of these cytokine patterns by different subsets has been borne out *in vivo*, in murine models of intracellular murine leishmania infection, in in-

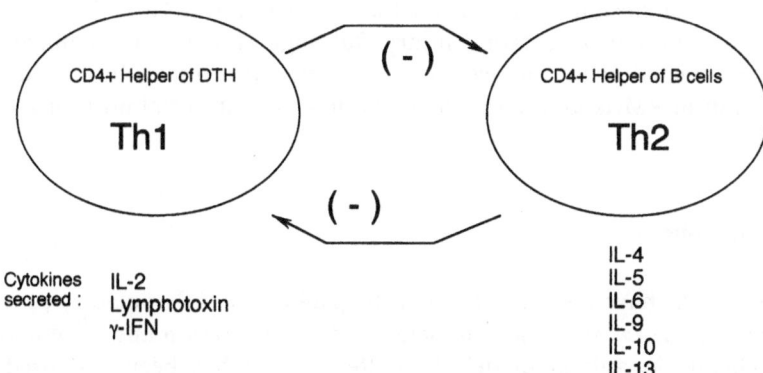

Fig. 6. Distinct profiles of cytokine patterns by T cell clones characterized two types of CD4 + helper T cells. The cytokines produced by Th1 and Th2 cells may negatively regulate each other, and may be important in the homeostatic regulation of immune responses. (From [25] with permission)

testinal parasite infections, and in human leprosy (reviewed in [23]). Thus, the Th0, Th1 and Th2 model correlating cytokine production and function has been important in dissecting and understanding the pathophysiology of disease. Depending on the antigenic challenge (infectious agent or organ transplantation), the genetic control of the immune response may be largely determined at the level of cytokines produced.

Neutrophils (Polymorphonuclear Leukocytes)

One of the central cell types that participate in the inflammatory response as a result of trauma, ischemia/reperfusion (I/R) and sepsis is the neutrophil or polymorphonuclear leukocyte (PMN). The majority of PMNs are in the peripheral blood and rarely in normal tissue, including the normal gut. However, as a result of tissue injury, PMNs transmigrate to the tissue site at risk, where they mature into functional effectors [27]. The ability of PMNs to release oxygen free radicals and other tissue-damaging molecules, underscores their major role in the sequelae of trauma and in the pathogenesis of multiple organ failure (MOF). The ability of neutrophils and other leukocytes to become activated, transmigrate and accumulate in the extravascular space depends on adhesive interactions between cell-surface molecules expressed on leukocytes and endothelial cells (reviewed in [28]). These adhesive interactions are determined by the cell surface expression of several families of cell adhesion molecules that are induced or 'upregulated' on leukocytes and endothelial cells in response to initial trauma, i.e. I/R, such as the selectins and the integrins (discussed below) [57].

One consequence of trauma at a remote site is reduced splanchnic flow to the intestine. Many animal models of I/R, including models of intestinal I/R, have implicated the neutrophil and its β2-integrin-dependent adhesion on subsequent tissue injury [29]. In low-flow intestinal I/R, the PMN was found to mediate local injury in the gut. However, in complete intestinal I/R, blocking of PMN adhesion by monoclonal antibodies to CD11b and CD18 reduced remote but not local intestinal injury [30], suggesting that mechanisms other than the activated neutrophil were responsible for this injury. Interestingly, the activation of PMNs appears to be a common feature of almost all models of I/R studied.

Mast Cells

Mast cells have been shown to participate in the inflammatory process following trauma i.e. they mediate neutrophil sequestration and edema after remote ischemia in animal models [31]. Recently, it has been proposed that mast cells may provide an important role as a 'sensor' of tissue damage in the body, which in turn induces the mast cell to release mediators (platelet activating factor (PAF), histamine) and other factors that recruit and activate other leukocytes, particularly the neutrophil, to the appropriate site at risk in the body [32].

Indeed, using intravital microscopy to visualize leukocyte-rolling flux and adhesion in rat mesenteric venules, it was shown that mast cell degranulation induced P-selectin rolling from histamine [32] and CD18-dependent leukocyte adhesion from PAF [32, 33]. Thus, mast cells are an important participant in the early phase of the inflammatory response induced by trauma.

Unique Structures in the Gut-associated Lymphoid Tissue (GALT)

Much of what we know about the immune system is related to the peripheral immune system which includes the peripheral blood, thymus, spleen and peripheral lymph nodes. We know less about the immune system in the gut, but to date, it appears that the GALT is qualitatively different, particularly with regard to oral tolerance, controlled inflammation and IgA production in a setting of systemic suppression. There are several structural features in the GALT that may help to explain differences in the immune system in the gut.

Peyer's Patches

Peyer's patches are unique lymphoid structures that are in close proximity to the intestinal lumen (Fig. 7). The structure of Peyer's patches shares common features with other antigen-trapping organs in the MALT, such as the lymph node, spleen and tonsil. Peyer's patches lie beneath specialized epithelial cells called M cells. M cells are thought to be the major site of antigen entry into the mucosal lymphoid follicles that are distributed along the small intestine. M cells can transport macromolecules, intact bacteria and virus from the lumen into the Peyer's patch [34]. Antigen is taken up by M cells and transported through the cell to the baso-lateral side where it is then taken up by tissue macrophages and dendritic cells, the APCs of Peyer's patches, which process and present antigen to T and B cells [35]. Cytokines are produced by APCs, T cells and B cells, and a GALT immune response ensues. The germinal center is a specialized site in Peyer's patches for B cell differentiation into mature plasma cells, primarily synthesizing IgA. Lymphocytes that recognize their cognate antigens are activated in the germinal center then migrate to mesenteric lymph nodes. Cells then transit to the thoracic duct where they empty into the vena cava and become part of the systemic circulation. Activated cells, particularly IgA + cells, usually "home" or migrate to the lamina propria, a loose connective tissue in the intestine and to other mucosal sites in the body such as the lung, lacrimal gland, salivary gland, lactating mammary gland, and uro-genital tract. This systemic "homing" or migration results in dissemination of protective IgA-producing B cells to other mucosal sites that may be vulnerable to pathogens.

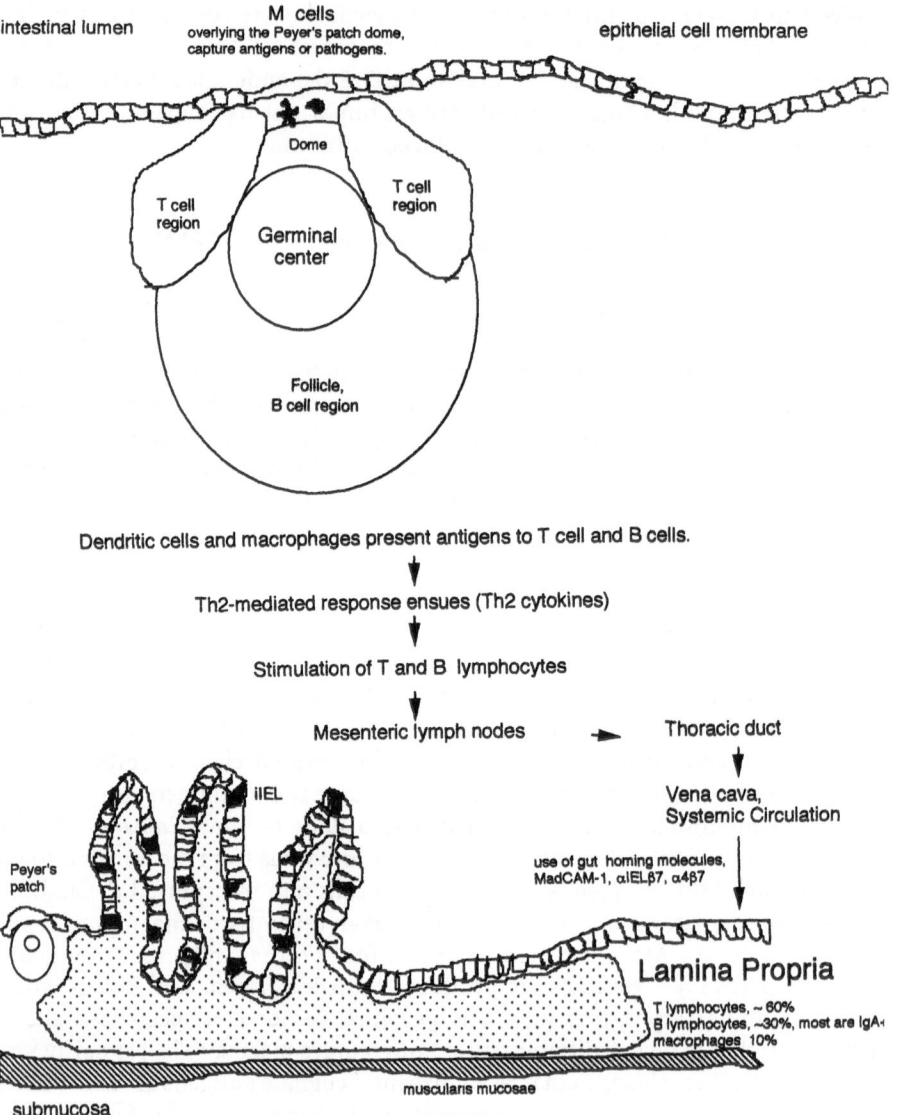

Fig. 7. Inductive (Peyer's patch) and effector (lamina propria) sites of an immune response in the GALT. (From [34] with permission)

Oral Tolerance

The physical characteristics and form of gut antigens (bacterial, viral, dietary) taken up by M cells, determine the quality and nature of the subsequent immune response. Most antigens that go through M cells result in Th2-mediated helper activity. In contrast the result of the oral route of immunization with antigen is a state of suppression of T cells expressing receptors for that antigen (reviewed in

[36]). This mechanism, called oral tolerance, is a general phenomena for antigens delivered by the oral route, i.e. dietary antigens [37]. In addition, antigen dose, type of APC and cytokine milieu influence the quality of the immune response. For example, high doses of antigen result in anergy of antigen-specific T cells, while low doses of antigen result in selective expression of cells producing regulatory cytokines (IL-10, TGF-β, IL-4) that result in T cell suppression [36]. Interestingly, the cytokines that promote immunosuppression also promote IgA production, suggesting that mucosal T cell tolerance and mucosal IgA responses are regulated in a similar way [38]. Oral tolerance is the basis for some types of vaccine development, and has implications for strategies aimed at dampening the immune response in autoimmune disorders for which there is no known etiological agent [36].

The precise mechanism for oral tolerance is not known but may be due to
1) anergy (T cell does not respond to subsequent stimulation through its antigen receptor [TCR/CD3 complex]);
2) deletion of antigen-reactive T cells; and/or
3) active suppression (probably mediated by cytokines).

Lamina Propria

The lamina propria (LP) is a loose connective tissue in the lamina propria compartment of the intestinal mucosa and in the epithelial layer that comprises the villous structure. LP consists of many cell types that include T cells, B cells, macrophages, eosinophils, mast cells, rare natural killer (NK) cells and fibroblasts. In contrast to the peripheral blood, and to other lymphoid compartments such as the spleen and tonsil, the normal LP lymphoid compartment is phenotypically distinct [39] and exhibits an enhanced state of activation [40, 41]. Intestinal mononuclear cells from normal small bowel and colon contain increased numbers of Ig-secreting plasma cells [40, 41], particularly of the IgA class. In addition, the state of activation of LP T cells is also enhanced [42]. The majority of T cells in LP are αβ TCR$^+$, CD3$^+$ and CD4$^+$ [39], suggesting that they interact with Class II-expressing cells (B cells, DCs and macrophages).

T cells can be stimulated by several biochemical pathways. Stimulation by anti-CD3 antibody is often used experimentally because it is directed towards the TCR/CD3 complex to mimic antigen recognition through the T cell receptor and results in proliferation [43] and cytokine production [44, 45]. Several studies have shown that while intestinal lymphocytes express an activation phenotype, they are defective in their ability to proliferate in vitro in response to TCR/ CD3 stimulation [42, 43]. In contrast to the hyporesponsiveness seen with anti-TCR/CD3 antibodies, stimulation of intestinal lymphocytes with antibodies to the CD2 and CD28 molecules generate substantial proliferation [20, 21, 45] and enhanced cytokine production [45, 46] compared to peripheral blood T cells from the same patient.

T cell accessory receptors such as CD2 and CD28 can initiate antigen-independent T cell activation with LFA-3 (CD58) and B7 respectively, as shown in Fig 5. Recent studies have demonstrated that CD2 appears to be unique in its ability to reverse the anergic or unresponsive state of T cells unable to be stimulated through TCR/CD3 [23]. This has important implications in the immune system in the intestine since the major phenotype of T cells in the intestinal mucosa (LP and intraepithelial lymphocytes) is unresponsive when stimulated through the TCR/CD3 complex, yet susceptible to proliferation and cytokine production by anti-CD2 stimulation [22, 45].

Intestinal Intra-epithelial Lymphocytes (iIELs)

The iIELs are a distinct population of T cells that can be distinguished from T cells in the peripheral blood and primary lymphoid organs in that the majority of iIELs express an activated phenotype [47]. The majority of IELs are TCR $\alpha\beta^+$, $CD3^+$ and $CD8^+$, however the remaining are TCR $\gamma\delta^+$, $CD3^+$ and $CD8^+$ [47, 48]. The spatial distribution of iIELs are ~ 1 iIEL/6 epithelial cells (Fig. 7). iIELs are difficult to stimulate with anti-CD3 antibodies but are maximally stimulated with anti-CD2 antibodies *in vitro* [43]. Thus, like lamina propria T cells, they may be anergized and not capable of being stimulated through their TCR/ CD3 signaling complex.

T Cell Repertoire of Human Intestinal T lymphocytes

Since the intestine is the major reservoir of lymphocytes in the human body and is in close proximity to diverse intestinal antigens, one might expect the T cell repertoire (the array of different antigen-recognition receptors on T cells) to be equally diverse, however this is not the case [49, 50]. DNA sequence analysis of the Vβ genes (*v*ariable region of the TCRβ gene that encodes the β chain of the αβTCR) in normal human intestinal biopsies showed that identical receptors could be found on T cells throughout the intestine of individual patients, suggesting that resident intestinal T cells were oligoclonal. In addition, no consistent pattern of TCR Vβ usage among donors could be detected [51, 52]. Other studies analysing the diversity of the intestinal Vδ genes (*v*ariable region of the TCR δ gene that encodes the δ chain of the γδ TCR) showed that this repertoire was also oligoclonal throughout the intestine and that it was stable over time [53]. Thus, the T cell repertoire in the intestine is biased or skewed toward expression of a limited number of different T cell receptors, suggesting that the antigens they recognize are also limited, or conserved.

   While IELs are oligoclonal, they have the capacity to mount immune responses to MHC Class I-restricted viral infections, to alloantigens, and to superantigens (bacterial toxins) (reviewed in [54]). Epithelial cells have been shown to express Class I and Class II molecules, and to express non-polymorphic MHC Class I-like molecules called CD1d, a member of the CD1 family (reviewed in [54]).

While CD1d is constitutively expressed on a large number of tissues, it is most highly expressed on intestinal epithelial cells, renal tubular epithelial cells and B cells. A precise role for CD1d in antigen presentation has not been elucidated but CD1d may play a role in selection or extrathymic education in the intestinal milieu (reviewed in [54]).

Intestinal Epithelial Cells

The epithelial cell membrane of the intestine is intimately involved in anti-bacterial host defenses that include several types of barriers:
1) physical barrier: comprised of junctional complexes between epithelial cells;
2) mechanical barrier: comprised of intestinal peristalsis, mucous production, epithelial desquamation;
3) chemical barrier: comprised of gastric acidity, bile salts, RES function, trefoils; and
4) immunological barrier: comprised of secretory IgA, GALT system.

In addition to these barriers that block pathogen invasion, epithelial cells have been shown to be an integral part of the immune system by several criteria: they have the capacity to
1) process and present antigen to T and B cells [35];
2) express Class II molecules [55];
3) express CD1d, a Class I-like molecule [54]; and
4) secrete cytokines in response to bacterial pathogens or their by-products (toxins) [56].

Indeed, recent studies have shown that invasion of epithelial cell lines or freshly isolated colonic epithelial cells by a panel of enteric pathogens resulted in coordinated enhanced expression of particular cytokines [56]. Thus, epithelial cells provide an early signaling system, by production of these cytokines, to immunoreactive cells in the underlying mucosa [56].

Cell Adhesion Molecules

Cell adhesion molecules, together with the antigen-recognition complex of molecules and co-stimulatory molecules on T cells and APCs, interact to optimize immune responses [18, 57].
  Cell adhesion molecules control a vast array of interactions between leukocytes, endothelial cells and other cells to regulate inflammation, leukocyte migration, activation and effector function.

The major structural families of cell adhesion molecules that participate in lymphocyte interactions are:
1) selectins;
2) certain members of the immunoglobulin superfamily (ICAMs, VCAMs);

3) integrins;
4) CD44, a mucin-like molecule; and
5) cadherins.

Characterization of the various families of cell adhesion molecules has been extensively studied (reviewed in [57]).

Effect of Inflammatory Mediators and Cytokines on Cellular Adhesion Molecules

While some cell adhesion molecules are constitutively expressed on cells, others are induced or "upregulated" in response to inflammatory mediators released from inflamed or damaged tissue. The inflammatory cytokine/cell adhesion cascade plays an important role in the transmigration of leukocytes, particularly neutrophils (PMNs), monocytes, and lymphocytes during inflammatory cascades from I/R injury; this cascade has been dissected at the molecular level into several stages in many *in vitro* and *in vivo* models (reviewed in [28, 57–59]). As shown in Fig. 8, tissue damage induces inflammatory mediators and cytokine production which induce P-selectin and E-selectin on endothelial cells and up-

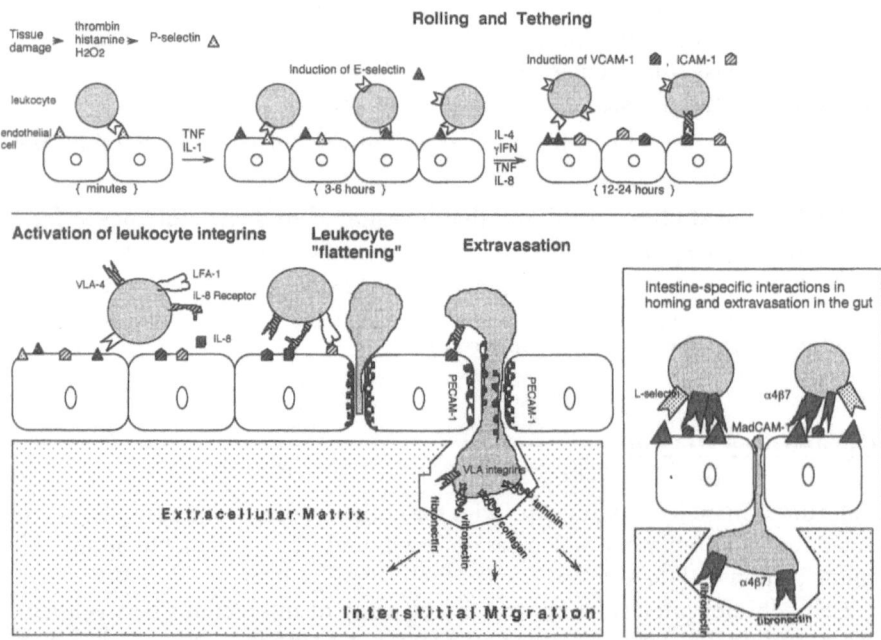

Fig. 8. Tissue damage induces an inflammatory cascade resulting in extravasation of cells (PMNs) from the blood into tissue. The inflammatory cascade has been dissected at the molecular level into several distinct stages. Intestine-specific homing and extravasation. α4β7 is selectively expressed on mucosal lymphocytes that colonize the intestine and GALT; it is the dominant receptor for MadCAM-1, the mucosal vascular addressin in the GALT. (From [57] with permission)

regulation of L-selectin on leukocytes. A second set of proinflammatory cytokines induce expression of ICAM-1 and VCAM-1. The leukocyte/endothelial cell interactions are intermittent ("tethering") and allow the leukocyte to "roll" along the vascular endothelium in the direction of blood flow. The interaction of cytokines with specific cytokine receptors (IL-8/IL-8R or MIP-1β-CD44/MIP-1βR) induces a conformational change in an integrin molecule making it a high affinity receptor for ICAM-1 and VCAM-1; this allows firm binding of the leukocyte to the endothelium. This site-specific adhesion allows leukocytes to squeeze between endothelial cells without disrupting vascular permeability. PECAM-1 (CD31) is expressed on both the leukocyte and endothelial cell and mediates extravasation by homotypic adhesion (diapedesis). This adhesion induces the expression of other integrin molecules on the leukocyte that allow it to interact with various extracellular matrix (ECM) proteins in the tissue (interstitial migration) [28, 57–59].

Intestine-specific homing and extravasation require specific cell adhesion molecules as shown in Fig 8. $\alpha 4\beta 7$ is selectively expressed on mucosal lymphocytes that colonize the intestine and GALT; it is the dominant receptor for Mad-CAM-1, the mucosal vascular addressin in the GALT. $\alpha 4\beta 7^+$ leukocytes, after extravasation, migrate into intestinal tissue by recognition of fibronectin [59] (reviewed in [57]).

Gut Dysfunction

The major conditions of critical illness that affect the immune system are shock and infection, and their complex sequelae. The role of the immune system in the GALT is pivotal in many aspects and stages of these broad conditions of stress.

Shock is a physiologic response characterized by decreased cardiac output, decreased blood flow and ischemia to involved organs, resulting in organ-specific ischemia or systemic ischemia. In animal models, reperfusion or restoration of blood volume results in a serious inflammatory response capable of causing a lethal septic-like syndrome in which failure of gut mucosal barrier integrity may contribute to mortality [60]. Thus, gut-derived endotoxin from translocated bacteria may be a link between gut failure (loss of mucosal barrier integrity) and multiple organ failure (MOF) in a septic-appearing patient without evidence of infection.

One common feature of many critically ill patients is the risk of translocation of enteric bacteria during "stressed" conditions such as shock and organ transplantation. Shock, with infectious complications, may involve secretion of increased quantities of cytokines induced by endotoxin challenge, compared to shock alone, particularly TNF, an important mediator of shock [61]. The production of cytokines therefore is critical to the pathogenic mechanisms of septic shock and injury. A model for how critical illness may develop from a variety of "stresses" on the gut and how infection may complicate this scenario is depicted in Fig. 9 [62–67].

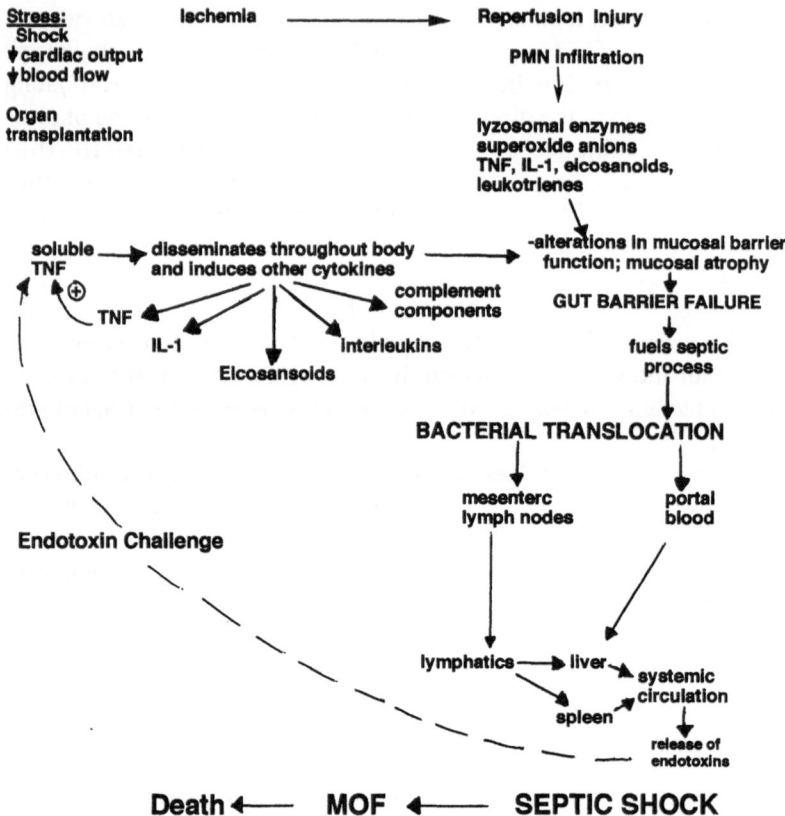

Fig. 9. Ischemia/reperfusion generates an inflammatory cascade resulting in tissue injury. Model for how ischemia/reperfusion injury results in the induction of potent inflammatory mediators and cytokines that may be neutrophil and non-neutrophil mediated. Mucosal barrier integrity may be altered allowing the translocation of enteric bacteria. This pathway may be exacerbated by endotoxin challenge from exogenous bacteria or from endogenous release of endotoxin, that may result in septic shock, MOF and death

Small Bowel Transplantation: A Paradigm of Gut Dysfunction

The gastrointestinal (GI) tract has a rich blood supply and any condition which reduces blood flow to the intestine may result in adverse sequelae. I/R injury is particularly relevant to organ transplantation. Organ transplants are ischemic/reperfused tissue that undergo the same initial tissue injury as ischemic/reperfused tissue in the body induced by shock (stress).

Increasing numbers of allogeneic small bowel transplants are being performed and most of these patients are treated in ICU for prolonged periods. There are many aspects of small bowel transplantation that make it unique among solid organ transplantation. As a result of ischemia and reperfusion of the graft, the small bowel is a target of the cytokine-induced alterations of the mucosal gut barrier and is a major site of bacterial translocation. In addition, since the small bowel is the major reservoir of lymphocytes in the human body, it is a major target of allograft rejection and of the development of graft-versus-host disease (GVHD) [68]. Thus, two distinct molecular scenarios may occur during small bowel transplantation: 1) I/R; and 2) immunologic rejection.

The sequelae of I/R is a non-specific, antigen-independent, largely PMN-mediated inflammatory cascade, while the sequelae of graft rejection is largely an alloantigen-dependent and T cell-dependent response. Both of these components of small bowel transplantation (SBT) require the participation of cell interaction molecules such as 1) cell adhesion molecules; 2) antigen recognition molecules; and 3) co-stimulatory molecules. At the inductive phase, the inflammatory cascade and T cell-mediated allograft response may be temporally and spatially distinct. Indeed, early histologic changes equivalent to those seen in graft rejection may occur within the first few days after autologous bowel transplantation [69] and may be due to I/R or to the trauma of surgery.

The non-specific, antigen-independent pathway activated during I/R is very effective in secreting cytokines (TNF) that upregulate cell adhesion molecules and promote extravasation of leukocytes from blood into tissue; in I/R in SBT, this extravasation is into intestinal tissue. Indeed, even in the presence of immunosuppressive agents that inhibit T cells, there is a large influx of cells into the mesenteric lymph node (MLN) [70], suggesting this may be independent of antigen recognition by T cells. Studies of a heterotopic rat model provided evidence that increased bacterial translocation occurred in isografts as well as allografts suggesting that the transplantation process itself affects intestinal permeability independently of T cell-mediated rejection [71]. However, later in the responses, cytokines and mediators induced by each "stress" may synergize and result in massive inflammatory cascades and increased T cell activity.

The alloantigen-dependent and T cell-dependent component of SBT may be comprised of at least two populations of T cells: 1) resident intestinal T lymphocytes; and 2) recirculating T cells that traffic through the gut. Both resident and recirculating T cells may mediate rejection. MLN and Peyer's patches are targets for immunologic "attack" during SBT [68]; in addition, they are the most responsive sites in the GALT during GVHD [72]. Thus, massive T cell activation, inflammation and subsequent rejection is a major therapeutic concern. The cellular interactions resulting from I/R injury in conjunction with vigorous T cell-mediated rejection of small bowel allografts can be devastating. Indeed, the poor outcome of SBT may be due to the plethora of cytokines and mediators secreted and cell interactions engendered in these two different cellular and immunologic responses.

The alloantigen-dependent pathway of T cell activation after SBT optimally requires all three set of cellular interaction molecules for T cell activation. The quality of the rejection response can be variable, however a major factor is the degree of histocompatibility disparity between the graft and the host i.e. differences in Class I loci [HLA-A, -B, or -C] and/or differences in Class II loci [HLA-DR, -DP or -DQ].

Understanding the contribution of each of these scenarios may help in dissecting the molecular basis of induction of acute or chronic allograft rejection. Despite the success rate of SBT with FK506 [73], and other solid organ transplantation with cyclosporin A in acute rejection, chronic rejection is the major cause of allograft loss within the first year following transplantation [74]. Chronic rejection of many allograft models are characterized by persistent perivascular inflammation and myointimal hyperplasia [74]. It is thought that initial injury to vascular endothelium in the graft, by immunologic or non-immunologic mechanisms, play a role in the development of chronic rejection [74]. Interestingly, blocking with FK506, which blocks T cell activation and clonal expansion, has no effect on chronic rejection suggesting that antigen-independent factors may be responsible for chronic rejection. Thus, prevention of initiation of the cytokine-cell adhesion molecule cascade is most important.

Diagnosis of Rejection

Infiltration of a graft by host cells is the basis of the histological diagnosis of rejection in solid organ allografts. However, this may not be feasible in SBT where the graft itself contains so many activated cells. Other functional tests have been used to detect acute rejection, but these are often measuring the results of loss of mucosal barrier function in the gut which does not provide histological evidence of rejection [68]. Thus, detection of qualitative and quantitative differences in cytokine production may provide a way to detect rejection in SBT. Indeed, the polymerase chain reaction has been used in animal models to detect *de novo* synthesis of cytokines [75].

Therapeutics for Small Bowel Transplantation

Many different immunosuppressive drugs are used for organ transplantation. Unfortunately, many of these drugs have side effects including malignancy. For small bowel transplants, FK506 alone or combined with other reagents have shown great therapeutic promise [73]. Monoclonal antibodies and peptides to some of the cell interaction molecules discussed previously are among the more specific immunosuppressives developed to induce long-term immunomodulation to effect organ tolerance and long-term survival without infectious or malignant complications [76]. However, most of these have been tested in other models of solid organ transplantation.

Future Directions

Trauma, I/R and subsequent inflammatory-mediated injury induce quantitative and qualitative changes in expression of many families of cell-interaction molecules including the cell adhesion molecules, antigen-recognition molecules, and the co-stimulatory molecules. Since cell adhesion molecules (selectins, integrins and others) play a central role in the inflammatory process immediately following trauma, antibodies to these molecules may be useful in trauma patients. Identification of inhibitors that block the production of pro-inflammatory cytokines, particularly TNF, would dampen this process; in addition, it may dampen both the antigen-independent and antigen-dependent pathways in organ transplantation, and other "stresses" that induce shock, loss of mucosal barrier function and MOF.

Since neutrophils are major participants in early events in critical illness, their migration from the blood to tissue could be blocked with antibodies to neutrophils (anti-CD18, anti-CD11b) or with antibodies to activated endothelial molecules. Indeed, in animal models of intestinal I/R, administration of monoclonal antibodies to CD11b or CD18 reduced remote but not local intestinal injury [29, 30].

While most therapies are given after reperfusion, it may be fruitful to administer therapies prior to or concommitant with reperfusion. Combination therapies that couple immunosuppressive or cytokine-suppressive drugs with monoclonal antibodies to cell interaction molecules may have useful clinical application and provide a successful therapeutic strategy for critical illness in man.

Conclusion

The activation state of immune cells in the intestine, in the lamina propria compartment and in the intraepithelial space are more activated compared to immune cells in the peripheral blood compartment, based on cell surface phenotype, cytokine production and functional effector capacity. While immune cells, particularly T and B lymphocytes, are in an activated state in the normal gut, they are systemically suppressed, as evidenced by the anergic state of T and B cells in the lamina propria compartment. Thus, the normal state of the intestine is controlled inflammation in the presence of systemic suppression.

Tissue injury from trauma at a remote site, particularly the production of cytokines and inflammatory mediators, may disseminate throughout the body and cause injury to other tissues. Alternatively, if trauma at a remote site significantly affects splanchnic blood flow to the gut, then gut injury may occur by cytokines and mediators from the remote site as well as from the influx of mononuclear cells (neutrophils, monocytes) from the blood into gut tissue that is ischemic/reperfused. Gut injury (damage to intestinal epithelial cells, for example) may be due to these cytokines directly, or to cytokines released from transmigrated leukocytes, or may be due to unchecked, inflammatory-mediated triggering of immune cells in the gut that are already in an activated state and poised for effector function. This may likely contribute to gut injury and gut dysfunction (hypermetabolism, stasis) in the critically ill patient.

Further basic research and clinical trials using novel approaches and therapies will bring us closer to understanding the cellular and molecular dynamics in trauma and gut dysfunction in critical illness.

References

1. Tonegawa S (1983) Somatic generation of antibody diversity. Nature 302:575–581
2. Kett K, Baklien K, Bakken A, Kral JG, Fausa O, Brandtzaeg P (1995) Intestinal B cell isotype response in relation to local bacterial load: Evidence for immunoglobulin A subclass adaptation. Gastroenterology 109:819–825
3. Koshland ME (1975) Structure and function of the J chain. Adv Immunol 20:41–51
4. Brantzaeg P, Prydz H (1984) Direct evidence for an integrated function of J chain and secretory component in epithelial transport of immunoglobulins. Nature 311:71–73
5. Kaetzle CS, Robinson JK, Chintalacharuvu KR, Vaerman JP, Lamm ME (1991) The polymeric immunoglobulin receptor (secretory component) mediates transport of immune complexes across epithelial cells: A local defense function for IgA. Proc Natl Acad Sci USA 88:8796–8800
6. Mostov KE, Deitcher DL (1986) Polymeric immunoglobulin receptor expressed in MDCK cells trancytoses IgA. Cell 46:613–621
7. Mazanec MB, Kaetzel CS, Lamm ME (1992) Intracellular neutralization of virus by immunoglobulin A antibodies. Proc Natl Acad Sci USA 89:6901–6905
8. Kaetzle CS, Robinson JK, Lamm ME (1994) Epithelial transcytosis of monomeric IgA and IgG cross-linked through antigen to polymeric IgA. A role for monomeric antibodies in the mucosal immune system. J Immunol 152:72–76
9. Weiss A, Stobo JD (1984) Requirement for the co-expression of T3 and T-cell antigen on a malignant T-cell line. J Exp Med 160:1284–1299
10. Weissman AM, Baniyash M, Hou D, Samelson LE, Burgess WH, Klausner RD (1988) Molecular cloning of the zeta chain of the T-cell antigen receptor. Science 239:1018–1021
11. Alarcon B, Berkhout B, Breitmeyer J, Terhorst C (1988) Assembly of the human T cell receptor-CD3 complex takes place in the endoplasmic reticulum and involves intermediary complexes between the CD3-γ,δ,ε core and single T cell receptor α and β chains. J Biol Chem 263:2953–2961
12. Sancho J, Chatila T, Wong CK, et al (1989) T cell antigen receptor (TCR)-ab heterodimer formation is prerequisite for association of CD3-z2 into functionally competent TCR/CD3 complexes. J Biol Chem 264:20760–20769
13. Janeway CA Jr (1992) The T-cell receptor is a multicomponent signaling machine: CD4/ CD8 coreceptors and CD45 in T-cell activation. Ann Rev Immunol 10:645–674
14. Shepherd JC, Schumacher TNM, Ashton-Rickardt PG, et al (1993) TAP-1-dependent peptide translocation in vitro is ATP-dependent and peptide selective. Cell 74:577–584
15. Lanzavecchia A, Reid PA, Watts C (1992) Irreversible association of peptides with class II MHC molecules in living cells. Nature 357:249–252
16. Schwartz RH (1990) A cell culture model for T lymphocyte clonal anergy. Science 248:1349–1356
17. Jenkins MK, Johnson JG (1993) Molecules involved in T-cell co-stimulation. Curr Opin Immunol 5:361–367
18. Guinan EC, Gribben JG, Boussiotis VA, Freeman GJ, Nadler LM (1994) Pivotal role of the B7:CD28 pathway in transplantation tolerance and tumor immunity. Blood 84:3261–3282
19. Tivol EA, Borriello F, Schweitzer AN, et al (1995) Loss of CTLA-4 leads to massive lymphoproliferation and fatal multiorgan tissue destruction, revealing a critical negative regulatory role for CTLA-4. Immunity 5:541–547
20. Pirzer UC, Schurmann G, Post S, Betzler M, Meuer S (1990) Differential responsiveness to CD3Ti vs CD2-dependent activation of human intestinal T lymphocytes. Eur J Immunol 20:2339–2342
21. Qiao L, Schurmann G, Betzler M, Meuer S (1991) Activation and signaling status of human lamina propria T lymphocytes. Gastroenterology 101:1529–1536
22. Ebert EC (1989) Proliferative responses of human intraepithelial lymphocytes to various T-cell stimuli. Gastroenterology 97:1372–1381
23. Boussiatis VA, Freeman GJ, Griffen JD, Gray CS, Gribben JG, Nadler LM (1994) CD2 is involved in maintenance and reversal of human alloantigen-specific clonal anergy. J Exp Med 180:1665–1673

24. Reinecker HC, Podolsky DK (1995) Human intestinal epithelial cells express functional cytokine receptors sharing the common γ chain of the interleukin-2 receptor. Proc Natl Acad Sci USA 92:8353–8357

25. Mosmann TR, Coffman RL (1989) Th1 and Th2 cells: Different patterns of lymphokine secretion lead to different functional properties. Ann Rev Immunol 7:145–173

26. Sad S, Marcotte R, Mosmann TR (1995) Cytokine-induced differentiation of precursor mouse CD8 + T cells into cytotoxic CD8 + T cells secreting Th1 or Th2 cytokines. Immunity 2:271–279

27. Van Furth R (1992) Development and distribution of mononuclear phagocytes. In: Gallin J, Goldstein I, Snyderman R (eds) Inflammation: Basic Principles and Clinical Correlates, 2nd edn., Raven Press, New York, pp 325–340

28. Kubes P (1993) Polymorphonuclear leukocyte-endothelium interactions: A role for pro-inflammatory and anti-inflammatory molecules. Can J Physiol Pharm 71:88–97

29. Simpson R, Alon R, Valeri CR, Shepro D, Hechtman HB (1993) Integrin-dependent neutrophil adhesion following gut ischemia and reperfusion. Behr Inst Mitt 92:210–217

30. Simpson R, Alon R, Kobzik L, Valeri CR, Shepro D, Hechtman HB (1993) Neutrophil and non-neutrophil-mediated injury in intestinal ischemia/reperfusion. Ann of Surg 218:444–454

31. Goldman G, Welbourne R, Klausner JM, et al (1992) Mast cells and leukotrienes mediate neutrophil sequestration and lung edema after remote ischemia in rodents. Surgery 112:578–586

32. Kubes P, Kanwar S (1994) Histamine induces leukocyte rolling in post-capillary venules. A P-selectin-mediated event. J Immunol 152:3570–3577

33. Gaboury JP, Johnston B, Niu XF, Kubes P (1995) Mechanisms underlining acute mast cell-induced leukocyte rolling and adhesion in vivo. J Immunol 154:804–813

34. Neutra MR, Kraehenbuhl JP (1993) The role of transepithelial transport by M cells in microbial invasion and host defense. J Cell Sci (Suppl) 17:209–215

35. Farstad IN, Halstensen TS, Fausa O, Brantzaeg P (1994) Heterogeneity of M-cell-associated B and T cells in human Peyer's patches. Immunology 83:457–464

36. Weiner HL, Friedman A, Miller A, et al (1993) Oral tolerance: Immunological mechanisms and treatment of murine and human organ specific autoimmune diseases by oral administration of autoantigens. Ann Rev Immunol 12:809–837

37. Mowat AM (1994) Oral tolerance and regulation of immunity to dietary antigens. In: Ogra PL, Mestecky J, Lamm ME, et al (eds) Handbook of Mucosal Immunology. Academic Press, San Diego, pp 185–201

38. Challacombe SJ, Tomasi TB Jr (1980) Systemic tolerance and secretory immunity after oral immunization. J Exp Med 152:1459–1472

39. James SP, Fiocchi C, Graeff AS, Strober W (1986) Phenotypic analysis of lamina propria lymphocytes: Predominance of helper-inducer and cytolytic T cell phenotypes and deficiency of suppressor-inducer phenotypes in Crohn's disease and control patients. Gastroenterology 91:1483–1489

40. Peters MG, Secrist H, Anders KR, et al (1989) Normal intestinal lymphocytes: Increased activation compared with peripheral blood. J Clin Invest 83:1827–1833

41. Pallone F, Fais S, Squarcia O, Biancone L, Boirivant A (1987) Activation of peripheral blood and intestinal lamina propria lymphocytes in Crohn's disease. In vivo state of activation and response to stimulation as defined by the expression of activation antigens. Gut 28:745–753

42. Zeitz M, Greene WC, Peffer NJ, James SP (1988) Lymphocytes isolated from the intestinal lamina propria of normal non-human primates have increased expression of genes associated with T-cell activation. Gastroenterology 94:647–655

43. Ebert EC (1989) Proliferative responses of human intraepithelial lymphocytes to various T-cell stimuli. Gastroenterology 97:1372–1381

44. Deem RL, Shanahan F, Targan SR (1991) Triggered human mucosal T cells release tumor necrosis factor-alpha and interferon-gamma which kill human colonic epithelial cells. Clin Exp Immunol 83:79–84

45. Targan SR, Deem RL, Liu M, Wang S, Nel A (1995) Definition of a lamina propria T cell responsive state: Enhanced cytokine responsiveness of T cells stimulated through the CD2 pathway. J Immunol 154:664–675
46. Thompson CB, Lindsten T, Ledbetter JA, et al (1989) CD28 activation pathway regulates the production of multiple T cell-derived lymphokines/cytokines. Proc Natl Acad Sci USA 86: 1333–1337
47. Ullrich R, Schieferdecker HL, Ziegler K, Riecken EO, Zeitz M (1990) Gamma/delta T cells in the human intestine express surface markers of activation and are preferentially located in the epithelium. Cell Immunol. 128:619–627
48. Deusch K, Pfeffer K, Reich K, et al (1991) Phenotypic and functional characterization of human TCRγδ+ intestinal intraepithelial lymphocytes. Curr Topics Micro Immunol 173:279–283
49. Balk SP, Ebert EC, Blumenthal RL, et al (1991) Oligoclonal expansion and CD1 recognition by human intestinal intraepithelial lymphocytes. Science 253:1411–1415
50. Van Kerckhove C, Russell GJ, Deusch K, et al (1992) Oligoclonality of human intestinal intraepithelial T cells. J Exp Med 175:57–63
51. Blumberg RS, Yockey CE, Gross GG, Ebert EC, Balk SP (1993) Human intestinal intraepithelial lymphocytes are derived from a limited number of T cell clones that utilize multiple Vβ T cell receptor genes. J Immunol 150:5144–5153
52. Gross GG, Schwartz VL, Stevens C, Ebert EC, Blumberg RS, Balk SP (1994) Distribution of dominant T cell receptor beta chains in human intestinal mucosa. J Exp Med 180: 1337–1344
53. Chowers Y, Holtmeier W, Harwood J, Morzycka-Wroblewska E, Kagnoff M (1994) The Vδ1 T cell receptor repertoire in human small intestine and colon. J Exp Med 180:183–190
54. Blumberg RS, Balk SP (1994) Intraepithelial lymphocytes and their recognition of non-classical MHC molecules. Int Rev Immunol 11:15–30
55. Panja A, Blumberg RS, Balk SP, Mayer L (1993) CD1d is involved in T cell/intestinal epithelial cell interactions J Exp Med 178:1115–1119
56. Eckmann L, Kagnoff MF, Fierer J (1993) Epithelial cells secrete the chemokine interleukin-8 in response to bacterial entry. Infection Immunity 61:4569–4574
57. Imhof BA, Dunon D (1995) Leukocyte migration and adhesion. Adv in Immunol 58: 345–410
58. Springer TA (1994) Traffic signals for lymphocyte recirculation and leukocyte migration: The multi-step paradigm. Cell 76:301–314
59. Bargatze RF, Jutila MA, Butcher EC (1995) Distinct roles of L-selectin and integrins α4β7 and LFA-1 in lymphocyte homing to Peyer's patch-HEV in situ: The multistep model confirmed and refined. Immunity 3:99–108
60. Deitch E (1990) The role of intestinal barrier failure and bacterial translocation in the development of systemic infection and multiple organ failure. Arch Surg 125:403–404
61. Jones WG II, Minei JP, Barber AE, et al (1990) Bacterial translocation and intestinal atrophy after injury and burn wounds sepsis. Ann Surg 211:399–405
62. Tracey KJ, Lowry SF (1990) The role of cytokine mediators in septic shock. Adv Surg 23: 21–56
63. Tracey KJ, Cerami A (1993) Tumor necrosis factor, other cytokines and disease. Annu Rev Cell Biol 9:317–343
64. Simpson R, Alan R, Kobzik L, Valeri R, Shepro D, Hechtman HB (1993) Neutrophil and non-neutrophil mediated injury in intestinal ischemia-reperfusion. Ann Surg 218:444–454
65. Wells CL (1990) Relationship between intestinal microecology and translocation of intestinal bacteria. J Anton van Leeuwen 58:87–93
66. Berg R (1992) Bacterial translocation from the gastrointestinal tract. J Med 23:217–244
67. Marshall J, Christou N, Horn R, Meakins J (1988) The microbiology of multiple organ failure. Arch Surg 123:309–315
68. Wood RFM, Ingham Clark CL (1994) Rejection and graft-versus-host disease. In: Grant DR, Wood RFM (eds) Small Bowel Transplantation. Edward Arnold Publishers, Great Britain, pp 30–42

69. Millard PR, Dennison A, Hughes DA, Collin J, Morris PJ (1986) Morphology of intestinal allograft rejection and the inadequacy of mucosal biopsies in its recognition. Br J Exp Pathol 67:687–698
70. Lear PA, Cunningham AJ, Crane PW, Wood RFM (1989) Lymphocyte migration patterns in small bowel transplants. Transplant Proc 21:2881–2882
71. Fabian MA, Bollinger RR (1992) Rapid translocation of bacteria in small bowel transplantation. Transplant Proc 24:1103–1104
72. Teitelbaum DH, Narasimhan, Chenault RH, Merion RM (1994) Lymphocyte immunologic interactions in intestinal transplantation. Transplant Proc 26:1521–1526
73. Hoffman AL, Makowa L, Banner B, et al (1990) The use of FK506 for small intestine allotransplantation. Transplantation 49:483–490
74. Azuma H, Tilney NL (1994) Chronic graft rejection. Curr Opin Immunol 6:770–776
75. McDiaramid SV, Farmer DG, Kuniyoshi JS, et al (1994) The correlation of intragraft cytokine expression with rejection in rat small intestine transplantation. Transplantation 58:690–697
76. Strom TB, Waldmann H (1994) Transplantation Editorial Review. Curr Opin Immunol 6:755–756

Mast Cells and Neutrophils in Intestinal Ischemia/Reperfusion

P. Kubes

Introduction

The key features of reperfusion of ischemic intestine associated with hemorrhage and other shock states include microvascular and mucosal alterations such as endothelial cell swelling, capillary plugging, a prolonged reduction in intestinal blood flow and mucosal barrier dysfunction [1–3]. The intestinal lesion becomes a very important factor inasmuch as loss of a restrictive lumenal barrier is strongly associated with toxic factors entering the circulation and causing sepsis and possibly multiple organ failure in patients otherwise recovering from shock [2]. There are many factors that likely contribute to ischemia/reperfusion (I/R)-induced intestinal dysfunction including reduced post-ischemic blood flow, increased production of reactive oxygen metabolites and various pro-inflammatory mediators as well as the activation and recruitment of inflammatory cells including mast cells and neutrophils [1, 2, 4–6]. In this review, we will focus on the growing body of evidence that mast cells recruit neutrophils and together these cells contribute to the pathogenesis of I/R in the intestine.

Mast Cells and the Post-Ischemic Intestine

Mast Cells are Activated in Post-Ischemic Intestine

There are numerous excellent reviews on the biology of the mast cells and therefore we will not dwell on this topic [7–9]. It is worthwhile mentioning however that mast cells are found in large numbers in close proximity to barriers that separate the internal milieu from the external environment, i.e. lungs, skin and the gastrointestinal (GI) tract. Moreover, these cells anatomically are also very closely apposed to microvessels suggesting that mast cells can directly modulate microvascular responses as well as mucosal barrier function. Once activated, mast cells are capable of releasing a myriad of inflammatory mediators including preformed cytokines, histamine, serotonin as well as newly synthesized platelet activating factor (PAF), leukotrienes, and many other mediators. Therefore, it is conceivable that the mast cell may be a first-line detector system during gross physiological changes such as I/R and may be the initiator of the inflammatory response. The first part of this review will focus on the potential role of the mast cell as a source of signaling molecules allowing neutrophils to infiltrate tissue.

There is increasing evidence that mast cells become activated and degranulate following I/R of the small intestine. Boros et al. [10] have reported increased histamine release from the post-ischemic intestine and anti-oxidants reduced this increase in histamine release. Since mast cells are a primary source of histamine in the small bowel, the authors proposed this observation to reflect increased mast cell degranulation in post-ischemic tissue [9]. More direct evidence to specifically implicate the mast cells in I/R was provided when elevated rat mast cell protease II (RMCP II) levels were measured in the systemic circulation in reperfused intestine [11]. RMCP II is a protease specific to mucosal (not connective tissue) mast cells and because it is released when mast cells are activated to degranulate, it serves as an excellent index of mast cell degranulation. Although RMCP II levels increased only 250% following intestinal I/R [11], this systemic increase in RMCP II is likely reflective of far greater increases in RMCP II levels locally in the blood draining the post-ischemic intestine. Kurose et al. [12] have reported a significant mast cell degranulation at 30 min of reperfusion further supporting the thesis that mast cells degranulate in I/R.

Mast Cells Recruit Neutrophils in I/R

Numerous pro-inflammatory mediators have been implicated to date in the neutrophil recruitment associated with I/R. These include PAF [13], leukotrienes [14, 15], and oxidants [16]. Interestingly, these mediators are produced by mast cells, suggesting perhaps that mast cells are indeed involved in the recruitment of neutrophils into post-ischemic vessels. Since other cells can produce the aforementioned mediators, a more direct method to test this hypothesis was needed. One approach is to stabilize mast cells with mast cell stabilizers to prevent mediator release from these immunocytes. Doxantrazole, a stabilizer of mast cells, prevented the systemic rise in protease II levels associated with I/R and also reduced the myeloperoxidase activity in post-ischemic intestine [11]. These data were interpreted to suggest that mast cells are an important source of mediators that contribute to neutrophil recruitment in post-ischemic venules.

Neutrophils infiltrate tissues via a multi-step mode of recruitment (described in neutrophil section), including neutrophil rolling, adhesion and emigration. To establish which phase of the neutrophil recruitment was affected by mast cells in I/R, intravital microscopy was performed and neutrophil rolling, adhesion and emigration were assessed in the cat post-ischemic mesenteric microvasculature in untreated animals and animals pretreated with a mast cell stabilizer [17]. Immediately upon reperfusion, there was a very dramatic rise in neutrophil rolling and adhesion which persisted for the next 60 min. Neutrophils emigrated throughout the 60-min reperfusion period. In sodium cromoglycate (mast cell stabilizer) pretreated animals, the flux of rolling neutrophils increased in the very early (5 min) reperfusion period, but by 10 min, the number of rolling neutrophils was significantly reduced. Sodium cromoglycate had little effect on neutrophil adhesion at the early time point but reduced adhesion by 50% at 60 min. Neutrophil emigration was almost entirely inhibited over the 60 min of reperfusion with sodium cromoglycate. These data suggest that interstitial mast cells are important mediators of the multi-step recruitment of neutrophils from blood to post-ischemic tissues, and based on the profound reduction in neutrophil emigration with sodium cromoglycate, raise the possibility that mast cells may set up a chemotactic gradient to draw neutrophils out of the vasculature. A criticism often levied against the mast cell stabilization approach is that these drugs may also affect neutrophil function directly. In our laboratory [17], we were not able to reduce stimulated neutrophil adhesion to human umbilical vein endothelium with any of the aforementioned mast cell stabilizers at concentrations that may represent those in the *in vivo* experiments. These data would not agree with a direct effect of these drugs on neutrophil adhesion *per se*. Further evidence to suggest that mast cells are important in I/R-induced neutrophil recruitment are preliminary data suggesting that mast cell-deficient mice have a blunted neutrophil response to I/R (unpublished observations).

Focus has also been put on the identity of the mediator that activates mast cells to degranulate in post-ischemic intestine. One possibility is the increased flux of oxidants at the onset of reperfusion [18]. Tandem administration of two antioxidants, superoxide dismutase and catalase, prevented the rise in plasma RMCP II levels suggesting that indeed oxidants (particularly superoxide and hydrogen peroxide), underlie the mucosal mast cell degranulation [11]. Although the source of the oxidants remains unknown, Boros et al. [19] demonstrated that allopurinol blocked by 87% the histamine release from post-ischemic gut. This observation suggests an important role for the oxidant-generating enzyme xanthine oxidase in I/R-induced mast cell activation. The oxidant-induced mast cell degranulation may also underlie the increased neutrophilic influx inasmuch as levels of superoxide dismutase and catalase that prevented mast cell degranulation also inhibited the rise in neutrophil recruitment [11].

Post-Ischemic Intestinal Dysfunction and the Role of Mast Cells

Evidence exists that mast cell degranulation contributes to the mucosal dysfunction in post-ischemic intestine. Stabilization of mucosal mast cells with doxantrazole greatly abrogated the rise in mucosal dysfunction [11]. It is possible that mast cells directly cause the mucosal barrier dysfunction inasmuch as many mast cell-derived mediators including histamine and PAF increase mucosal permeability. However neither a PAF-receptor antagonist (WEB 2086) nor an H_1-receptor antagonist (diphenhydramine) had any effect on the mucosal dysfunction raising doubts about these mediators as important in the pathogenesis of the mucosa in I/R [11]. The role of other mediators including serotonin have not been tested to date and therefore, a direct effect of mast cells on the mucosal barrier cannot be entirely eliminated. Finally, the aforementioned data should not be interpreted as indicating that mast cells contribute to all aspects of I/R-induced intestinal injury. Although a close correlation exists between mast cell degranulation and microvascular dysfunction, no evidence exists to date to link the two events.

Neutrophils and the Post-Ischemic Intestine

There is a growing body of evidence suggesting an important role for polymorphonuclear leukocytes (PMN) or neutrophils in mediating the tissue injury and dysfunction associated with I/R of the GI tract. The evidence to support this contention includes the fact that neutrophils infiltrate into post-ischemic intestinal tissues, and preventing neutrophil infiltration in part prevents the tissue injury. In the second section of this review, I will summarize the data demonstrating that neutrophils infiltrate into the post-ischemic intestine and discuss the mechanisms by which this process may occur.

Neutrophils Infiltrate the Post-Ischemic Intestine

The first evidence to demonstrate that neutrophils do indeed infiltrate into post-ischemic intestine was based on tissue myeloperoxidase (MPO) measurements [20, 21], a direct index of neutrophil levels within the afflicted tissue. The MPO activity in the intestinal mucosa doubled during ischemia and increased fourfold during reperfusion, suggesting a profound influx of neutrophils into this layer of the small bowel. Other layers of the bowel can also be examined using the MPO assay; MPO levels also increased in the submucosa but only during reperfusion (3.5-fold). The intestinal muscle tissue seemed most sensitive to I/R-induced neutrophil infiltration as MPO activity increased sixfold and tenfold during ischemia and reperfusion, respectively. It should however be noted that baseline mucosal MPO levels are far greater in the mucosa than in other layers of the intestine. Therefore, the fold increase in neutrophil recruitment during reperfusion may be greatest in muscle, but the net neutrophil recruitment is by far largest in the mucosa, the layer that serves as the barrier to the external environment. The large baseline level of neutrophils in the mucosal barrier under normal conditions may reflect an ongoing function for these cells in the intact intestine. Finally, a similar pattern of neutrophil recruitment was observed in the post-ischemic mesenteric tissue as the post-ischemic mucosa [22]. This is a very important point inasmuch as the mesentery is used for intravital microscopy to directly visualize neutrophil recruitment and the data are often used to reflect events in the mucosal tissue.

Neutrophil efflux out of the vasculature is a complex series of events that includes
1) initial contact with the endothelium;
2) rolling;
3) firm adhesion; and
4) emigration into surrounding tissue.

Directly visualizing neutrophil influx into post-ischemic tissue using intravital microscopy permits observation of the multi-step recruitment of neutrophils into post-ischemic vessels (technique described elsewhere [23]). Following the induction of I/R in for example the cat intestine, a very dramatic increase in neutrophil rolling, adhesion and ultimately neutrophil emigration into the tissue is observed [17, 24]. This technique has permitted identification of the adhesion molecules that contribute to the multi-step recruitment of neutrophils. First, neutrophils moving at very high speeds in the mainstream of blood make initial contact with the endothelial cells lining the vessel wall and roll along the vessel at a greatly reduced velocity relative to red blood cells [25, 26]. This initial neutrophil-endothelial cell interaction is termed neutrophil rolling and is entirely dependent upon the selectin family of adhesion molecules [27, 28]. L-selectin is constitutively expressed on the surface of neutrophils and appears to be essential for the ability of neutrophils to initiate rolling in the microcirculation. Two other selectins, P-selectin (induced in minutes) and E-selectin (4–6 h for maximal induction) expressed on activated endothelium also, contribute significantly to the rolling event. When activated, the rolling neutrophils firmly adhere to the endothelium and ultimately emigrate out of the vasculature. This event is mediated by the integrins, and in the case of neutrophils the β_2-integrin (CD11/CD18). There are three important assumptions made when considering this scheme for neutrophil recruitment. First, this is an inter-related cascade of events and therefore the rolling event is a necessary prerequisite to neutrophil adhesion and subsequent emigration. Secondly, the rolling, adhesion and emigration transpire primarily within the post-capillary venules and very rarely do investigators observe neutrophil-endothelial cell interactions in other vessels. A final point that should be made is that histological assessment has established the phenotype of adhering and emigrating cells as neutrophils. Although it is tempting to conclude that the rolling cells are also neutrophils, to date it has been impossible to determine the phenotype of the rolling population(s) of leukocytes. Nevertheless, the adhesion and emigration data are strongly suggestive that some of the rolling cells must be neutrophils.

Selectins Mediate I/R-Induced Leukocyte Rolling

Using intravital microscopy, it was observed that the L- and P-selectin-binding carbohydrate, fucoidin, essentially abolished (>90%) leukocyte rolling in post-ischemic vessels (Fig. 1) [24]. Antibodies against either P-selectin (PB 1.3) or L-selectin (DREG 200) reduced the number of rolling leukocytes by approximately 60% at both 10 and 60 min of reperfusion. Leukocyte rolling was not decreased further in animals given both anti-L-selectin and anti-P-selectin antibody; a 60% reduction in rolling was still observed (Fig. 1). The lack of additive effect of tandem antibody therapy suggests either that P-selectin and L-selectin pathways worked in concert, i.e. as counter-ligands, or that they mediate different components of leukocyte rolling in a sequential manner so that one is dependent upon the other [29]. Moreover, based on the L- and P-selectin antibody

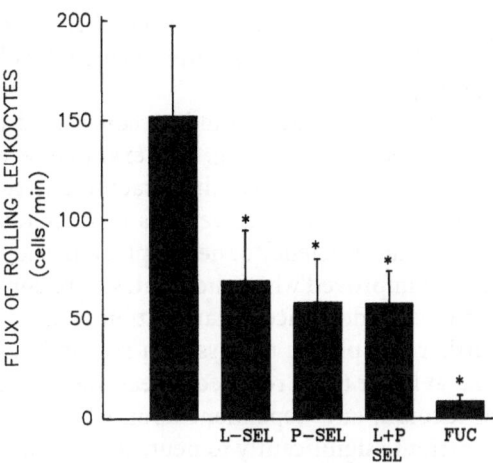

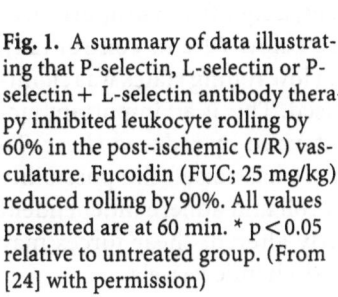

Fig. 1. A summary of data illustrating that P-selectin, L-selectin or P-selectin + L-selectin antibody therapy inhibited leukocyte rolling by 60% in the post-ischemic (I/R) vasculature. Fucoidin (FUC; 25 mg/kg) reduced rolling by 90%. All values presented are at 60 min. * p < 0.05 relative to untreated group. (From [24] with permission)

studies and the fucoidin study, these data may suggest that there exists an L- and P-selectin-independent fucoidin-inhibitable rolling pathway during reperfusion. Although each of the reagents was used at optimal concentrations, it is also possible that fucoidin simply blocks P-selectin and L-selectin more effectively than the antibodies.

The third selectin, E-selectin, may also induce leukocyte rolling [30, 31] in post-ischemic vessels. However, it is unlikely that E-selectin plays a role in the first 60 min of reperfusion inasmuch as induction of this molecule on the surface of endothelium is thought to require at least 3 h of reperfusion. Only very small numbers of vessels demonstrated E-selectin expression (15–20% of all vessels) in post-ischemic vasculature [32]. Moreover, the leukocyte rolling in the feline intravital microscopy study was abolished by fucoidin, yet fucoidin has been shown not to bind to E-selectin [27, 33].

Fucoidin, a heavily sulfated polysaccharide, may interfere with the ability of leukocytes to interact with other potential adhesive mechanisms. For example, fucoidin may compete for binding sites with sulfate-containing proteoglycans on the surface of vascular endothelium. Although the possibility that these molecules contribute to rolling is purely speculative, various other sulfated molecules have been shown to strongly interfere with leukocyte rolling *in vivo* [34–36] and leukocyte adhesion *in vitro* [37].

Based on the contention that a reduction in neutrophil rolling will reduce neutrophil adhesion, it is surprising that the 60% reduction in neutrophil rolling flux with the anti-selectin antibodies failed to reduce neutrophil adhesion. However, there is a surplus of rolling cells in post-ischemic vessels, i.e. approximately 1 in every 100 rolling neutrophils adheres. Therefore, it is conceivable that the reduction in neutrophil rolling has to reach a critical level to impact on adhesion. Indeed, an observation that supports this hypothesis is the fact that the 90% reduction in rolling with fucoidin only reduced neutrophil adhesion by approximately 50%. Therefore, anti-selectin therapy requires a very high level of efficiency in this particular model of I/R before adhesion is affected. It is therefore not surprising that others have demonstrated protection from PAF-induced intestinal injury by depleting circulating neutrophils but not by treating animals with fucoidin [38].

A final point that should be considered is the role of shear forces in I/R-induced neutrophil rolling. For example, even when neutrophil rolling was reduced by 90% with fucoidin in cat mesenteric venules, a significant proportion of neutrophils adhered in venules if shear rates were below 70% of control [24]. Clearly, the efficiency of neutrophil adhesion during low rolling states was significantly improved when shear rates were compromised. This is an important factor to consider since inflammation is often characterized by reduced shear. To further complicate this issue, a recent *in vivo* report has raised the possibility that at lower (50% reduced) shear, neutrophils can roll and adhere independent of fucoidin and dependent upon CD18 [39]. Clearly altered, shear forces may contribute significantly to neutrophil influx in post-ischemic vessels.

The β_2-Integrin (CD11/CD18) Mediates Neutrophil Adhesion and Emigration

Both MPO as an index of neutrophil influx and intravital microscopy revealed that functional CD11/CD18 was essential for reperfusion-induced neutrophil adhesion and emigration [22]. Acute treatment with a monoclonal antibody (MoAb IB$_4$) which immunoneutralized the β-subunit (CD18) of the CD11/CD18 adhesion glycoprotein complex prevented the reperfusion-induced increase in MPO levels in all of the intestine, implicating a CD18-dependent mechanism of neutrophil recruitment during I/R. Additionally, MoAb IB$_4$ completely prevented the reperfusion-induced increase in neutrophil adhesion as visualized by intravital microscopy [40]. These results suggested that the adhesion was entirely mediated by the CD18 glycoprotein complex. Although neutrophil emigration was also completely prevented, whether the emigration was dependent on CD18 or simply on the inability of the neutrophils to adequately adhere remains unclear. A clinically-relevant observation is that administration of MoAb IB$_4$ at 60 min of reperfusion almost immediately reversed the adhesion of neutrophils to postcapillary venules [41]. Clearly the neutrophil-endothelial cell interaction could be interrupted. Post-treatment with MoAb IB$_4$ at 1 h of reperfusion immediately reduced MPO activity by 40, 35 and 20% in the mucosa, submucosa, and mesentery, respectively. Since post-treatment reverses the adhesion within venules, the change in MPO values of whole tissue following MoAb IB$_4$ likely represents the contribution of adherent cells within the vasculature to the total MPO activity of the tissue.

Similar results have been observed in the rat mesentery and furthered by the availability of antibodies against other adhesion molecules [42]. Antibodies against either CD18 (MoAb CL26), the CD11b subunit of CD11/CD18 adhesion complex (MoAb 1B6c) or against endothelial ICAM-1 (MoAb 1A29), a ligand for CD18, also significantly reduced reperfusion-induced neutrophil adhesion and emigration. The ICAM-1 data were recently confirmed in a cat model of I/R using the monoclonal antibody RR1/1 [43].

Neutrophils Mediate I/R-Induced Intestinal Injury

The key study illustrating that neutrophils contributed to post-ischemic intestinal injury made use of a polyclonal antiserum to remove neutrophils from the circulation. Depletion of neutrophils significantly attenuated the increased microvascular permeability associated with I/R [20]. Similar protective effects were reported in reperfusion-induced gastric bleeding in a model of hemorrhagic shock [44]. These data suggested that neutrophils were responsible for a significant portion of the injury in post-ischemic tissues of the GI tract. Prevention of neutrophil adhesion to postcapillary venules in the cat intestinal circulation with anti-CD18 antibodies (MoAb 60.3 or IB$_4$), attenuated the increased microvascular permeability associated with I/R [20, 45]. These data suggested that neutrophil adherence or a neutrophil-adherence-dependent event (eg emigration) was a rate-limiting step in neutrophil-mediated microvascular dysfunction.

The role of adhering neutrophils as mediators of microvascular dysfunction has recently been confirmed with FITC-albumin leakage from single venules in the rat mesenteric vasculature. Kurose et al. [42] found that vascular protein leakage of FITC-albumin was highly correlated with both the number of adherent cells in post-capillary venules and the number of cells emigrated from the vasculature. Treatment of animals with MoAb's against CD18 (CL26), CD11b (1B6c) or ICAM-1 (1A29) significantly prevented reperfusion-induced increases in PMN adhesion, emigration and FITC-albumin leakage. These data again provide strong evidence that vascular protein leakage was a secondary response to leukocyte adherence and/or emigration. It should be noted that in all of these experiments, some injury to the vasculature was consistently evident suggesting perhaps a neutrophil-independent component to the I/R-induced vascular dysfunction.

The aforementioned data refer to microvascular permeability alterations. Interestingly, similar results were not obtained for mucosal dysfunction when neutrophil recruitment was impaired. Associated with the increased neutrophil accumulation within the mucosa and the increased edema formation following reperfusion of the ischemic intestine, there was a reduction in villus height and crypt depth as well as a reduction in mucosal thickness with epithelial lifting down the sides of the villi and a disruption of the lamina propria [46]. These morphological alterations translated into a dramatic increase in mucosal permeability (barrier dysfunction) to ^{51}Cr-EDTA a marker of epithelial permeability [47]. Surprisingly, we found that acute treatment of cats with MoAb IB$_4$ did not prevent fluid and protein leakage into the lumen of the small bowel. These data suggest that adhesion of intravascular neutrophils to venules is not responsible for the I/R-induced mucosal dysfunction.

Significant MPO levels are always noted in the normal cat intestine suggesting that some neutrophils reside temporarily (half-life less than 2 days) within the intestinal tissue before they are either destroyed or emigrate into the bowel lumen. These neutrophils would not be affected within 60 min by a single acute dose of MoAb IB$_4$. In other words, despite inhibition of neutrophil adhesion and emigration from the vasculature, the intestinal mucosa already has a significant level of neutrophils regardless of anti-adhesion therapy. To test the possibility that these transiently resident tissue neutrophils were responsible for the mucosal dysfunction, cats were pretreated with chronic (3 day) administration of MoAb IB_4. This approach blocks the continuous flux of neutrophils out of the vasculature [47] and thereby depletes the transient population of neutrophils within the mucosal interstitium. This contention is based on the concept that the half-life of neutrophils within tissue is less than 48 h. Indeed, the 3-day regimen of MoAb IB_4: 1) greatly attenuated the baseline MPO level; and 2) abolished the I/R-induced mucosal dysfunction [47]. Clearly, neutrophils within post-ischemic mucosal tissue are activated to induce a significant portion of the intestinal barrier dysfunction. The mechanism that activates these resident neutrophils remains unclear but may be also related to mast cells found in the interstitium. This is an area that clearly requires additional work.

Based on all of the data to date, our working hypothesis is that following the reperfusion of the ischemic intestine, oxidants (perhaps from xanthine oxidase) cause mast cell degranulation and thereby recruit neutrophils to the post-ischemic tissue. As the neutrophils adhere and emigrate they directly impact on the integrity of the microvascular barrier. Since mucosal barrier dysfunction can be inhibited by manipulation of either interstitial neutrophils or mucosal mast cells, it is possible that these cells may interact with each other in a sequential order to induce the mucosal dysfunction. The technology is presently not available to test the contention that mast cells activate resident granulocytes, however based on the strong evidence that mast cell degranulation recruits and activates circulating neutrophils [48], a similar scenario may exist in the interstitial space (Fig. 2).

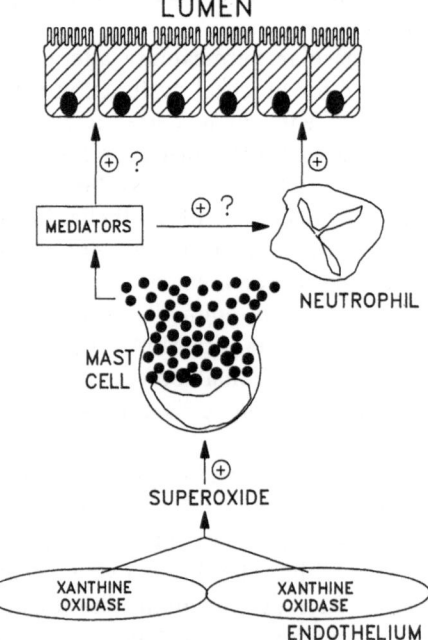

Fig. 2. A schematic summarizing the potential role of mast cells and resident granulocytes in I/R-induced mucosal barrier dysfunction

Conclusion

There are numerous avenues of research that will further our understanding of the events that comprise the pathogenesis of ischemia/reperfusion. There is a growing body of evidence that tissues produce endogenous anti-adhesive molecules to regulate and perhaps turn off the inflammatory response. These include nitric oxide, adenosine and interleukin-10 and these reagents are being studied avidly. Nitric oxide donors, adenosine analogs and interleukin-10 may have significant potential as anti-inflammatory molecules in this setting. Moreover, development of reagents that selectively target human mast cells and prevent the release of some or most mast cell-derived mediators may be useful therapeutically. Presently, many of the mast cell stabilizers have potent effects on rat connective tissue mast cells but lesser effects on human mast cells. Finally, the interplay between mast cell degranulation and adhesion molecule expression needs to be better understood to more selectively target the adhesion molecules involved in the recruitment of neutrophils at the time of reperfusion.

Acknowledgements: This work was supported by a grant from the Alberta Heritage Foundation for Medical Research (AHFMR) and the Crohn's and Colitis Foundation of Canada (CCFC).

References

1. Schoenberg MH, Muhl E, Sellin D, Younes M, Schildberg FW, Haglund U (1984) Posthypotensive generation of superoxide free radicals: Possible role in the pathogenesis of the intestinal mucosal damage. Acta Chir Scand 150:301–309
2. Haglund U, Bulkley GB, Granger DN (1987) On the pathophysiology of intestinal ischemic injury. Clinical review. Acta Chir Scand 153:321–324
3. Granger DN, Hollwarth ME, Parks DA (1986) Ischemia-reperfusion injury: Role of oxygen-derived free radicals. Acta Physiol Scand (Suppl) 548:47–63
4. Kubes P, Suzuki M, Granger DN (1991) Nitric oxide: An endogenous modulator of leukocyte adhesion. Proc Natl Acad Sci USA 88:4651–4655
5. Granger DN, Sennett M, McElearney PM, Taylor AE (1980) Effect of local arterial hypotension on cat intestinal capillary permeability. Gastroenterology 79:474–480
6. Granger DN (1988) Role of xanthine oxidase and granulocytes in ischemia-reperfusion injury. Am J Physiol 255:H1269–H1275
7. Galli SJ (1993) New concepts about the mast cell. N Engl J Med 328:257–265
8. Metcalfe DD, Costa JJ, Burd PR (1992) Mast cells and basophils. In: Gallin JI, Goldstein IM, Snyderman R (eds) Inflammation basic principles and clinical correlates. Raven Press, New York, pp 709–725
9. Crowe SE, Perdue MH (1992) Gastrointestinal food hypersensitivity: Basic mechanisms of pathophysiology. Gastroenterology 103:1075–1095
10. Boros M, Kaszaki J, Nagy S (1991) Histamine release during intestinal ischemia-reperfusion: Role of iron ions and hydrogen peroxide. Circ Shock 35:174–180
11. Kanwar S, Kubes P (1994) Mast cells contribute to ischemia/reperfusion-induced granulocyte infiltration and intestinal dysfunction. Am J Physiol 267:G316–G321
12. Kurose I, Wolf R, Grisham MB, Granger DN (1994) Modulation of ischemia/reperfusion-induced microvascular dysfunction by nitric oxide. Circ Res 74:376–382
13. Kubes P, Ibbotson G, Russell JM, Wallace JL, Granger DN (1990) Role of platelet activating factor in ischemia/reperfusion-induced leukocyte adherence. Am J Physiol 259:G300–G305

14. Lehr HA, Guhlmann A, Nolte D, Keppler D, Messmer K (1991) Leukotrienes as mediators in ischemia-reperfusion injury in a microcirculation model in the hamster. J Clin Invest 87: 2036–2041
15. Zimmerman BJ, Guillory DJ, Grisham MB, Gaginella TS, Granger DN (1993) Role of leuko-triene B₄ in granulocyte infiltration into the post-ischemic feline intestine. Gastroenterology 99:1–6
16. Zimmerman BJ, Grisham MB, Granger DN (1990) Xanthine oxidase-derived oxidants: Role in ischemia/reperfusion-induced granulocyte infiltration. Am J Physiol 258:G185–G190
17. Kanwar S, Kubes P (1994) Ischemia/reperfusion-induced granulocyte influx is a multistep process mediated by mast cells. Microcirc 1:175–182
18. Blum H, Sommers JJ, Schnall MD, et al (1986) Acute intestinal ischemia studies by phos-phorous nuclear magnetic resonance spectroscopy. Ann Surg 204:83–88
19. Boros M, Kaszaki J, Nagy S (1989) Oxygen free radical-induced histamine release during intestinal ischemia and reperfusion. Eur Surg Res 21:297–304
20. Hernandez LA, Grisham MB, Twohig B, Arfors KE, Harlan JM, Granger DN (1987) Role of neutrophils in ischemia-reperfusion-induced microvascular injury. Am J Physiol 253: H699–H703
21. Grisham MB, Hernandez LA, Granger DN (1986) Xanthine oxidase and neutrophil infiltra-tion in intestinal ischemia. Am J Physiol 251:G567–G574
22. Kurtel H, Zhang S, Tso P, Granger DN (1991) Granulocyte accumulation in different layers of small intestine during ischemia-reperfusion (I/R): Role of leukocyte adhesion glycopro-tein CD11/CD18. Am J Physiol 262:G878–G882
23. Granger DN, Kubes P (1994) The microcirculation and inflammation: Modulation of leuko-cyte-endothelial cell adhesion. J Leukocyte Biol 55:662–675
24. Kubes P, Jutila M, Payne D (1995) Therapeutic potential of inhibiting leukocyte rolling in ischemia/reperfusion. J Clin Invest 95:2510–2519
25. Von Andrian UH, Chambers JD, McEvoy LM, Bargatze RF, Arfors KE, Butcher EC (1991) Two-step model of leukocyte-endothelial cell interaction in inflammation: Distinct roles for LECAM-1 and the leukocyte β₂ integrins in vivo. Proc Natl Acad Sci USA 88:7538–7542
26. Ley K, Gaehtgens P, Fennie C, Singer MS, Lasky LA, Rosen SD (1991) Lectin-like cell adhe-sion molecule 1 mediates leukocyte rolling in mesenteric venules in vivo. Blood 77: 2553–2555
27. Bevilacqua MP, Nelson RM (1993) Selectins. J Clin Invest 91:379–387
28. Springer TA (1994) Traffic signals of lymphocyte recirculation and leukocyte emigration: The multistep paradigm. Cell 76:301–314
29. Lawrence MB, Bainton DF, Springer TA (1994) Neutrophil tethering to and rolling on E-se-lectin are separable by requirement for L-selectin. Immunity 1:137–145
30. Lawrence MB, Springer TA (1993) Neutrophils roll on E-selectin. J Immunol 151:6338–6346
31. Kishimoto TK, Warnock RA, Jutila MA, et al (1991) Antibodies against human neutrophil LECAM-1 (LAM-1/Leu-8/DREG-56 antigen) and endothelial cell ELAM-1 inhibit a common CD18-independent adhesion pathway in vitro. Blood 78:805–811
32. Albertine KH, Weyrich AS, Ma X, Lefer DJ, Becker LC, Lefer AM (1994) Quantification of neutrophil migration following myocardial ischemia and reperfusion in cats and dogs. J Leukoc Biol 55:557–566
33. Nelson RM, Dolich S, Aruffo A, Cecconi O, Bevilacqua MP (1993) Higher-affinity oligosac-charide ligands for E-selectin. J Clin Invest 91:1157–1166
34. Arfors KE, Ley K (1993) Sulfated polysaccharides in inflammation. J Lab Clin Med 121: 201–202
35. Ley K, Cerrito M, Arfors KE (1991) Sulfated polysaccharides inhibit leukocyte rolling in rab-bit mesentery venules. Am J Physiol 260:H1667–H1673
36. Tangelder GJ, Arfors KE (1991) Inhibition of leukocyte rolling in venules by protamin and sulfated polysaccharides. Blood 77:1565–1571
37. Cecconi O, Nelson RM, Roberts WG, et al (1994) Inositol polyanions: Noncarbohydrate in-hibitors of L-selectin and P-selectin that block inflammation. J Biol Chem 269:15060–15066
38. Sun X, Qu X, Huang W, Granger DN, Bree M, Hsueh W (1995) The role of leukocyte beta 2-integrin PAF-induced shock and intestinal injury. Am J Physiol 270:G184–G190

39. Gaboury JP, Kubes P (1994) Reductions in physiologic shear rates lead to CD11/CD18-de-pendent, selectin-independent leukocyte rolling *in vivo*. Blood 83:345–350
40. Granger DN, Benoit JN, Suzuki M, Grisham MB (1989) Leukocyte adherence to venular endothelium during ischemia-reperfusion. Am J Physiol 257:G683–G688
41. Suzuki M, Inauen W, Kvietys PR, et al (1989) Superoxide mediates reperfusion-induced leukocyte-endothelial cell interactions. Am J Physiol 257:H1740–H1745
42. Kurose I, Anderson DC, Miyasaka M, et al (1994) Molecular determinants of reperfusion-induced leukocyte adhesion and vascular protein leakage. Circ Res 74:336–343
43. Kubes P, Kurose I, Granger DN (1994) NO donors prevent integrin-induced leukocyte adhesion, but not P-selectin-dependent rolling in post-ischemic venules. Am J Physiol 267:H931–H937
44. Smith SM, Holm-Rutili L, Perry MA, et al (1987) Role of neutrophils in hemorrhagic shock-induced gastric mucosal injury in the rat. Gastroenterology 93:466–471
45. Kubes P, Granger DN (1989) Interaction between circulating granulocytes and xanthine oxidase-derived oxidants in the post-ischemic intestine. In: Reinhart K, Eyrich K (eds.) Clinical Aspects of O_2 Transport and Tissue Oxygenation. Springer-Verlag, Berlin Heidelberg, pp 133–147
46. Parks DA, Granger DN (1986) Contributions of ischemia and reperfusion to mucosal lesion formation. Am J Physiol 250:G749–G753
47. Kubes P, Hunter JA, Granger DN (1992) Ischemia/reperfusion-induced feline intestinal dysfunction: Importance of granulocyte recruitment. Gastroenterology 103:807–812
48. Gaboury JP, Johnston B, Niu XF, Kubes P (1995) Mechanisms underlying acute mast cell-induced leukocyte rolling and adhesion *in vivo*. J Immunol 154:804–813

Clinical Markers of Gastrointestinal Dysfunction

J. C. Marshall

Introduction

Physiologic support of failing vital organ function is the "raison d'être" of the intensive care unit (ICU). The development of individual organ dysfunction in the critically ill patient describes a clinical syndrome and defines a series of therapeutic challenges. The challenge of pulmonary failure, manifested as the acute respiratory distress syndrome (ARDS), is to support optimal gas exchange without inducing further iatrogenic lung injury, while that of acute renal failure is to optimize fluid and electrolyte homeostasis without adversely affecting systemic hemodynamic function. In aggregate, graded degrees of vital organ dysfunction comprise the multiple organ dysfunction syndrome (MODS), the leading cause of ICU morbidity and mortality, and the embodiment of the unsolved obstacles to recovery from critical illness [14].

Gastrointestinal (GI) dysfunction is common in critical illness, yet it has proven particularly difficult to characterize. The gut, moreover, is widely believed to be not only a *target*, but also a *mechanism* contributing to the evolution and persistence of MODS [5–7]. Attempts to describe gut dysfunction, or to estimate its prevalence, must consider not only manifestations of gut injury, but also the changes in gut homeostatic mechanisms that may predispose to organ injury at remote sites. The former task is rendered difficult because functional changes in the gut are not readily apparent using conventional ICU monitoring techniques; the latter task is complicated by the intrinsic difficulties in establishing a pathogenetic role for the gut in human MODS.

What Constitutes Organ Dysfunction in Critical Illness?

Prior to embarking on a systematic consideration of the various manifestations of gut dysfunction in critical illness, it is important to consider what, in generic terms, characterizes organ system dysfunction in the ICU setting. Delineation of these principles will provide an objective basis to evaluate potential manifestations of gut dysfunction, and to determine which variables are best used for its description.

Organ dysfunction in critical illness is generally considered to be an acute, but potentially reversible state of physiologic dysfunction that arises following resuscitation from a life-threatening insult [1]. Such a definition excludes pre-existing chronic organ system dysfunction such as might be present in advanced cirrhosis or chronic renal failure, as well as the acute *irreversible* structural injury that occurs following massive head injury or extensive pulmonary resection. Organ injury in MODS is generally believed to result from the activation of endogenous host inflammatory mediator systems; therefore the syndrome arises in clinical settings where such activation might occur including infection, injury, ischemia, sterile inflammation, and immunologic activation.

The dysfunction of any given organ system can be characterized in one of three ways. First, it can be described by graded degrees of abnormality in a single variable that reflects function in the system of interest: description of pulmonary dysfunction using the PO_2/FiO_2 ratio is an example of this approach. Secondly, organ system dysfunction may be described by variables reflecting the therapeutic response evoked by the physiologic derangement: such an approach is examplified by the description of pulmonary dysfunction as the need for mechanical ventilation, or the level of PEEP employed. Finally, organ dysfunction can be characterized as a syndrome, whose presence is established by the presence of a combination of variables: characterization of pulmonary dysfunction as ARDS defined as the presence of a PO_2/FiO_2 ratio of less than 200, in association with radiographic evidence of bilateral pulmonary infiltrates and a pulmonary capillary wedge pressure of less than 18 mmHg. Each descriptive model has its merits and disadvantages, and all are widely and interchangeably used in published descriptions of MODS.

The criteria used to define MODS vary widely in the published literature, and such variability inevitably contributes to divergent estimates of prevalence and prognostic impact. The characteristics of the ideal descriptor of dysfunction for a given organ system have been previously elaborated [8]. Such a descriptor should above all be simple, and should be readily, reliably, and reproducibly measured. It should be objective, and independent of clinical judgment. It should be both specific for the function of the system of interest, and comprehensive in its ability to describe the entire spectrum of abnormality within that system. It should be only minimally altered by transient abnormalities associated with resuscitation and therapy, and should be maximally abnormal after resuscitation is complete. It should mirror acute reversible physiologic changes, rather than the sequelae of chronic disease. Finally to optimize its utility, it should be a single continuous variable, whose abnormality is unidirectional.

Published Descriptors of Gastrointestinal Dysfunction in MODS

A systematic and comprehensive review of reports of MODS or multiple organ failure (MOF) published prior to 1994, identified 30 publications in which unique criteria for organ failure or dysfunction were articulated and applied to the study of critically ill patients [8]. GI dysfunction was included as a component of the clinical syndrome in 21 of these; the criteria used to define gut dysfunction are summarized in Table 1.

Table 1. Published criteria for gut dysfunction in MODS

Criterion	Number of reports employing
Upper or lower GI stress bleeding	21
Ischemia/necrotizing enterocolitis	4
Ileus	3
GI perforation	2
Intolerance of enteral feeds	2
Mechanical obstruction	1
Acalculous cholecystitis	4
Gall bladder perforation	1
Pancreatitis	7

GI bleeding was the most commonly used variable, although the diagnostic criteria varied with respect to the volume of bleeding, and the need for endoscopic confirmation. A fall in hemoglobin of 20 g/L or more and/or a requirement for at least two units of blood to be transfused in 24 h was typically selected as a cut-off to define clinically significant bleeding. Other variables were used less frequently, and with less precise diagnostic criteria. In three reports, intestinal infarction or necrotizing enterocolitis was considered a manifestation of the gut dysfunction of MODS, while two reports included gut perforation, and one each specified ileus or obstruction as a diagnostic criterion. Extraintestinal processes considered to be reflective of gut dysfunction were acalculous cholecystitis (with or without perforation) and acute pancreatitis.

Although GI stress bleeding has been the classic manifestation of organ dysfunction in MODS, this variable alone is unsatisfactory as representative of the spectrum of gut dysfunction in MODS for a number of reasons. In the first place, it is not truly a reflection of physiologic dysfunction but rather of acute injury. Clinically significant GI bleeding has become an uncommon occurrence in contemporary ICUs, with prevalence rates of less than 4% in mixed ICUs [9]; moreover bleeding in these patients commonly arises from sources other than stress ulceration. Finally, reliable and reproducible quantification of the magnitude of stress bleeding is difficult.

Alternate methods of describing gut dysfunction in critical illness may be possible, and their availability would aid in the monitoring and support of gut function in the ICU. Characterization of these methods requires consideration of the spectrum of normal gut function, and how it is altered in critical illness.

Gut Function in Health and Disease

The GI tract is a deceptively complex organ. In addition to its obvious role in degrading biologic foodstuffs into nutrients that can be absorbed into the body, the gut subserves a selective barrier function, detoxifying potentially harmful substances that have been ingested, and preventing the entry into the host of macro-molecules and microorganisms from the environment. It functions as a conduit for the elimination of wastes that have been excreted in bile, and of components of ingested food that have not been degraded, and through the reabsorption of water and electrolytes in the colon, plays a role in fluid and electrolyte homeostasis.

Beyond its function in metabolic homeostasis, the gut also plays an important role in the maturation and expression of systemic immunity. The gut houses a remarkably diverse and stable microbial flora, that has been shown to be essential for the normal expression of a number of immunologic phenomena. Moreover, the gut is composed of a multilayered network of immune cells that modulate the expression of systemic immunity to antigens of gut origin, and that interact in a complex neuroendocrine axis to regulate local gut function.

Finally the gut is vulnerable to the systemic derangements of critical illness, particularly ischemia resulting from altered regional blood flow, and ileus resulting, in part, from sympathetic overactivity. This vulnerability accounts for some of the most obvious phenotypic manifestations of gut dysfunction in the ICU.

Ischemia and Its Consequences as Manifestations of Gut Dysfunction

Splanchnic blood flow is selectively and acutely reduced following hemorrhage and sepsis in both animal models [10] and humans [11–13]. Transient ischemia of the kidney induced by the same stimuli is an important factor in the pathogenesis of acute renal failure, and manifested as impairment of the ability of the kidney to clear fluids, electrolytes, and metabolic byproducts, notable creatinine. While renal ischemia produces readily detectable functional impairment, acute ischemia of the gut is evident primarily through its effects on morphology and structural integrity.

Clinical Syndromes of Gut Ischemia

Stress Ulceration. Stress ulceration was originally described as a complication of burns [14] and head injury [15]. With the development of ICU, GI bleeding from diffuse erosive gastritis became a common clinical problem; indeed the earliest formulation of the concept of MOF was a clinical report of patients with stress ulceration who developed liver, pulmonary, and cardiovascular failure [16]. Reported rates of stress bleeding in the ICU vary with the population studied and the criteria used to define bleeding, however there is a general consensus that the prevalence of bleeding has declined over the past several decades, independent of the use of prophylactic regimens. Several recent studies suggest that the rate of clinically important bleeding in the contemporary ICU is no more than 6%, and that routine prophylactic measures can safely be withheld in the majority of patients [9, 17].

The ability of antacids or histamine type 2 blockers to reduce the frequency of stress-related GI bleeding [18, 19] suggested that hyperacidity was the predominant pathologic problem. It has been shown that the risk of bleeding correlates better with measures of mucosal acidosis than measures of gastric luminal hyperacidity [20], and contemporary theories of pathogenesis have emphasized the role of gastric mucosal ischemia [21]. Accordingly, improvements in resuscitation and hemodynamic support may well explain the declining incidence of this once-feared complication.

Necrotizing Enterocolitis and Intestinal Infarction. Mucosal ischemia in the critically ill adult can result in bleeding at any level of the GI tract [22], although the stomach is the most common site. For the most part, GI ischemia is a morphologically minor phenomenon whose significance is reflected more in functional changes, principally impairment of barrier function. Ischemic changes are usually limited to the mucosa and are most pronounced at the tip of the villus [23]; rapid re-epithelialization occurs as the patient improves.

More severe syndromes of intestinal ischemia have been described in the critically ill, although these are decidedly less common. Desai et al. [24] reviewed the *post mortem* findings of a group of patients dying of thermal injury, and found a spectrum of ischemic changes in the gut, ranging from superficial mucosal changes to full thickness necrosis. Changes were evident in more than half of the autopsy specimens, and 80% of patients had infectious complications with enteric organisms [24]. Although intestinal infarction is considered a manifestation of the gut dysfunction of MODS by some authors [25–27], the prevalence of such changes in an heterogeneous group of ICU patients is unknown. Necrotizing enterocolitis in the neonate may be considered as a manifestation of gut ischemia in MODS. However the pathogenesis of this entity is not well understood [28], and the absence of an adult correlate may suggest that the developmental immaturity is the cornerstone of the disorder.

Intestinal ischemia or infarction as a consequence of thrombosis or embolism is a not uncommon indication for admission to ICU, and a predisposing factor to the development of MODS [29]; however these disorders represent primary disease processes rather than their complications, and are not appropriately viewed as manifestations of MODS.

Acalculous Cholecystitis and Pancreatitis. Acute acalculous cholecystitis is a well recognized complication of trauma, burns, and other forms of critical illness [30, 31]. Diagnostic criteria are not well established, and its prevalence in the contemporary ICU is unknown [32]. One small prospective study of severely traumatized patients documented an incidence of acute acalculous cholecystitis (as defined by sonographic findings of hydrops of the gall bladder, increased wall thickness, and sludge) of 18% [33]. Most of these resolved with non-operative management, and their clinical significance is uncertain. Risk factors included the severity of injury, number of blood transfusions, and use of narcotics.

Acute pancreatitis occurs as a complication of critical illness, although prevalence rates are unknown. Multiple factors including ischemia, trauma, and drug effects contribute to its pathogenesis [34]. Hyperamylasemia has been described in up to half of patients admitted to ICU, although in the majority of cases, the amylase appears to be of salivary gland origin [35].

Although both cholecystitis and pancreatitis have been considered to be manifestations of gut dysfunction in MODS, the problems associated with the satisfactory diagnosis of these entities in critically ill patients, and the inherent difficulty in differentiating an ICU-acquired complication from a primary disorder make them unsatisfactory as markers of gut dysfunction.

Quantification of Gut Ischemia in Critical Illness

A reliable method of detecting otherwise occult GI ischemia, gastric tonometry, has found variable utility as a method of monitoring splanchnic resuscitation. The technique involves the placement in the stomach of a modified nasogastric tube or tonometer, containing a balloon that is permeable to carbon dioxide. After a suitable interval to permit equilibration of the CO_2 in the saline-filled balloon with that of the stomach lumen, simultaneous blood gas analyses are performed on the balloon contents and a sample of arterial blood. Since the arterial blood sample is representative of arterial blood in the gastric wall, and CO_2 levels in the gastric lumen are in equilibrium with levels in the gastric wall, gastric mucosal pH (pHi) can be calculated using the Henderson-Hasselbalch equation.

Mucosal acidosis as diagnosed tonometrically demonstrates a convincing correlation with ICU prognosis [36] and appears to reliably reflect splanchnic oxygenation [37]. Vasoactive agents such as dobutamine have been shown to increase pHi suggesting that pHi can be used as a valid outcome measure in descriptive or interventional studies [38]. Moreover, the use of tonometry to monitor the resuscitation and hemodynamic stabilization of the critically ill patient has been shown to lead to an improved clinical outcome [39]. However, it is not clear that the tonometer provides additional information beyond that already available with routine blood gas analysis [40]. The device is expensive, making it impractical for the routine monitoring of all but the most unstable ICU patients. Although measurements of pHi or intramural pCO_2 provide information of prognostic value in septic patients [41], they reflect a cause of gut dysfunction, rather than the resultant dysfunction itself.

Altered Nutrient Absorption and Barrier Function as Markers of Gut Dysfunction

The normal GI tract subserves a complex role in nutrient homeostasis, selectively absorbing low molecular weight nutrients such as sugars and amino acids against a concentration gradient, while excluding larger molecular weight substances and bacteria. The lumen of the gut contains a large number of potentially immunogenic substances, while the gut wall is richly endowed with lymphatic tissue; therefore, the reciprocal processes of nutrient absorption and barrier function must be expressed without evolving a potentially injurious local response.

Impaired Nutrient Absorption

Nutrient absorption is a complex process, potentially affected by a variety of factors including the concentration of the nutrient in the succus entericus, the transit time through the small bowel, the availability of gastric acid, bile salts, and pancreatic secretions to aid in the degradation and absorption of foodstuffs, the total area of the gut mucosal surface, and the metabolic activity of the enterocyte. Both the route [42] and the composition [43] of nutritional support may influence clinical outcome in critical illness; therefore, it is difficult in evaluating the clinical literature to differentiate abnormalities resulting from intrinsic gut dysfunction from those resulting from the strategy used for nutritional support.

Impairment of the absorption of a specific marker substance has not been evaluated as a marker of gut dysfunction in critical illness, although the concept is theoretically attractive. Rather, absorptive function has been described through the use of presumed surrogate markers. Intolerance of enteral feeding is perhaps the most intuitively appealing measure of impaired gut absorptive function. The inability to feed a patient enterally, independent of global illness severity as reflected in APACHE II score, identifies a group of patients at significantly increased risk of ICU morbidity and mortality [44]. However, intolerance of enteral feeding is difficult to quantify objectively, and the concept incorporates a spectrum of physiologic abnormalities including diarrhea, ileus, or impaired gastric emptying. Moreover, it may be significantly affected by the timing and route of institution of enteral support.

Hypoalbuminemia induced by volume expansion alone results in impairment of protein uptake and increased water secretion into the gut lumen of the experimental animal [45]; whether this mechanism contributes to the development of diarrhea following the initiation of enteral feeding in the critically ill patient is speculative [46]. In ICU patients, the development of diarrhea following attempted enteral feeding is most strongly associated with the use of antimicrobial agents [47], and likely mirrors a biologic process mediated indirectly through changes in gut flora [48], rather than directly through nutritional influences on the enterocyte. Intestinal transit has not been reliably evaluated in the ICU setting, however critically ill patients are known to develop a significant delay in rates of gastric emptying [49].

Altered Intestinal Barrier Function

The normal GI tract is essentially impermeable to macromolecules and microorganisms. Nutrient absorption generally occurs by an active process across the enterocyte; tight junctions between the enterocytes prevent the passive absorption of large molecules. In addition, immune cells of the gut mucosa, particularly macrophages and Paneth cells, both phagocytose bacteria that have passed across the gut wall, and elaborate soluble antimicrobial mediators including cytokines, defensins [50], and nitric oxide [51]. Local structural changes resulting from ischemia or inflammation can impair gut barrier function.

Increased Permeability to Macromolecules. The normal intestine is impermeable to enterally-administered lactulose. Increases in the ratio of urinary lactulose to mannitol reflect increased permeability at the level of the paracellular tight junctions in the intestinal crypts [52], and have been used as a measure of gut permeability in the critically ill patient. These studies have demonstrated that gut permeability is increased following multiple trauma [52] and burn injury [53], particularly when infectious complications supervene [54]. Although the lactulose/mannitol ratio has proven useful as a measure of impaired intestinal barrier function in descriptive studies, the lack of a simple assay for urinary mannitol and lactulose limits its utility in routine clinical practice.

D-lactate, a byproduct of bacterial metabolism, can be detected in the systemic circulation in patients with acute mesenteric ischemia or bowel obstruction [55], and in some patients with short gut syndrome and gut microbial overgrowth [56]. It has not been evaluated as a marker of altered permeability in a general ICU population.

Systemic endotoxemia, presumably of gut origin and a reflection of impaired barrier function, has been demonstrated in patients with burn injury; endotoxin levels correlate well with burn size [57]. Endotoxin can also be detected in blood from patients undergoing cardiopulmonary bypass [58] and/or having active inflammatory bowel disease [59], while levels of enterobacterial common antigen are increased in patients with pancreatitis [60]. Endotoxemia, however, is not specific for gut barrier dysfunction, and the lack of a simple assay renders its measurement impractical for routine clinical use. Furthermore, other investigators have been unable to demonstrate significant systemic endotoxemia in disorders such as hemorrhagic shock where gut origin endotoxemia might be expected to occur [61].

Bacterial Translocation as a Marker of Intestinal Barrier Failure. Bacterial translocation, the passage of intact microorganisms through the gut wall and into mesenteric lymph nodes, the peritoneal cavity, and portal and systemic blood, is readily demonstrable in a variety of animal models of acute illness including trauma, hemorrhage, thermal injury, peritonitis, endotoxemia, malnutrition, and gut bacterial overgrowth [62].

Evidence that translocation occurs in humans is largely indirect and circumstantial, but nevertheless, convincing. Sedman and colleagues [63] demonstrated that translocating microorganisms can be cultured from the intestinal serosa or mesenteric lymph nodes of approximately 10% of 267 patients undergoing laparotomy, and that infectious complications are twice as frequent in these patients, although mortality rates are unaffected. Perhaps the most compelling evidence that viable organisms can translocate across an intact human gut was provided by an intrepid German surgeon who swallowed 180 g of live *Candida* (roughly 10^{12} organisms), and rapidly became acutely ill with both *Candidemia* and *Candiduria* [64]. Systemic bacteremia with enteric organisms has been demonstrated in patients with sigmoid ischemia [65], and in one third of patients resuscitated from a cardiac arrest [66]. Nosocomial bacteremias have been traced to contaminated enteral feeding solutions [67]. In contrast to these observations, however, Moore and coworkers [68] were unable to document portal bacteremia or endotoxemia over a period of 5 days in a group of multiply-traumatized patients who had portal venous catheters placed at the time of laparotomy. In a descriptive study of proximal gut colonization in critically ill surgical patients, we found [69] a striking association between proximal gut flora and isolates from concomitant episodes of pneumonia, urinary tract infection, recurrent peritonitis, and bacteremia. The development of nosocomial infection with *Candida* [70] and the enterococcus [71] has been postulated by others to be a consequence of bacterial translocation from the gut.

The relative inaccessibility of the gut for regular microbial surveillance, and the need for more sophisticated molecular techniques to document that an organism isolated from a focus of invasive infection is the same as one cultured from the gut, make definitive documentation of translocation difficult.

Altered Gut Microbial Ecology and Immunity as Markers of Gut Dysfunction

The microbial flora of the normal gut is complex, comprising in excess of 400 separate species [72]. Patterns of colonization vary strikingly at different levels of the gut, yet are remarkably stable over time in any given individual [73]. Factors contributing to the stability of the normal flora are many, however the competitive and symbiotic interactions of the organisms themselves play a leading role [74]. The indigenous flora exerts multiple influences on normal immunologic and metabolic homeostasis, therefore it is conceptually appropriate to consider the maintenance of stable patterns of microbial growth as evidence of the normal functioning of the gut.

Changes in the composition of the colonic flora are difficult to evaluate, if only because of the prodigious variety and number of organisms present. On the other hand, the proximal gut is normally sterile, or lightly populated with relatively avirulent species, and changes are much more readily detectable.

Gram-negative organisms are readily killed in an acid environment, and the normal production of hydrochloric acid by the stomach is an important mechanism inhibiting their growth in the proximal gut [75]. It is not surprising, therefore, that gastric overgrowth with gram-negative organisms has been recognized in critically ill patients receiving stress ulcer prophylaxis [76]. However, gastric overgrowth with acid-resistant gram-positive organisms and fungi is also apparent in the critically ill patient [69, 77], suggesting that other mechanisms must play a role in the antimicrobial defenses of the normal stomach. Clinical trials of strategies targeting proximal gut bacterial overgrowth, including selective decontamination of the digestive tract and the use of cytoprotective agents for stress ulcer prophylaxis, strongly suggest that proximal gut colonization with gram-negative organisms is a cause of nosocomial pneumonia in the critically ill patient [78].

The evidence that gut colonization leads to systemic infections at other sites is less rigorous, but as discussed earlier, convincing. It has been shown that the most common species colonizing the proximal gut of the critically ill surgical patient, *S. epidermidis, Candida, Pseudomonas*, and the enterococcus [69] are also the most common isolates from nosocomial ICU-acquired infections in these patients [79]. Moreover, patients who are colonized with *Pseudomonas* or the enterococcus have a significantly increased risk of ICU mortality, and patients colonized with the enterococcus develop significantly greater degrees of organ dysfunction [69].

Animal studies have shown that the normal flora of the gut exerts a significant protective role in inhibiting colonization and overgrowth with both *Pseudomonas* and *Candida*; thus it is plausible to consider gut colonization, or even nosocomial infection with the typical microbial flora of ICU-acquired infection as evidence of dysfunction of normal gut microbial defenses. However, although both gut colonization and ICU-acquired infection correlate convincingly with adverse outcome, the association of nosocomial infection with gut dysfunction is not sufficiently specific to justify its use as a marker of gut dysfunction, in the absence of microbial surveillance studies. The latter are costly, time-consuming, and not readily amenable to performance as a routine evaluation in critically ill patients.

Disruption of normal patterns of the indigenous gut flora, with overgrowth by potentially pathogenic species, is the most readily evident manifestation of altered gut immunity in the critically ill patient. Other markers of deranged gut immunity have not been evaluated in humans.

Markers of Gut Dysfunction: A Critical Overview

Gut dysfunction is a common problem in critical illness; its prevalence varies depending on the population studied and the criteria used to define dysfunction. Accurate description is rendered difficult by the complexity of the physiologic roles played by the gut, and by the relative inaccessibility of the gut to routinely applicable monitoring techniques. Dysfunction of the gut can be described from the perspective of absorptive or barrier function, regional immunity, and impairment of regional blood flow, however none of the readily available measures of these is satisfactory as a single measure of gut dysfunction (Table 2).

The most widely used markers of gut dysfunction are those reflecting relative splanchnic ischemia, principally stress bleeding, but also reductions in mucosal pHi, and the development of acalculous cholecystitis or pancreatitis. A major failing of this approach is that it measures not gut dysfunction *per se*, but a physiologic abnormality that may produce dysfunction. Indeed the reduction in rates of clinically important stress bleeding in the contemporary ICU likely reflects improvements in hemodynamic monitoring and management, rather than a true reduction in the prevalence of gut physiologic dysfunction. Only tono-

Table 2. Markers of gut dysfunction in critical illness

Physiologic process	Functional markers
Nutrient absorption	Intolerance of enteral feeding Need for parenteral feeding Diarrhea ? Impaired uptake of marker
Barrier function	Lactulose/mannitol ratio Endotoxin levels D-(-lactate) levels ? Bacterial translocation
Gut immunity	Microbial overgrowth Diarrhea ? ICU-acquired infection ? Translocation
Splanchnic blood flow	Stress bleeding Tonometrically-measured pHi or pCO_2 Mesenteric ischemia, acalculous cholecystitis, pancreatitis

metry provides a graded quantitative measure of gut ischemia, and this technique suffers from being costly, invasive, and most abnormal prior to successful resuscitation.

Measures of gut absorptive function would comprise the most appealing markers of gut function. Unfortunately, there is no simple marker substance whose levels can reliably detect derangements of gut absorptive function in the ICU setting. The development of such a marker, particularly one whose use would be inexpensive and routinely applicable, would be a significant advance in the monitoring of gut dysfunction in the critically ill patient. Although intolerance of enteral feeding is a relevant clinical manifestation of gut dysfunction, there are no objective measures to permit its evaluation. Furthermore, feeding tolerance is affected by patterns of clinical practice, reducing the generalizability of the measure across differing ICUs.

Demonstration of altered intestinal barrier function to experimental macromolecules such as lactulose and mannitol, or to microbial products such as endotoxin or D-lactate has served as a marker of altered gut function in descriptive and interventional studies in the ICU setting. The relative complexity and cost of the techniques has limited their utility for routine clinical purposes.

Changes in gut microbial ecology, and even the development of nosocomial infection, can reflect altered gut immune function. Quantitative monitoring of proximal gut flora is difficult, however semi-quantitative or qualitative techniques may be more feasible. Therapeutic measures such as selective decontamination of the digestive tract may alter gut flora without correcting the underlying dysfunction, and therefore affect the interpretation of such changes. The development of nosocomial infection is an attractive marker of organ dysfunction, however it obviously lacks specificity as a measure of gut dysfunction.

Conclusions

Although gut dysfunction is common in the ICU, a satisfactory measure is not available for routine clinical use. Measures reflecting altered regional blood flow, local immune homeostasis, or increased permeability are the best markers currently available, but remain incompletely validated and difficult to use. The availability of a single biochemical marker reflecting impaired absorption, or the effects of changed gut homeostasis on another organ (an acute phase reactant produced by the liver, for example) would be a valuable tool to assist in the characterization and monitoring of gut dysfunction in the critically ill patient. The absence of a comprehensive, generic descriptor makes the evaluation of gut dysfunction as a component of the multiple organ dysfunction syndrome difficult. More sophisticated measures of gut permeability or blood flow can serve as useful markers of specific aspects of GI function for use in experimental studies.

References

1. Marshall JC (1991) Multiorgan failure. In: Wilmore DW, Brennan MF, Harken AH, et al (eds) Scientific American Surgery Vol 1 Critical Care, Holcroft J, Meakins JL (eds), Scientific American Medicine, New York, pp 13.1–13.20
2. Bone R, Balk R,. Cerra F, Dellinger RP, et al (1992) Definitions for sepsis and organ failure and guidelines for the use of innovative therapies in sepsis. Chest 101:1644–1655
3. Deitch EA (1992) Multiple organ failure. Pathophysiology and potential future therapy. Ann Surg 216:117–134
4. Beat AL, Cerra FB (1994) Multiple organ failure syndrome in the 1990's. Systemic inflammatory response and organ dysfunction. JAMA 271:226–233
5. Carrico CJ, Meakins JL, Marshall JC, Fry D, Maier RV (1986) Multiple organ failure syndrome. The gastrointestinal tract: The 'motor' of MOF. Arch Surg 121:196–208
6. Wilmore DW, Smith RJ, O'Dwyer ST, Jacobs DO, Ziegler TR, Wang XD (1988) The gut: A central organ after surgical stress. Surgery 104:917–923
7. Deitch EA (1990) The role of intestinal barrier failure and bacterial translocation in the development of systemic infection and multiple organ failure. Arch Surg 125:403–404
8. Marshall JC (1995) Multiple organ dysfunction syndrome (MODS). In: Sibbald WJ, Vincent JL (eds) Clinical Trials for the Treatment of Sepsis. Springer-Verlag, Berlin, pp 122–138
9. Cook DJ, Fuller H, Guyatt GH, et al (1994) Risk factors for gastrointestinal bleeding in critically ill patients. N Engl J Med 330:377–381
10. Arvidsson D, Rasmussen I, Almqvist P, Niklasson F, Haglund U (1991) Splanchnic oxygen consumption in septic and hemorrhagic shock. Surgery 109:190–197
11. Price HL, Deutsch S, Marshall BE, Stephen GW, Behar MG, Neufeld GR (1966) Hemodynamic and metabolic effects of hemorrhage in man with particular reference to the splanchnic circulation. Circ Res 18:469–474
12. Gump FE, Price JB, Kinney JM (1970) Whole body and splanchnic blood flow and oxygen consumption measurements in patients with intraperitoneal infection. Ann Surg 171:321–328
13. Gottlieb ME, Sarfeh IJ, Stratton H, Goldman ML, Newell JC, Shah DM (1983) Hepatic perfusion and splanchnic oxygen consumption in patients postinjury. J Trauma 23:836–843
14. Curling TB (1842) On acute ulceration of the duodenum in cases of burns. Med Chir Tr London 25:260
15. Cushing H (1932) Peptic ulcers and interbrain. Surg Gynecol Obstet 55:1–34

16. Skillman JJ, Bushnell LS, Goldman H, Silen W (1969) Respiratory failure, hypotension, sepsis, and jaundice. A clinical syndrome associated with lethal hemorrhage and acute stress ulceration in the stomach. Am J Surg 117:523–530
17. Ben-Menachem T, Fogel R, Patel RV, et al (1994) Prophylaxis for stress-related gastric hemorrhage in the medical intensive care unit. A randomized, controlled, single-blind study. Ann Intern Med 121:568–575
18. Priebe HJ, Skillman JJ, Bushnell LS, Long PC, Silen W (1980) Antacid versus cimetidine in preventing acute gastrointestinal bleeding. A randomized trial in 75 critically ill patients. N Engl J Med 302:424–430
19. Cook DJ, Witt LG, Cook RJ, Guyatt GH (1991) Stress ulcer prophylaxis in the critically ill: A meta-analysis. Am J Med 91:519–527
20. Fiddian-Green RG, McGough E, Pittenger G, Rothman E (1983) Predictive value of intramural pH and other risk factors for massive bleeding from stress ulceration. Gastroenterology 85:613
21. Navab F, Steingrub J (1995) Stress ulcer: Is routine prophylaxis necessary? Am J Gastroenterology 90:708–712
22. Perey BJ (1983) Acute necrosis of the gastrointestinal tract: A unified view. Can J Surg 26:203–204
23. Haglund U (1994) Gut ischemia. Gut 35:S73–S76
24. Desai MH, Herndon DN, Rutan RL, Abston S, Linares HA (1991) Ischemic intestinal complications in patients with burns. Surg Gynecol Obstet 172:257–261
25. Bell RC, Coalson JJ, Smith JD, Johanson WG (1983) Multiple organ system failure and infection in adult respiratory distress syndrome. Ann Intern Med 99:293–298
26. Goris RJA, te Boekhorst TPA, Nuytinck JKS, Gimbrere JSF (1985) Multiple organ failure. Generalized autodestructive inflammation? Arch Surg 120:1109–1115
27. Tran DD, Groeneveld ABJ, Van der Meulen J, Nauta JJP, Strack van Schijndel RJM, Thijs LG (1990) Age, chronic disease, sepsis, organ system failure, and mortality in a medical intensive care unit. Crit Care Med 18:474–479
28. Nowicki PT, Nankervis CA (1994) The role of the circulation in the pathogenesis of necrotizing enterocolitis. Clin Perinatol 21:219–234
29. Harward TR, Brooks DL, Flynn TC, Seeger JM (1993) Multiple organ dysfunction after mesenteric artery revascularization. J Vasc Surg 18:459–467
30. Glenn F, Becker CG (1982) Acute acalculous cholecystitis. An increasing entity. Ann Surg 195:131–136
31. Howard RJ (1981) Acute acalculous cholecystitis. Am J Surg 141:194–198
32. Boland G, Lee MJ, Mueller PR (1993) Acute cholecystitis in the intensive care unit. New Horizons 1:246–260
33. Raunest J, Imhof M, Rauen U, Ohmann C, Thon KP, Burrig KF (1992) Acute cholecystitis: A complication in severely injured intensive care patients. J Trauma 32:433–440
34. Steinberg W, Tenner S (1994) Acute pancreatitis. N Engl J Med 330:1198–1210
35. Kameya S, Hayakawa T, Kameya A, Watanabe T (1986) Hyperamylasemia in patients in an intensive care unit. J Clin Gastroenterol 8:438–462
36. Doglio DR, Pusajo JF, Egurrola MA, et al (1991) Gastric mucosal pH as a prognostic index of mortality in critically ill patients. Crit Care Med 19:1037–1040
37. Maynard N, Bihari D, Beale R, et al (1993) Assessment of splanchnic oxygenation by gastric tonometry in patients with acute circulatory failure. JAMA 270:1203–1210
38. Gutierrez G, Clark C, Brown SD, Price K, Ortiz L, Nelson C (1994) Effect of dobutamine on oxygen consumption and gastric mucosal pH in septic patients. Am J Resp Crit Care Med 150:324–329
39. Gutierrez G, Palizas F, Doglio G, et al (1992) Gastric intramucosal pH as a therapeutic index of tissue oxygenation in critically ill patients. Lancet 339:195–199
40. Boyd O, MacKay CJ, Lamb G, Bland JM, Grounds RM, Bennett ED (1993) Comparison of clinical information gained from routine blood gas analysis and from gastric tonometry for intramural pH. Lancet 341:142–146
41. Friedman G, Berlot G, Kahn RJ, Vincent JL (1995) Combined measurements of blood lactate concentrations and gastric intramucosal pH in patients with severe sepsis. Crit Care Med 23:1184–1193

42. Moore FA, Feliciano DV, Andrassy RJ, et al (1992) Early enteral feeding, compared with parenteral, reduces postoperative septic complications. The results of a meta-analysis. Ann Surg 216:172-183
43. Heyland DK, Cook DJ, Guyatt GH (1994) Does the formulation of enteral feeding products influence infectious morbidity and mortality rates in the critically ill patient? A critical review of the evidence. Crit Care Med 22:1192-1202
44. Chang RWS, Jacob S, Lee B (1987) Gastrointestinal dysfunction among intensive care unit patients. Crit Care Med 15:909
45. Brinson RR, Pitts VL, Taylor AE (1989) Intestinal absorption of peptide enteral formulas in hypoproteinemic (volume expanded) rats: A paired analysis. Crit Care Med 17:657-660
46. Brinson RR, Curtis WD, Singh M (1987) Diarrhea in the intensive care unit: The role of hypoalbuminemia and the response to a chemically defined diet (case reports and review of the literature). J Am Coll Nutr 6:517-523
47. Guenter PA, Settle RG, Perlmutter S, Marino PL, DeSimone GA, Rolandelli RH (1991) Tube feeding-related diarrhea in acutely ill patients. J Parent Enteral Nutr 15:277-280
48. Wanke CA, Guerrant RL (1987) Small bowel colonization alone is a cause of diarrhea. Infect Immun 55:1924-1926
49. Spapen HD, Duinslaeger L, Diltoer M, Gillet R, Bossuyt A, Huyghens LP (1995) Gastric emptying in critically ill patients is accelerated by adding cisapride to a standard enteral feeding protocol: Results of a prospective, randomized, controlled trial. Crit Care Med 23:481-485
50. Ouellette AJ, Hsieh MM, Nosek MT, et al (1994) Mouse Paneth cell defensins: Primary structures and antibacterial activities of numerous cryptidin isoforms. Infect Immun 62:5040-5047
51. Tepperman BL, Brown JF, Whittle BJR (1993) Nitric oxide synthase induction and intestinal epithelial cell viability in rats. Am J Physiol 265:G214-G218
52. Langkamp-Henken B, Donovan TB, Pate LM, Maull CD, Kudsk KA (1995) Increased intestinal permeability following blunt and penetrating trauma. Crit Care Med 23:660-664
53. Deitch EA (1990) Intestinal permeability is increased in burn patients shortly after injury. Surgery 107:411-416
54. Ziegler TR, Smith RJ, O'Dwyer ST, Demling RH, Wilmore DW (1988) Increased intestinal permeability associated with infection in burn patients. Arch Surg 123:1313-1319
55. Murray MJ, Gonze MD, Nowak LR, Cobb CF (1994) Serum D(−)-lactate levels as an aid to diagnosing acute intestinal ischemia. Am Surg 167:575-578
56. Hove H, Mortensen PB (1995) Colonic lactate metabolism and D-lactic acidosis. Dig Dis Sci 40:320-330
57. Winchurch RA, Thupari JN, Munster AM (1987) Endotoxemia in burn patients:Levels of circulating endotoxins are related to burn size. Surgery 102:808-812
58. Martinez-Pellus AE, Merino P, Bru M, et al (1993) Can selective digestive decontamination avoid the endotoxemia and cytokine activation promoted by cardiopulmonary bypass? Crit Care Med 21:1684-1691
59. Van Deventer SJH, Ten Cate JW, Tytgat GNJ (1988) Intestinal endotoxemia. Clinical significance. Gastroenterology 94:825-831
60. Kivilaakso E, Valtonen VV, Malkamaki M, et al (1984) Endotoxemia and acute pancreatitis: Correlation between the severity of the disease and the anti-enterobacterial common antigen antibody titre. Gut 25:1065-1070
61. Endo S, Inada K, Yamada Y, et al (1994) Plasma endotoxin and cytokine concentrations in patients with hemorrhagic shock. Crit Care Med 22:949-955
62. Wells CL, Maddaus MA, Simmons RL (1988) Proposed mechanisms for the translocation of intestinal bacteria. Rev Infect Dis 10:958-979
63. Sedman PC, Macfie J, Sagar P, et al (1994) The prevalence of gut translocation in humans. Gastroenterology 107:643-649
64. Krause W, Matheis H, Wulf K (1969) Fungaemia and funguria after oral administration of Candida albicans. Lancet 1:598-599
65. Fiddian-Green RG, Gantz NM (1987) Transient episodes of sigmoid ischemia and their relation to infection from intestinal organisms after abdominal aortic operations. Crit Care Med 15:835-839

66. Gaussorgues Ph, Gueugniaud PY, Vedrinne JM, Salord F, Mercatello A, Robert D (1986) Septicémies dans les suites immédiates des arrêts cardio-circulatoires. Réan Soins Intens Med Urg 2:67-68

67. Levy J, Van Laethem Y, Verhaegen G, Perpete C, Butzler JP, Wenzel RP (1989) Contaminated enteral nutrition solutions as a cause of nosocomial bloodstream infection: A study using plasmid fingerprinting. J Parent Enteral Nutr 13:228-234

68. Moore FA, Moore EE, Poggetti R, et al (1991) Gut bacterial translocation via the portal vein: A clinical perspective with major torso trauma. J Trauma 31:629-638

69. Marshall JC, Christou NV, Meakins JL (1993) The gastrointestinal tract. The "undrained abscess" of multiple organ failure. Ann Surg 218:111-119

70. Dyess DL, Garrison RN, Fry DE (1985) Candida sepsis. Implications of polymicrobial blood borne infection. Arch Surg 120:345-348

71. Garrison RN, Fry DE, Berberich S, Polk HC (1982) Enterococcal bacteremia. Clinical implications and determinants of death. Ann Surg 196:43-47

72. Moore WEC, Holdeman LV (1974) Human fecal flora: The normal flora of 20 Japanese-Hawaiians. Appl Microbiol 27:961-979

73. Gorbach SL, Nahas L, Lerner PI, Weinstein L (1967) Studies of intestinal microflora. I. Effects of diet, age, and periodic sampling on numbers of fecal microorganisms in man. Gastroenterology 53:845-855

74. Van Der Waaij D (1989) The ecology of the human intestine and its consequences for overgrowth by pathogens such as Clostridium difficile. Ann Rev Microbiol 43:69-87

75. Giannella RA, Broitman SA, Zamcheck N (1972) Gastric acid barrier to ingested microorganisms in man: Studies in vivo and in vitro. Gut 13:251-256

76. Du Moulin GC, Hedley-Whyte J, Paterson DG, Lisbon A (1982) Aspiration of gastric bacteria in antacid treated patients: A frequent cause of postoperative colonisation of the airway. Lancet 1:242-245

77. Garvey BM, McCambley JA, Tuxen DV (1989) Effects of gastric alkalization on bacterial colonization in critically ill patients. Crit Care Med 17:211-216

78. Heyland D, Mandell LA (1992) Gastric colonization by gram-negative bacilli and nosocomial pneumonia in the intensive care unit patient. Evidence for causation. Chest 101:187-193

79. Marshall JC, Christou NV, Horn R, Meakins JL (1988) The microbiology of multiple organ failure. The proximal GI tract as an occult reservoir of pathogens. Arch Surg 123:309-315

Bacterial Translocation

Bacterial Translocation: Intestinal Epithelial Permeability

C. L. Wells and S. L. Erlandsen

Introduction

In its broadest terms, intestinal bacterial translocation can be defined as the passage of bacteria (both live and dead) and bacterial products (such as exotoxins, endotoxins, and cell wall fragments) from the intestinal lumen to otherwise sterile extraintestinal sites. Investigators studying immune mechanisms at mucosal surfaces have long recognized that epithelial uptake and processing of intestinal antigens is a complex process, needed not only to establish the immune status of the host, but to continually regulate the immune response (both inductive and suppressive) to intestinal antigens [1]. The transmigration of intestinal bacteria was initially viewed with skepticism by many physicians; however, in recent years, the existence of bacterial translocation (BT) has become generally accepted among clinicians, although the clinical significance of this process remains a subject of debate.

Clarification of the mechanisms involved in BT has become a popular area of research, and a search of the recent literature revealed at least 500 journal articles devoted to this topic in the last five years. This level of interest is due, at least in part, to the fact that results from this research can often be directly applied to the clinical setting. The aims of the present manuscript are
1) to clarify the clinical relevance of bacterial translocation;
2) to describe the intestinal epithelial barrier and how alterations in this barrier affect epithelial permeability;
3) to describe the relationship between increased epithelial permeability and BT; and
4) to suggest future areas of research that may help target novel treatment regimens to decrease the costly morbidity associated with complicating infections caused by translocating intestinal bacteria.

Evidence for Bacterial Translocation in the Clinical Setting

Although endogenous bacteria can theoretical penetrate any mucosal surface to gain access to deeper bodily tissues, the term BT is generally applied to the process by which endogenous microbes migrate out of the intestinal tract. Bacterial penetration of the intestinal epithelium is not an abnormal process; antigen sampling at mucosal surfaces is a critical element in the initiation of normal immune responses to intestinal antigens. However, under certain conditions, translocating microflora can initiate systemic infection, but this latter scenario is typically seen only in specific patient populations. Patients at greatest risk for complicating infections caused by enteric bacteria include postsurgical patients, trauma patients, and immunosuppressed patients such as organ transplant recipients and cancer patients [2]. The economic impact of translocating microbes may be substantial. For example, in the United States, as many as 10% of hospitalized patients develop a complicating infection, estimated to annually involve more than 2 million patients (and 58 000 deaths), and cost more than 4.5 billion American dollars [3, 4]. In decreasing order of frequency, nosocomial infections include urinary tract infections, surgical site infections, and blood stream infections; the bacteria most frequently isolated are *Escherichia coli*, *Staphylococcus aureus*, coagulase-negative staphylococci, *Enterococcus* species, and *Pseudomonas aeruginosa* [3]. Although many nosocomial infections are exogenously acquired (eg microbial contamination of a cutaneous wound), many have an undefined focus and are attributed to translocating enteric bacteria.

Nearly all the direct evidence for BT has been obtained from experimental animals, where it is possible to monitor bacterial migration using tissue histology, microbial culture of internal organs, and dissemination of specifically labelled (eg radiolabelled) intestinal bacteria. These techniques are generally impractical, if not impossible, to perform in humans. Consequently, much of the evidence for BT in humans is indirect and anecdotal. However, this body of literature contains substantial information consistent with the more direct evidence obtained from animal models. Below is some of the evidence for BT in the clinical setting.

Association between Intestinal Bacteria and Systemic Infection

Several prospective studies have reported that a predominant strain of fecal bacteria is often the agent of subsequent systemic infection. These studies are cumbersome, necessitating careful prospective characterization of the fecal flora of high risk patients, storage of individual bacterial isolates, and subsequent identification of patients who develop systemic infection; the etiologic agent of infection is then tested to determine if it is the same bacterial strain previously isolated from fecal flora. Using this technique, Tancrede and Andremont [5] identified and quantified bacteria in 4347 stool specimens from 688 cancer patients receiving no antimicrobial therapy; 60 patients developed 64 episodes of gram-negative bacteremia that appeared to be caused by a dominant fecal organism that translocated from the intestinal tract during a period of severe granulocytopenia. Wells et al. [6, 7] similarly found evidence of prior fecal carriage in organ transplant recipients who developed gram-negative bacteremia and in hospitalized medical/surgical patients who developed infections with vancomycin-resistant enterococci.

Several investigators have monitored the incidence of enteric bacteria in nosocomial infections as an indirect assessment of the incidence of BT. For example,

Ford et al. [8] reported that 329 patients developed 55 postoperative infections after coronary artery revascularization; the vast majority of these infections (75%) involved gram-negative enteric bacteria presumed to translocate from the intestinal tract, with the most significant risk factor being the length of gastrointestinal disuse. After numerous studies involving multiple trauma and shock, Schlag et al. [9] concluded that the intestine is one of the first of the organs involved in shock, causing BT and releasing endotoxin which activates humoral and cellular systems, causing intravascular coagulation and microthrombosis, leading to organ failure. Tran et al. [10] noted that multiple organ failure (MOF) developed in 88 of 538 consecutive surgical intensive care patients; infection was documented in 65% of these 88 patients, of whom 34% had bacteremia and 52% had intraabdominal infection; a species of *Enterobacteriaceae* was isolated from a majority (60%) of infected patients, implicating the intestinal tract as the source of the infection as well as the subsequent MOF. Tran et al. [19] concluded that translocation of bacteria and endotoxin might be important in evolution and perpetuation of MOF, and that future therapies should focus on maintenance of gut barrier function and normal ecology of the intestinal tract, as well as elimination of harmful intestinal pathogens and endotoxin.

In contrast to the above investigators, Moore et al. [11] concluded that BT was not a frequent result of injury, largely because they failed to detect endotoxin or enteric bacteria in the blood of trauma patients undergoing emergency laparotomy. Moore et al. [11] concluded that systemic bacteremia was a rare occurrence in their trauma patients. In contrast, Rush et al. [12] reported that blood cultures were positive in 56% (n = 18) of trauma patients who had an admitting systolic blood pressure < 80 mmHg and who were tested within 3 h of admission to a trauma unit. Unfortunately, in this latter study, most bacteria were gram-positive and were not further identified, making it impossible to determine if these bacteria were likely skin flora (eg coagulase-negative staphylococci) or enteric flora (eg enterococci).

Thus, epidemiological studies have documented that enteric bacteria frequently cause complicating infections in high risk hospitalized patients. And, prospective studies have documented that bacteria carried in the fecal flora are typically the same strains isolated from complicating infections in hospitalized patients. Depending on the study design and the patient population, attempts to recover translocating bacteria from blood culture did not consistently yield positive results. (However, blood culture might not accurately reflect BT due to the relatively small volume of blood that is sampled.) More consistent results can be obtained using animal models where quantitative culture of extraintestinal tissue (rather than blood culture) is likely a more sensitive indicator of extraintestinal dissemination of enteric bacteria.

Efficacy of Selective Digestive Decontamination

Clinicians have attempted to decrease the incidence of nosocomial infections using antimicrobial therapy designed to selectively eliminate the enteric species most frequently involved in complicating infections. This approach has been termed selective digestive decontamination (SDD). Over the last 20 years, specific groups of high risk patients (usually immunosuppressed, surgical, or trauma patients) have been treated with antibiotic regimens carefully designed to prevent oropharyngeal/gastrointestinal colonization with potentially pathogenic microbes. Here, potential pathogens include aerobic and facultative gram-negative bacilli (such as *E. coli*, other Enterobacteriaceae, *Pseudomonas* species) and often yeast. According to the basic tenet of SDD, enteric gram-negative bacteria should be selectively eliminated, while maintaining the populations of strictly anaerobic bacteria. This approach is based on the theory of "colonization resistance". According to this theory, intestinal anaerobic bacteria are considered relatively non-invasive, and are thought to play a pivotal role in limiting the intestinal colonization and subsequent dissemination of *E. coli* and other potentially pathogenic enteric bacteria [13]. It is widely accepted that the ideal agent for prophylactic gut decontamination is one that preserves the integrity of the anaerobic microflora while eliminating potential pathogens such as *E. coli* and other Enterobacteriaceae.

A majority of investigators have reported that SDD causes a significant decrease in the incidence of complicating infections, but some investigators do not agree; some investigators report that SDD causes a significant decrease in mortality, but most investigators do not agree [14, 15]. The efficacy of SDD is controversial, and this situation is not likely to change in the near future due to the difficulties involved in designing a definitive, objective study. For example, bacterial colonization, infection, and mortality should all be monitored. However, it is often difficult to distinguish infection from colonization, or to distinguish preexisting infection from infection acquired after the onset of SDD. In fact, the definition of infection is itself controversial. Some claim that infection is a condition that must be documented by microbial culture, but that is often not possible. In addition, it has been estimated that at least 600 patients would be needed to show a statistically significant decrease in respiratory tract infections from a baseline value of 20 to 12% [14]. Mortality is the most unambiguous outcome variable of SDD, but identifying mortality attributable to infection is difficult, and some stratification (eg APACHE II score) is clearly needed to eliminate those patients whose death is related to prognosis or underlying condition, rather than infection. Some clinical trials have shown a positive effect of SDD on mortality when infection-related mortality is considered, rather than overall mortality [15]. Most investigators agree that the ideal patient population for an SDD trial should be previously healthy individuals with acute to moderate disease and a good prognosis in the absence of infectious complications. However, it has been calculated that approximately 2000 patients would be needed to show a realistic 10–20% reduction (3–5% absolute difference) in mortality [16], and the European Consensus Conference concluded that approximately 1500 patients would be needed to show a 3–6% reduction in mortality, and that patient follow-up should last approximately six months [14]. Failure to detect differences in mortality associated with SDD may therefore reflect the study design, the types of patients included, the sample size, or the type of analysis undertaken.

A summary of 9 review articles on SDD indicates that a decreased incidence of infection is achievable in most high risk patient populations, and that decreased mortality may be possible in selected groups of patients [15]. In other words, SDD has little affect on mortality, but seems useful in preventing infection; it seems premature to ignore the potential benefits of SDD in selected patients at greatest risk for developing systemic infection due to translocating bacteria. Regardless, data from SDD trials indicate that normal intestinal bacteria migrate out of the intestinal lumen and cause systemic infection, and that elimination of these potentially pathogenic enteric bacteria results in decreased numbers of complicating infections.

Recovery of Viable Enteric Bacteria from Mesenteric Lymph Nodes

Recovery of viable enteric bacteria from mesenteric lymph nodes (MLN) is considered one of the most sensitive methods to detect BT in experimental animals. Although MLN are relatively easy to obtain from laboratory animals, this tissue is not as easily obtained from hospitalized patients. However, a number of clinicians have cultured MLN excised from patients undergoing various surgical procedures. This literature confirms that enteric bacteria are often recovered from the MLN of patients at high risk for BT (Table 1). Because perioperative anti-

Table 1. Clinical studies documenting the recovery of viable enteric bacteria from mesenteric lymph nodes (MLN) excised during surgery

Reason for surgery	No. of patients	% of patients with MLN bacteria	Reference
Crohn's disease	46	33	[17]
other elective abdominal surgery	43	5	
Crohn's disease	28	25	[18]
Colorectal cancer	20	65	[19]
other digestive diseases	20	30	
Intestinal obstruction without necrosis	17	59	[20]
other abdominal surgery	25	4	
Laparotomy for intestinal disease	4	75	[21]
laparotomy following trauma	25	0	
Colorectal carcinoma	22	64	[22]
General surgery patients	267	10[a]	[23]
Laparotomy following trauma	20	20[b]	[24]
Laparotomy following trauma	16	25	[25]
Organ donors	21	67[c]	[26]

[a] Includes cultures of intestinal serosa.
[b] Includes cultures of portal blood obtained during surgery.
[c] Includes three patients with bacteria recovered from lung but not MLN.

biotics were used in some patients, the recovery of viable bacteria is likely underestimated, but these data provide direct evidence for the existence (but not the significance) of bacterial migration from the intestinal lumen to the draining MLN in the clinical setting.

Several clinicians have attempted, not only to document the existence of BT, but to associate this phenomenon with clinical outcome. For example, in 267 consecutive general surgical patients, *E. coli* was the predominate translocating organism recovered from MLN; postoperative septic complications were twice as common in patients with translocation as in those without translocation, but no difference in mortality was noted [23]. Peitzman et al. [21] sampled MLN of 25 trauma patients during laparotomy; although enteric bacteria were never recovered from MLN, 28% of these patients developed infection, the majority of which were caused by gram-negative enteric bacteria. Peitzman et al. [21] concluded that BT to the MLN was not common in trauma patients, yet infections caused by enteric pathogens were frequent complications. Here, it seems appropriate to mention that results from animal models have documented that enteric bacteria can translocate out of the intestinal tract either via the MLN or the portal blood [27, 28], and there is some evidence that the portal blood may be the major route of translocation [28]. Thus, while recovery of enteric bacteria from MLN provides direct evidence of bacterial migration out of the intestinal tract, this type of testing likely underestimates the incidence of extraintestinal dissemination of enteric bacteria.

Observations from Clinical Studies

In conclusion, results from diverse clinical studies are consistent with the hypothesis that bacteria translocate out of the intestinal tract and initiate complicating systemic infections. This conclusion is based on data documenting that: 1) enteric bacteria are often involved in complicating infections in high risk hospitalized patients; 2) bacteria carried in the fecal flora are often the same bacterial strains isolated from systemic infections; 3) the incidence of complicating infections can often be decreased by administering antimicrobial agents compatible with the guidelines of SDD; and 4) migrating enteric bacteria can often be recovered from the draining MLN of high risk patients. These data are largely circumstantial. However, these data are not compatible with the conclusion that BT is an irrelevant phenomenon in hospitalized patients. Rather, these data, derived from a number of different experimental protocols, are consistent with the conclusion that BT is relevant in the development of systemic infection in selected populations of high risk patients.

Intestinal Epithelial Permeability and Bacterial Translocation across the Epithelial Barrier

The gut mucosal barrier is not well defined nor understood. According to Madara [29], this barrier has extrinsic and intrinsic components. The extrinsic barrier (within the intestinal lumen) stabilizes the microenvironment at the intestinal epithelial surface and consists of mucus, secretory IgA, and the so-called unstirred layer overlying the epithelium. The intrinsic barrier (intrinsic to the epithelium) consists of epithelial cells and spaces around the epithelial cells. Molecules and particles can traverse the epithelial barrier by either the transcellular route (through epithelial cells) or the paracellular route (between epithelial cells), as diagrammed in Fig. 1. The paracellular pathway includes the apical junctional complex consisting of the tight junction, intermediate junction, and spot desmosome, as well as the subjunctional space [29]. Electrical resistance across a biological membrane, such as the apical enterocyte membrane, is 10^3 to 10^4 ohm/cm^2, while resistance across the small intestine is only approximately 10^2 ohm/cm^2; thus, the major permeation pathway across the intestinal epithelium is paracellular [29]. While the intermediate junction (zonula adherens) and desmosomes function primarily in cell-cell adhesion, the tight junction (zonula occludens) is the major permeability barrier limiting the paracellular movement of particles from the apical to the basolateral compartments of the extracellular milieu. Under certain circumstances these tight junctions become "leaky", facilitating the paracellular penetration of macromolecules, including enteric bacteria (Fig. 1). As explained below, increased intestinal epithelial permeability, ac-

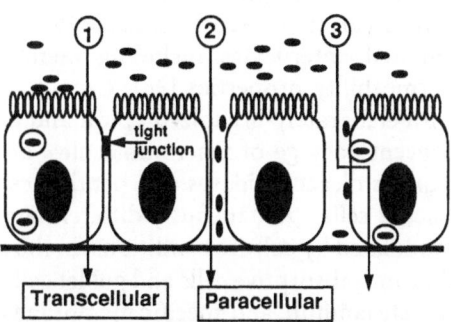

Fig. 1. Diagrammatic representation of three postulated routes of bacterial movement across the intestinal epithelial barrier. (1) Bacterial uptake by the apical enterocyte membrane followed by bacterial internalization in a membrane-bound cytoplasmic vacuole and transcellular bacterial migration through the enterocyte cytoplasm. (2) Opening of the enterocyte tight junction and paracellular bacterial penetration between enterocytes. (3) Opening of the enterocyte tight junction and subsequent bacterial uptake at the enterocyte lateral membrane following, and subsequent transcellular bacterial migration through the enterocyte cytoplasm. The literature contains evidence supporting the engulfment of bacteria through the apical enterocyte membrane, the facilitated bacterial entry through the enterocyte lateral surface following opening of the tight junction, and the existence of intracellular bacteria within membrane-bound vacuoles (see text). These routes assume that bacteria penetrate the enterocyte basement membrane, but the mechanism for this is unknown

companied by paracellular penetration of enteric bacteria, may be a common mechanism facilitating BT in the diverse patient populations at high risk for BT.

Enterocyte as a Portal of Entry for Translocating Bacteria

There is microscopic evidence from both *in vivo* (laboratory animals) and *in vitro* (cultured enterocytes) experiments documenting that the absorptive enterocyte is at least one portal of entry for translocating enteric bacteria. Using rodent models of microbial translocation, *Candida albicans, E. coli, Proteus mirabilis*, and *Enterococcus faecalis* have been visualized within intact intestinal epithelial cells [30–33], and bacterial uptake by these "non-professional phagocytes" is becoming a widely studied mechanism of bacterial invasion [34]. *In vivo* observations of bacterial entry into the intestinal epithelium are few due to the sampling problem. For example, if the number of viable bacteria recovered from MLN is a reliable indicator of the number of translocating microbes [32, 33], one can anticipate approximately 100 to 1000 transmigrating bacteria in a small intestine approximately 20 feet long with an inner surface area of approximately 15 m^2 in the adult human [35]. Locating one micron bacterial particles in this cellular area is a formidable task using traditional microscopic techniques.

Cultured intestinal epithelium is an attractive alternative to *in vivo* testing, and there is an expanding literature describing the interactions of enteric pathogens with cultured enterocytes. For the past several years, our laboratory has studied the interactions of enteric bacteria with cultured enterocytes, namely Caco-2 and HT-29 cells. Although there are literally hundreds of enterocytes available for *in vitro* culture, only a few cell lines differentiate to resemble mature, polarized enterocytes. Caco-2 and HT-29 cells have many features of differentiated enterocytes including membrane potential, ion conductance, and permeability properties [36]. Caco-2 and HT-29 cells have structural polarity with elaborately-organized apical and basolateral domains, tight junctions that prevent passage of macromolecules, and well developed apical microvilli that express disaccharidases and peptidases typical of small intestinal villous cells. Caco-2 cells spontaneously differentiate, but HT-29 differentiation cells can be modulated by culture conditions; in the absence of glucose, HT-29 cells differentiate into absorptive cells and goblet cells containing mucin granules. HT-29 cells secrete laminin, and specific membrane components (Na, K-ATPase, transferrin receptor, polymeric IgA receptor, histocompatibility antigen) are synthesized and appropriately delivered to the basolateral domain. Caco-2 and HT-29 cells have been used to document enterocyte interactions with *E. coli, Vibrio cholerae, Salmonella* species, *Listeria* species, *Shigella flexneri, Clostridium difficile, Bacteroides fragilis, Cryptosporidium parvum, Entamoeba histolytica*, and several viruses, and *in vitro* interactions have been shown to have *in vivo* relevance [34, 36].

As expected, invasive enteric bacteria, such as salmonella and listeria, are readily internalized by Caco-2 and HT-29 enterocytes; however, normal enteric flora such as *E. coli, P. mirabilis*, and *E. faecalis* are internalized as well, although in relatively few numbers [37–39]. Bacterial adherence to enterocyte apical mi-

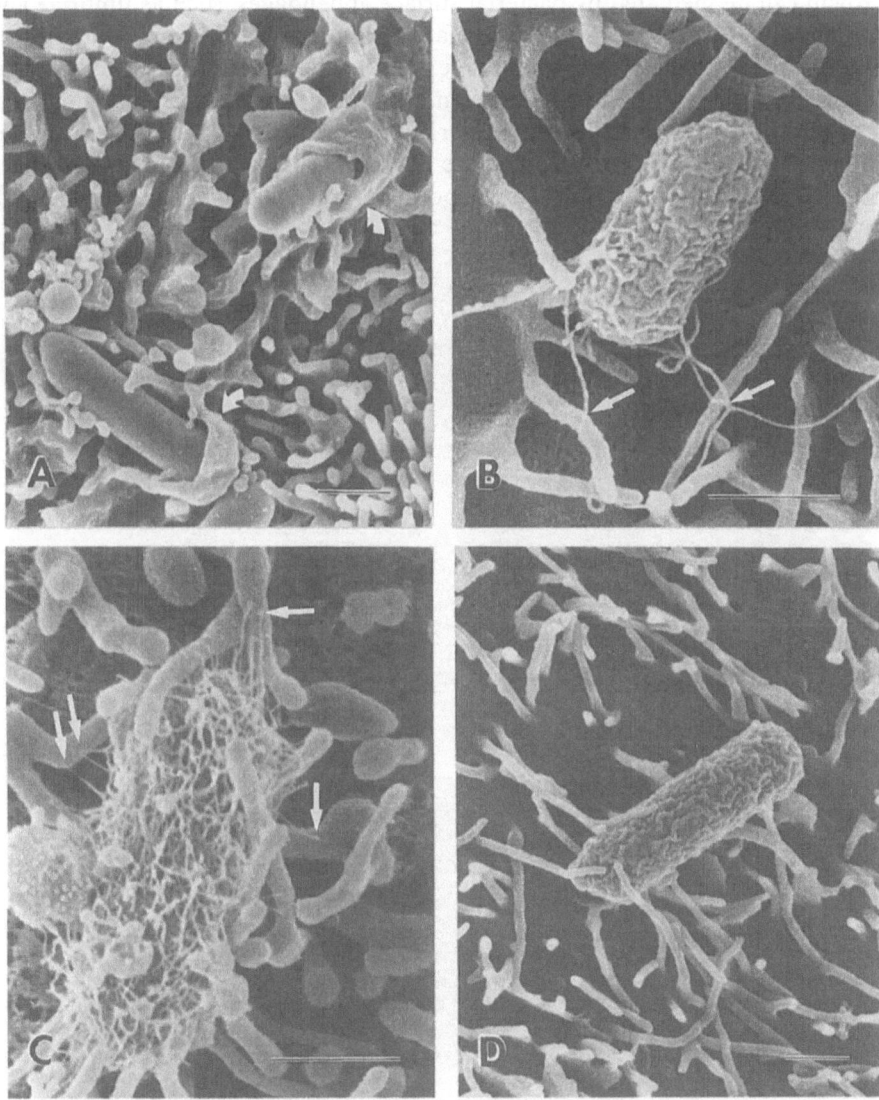

Fig. 2. Interactions of enteric bacteria with the apical surface of cultured intestinal epithelial cells viewed with low voltage (3.5–4.0 kV), field emission, scanning electron microscopy. **A** *Listeria monocytogenes* ATCC 43249 deeply entwined in the apical microvilli of HT-29 enterocytes, with veil-like structures termed lamellapodia (curved white arrows) engulfing rod-shaped listeria; **B** *Salmonella typhimurium* ATCC 14028, with flagella mediating adherence to microvilli (*arrows*) of Caco-2 enterocyte; **C** *Proteus mirabilis* M13, with fimbriae mediating adherence to microvilli (*arrows*) of Caco-2 enterocyte; **D** *Escherichia coli* M21, devoid of surface appendages, yet firmly adherent to HT-29 apical microvilli. Scale bars: 0.5 microns

crovilli can be mediated by bacterial surface appendages, such as fimbriae and flagella, although bacteria without surface appendages can become anchored by enterocyte microvilli (Fig. 2). Despite extensive efforts, the process of bacterial internalization by enterocytes has been only rarely observed by scanning electron microscopy, suggesting that bacterial uptake must be a rapid event, similar to bacterial endocytosis by leukocytes [40]. Enterocyte apical microvilli have been observed to flatten into lamellapodia, or veil-like structures, that engulf

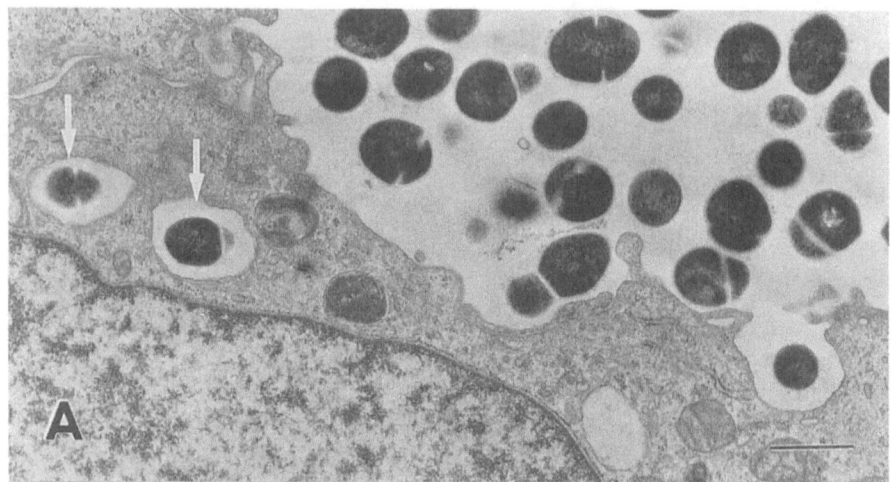

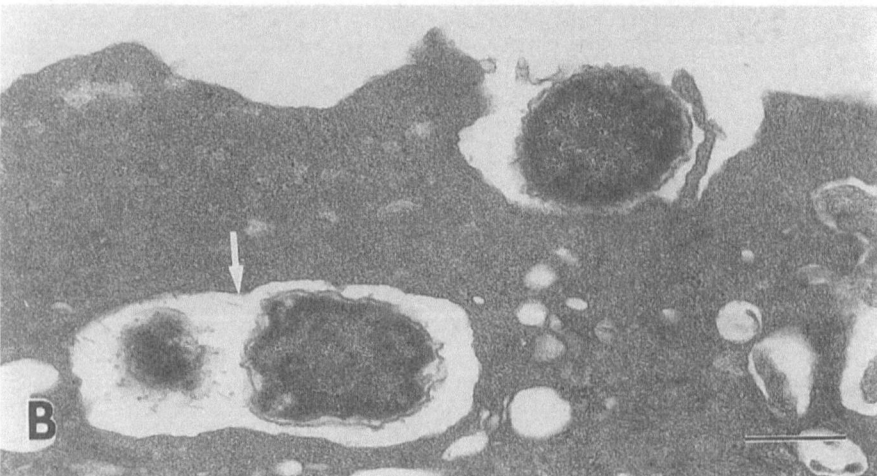

Fig. 3. Transmission electron micrographs of enteric bacteria in membrane-bound vacuoles (*arrows*) in the apical cytoplasm of cultured intestinal epithelial cells. **A** *Enterococcus faecalis* OG1RF pINY1801 interacting with the apical surface of an HT-29 enterocyte, with the enterocyte containing enterococci within two membrane-bound cytoplasmic vacuoles; **B** *Salmonella typhimurium* ATCC 14028 interacting with the apical surface of a Caco-2 enterocyte, with a membrane-bound cytoplasmic vacuole containing two salmonella cells as well as bacterial flagella cut in cross-section and longitudinal section. Scale bars: **A** 2.5 microns; **B** 0.5 microns

bacterial cells (Fig. 2A). Lamellapodia may mimic the "zipper mechanism" of leukocytes where advancing pseudopodia fuse to form a membrane-bound vacuole [40]. Once internalized, enteric bacteria have been localized within cytoplasmic membrane-bound vacuoles [37–39], a phenomenon similar to the fate of intracellular bacteria within leukocytes [40]. Fig. 3 presents examples of intracellular *Salmonella typhimurium* and *Enterococcus faecalis*. Thus, normal enteric bacteria, such as *E. coli* and enterococci, can be internalized by intestinal epithelial cells, and bacterial internalization by these "non-professional phagocytes" has mechanistic similarities with bacterial phagocytosis by leukocytes.

Bacterial Internalization Facilitated by Opening Enterocyte Tight Junctions

In clinical conditions associated with increased intestinal permeability, intercellular junctions are a likely target for injury, and there is recent *in vitro* evidence that opening of enterocyte tight junctions causes increased bacterial penetration of the intestinal epithelial barrier. This evidence is derived from *in vitro* models that involve opening of enterocyte tight junctions following exposure of confluent enterocyte cultures to low extracellular calcium [41] or to a purified bacterial toxin [42].

Depletion of extracellular calcium from cultures of confluent, polarized epithelial cells causes the following: 1) a decrease in transepithelial electrical resistance, implying an opening of the tight junctions [43], 2) alterations in the distribution of the tight junction-associated protein ZO-1 [44], and 3) individual epithelial cells to pull apart [45]. For example, calcium chelation of rabbit tracheal epithelium decreases the transepithelial electrical resistance and increases the transepithelial flux of radiolabelled mannitol, a marker of paracellular permeability [46]. There is *in vivo* evidence that irradiation causes a reversible increase in the permeability of the mouse small intestine junctional complex by a calcium-dependent mechanism [47]. Thus, the integrity of the intercellular junctions appears calcium-dependent.

In a recent study, depletion of extracellular calcium had no apparent effect on the viability of confluent, polarized HT-29 enterocytes, but transepithelial electrical resistance was significantly decreased and the enterocytes pulled apart [41]. Enteric bacteria appeared preferentially adherent on the exposed lateral enterocyte surface (Fig. 4), and the numbers of bacteria (represented by *S. typhimurium, P. mirabilis, E. coli, E. faecalis*) internalized by these enterocytes were significantly increased [41]. Interestingly, the effects of extracellular calcium depletion on HT-29 morphology (cell rounding) and enterocyte function (bacterial uptake) were reversible following restoration of normal growth medium to HT-29 cultures, and others have also noted that opening of enterocytes tight junctions can be a reversible defect in the epithelial barrier [29, 43]. Although extremely low concentrations of extracellular calcium might not occur *in vivo*, subtle variations in calcium concentration may be a significant modulatory signal *in vivo*, and under physiological conditions, this same pathway could be activated by other factor(s) controlling epithelial integrity.

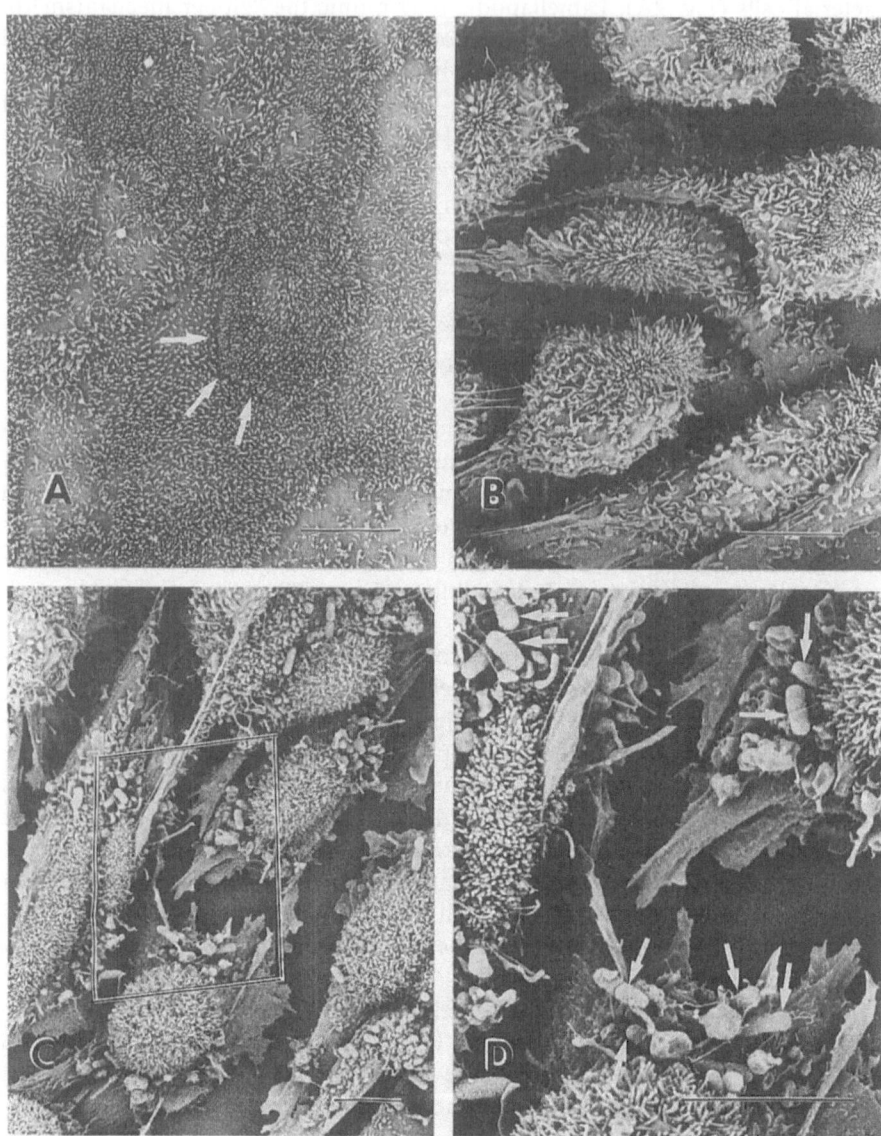

Fig. 4. Effect of low extracellular calcium on bacterial adherence to cultured HT-29 enterocytes viewed with low voltage (3.5 kV), field emission, scanning electron microscopy. A Enterocytes cultivated in normal tissue culture medium, showing a confluent cellular layer with closely apposed intercellular junctions between individual enterocytes (one junction highlighted with *white arrows*): B Enterocytes incubated for 1 h in calcium-free medium, showing separation and rounding of individual enterocytes; C Low magnification of enterocytes treated for 1 h with calcium-free medium, followed by 1 h incubation with *Salmonella typhimurium* ATCC 14028 showing salmonella preferentially adherent to the lateral enterocyte surface, and with the apical enterocyte surface relatively devoid of adherent bacteria; D High magnification of boxed area in (C), where adherent bacteria (some highlighted with *white arrows*) are more clearly visualized. Scale bars: 5.0 microns

In a companion study, HT-29 enterocytes were used to study the effect of *Bacteroides fragilis* enterotoxin on bacteria-enterocyte interactions. *B. fragilis* comprises 1 to 2% of the normal human colonic flora, and is the anaerobic species most commonly isolated from human clinical specimens. A widely known virulence factor is a capsular polysaccharide that induces abscess formation and may be antiphagocytic. However, recent attention has focused on an enterotoxin. *B. fragilis* enterotoxin causes fluid accumulation in ligated ileal loops of experimental animals, and has been implicated in diarrhea in children between 1 and 5 years of age; there is also preliminary evidence that enterotoxigenic strains may be prevalent in clinical isolates (reviewed in [42]). *B. fragilis* enterotoxin has been purified to homogeneity, has a molecular weight of approximately 20 000, and has a cytopathic effect characterized by separation and rounding of HT-29 enterocytes with no detectable loss in enterocyte viability [48]. We recently noted that purified enterotoxin enhanced enterocyte internalization of *S. typhimurium*, *P. mirabilis*, *E. coli*, and *E. faecalis*, and that these bacteria appeared preferentially adherent on the exposed enterocyte lateral membrane [42].

Results of the above study with *B. fragilis* enterotoxin did not prove that the increased internalization of enteric bacteria by HT-29 cells was due to exposure of the enterocyte lateral membranes. However, the almost exact correlation of data obtained with *B. fragilis* enterotoxin with that obtained using low extracellular calcium suggests that exposure of the enterocyte lateral membranes is the most likely explanation. Mounier et al. [49] were the first to suggest that bacteria entering intestinal epithelial cells might not always enter through the apical surface. They showed that *Shigella flexneri* preferentially bound to the lateral membranes of polarized Caco-2 enterocytes when these membranes were artificially exposed by chelation of calcium, and that these adherent bacteria more easily invaded the enterocytes. At this time, it seems reasonable to speculate that compromised intestinal barrier function, i.e. opening of the enterocyte tight junctions, exposes the enterocyte lateral membranes, and may increase the translocation of enteroinvasive bacteria in compromised patients. This speculative hypothesis can only be proven or disproven by careful clinical studies, and such studies will be done only if clinicians become aware of the possible association between compromised intestinal barrier function and increased BT.

Intestinal Epithelial Permeability

Using experimental animals, many investigators have helped clarify the clinical conditions that facilitate BT. These clinical conditions are diverse, and include enteric overgrowth, mesenteric ischemia, hemorrhagic shock, burn wounds and other trauma, surgery, liquid alimentation, bowel stasis, and immunosuppression [2, 9, 10, 23, 50, 51]. Patients at highest risk for increased incidences of BT include immunosuppressed patients, postsurgical patients, and trauma patients. An emerging body of literature supports the hypothesis that compromised gut barrier function, accompanied by increased intestinal epithelial permeability, may be a common mechanism predisposing to BT. Intestinal permeability can be assessed *in vivo* by a variety of techniques that include: 1) urinary excretion of orally administered non-metabolizable sugars, such as lactulose and mannitol known to pass either paracellularly or transcellularly through the intestinal epithelium; and 2) plasma-to-intestinal luminal clearance of radiolabelled tracer molecules, such as ^{51}Cr-ethylene-diamine-tetra-acetic acid (EDTA).

Many investigators have quantitatively assessed gut barrier function (i.e. intestinal epithelial permeability) in experimental animals and in humans with clinical conditions typical of those reported to facilitate BT (Table 2). Interestingly, some investigators have concurrently assessed BT, and have reported increased incidence of translocation associated with concurrent increase in intestinal permeability. These latter reports include rat models of burn injury [53–55], dexamethasone-induced epithelial adherence of enteric flora [89, 90], hemorrhagic shock [66], indomethacin treatment [71], and administration of morphine plus tumor necrosis factor [88]. In addition, administration of parenteral endotoxin has been noted to simultaneously increase BT and intestinal epithelial permeability in mice, rats, and pigs [73–78]. As mentioned above, increased paracellular permeability and increased enterocyte endocytosis of viable bacteria caused by low extracellular calcium was reversible within 24 h [41]; similarly, several animal models associated with increased intestinal permeability, namely parenteral endotoxin and burn wounds, have a transient increase in BT that peaks at 24 h and then reverts to normal levels [90, 91]. Therefore, a speculative hypothesis is that increased intestinal permeability associated with endotoxin and burn wounds might involve a mechanism that is similar to the reversible epithelial permeability caused by low concentrations of extracellular calcium. To summarize, *in vivo* loss of intestinal barrier integrity has been reported in essentially all the diverse clinical conditions associated with BT. A body of literature is emerging supporting the hypothesis that compromised gut barrier

Table 2. Selected reports of increased intestinal permeability in humans and animals

Treatment or clinical condition	Species	References
Burn trauma or multiple trauma	human, rat	[52–61]
Major surgery	human, rat	[62–65]
Hemorrhagic shock	human, rat	[66–67]
Ischemia-reperfusion injury	rat	[68–69]
Indomethacin	human, rat	[70–72]
Parenteral endotoxin	human, mouse, rat, pig	[64, 73–79]
Intensive care patients	human	[80]
Pancreatitis	rat	[81]
Intestinal bacterial overgrowth	dog	[63, 82]
Liquid diet	rat	[83–85]
Small bowel transplant	rat	[86]
Experimental colitis	rat	[87]
Morphine plus tumor necrosis factor	rat	[88]
Dexamethasone	rat	[89–90]

function may be a common factor in the diverse clinical conditions that predispose to BT.

Conclusion

Bacterial translocation is a major factor in the development of systemic infection in hospitalized immunosuppressed, postsurgical, and trauma patients. This statement is based on ample evidence in the literature documenting extraintestinal dissemination of enteric bacteria in complicating infections in high risk hospitalized patients, as well as in a variety of animal models such as enteric overgrowth, mesenteric ischemia, hemorrhagic shock, burn wounds and other trauma, surgery, liquid alimentation, bowel stasis, small bowel transplantation, liver resection, parenteral endotoxin, immunosuppression. There is also evidence in the literature that altered intestinal epithelial permeability may be a common mechanism in the diverse clinical conditions associated with increased incidence of bacterial translocation. This observation requires further confirmation with appropriately designed experiments. However, this observation suggests that novel treatment regimens, eg epithelial barrier-sustaining agents, may be effective in decreasing the costly morbidity associated with complicating infections caused by translocating intestinal bacteria.

Acknowledgement: This work was supported by grant AI-23484 from the National Institutes of Health, USA.

References

1. Bland PW, Kambarage DM (1991) Antigen handling by the epithelium and lamina propria macrophages. In: MacDermott RP, Elson CO (eds) Gastroenterology Clinics of North America, WB Saunders, Philadelphia, pp 577-596
2. Carter L (1994) Bacterial translocation: Nursing implications in the care of patients with neutropenia. Oncology Nursing Forum 21:857-865
3. Emori TG, Gaynes RP (1993) An overview of nosocomial infections, including the role of the microbiology laboratory. Clin Microbiol Rev 6:428-444
4. Centers for Disease Control (1992) Public health focus: Surveillance, prevention, and control of nosocomial infections. Morbidity and Mortality Weekly Reports 41:783-787
5. Tancrede CH, Andremont AO (1985) Bacterial translocation and gram-negative bacteremia in patients with hematological malignancies. J Infect Dis 152:99-103
6. Wells CL, Podzorski RP, Peterson PK, Ramsay NK, Simmons RL, Rhame FS (1984) Incidence of trimethoprim-sulfamethoxazole resistant enterobacteriaceae among transplant recipients. J Infect Dis 150:699-706
7. Wells CL, Juni BA, Cameron SB, Mason KR, Ferrieri P, Rhame FR (1995) Stool carriage, clinical isolation, and mortality during an outbreak of vancomycin-resistant enterococcal infections in hospitalized medical/surgical patients. Clin Infect Dis 21:45-50
8. Ford EG, Baisden CE, Matteson ML, Picone AL (1991) Sepsis after coronary bypass grafting: Evidence for loss of the gut mucosal barrier. Ann Thorac Surg 52:514-517
9. Schlag G, Redl H, Hallstrom S (1991) The cell in shock: The origin of multiple organ failure. Resuscitation 21:137-180

10. Tran DD, van Onselen EBH, Wensink AJF, Cuesta MA (1994) Factors related to multiple organ system failure and mortality in a surgical intensive care unit. Nephrol Dialysis Transplant 9 (Suppl 4):172–178
11. Moore FA, Moore EE, Paggetti R, et al (1991) Gut bacterial translocation via the portal vein: A clinical perspective with major torso trauma. J Trauma 31:629–638
12. Rush BF, Sori AJ, Murphy TF, Smith S, Flanagan JJ, Machiedo GW (1988) Endotoxemia and bacteremia during hemorrhagic shock. The link between trauma and sepsis? Ann Surg 207: 549–554
13. Van der Waaij DJM, Berghuis-de Vries JM, Lekkerkerk-van der Wees JEC (1971) Colonization resistance of the digestive tract and the spread of bacteria to the lymphatic organs in mice. J Hyg 70:335–342
14. Loirat Ph, Johanson WG, Van Saene HKF (1992) First European consensus conference in intensive care medicine: Selective decontamination of the digestive tract in intensive care and emergency medicine. Intensive Care Med 18:182–188
15. Wells CL (1993) A decade of selective decontamination of the digestive tract as prophylaxis for infections in ICU patients: What have we learned? (editorial) Clin Infect Dis 17: 1055–1057
16. Boom SJ, Ramsay G (1992) Selective decontamination of the digestive tract in intensive care. Epidemiol Infect 109:337–347
17. Ambrose NS, Johnson M, Burdon DW, Keighley MRB (1984) Incidence of pathogenic bacteria from mesenteric lymph nodes and ileal serosa during Crohn's disease surgery. Br J Surg 71:623–625
18. Laffineur G, Lescut D, Vincent P, Quandalle P, Wurtz A, Colombel JF (1992) Bacterial translocation in Crohn's disease. Gastroenterol Clin Biol 16:777–781
19. Vincent P, Colombel JF, Lescut D, et al (1988) Bacterial translocation in patients with colorectal cancer. J Infect Dis 158:1395–1396
20. Deitch EA (1989) Simple intestinal obstruction causes bacterial translocation in man. Arch Surg 124:699–701
21. Peitzman AB, Odekwu AO, Ochoa J, Smith A (1991) Bacterial translocation in trauma patients. J Trauma 31:1083–1087
22. Koha M, Brismar B, Wikstrom B, Ewrth S, Nord CE (1992) Bacterial colonization and translocation in colorectal carcinoma. Med Microbiol Lett 1:168–176
23. Sedman PC, Macfie J, Sagar P, et al (1994) The prevalence of gut translocation in humans. Gastroenterol 107:643–649
24. Brathwaite CEM, Ross SE, Nagele R, Mure AJ, O'Malley KF, Garcia-Perez FA (1993) Bacterial translocation occurs in humans after traumatic injury: Evidence using immunofluorescence. J Trauma 34:586–590
25. Reed LL, Martin M, Manglano R, Newson B, Kocka F, Barrett J (1994) Bacterial translocation following abdominal trauma in humans. Circ Shock 42:1–6
26. van Goor H, Rosman C, Ground J, Kooi K, Wubbels GH, Bleichrodt RP (1994) Translocation of bacteria and endotoxin in organ donors. Arch Surg 129:1063–1066
27. Wells CL, Jechorek RP, Erlandsen SL (1990) Evidence for the translocation of *Enterococcus faecalis* across the mouse intestinal tract. J Infect Dis 162:82–90
28. Mainous MR, Tso P, Berg RD, Deitch EA (1991) Studies of the route, magnitude, and time course of bacterial translocation in a model of systemic inflammation. Arch Surg 126: 33–37
29. Madara JL (1990) Pathobiology of the intestinal epithelial barrier. Am J Pathol 137: 1273–1281
30. Alexander JW, Boyce ST, Babcock GF, et al (1990) The process of microbial translocation. Surgery 212:496–512
31. Cole GT, Seshan KR, Pope LM, Vancey RJ (1988) Morphological analysis of gastrointestinal tract invasion by *Candida albicans* in the infant mouse. J Med Vet Mycol 26:173–185
32. Wells CL, Erlandsen SL (1991) Localization of translocating *Escherichia coli*, *Proteus mirabilis*, and *Enterococcus faecalis* within cecal and colonic tissue of monoassociated mice. Infect Immun 59:4693–4697

33. Wells CL, Jechorek RP, Erlandsen SL (1990) Evidence for the translocation of *Enterococcus faecalis* across the mouse intestinal tract. J Infect Dis 162:82-90
34. Falkow S, Isberg RR, Portnoy DA (1992) The interaction of bacteria with mammalian cells. Annu Rev Cell Biol 8:333-363
35. Brandtzaeg P (1989) Overview of the mucosal immune system. Curr Topics Microbiol Immunol 146:13-25
36. Neutra M, Louvard D (1989) Differentiation of intestinal epithelial cells *in vitro*. In: Satir BH (ed) Functional epithelial cells in culture. Alan R Liss, New York, pp 363-398
37. Wells CL, Jechorek RP, Olmsted SB, Erlandsen SL (1993) Effect of LPS on epithelial integrity and bacterial uptake in the polarized human enterocyte-like cell line Caco-2. Circ Shock 40:276-288
38. Wells CL, Jechorek RP, Olmsted SB, Erlandsen SL (1994) Bacterial translocation in cultured enterocytes: Magnitude, specificity, and electron microscopic observations of endocytosis. Shock 1:443-451
39. Olmsted SB, Dunny GM, Erlandsen SL, Wells CL (1994) A plasmid-encoded surface protein on *Enterococcus faecalis* augments its internalisation by cultured intestinal epithelial cells. J Infect Dis 170:1549-1556
40. Griffin FM Jr, Griffin JA, Silverstein SC (1975) Studies on the mechanism of phagocytosis. I. Requirements for circumferential attachment of particle-bound ligands to specific receptors on the macrophage plasma membrane. J Exp Med 142:1263-1282
41. Wells CL, van de Westerlo EMA, Jechorek RP, Erlandsen SL (1995) Exposure of the lateral enterocyte membrane by dissociation of calcium-dependent junctional complex augments endocytosis of enteric bacteria. Shock 4:204-210
42. Wells CL, van de Westerlo EMA, Jechorek RP, Feltis BA, Wilkins TD, Erlandsen SL (1996) *Bacteroides fragilis* enterotoxin modulates epithelial permeability and bacterial internalization by HT-29 enterocytes. Gastroenterol (In press)
43. Armitage WJ, Juss BK, Easty DL (1994) Response of epithelial (MDCK) cell junctions to calcium removal and osmotic stress is influenced by temperature. Cryobiology 31:453-460
44. Howarth AG, Singer KL, Stevenson BR (1994) Analysis of the distribution and phosphorylation state of ZO-1 in MDCK and non-epithelial cells. J Membrane Biol 137:261-270
45. Citi S (1992) Protein kinase inhibitors prevent junction dissociation induced by low extracellular calcium in MDCK epithelial cells. J Cell Biol 117:169-178
46. Bhat M, Toledo-Velasquez D, Wang L, Malanga CJ, Ma JK, Rojanasakul Y (1993) Regulation of tight junction permeability by calcium mediators and cell cytoskeleton in rabbit tracheal epithelium. Pharmaceutical Res 10:991-997
47. Somosy Z, Kovacs J, Siklos L, Koteles GJ (1993) Morphological and histochemical changes in intercellular junctional complexes in epithelial cells of mouse small intestine upon X-irradiation: Changes of ruthenium red permeability and calcium content. Scanning Microscopy 7:961-971
48. Moncrief JS, Obiso R Jr, Barroso LA, et al (1995) The enterotoxin of *Bacteroides fragilis* is a metalloprotease. Infect Immun 63:175-181
49. Mounier J, Vasselon T, Hellio R, Lesourd M, Sansonetti PJ (1992) *Shigella flexneri* enters human colonic Caco-2 epithelial cells through the basolateral pole. Infect Immun 60:237-248
50. Edmiston CE, Condon RE (1991) Bacterial translocation. Surg Gyn Obstetrics 173:73-83
51. Van Leeuwen PA, Boermeester MA, Houdijk AP, et al (1994) Clinical significance of translocation. Gut 35:S28-S34
52. Ryan CM, Bailey SH, Carter EA, Schoenfeld DA, Tompkins RG (1994) Additive effects of thermal injury and infection on gut permeability. Arch Surg 129:325-328
53. Berthiaume F, Ezzell RM, Toner M, Yarmush ML, Tompkins RG (1994) Transport of fluorescent dextrans across the rat ileum after cutaneous thermal injury. Crit Care Med 22:455-464
54. Horton JW (1994) Bacterial translocation after burn injury: The contribution of ischemia and permeability changes. Shock 1:286-290
55. Messick WJ, Koruda M, Meyer A, Zimmerman K (1994) Differential changes in intestinal permeability following burn injury. J Trauma 36:306-311

56. Rhodes RS, Karnovsky MJ (1971) Loss of macromolecular barrier function associated with surgical trauma to the intestine. Lab Invest 25:220–229
57. Ziegler TR, Smith RJ, O'Dwyer ST, Demling RH, Wilmore DW (1988) Increased intestinal permeability associated with infection in burn patients. Arch Surg 123:1313–1319
58. Deitch EA (1990) Intestinal permeability is increased in burn patients shortly after injury. Surg 107:411–416
59. Ryan CM, Yarmush ML, Burke JF, Tompkins (1992) Increased gut permeability early after burns correlates with the extent of burn injury. Crit Care Med 20:1508–1512
60. Pape HC, Dweger A, Regel G, et al (1994) Increased gut permeability after multiple trauma. Br J Surg 81:850–852
61. Langkamp-Henken B, Donovan TB, Pate LM, Maull CD, Kudsk KA (1995) Increased intestinal permeability following blunt and penetrating trauma. Crit Care Med 23:660–664
62. Wang XD, Parsson H, Andersson R, Soltesz V, Johansson K, Bengmark S (1994) Bacterial translocation, intestinal ultrastructure and cell membrane permeability early after major liver resection in the rat. Br J Surg 81:579–584
63. Morris TH, Sorensen SH, Turkington J, Batt RM (1994) Diarrhoea and increased intestinal permeability in laboratory beagles associated with proximal small intestinal bacterial overgrowth. Lab Animals 28:313–319
64. Herlbert DJ, Zhong R, Wang P (1989) Intestinal permeability with hemorrhagic shock, surgical trauma, and endotoxemia. Surg Forum 40:93–95
65. Roumen RM, van der Vliet JA, Wevers RA, Goris JA (1993) Intestinal permeability is increased after major vascular surgery. J Vascular Surg 17:734–737
66. Deitch EA, Morrison J, Berg RD, Specian RD (1990) Effect of hemorrhagic shock on bacterial translocation, intestinal morphology, and intestinal permeability in conventional and antibiotic-decontaminated rats. Crit Care Med 18:529–536
67. Roumen RM, Hendriks T, Wevers RA, Goris JA (1993) Intestinal permeability after severe trauma and hemorrhagic shock is increased without relation to septic complications. Arch Surg 128:453–457
68. Horton JW, Walker PB (1993) Oxygen radicals, lipid peroxidation, and permeability changes after intestinal ischemia and reperfusion. J Appl Physiol 74:1515–1520
69. Vaughn WG, Horton JW, Walker PB (1992) Allopurinol prevents intestinal permeability changes after ischemia-reperfusion injury. J Pedr Surg 27:968–972
70. Mion F, Cuber JC, Minaire Y, Chayvialle JA (1994) Short-term effects of indomethacin on rat small intestinal permeability. Role of eicosanoids and platelet activating factor. Gut 35:490–495
71. Yamada T, Deitch E, Specian RD, Perry MA, Sartor RB, Grisham MB (1993) Mechanisms of acute and chronic intestinal inflammation induced by indomethacin. Inflammation 17:641–662
72. Davies GR, Wilkie ME, Prampton DS (1993) Effects of metronidazole and misoprostol on indomethacin-induced changes in intestinal permeability. Dig Dis Sci 38:417–425
73. Salzman AL, Wang H, Wollert PS, et al (1994) Endotoxin-induced ileal mucosal hyperpermeability in pigs: Role of tissue acidosis. Am J Physiol 266:G633–G646
74. Xu D, Qi L, Guillory D, Cruz N, Berg R, Deitch EA (1993) Mechanisms of endotoxin-induced intestinal injury in a hyperdynamic model of sepsis. J Trauma 34:676–682
75. Walker RI, Porvaznik MJ (1978) Disruption of the permeability barrier (zonula occludens) between intestinal epithelial cells by lethal doses of endotoxin. Infect Immun 21:655–658
76. Fink MP, Antonsson JB, Wang H, Rothschild HR (1991) Increased intestinal permeability in endotoxic pigs. Arch Surg 126:211–218
77. Fink MP, Kaups KL, Wang HL, Rothschild HR (1991) Maintenance of superior mesenteric arterial perfusion prevents increased intestinal permeability in endotoxic pigs. Surg 110:154–160
78. Deitch EA, Specian RD, Berg RD (1991) Endotoxin-induced bacterial translocation and mucosal permeability: Role of xanthine oxidase, complement activation, and macrophage products. Crit Care Med 19:785–789
79. O'Dwyer ST, Michie HR, Ziegler TR, Revhaug A, Smith RJ, Wilmore DW (1988) A single dose of endotoxin increases intestinal permeability in healthy humans. Arch Surg 123:1459–1464

80. Harris CE, Griffiths RD, Freestone N, Billington D, Atherton ST, Macmillan RR (1992) Intestinal permeability in the critically ill. Intensive Care Med 18:38–41
81. Ryan CM, Schmidt J, Lewandrowski K, et al (1993) Gut macromolecular permeability in pancreatitis correlates with severity of disease in rats. Gastroenterol 105:956–957
82. Batt RM, Hall EJ, McLean L, Simpson KW (1992) Small intestinal bacterial overgrowth and enhanced intestinal permeability in healthy beagles. Am J Vet Res 53:1935–1940
83. Spaeth G, Gottwald T, Specian RD, Mainous MR, Berg RD, Deitch EA (1994) Secretory immunoglobulin A, intestinal mucin, and mucosal permeability in nutritionally-induced bacterial translocation in rats. Ann Surg 220:798–808
84. Li J, Langkamp-Henken B, Suzuki K, Stahlgren LH (1994) Glutamine prevents parenteral nutrition-induced increases in intestinal permeability. J Parent Enteral Nutr 18:289–290
85. Illig KA, Ryan CK, Hardy DJ, Rhodes J, Locke W, Sax HC (1992) Total parenteral nutrition-induced changes in gut mucosal function: Atropy alone is not the issue. Surg 112:631–637
86. Grant D, Hurlbut D, Zhong R, et al (1991) Intestinal permeability and bacterial translocation following small bowel transplantation in the rat. Transplantation 52:221–224
87. Pantzar N, Ekstrom GM, Wang Q, Westrom BR (1994) Mechanisms of increased intestinal CrEDTA absorption during experimental colitis in the rat. Dig Dis Sci 39:2327–2333
88. Leslie KA, Behme R, Clift A, Martin S, Grant D, Duff JH (1994) Synergistic effects of tumor necrosis factor and morphine on gut barrier function. Can J Surg 37:143–147
89. Spitz J, Hecht G, Taveras M, Aoys E, Alverdy J (1994) The effect of dexamethasone administration on rat intestinal permeability: The role of bacterial adherence. Gastroenterology 106:35–41
90. Alverdy J, Aoys E (1991) The effect of glucocorticoid administration on bacterial translocation. Evidence for an acquired mucosal immunodeficient state. Ann Surg 214:719–723
91. Wells CL, Barton RG, Erlandsen SL, Cerra FB, Jechorek RP, Dunn D (1990) Parenteral endotoxin and intestinal function. In: Nowotny A, Spitzer JJ, Ziegler EJ (eds) Cellular and molecular aspects of endotoxin reactions. Endotoxin research series, vol 1, Elsevier, New York, pp 509–519
92. Jones WG, Minei JP, Richardson RP, et al (1990) Pathophysiologic glucocorticoid elevations promote bacterial translocation after thermal injury. Infect Immun 58:3257–3261

Is Bacterial Translocation Clinically Relevant?

H. Redl, S. Bahrami, and G. Schlag

Introduction

Endotoxin, derived from the cell wall of gram-negative organisms, may be responsible for much of the pathophysiology found in patients in an intensive care unit. It has been suggested that the intestine is the source of endotoxin (eg lipopolysaccharide (LPS)) in a number of clinical conditions [1]:
1) when the gut barrier function is lost in critical illness [2]; and
2) when bacterial/endotoxin translocation (BT) occurs with subsequent endotoxemia and bacteremia [3, 4].

This hypothesis is a possible explanation of the hitherto unknown pathogenesis of septic events where no focus of organisms has been identified.

Both hypoxic damage itself [5] and reperfusion damage might be responsible for intestinal injury that may result in increased translocation [6]. It should however be kept in mind that reduced elimination during shock [7] without any change in the real translocation rate might also lead to the observation of "increased BT" during shock [8].

In order to deal with the question of the relevance of BT, one can approach the problem from four different directions (Fig. 1).

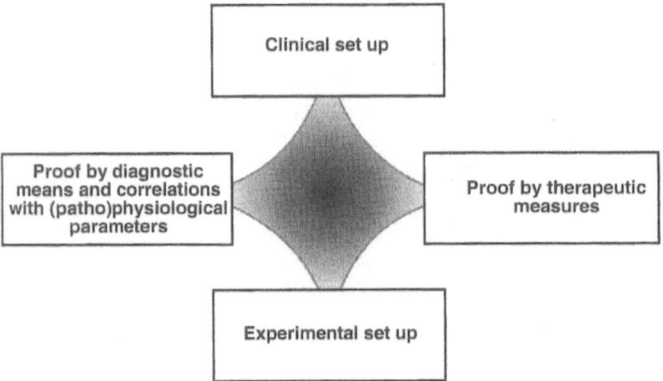

Fig. 1. Different approaches to study the relevance of bacterial translocation

Detection of Bacterial Translocation

The direct detection of BT is hampered by several factors such as the difficulty to detect positive blood cultures especially with small sample volumes, and the failure to detect bacteria in organs using culture techniques (= only live bacteria). On the other hand, the detection of endotoxin (just as of bacteria) is hampered by fast clearance, non-continuous release, and insensitive detection systems, which may lead to false negative results regarding BT.

After the first passage through the epithelial layer, bacteria and toxins pass the lamina propria, where immunologically active cells of the gut-associated lymphatic tissues (GALT) are located. Bacteria or endotoxin might be scavenged in this layer, in which case they would no longer be detectable but could induce local cytokine formation as suggested by the work of several groups [9–12]. Detection of cytokine formation could then be used as one of the factors permitting indirect proof of BT (Fig. 2).

In an experimental study [13], it was determined that tumor necrosis factor (TNF) increased faster in the portal than in the systemic circulation and that the maximum levels were higher. Cabie et al. [14] reported similar results in patients, finding significantly higher levels of TNF in the portal vein than in systemic samples. Further, Shenkar and Abraham [10] found the first induction of cytokine mRNA after hemorrhage in the gut. This leads us to hypothesize that when LPS or bacteria reach the lamina propria, macrophages might locally produce cytokines without it being necessary to transport endotoxin via portal vein (consequently, without detection of LPS) and to the liver to provoke a cytokine response [11]. Local TNF production is also a possible explanation for why TNF, but not endotoxin, could be detected after hemorrhagic shock in some studies (eg Ayala et al. [15]). It should also be taken into consideration that the source of post-hemorrhagic inflammatory cytokines could also be Kupffer cells, some of which might be activated by shock-related hypoxia [16].

Another possible means of indirect proof of BT is the measurement of gut wall permeability by means of tracers (eg lactulose/mannitol, used eg in trauma pa-

Indirect - primary reactions	Flow mesenteric artery / pHi Permeability - tracer	
Direct	Live bacteria Live or dead bacteria Bacterial toxins D-lactate	*Where ?* • Organs • Systemic Portal ⟩ Blood • Lymph
Indirect - secondary reactions	Cytokines	

Fig. 2. Direct and indirect indicators of bacterial translocation

tients [7, 17]), but which, of course, is not equivalent to the measurement of LPS or bacterial cultures.

Viable or Non-Viable Bacteria

The low sensitivity to detect bacteria in blood might be due to the rapid clearance by the body's reticular endothelial system (RES). In an experimental setting, a blood concentration of 1×10^5 CFU *E. coli*/mL was reduced to 0 within 15 min when the infusion of *E. coli* was stopped [18].

Several measures have been taken to overcome the measurement problem such as by feeding animals radioactively labelled bacteria and by tracing radio-activity in the blood [19, 20]. Another approach was taken to detect bacteria in organs, using antibodies to bacteria constituents in order to detect both viable and non-viable bacteria [20, 21]. With such techniques, Alexander et al. [20] found that less than 1% of translocating bacteria were viable. This is consistent with a recent patient study in which the macrophages of bacterial culture-negative mesenteric lymph nodes were found to contain *E. coli* β-galactosid-ase, indicating the presence of non-viable phagocytized bacteria [22]. Further-more, electron microscopic evaluation of mesenteric lymph nodes demonstrated that the incidence of translocation is greater than anticipated by culture alone [23].

Endotoxin

Despite the generally good quality of commercially available test systems, poten-tial sources of error still exist. The test is not absolutely specific (even when a fac-tor G free lysate preparation is used). One major source of error is the blood (plasma) sampling procedure, because commercially available blood collection tubes may be contaminated with endotoxin. Plasma separation and storage may generate cytokines, and blood collection tubes may adsorb endotoxin to the tube walls. To preclude error in blood sampling and handling, new blood collection tubes have been developed [24]. These tubes are sterile and pyrogen-free and al-low samples to be stored and transported for further analysis while avoiding common sources of contamination. Various sample treatment methods are sug-gested to eliminate interference from proteases, some of which are very un-reliable. Combined dilution and heat treatment is the most convenient and use-ful method for treating plasma samples.

The absence of measurable amounts of circulating endotoxin (at specific time points) is not absolute proof of the absence of bacteria in sepsis. Usually, the de-tection of endotoxin is only possible in a certain percentage of subjects, eg 61% in Cabie's study [14]. Detection might be made impossible by the endotoxin re-lease kinetics (short peaks), insensitive measurement techniques, or very high (local) potency of the endotoxins even at extremely low non-detectable systemic concentrations. The presence of measurable amounts of endotoxin in the systemic circulation is probably just an indication of an exhaustion of RES, which can no longer provide full clearance capacity. This conclusion stems from experimental settings where LPS is only detectable in the systemic circulation after partial resection of the liver in a gut ischemia-reperfusion (I/R) situation [25] or from liver transplantation studies [26]. The liver's capacity to clear endotoxin has been reported to be 1–5 µg/g liver/h in rats [3], and Nakao et al. [27] demonstrated that 98–99.9% of endotoxin could be eliminated within 5 min of intravenous injection.

Detection problems might be the cause of the failure of the diagnostic approach to detect BT in experimental hemorrhagic shock [16, 28].

D(−)-Lactate

D(−)-lactate is produced by indigenous bacteria found in the gastrointestinal tract, and mammals do not possess the enzyme systems to rapidly metabolize it [29]. An increase in D(−)-lactate may therefore reflect an efflux of bacteria and/or its products into circulation due to mucosal injury. Recently, there have been reports of increased serum D(−)-lactate in animal models of acute intestinal ischemia and simple obstruction [30] and in I/R of the small bowel associated with failure of the intestinal mucosal barrier. Prophylactic intervention with neutralizing antibody to TNF significantly ameliorated intestinal lesions and attenuated the increase in plasma D(−)-lactate [31]. Moreover, in a clinical study, Murray et al. [32] demonstrated that patients found to have mesenteric ischemia at laparotomy had significantly elevated D(−)-lactate levels in peripheral blood compared with patients with either an acute or normal abdomen. Plasma D(−)-lactate levels can be measured by an enzymatic spectrophotometric assay [33] with a slight modification using a centrifugal analyzer [31] and could thus help to achieve easy non-invasive detection of BT.

Clinical Setup – Diagnostic Means

A serious limitation in research on BT is that human data are extremely limited, but in the following section a few examples are reviewed.

Ischemia/Reperfusion (I/R)

An intraoperative increase in the level of plasma endotoxin primarily occurs after initiation of cardiopulmonary bypass and the removal of the aortic cross clamp [34]. In another study, Schlag et al. [35] were also able to detect endotoxin in the systemic circulation during cardiopulmonary bypass; they also reported the release of cytokines and especially of soluble cytokine receptors such as TNF receptors.

154   H. Redl, S. Bahrami, and G. Schlag

Shock, Trauma and Critically Ill Patients

One study with 50 polytraumatized patients [36] revealed positive blood cultures in 26% of the trauma victims within 3 h of trauma. In another trauma study [37], no positive blood cultures were found in samples obtained from portal vein catheters. Similarily, Endo et al. [38] failed to find elevated LPS levels in 29 patients with hemorrhagic shock, but Roumen et al. [39] reported systemic endotoxemia to be a common finding in patients after major vascular operation and hemorrhagic shock. Braithwaite et al. [22] found bacteria in the lymph nodes of trauma patients using histochemical techniques, and most recently it has been shown that severe injury leads to increased intestinal permeability lasting several days [40]. A correlation between increased permeability and translocation was not shown, however. In patients undergoing elective surgery, Deitch [41] found that only 4% of the mesenteric lymph nodes (MLN) contain bacteria; in contrast, he detected bacteria among MLN in 59% of patients undergoing surgery for small bowel obstructions [42]. In another series of 267 general surgical patients, translocation occurred in 10.3% of the patients overall [43].

In a study measuring endotoxin and cytokines in the systemic and portal blood of patients undergoing abdominal aortic surgery [9], portal LPS was detected after bowel manipulation in 36% and during the reperfusion phase in 71% of the cases. In contrast to endotoxin, positive blood cultures could not be found in either the portal or in the systemic circulation. The absorption of BT and LPS is also frequent among organ donors and may adversely influence organ function in transplant recipients and other critically ill patients [44].

Using a limulus test with a high sensitivity of 0.02 EU/mL, Berger and Beger [45] studied several aspects of postoperative endotoxemia. In 13 patients with peritonitis and operative treatment on continuous peritoneal lavage, they found maximum levels of LPS 1 day after the operation. Endotoxin plasma levels decreased over the next 4–5 days. They also asked whether patients undergoing elective surgery not involving the gut region would develop endotoxemia as a result of BT. They again found significantly increased levels of LPS in plasma on the first postoperative day, even in patients with strumectomy only. With sufficiently sensitive LPS assays, it is probable that more interesting data will be collected, which should help us answer the question as to the significance of LPS monitoring in patients.

Burns

In patients with extensive burns, early increases (7–12 h and 3–4 days post-burn) in plasma endotoxin have been reported by Winchurch et al. [46] and Dobke et al. [47]. These increases were not attributed to the burn wound itself, but to BT. In a group of extensively burned patients (more than 70% TBSA), endotoxemia was not only common in the immediate post-injury period but also strongly associated with the development of multiple organ failure and an adverse outcome [48]. In addition, there have been reports that intestinal permeability be increased shortly after injury [49–51].

In summary, clinical studies provide both positive and negative findings in BT, the differences depending partly on the measurement technique used and partly on the specific clinical setting. It is difficult, however to draw any conclusions relevant to clinical outcome from the abovementioned studies.

Experimental Setup – Diagnostic Means

Ischemia/Reperfusion

Studies on the route of LPS translocation from the gut have primarily focused on superior mesenteric artery occlusion shock. Based on these studies, it has been suggested that gut-derived LPS enters the systemic circulation mainly via the portal vein during intestinal ischemia [52, 53]. The accompanying BT is also associated with cytokine (TNF and interleukin (IL)-6) formation mainly after reperfusion [31, 54].

Such studies raise the question as to the exact cause of epithelial damage: hypoxia, reperfusion injury, or both? Haglund et al. [55] have performed extensive experimental studies on hypoxia and gut damage during hypotension and shock. They observed that mucosal alterations developed during arterial hypotension secondary to increased oxygen "shunting" in the countercurrent exchanger [56].

Hemorrhagic Shock

Endotoxemia and also bacteremia together with penetrating bacteria in the intestinal wall have been detected after hemorrhagic shock in rats [13, 36]. By comparing the portal and systemic endotoxin levels, it was noted that the significant rise in the portal circulation took place half an hour before that in the systemic circulation. The LPS levels were higher in the portal than in the systemic circulation throughout the experiment [13]. In the baboon trauma model of Schlag et al. [18], LPS and bacteremia were also found systemically, similar to previous studies [57].

There have also been reports of failures to detect positive LPS or bacteria levels [15, 28]. In this respect, it is evident that the experimental set up (eg species differences and the age of animals, type and depth of anesthesia, animal temperature, duration of shock and type of resuscitation) might also influence BT [58].

Burns

Using a non-lethal burn injury model, Deitch et al. [59] found that 44% of the rats with a 40% TBSA burn had viable, gram-negative bacteria in the MLN. The combination of trauma and intestinal overgrowth with gram-negative enteric bacilli or *Candida* may result in the synergistic spread of bacteria from the gut to systemic organs, such as the spleen and liver [59, 60]. It was also shown that burn injury followed by wound infection with *Pseudomonas* caused prolonged and enhanced BT [61]. On the other hand, using a radionuclide probe of a specific organism or endotoxin, Alexander et al. [20] reported that both organism and endotoxin translocated very early (within 1 h) after burn injury. BT has also been shown to take place in large animals subject to thermal injury. In a series of experiments in awake sheep, Morris et al. [62] found translocation after thermal injury, smoke inhalation, and a combination of the two.

Relevance

As with all factors that can be identified, the basic question remains whether BT is clinically relevant. The few interesting correlations between BT parameters and clinical variables are no final proof. It is necessary to therapeutically interfere with gut permeability or potentially translocated bacteria/endotoxin and determine the therapeutic effect on secondary organ dysfunction and mortality (without necessarily being able to detect either bacteria or endotoxin) in order to obtain a final answer.

Clinical Setup – Therapeutic Means

When the gut is suspected of being the source of bacteria causing systemic infections, the most logical approach is to reduce the amount of bacteria in the gut lumen and minimize the chance for BT. Since it is almost impossible to sterilize the gut, the regimen of selective digestive decontamination (SDD) with antibiotics was developed [63]. Several clinical trials with SDD have been performed with the rather consistent finding of decreased nosocomial infections, but with only one study demonstrating clinical benefits in terms of survival [64].

There are several reasons why such therapy might not be successful. Especially in the case of trauma, the onset of therapy is too late. Also it is probably not the whole bacteria, but especially bacterial toxins such as endotoxin, that induce the host response, and SDD is usually not designed to neutralize endotoxin. A logical consequence would be a direct anti-LPS approach (either in the gut lumen or systemic) [65], but this is usually not realized in the clinical setting. In one case, early post-burn translocational endotoxemia was treated with polymyxin B, but this did not influence the cytokine cascade or the mortality rate [66]. A trauma study with a probably more potent anti-LPS agent (BPI-21) is currently under way in the US. The lack of clinical data compels us to rely on experimental studies.

Finally, there are also therapeutic approaches to support the gut wall by the appropriate (mainly enteral) nutrition. For instance enteral nutrition in critically ill patients improved the GI tract dysfunction (= permeability) [67] measured by urinary recovery of tracers. According to a recent review, there is no direct evidence suggesting that enteral nutrition prevents or modifies BT in humans [68].

Experimental Setup – Therapeutic Means

Many different approaches can be taken to reduce BT and thus improve the 'clinical' conditions of test animals. The wide variety of strategies has recently been summarized [65], and includes 'maintenance' of the gut wall with a resultant lower permeability, in addition to anti-LPS therapy or SDD (Fig. 3).

If invading enteric bacteria and especially endotoxin are indeed the reason for sepsis to develop, then germ-free animals [69] or animals treated with agents to eliminate bacterial endotoxin should be more resistant, for example to hemorrhagic insult. In fact, such protective effects have been reported from studies using different approaches. Donahue et al. [70] reported that late survival in their rat hemorrhagic shock model was significantly improved when antibiotics against translocated bacteria were given to the animals in the post-shock period. Because of its LPS-binding, lactoferrin has been reported to result in decreased [21] cytokine production. Lactoferrin was given orally [71] in a rat hemorrhagic shock model. A dose-dependent reduction in endotoxin transfer from the intestinal tract was measured in the therapy group receiving lactoferrin.

In an experiment in which rabbits were subject to hemorrhagic shock after they had been previously fed with *E. coli*, bacterial and endotoxin translocation was detected. In this model, the incidence of multiorgan failure was significantly reduced and survival rate was increased in animals pretreated with an anticore endotoxin antiserum [72].

A murine monoclonal antibody, which is widely cross reactive and protective against smooth and rough LPS from members of *Enterobacteriacae*, was employed in a rat model of prolonged hemorrhagic shock [73]. This treatment resulted in a significant reduction in 48 h mortality, which was 79% in the control group and 27% in the treatment group. Histopathological examinations also re-

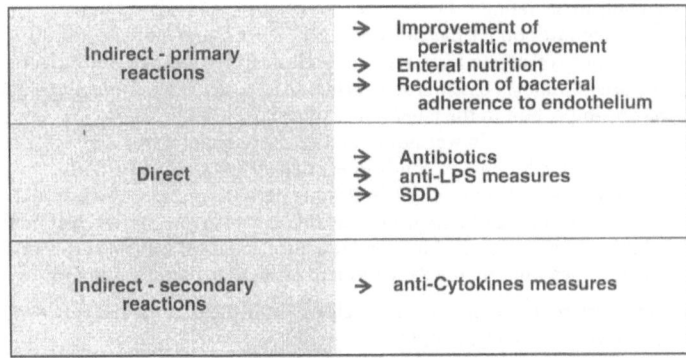

Fig. 3. Possible therapeutic approaches to deal with bacterial translocation

vealed significantly less damage to various organs in the treatment group. These studies, together with previous ones [74, 75], suggest the importance of endogenous endotoxemia after shock/trauma and indicate that, at least in rat, *Enterobacteriacae* might provide the main source of bacterial endotoxin [73]. It is important to know that treatment with the anti-LPS antibody not only neutralized systemic endotoxemia and protected the animals but also significantly reduced the incidence of BT in the intestinal wall, which supports the assumption that endotoxin itself might induce a feedback mechanism further enhancing the translocation process.

A protein from human neutrophils – bactericidal permeability increasing protein (BPI) – was initially characterized as an antibiotic protein only later to be found a homologous protein to lipopolysaccharide binding protein (LBP). Similar to LBP, BPI binds endotoxin, but in contrast to LBP it inhibits CD14-mediated stimulation of leukocytes [76–78]. BPI was demonstrated to blocking endotoxin (translocated during or after hemorrhagic shock) by Bahrami et al. with BPI23 [22] and BPI21 [79].

Results from both the BPI and the endotoxin antibody experiments as well as older [80] and more recent successful hemorrhagic shock experiments with LPS-tolerant animals [81] indicate that endotoxin is an important factor in organ dysfunction and survival after hemorrhagic shock. Nevertheless, it is probably not the only factor since some of the animals are not fully protected with the anti-endotoxin regimen. This could be due either to insufficient treatment protocols or to mediators other than endotoxin, eg hypovolemia-associated ischemia and hypoxia, being at least partially responsible for organ dysfunction and mortality.

Despite the differences in the models, the common theme is that BT is clearly evident, not only demonstrated by the less reliable diagnostic techniques, but also by the results of therapeutic studies (Table 1). The therapeutic approach also

Table 1. Current view on the relevance of human BT

	Ref.
– Translocation occurs as a spontaneous event in humans, but its clinical significance remains to be defined	[43]
– Extensive work on BT has been performed in animal models. It is difficult to extrapolate these results to humans and its clinical significance is not clear	[82]
– The predominance of *Enterobacteriaceae* in patients with infection suggests that BT may be important in the late MOF septic state	[83]
– Circulating endotoxin was not related to subsequent adverse effects of either the patients treated for acute conditions or electively treated patients	[39]
– The clinical significance of BT in trauma patients remains unclear	[22]
– Convincing data to establish a causal link between gut barrier dysfunction and organ failure in humans are lacking, and the importance of translocation and/or mucosal hyperpermeability on the development of MOF in patients remains to be elucidated	[84]

In summary these statements pretty clearly indicate that the relevance of BT in humans is far from being widely accepted

MOF: multiple organ failure

proves the importance of translocation events for organ dysfunction and survival, at least in rodents (which hopefully will be corroborated by forthcoming primate studies).

Conclusion

There is good data on the role of BT in the experimental (including non-human primates) and clinical settings despite the many limitations inherent in the current measurement techniques. Data on its *relevance* can only be obtained, however, by therapeutic approaches, which so far have been largely limited to the experimental arena. This leaves the question regarding the relevance in humans open until adequate clinical studies with improved therapeutic agents can be performed. The interesting positive results in animals suggest that potential beneficial aspects are to be expected from forthcoming clinical trials.

Acknowledgement: Parts of cited projects are supported by Lorenz Böhler Fond.

References

1. Fine J, Ruteburg SH, Schweinburg FB (1959) The role of the RES in hemorrhagic shock. J Exp Med 110:547–551
2. Carrico CJ, Meakins JL, Marshall JC, Fry D, Maier RV (1986) Multiple organ failure syndrome. The gastrointestinal tract: The "motor" of MOF. Arch Surg 121:196–208
3. Berg RD, Wommack E, Deitch EA (1988) Immunosuppression and intestinal bacterial overgrowth synergistically promote bacterial translocation. Arch Surg 123:1359–1364
4. Deitch EA, Berg RD (1987) Endotoxin but not malnutrition promotes bacterial translocation of the gut flora in burned mice. J Trauma 27:161–166
5. Haglund U (1993) Hypoxic damage. In: Schlag G, Redl H (eds) Pathophysiology of shock, sepsis, and organ failure. Springer-Verlag, Berlin Heidelberg New York, pp 314–321
6. Granger DN (1988) Role of xanthine oxidase and granulocytes in ischemia-reperfusion injury. Am J Physiol 255:H1269–H1275
7. Pape HC, Dwenger A, Regel G, et al (1994) Increased gut permeability after multiple trauma. Br J Surg 81:850–852
8. Cruz N, Lu Q, Alvarez X, Deitch EA (1994) Bacterial translocation is bacterial species dependent: Results using the human Caco-2 intestinal cell line. J Trauma 36:612–616
9. Yao YM, Tian HM, Sheng ZY, Wang YP, Shi ZG, Lan FS (1992) The role of endotoxin in the pathogenesis of experimental multiple system organ failure: A preliminary report. Chin Med Sci J 7:161–165
10. Shenkar R, Abraham E (1993) Effects of hemorrhage on cytokine gene transcription. Lymphokine Cytokine Res 12:237–247
11. Bahrami S, Yao YM, Leichtfried G, Redl H, Schlag G, Foulkes R (1994) Efficacy of monoclonal antibody (mab) to tumor necrosis factor (TNF) against hemorrhage-induced mortality in rats. Intensive Care Med 20:S61 (Abstract)
12. Sanderson PJ (1989) Selective decontamination of the digestive tract. Br Med J 299:1413–1414
13. Jiang JX, Bahrami S, Leichtfried G, Redl H, Oehlinger W, Schlag G (1995) Kinetics of endotoxin and tumor necrosis factor appearence in portal and systemic circulation following hemorrhagic shock in rats. Ann Surg 221:100–106
14. Cabie A, Farkas JC, Fitting C, et al (1993) High levels of portal TNF-α during abdominal aortic surgery in man. Cytokine 5:448–453

15. Ayala A, Perrin MM, Meldrum DR, Ertel W, Chaudry IH (1990) Hemorrhage induces an increase in serum TNF which is not associated with elevated levels of endotoxins. Cytokine 2:170–174
16. Chaudry IH, Ertel W, Ayala A (1993) Alterations in inflammatory cytokine production following hemorrhage and resuscitation. In: Schlag G, Redl H, Traber DL (eds) Third Wiggers Bernard conference-cytokine network. Springer-Verlag, Berlin Heidelberg New York, pp 72–127
17. Roumen RM, Hendriks T, Wevers RA, Goris JA (1993) Intestinal permeability after severe trauma and hemorrhagic shock is increased without relation to septic complications. Arch Surg 128:453–457
18. Schlag G, Redl H, Dinges HP, Radmore K (1991) Bacterial translocation in a baboon model of hypovolemic-traumatic shock. In: Schlag G, Redl H, Siegel JH, Traber DL (eds) Shock, Sepsis, and Organ Failure. Second Wiggers Bernard Conference. Springer-Verlag, Berlin Heidelberg New York, pp 53–90
19. Sori AJ, Rush BF Jr, Lysz TW, Smith S, Machiedo GW (1988) The gut as source of sepsis after hemorrhagic shock. Am J Surg 155:187–192
20. Alexander JW, Gianotti L, Pyles T, Carey MA, Babcock GF (1991) Distribution and survival of *Escherichia coli* translocating from the intestine after thermal injury. Ann Surg 213:558–566
21. Siegfried MR, Ma X, Lefer AM (1992) Splanchnic vascular endothelial dysfunction in rat endotoxemia: Role of superoxide radicals. Eur J Pharmacol 212:171–176
22. Brathwaite CEM, Ross SE, Nagele R, Mure JA, O'Malley KF, Garcia-Perez FA (1993) Bacterial translocation occurs in humans after traumatic injury: Evidence using immunofluorescence. J Trauma 34:586–589
23. Reed LL, Martin M, Manglano R, Newson B, Kocka F, Barrett J (1994) Bacterial translocation following abdominal trauma in humans. Circ Shock 42:1–6
24. Redl H, Bahrami S, Leichtfried G, Schlag G (1992) Special collection and storage tubes for blood endotoxin and cytokine measurements. Clin Chem 38:764–765
25. van Leeuwen PAM, Hong RW, Rounds JD (1991) Hepatic failure and coma following liver resection is reversed by manipulation of gut contents: The role of endotoxin. Eur Surg Res (Suppl) 23:59 (Abst)
26. Steininger R, Függer R, Hackl W (1990) Immediate graft function after orthotopic liver transplantation clears endotoxin. Transplant Proc 22:1544–1546
27. Nakao A, Shimohara M (1985) Changes of circulating blood endotoxin analyzed by quantitative assay after intravenous administration of endotoxin. Jap J Gastroenterol 82:296–300
28. Thiemermann C, Szabo C, Mitchell JA, Vane JR (1993) Vascular hyporeactivity to vasoconstrictor agents and hemodynamic decompensation in hemorrhagic shock is mediated by nitric oxide. Proc Natl Acad Sci 90:267–271
29. Smith SM, Eng RH, Buccini F (1986) Use of D-lactic acid measurements in the diagnosis of bacterial infections. J Infect Dis 154:658–664
30. Murray MJ, Barbose JJ, Cobb CF (1993) Serum D(−)-lactate levels as a predictor of acute intestinal ischemia in a rat model. J Surg Res 54:507–509
31. Yao YM, Bahrami S, Leichtfried G, Schiesser A, Redl H, Schlag G (1996) Elevated plasma D(−)-lactate correlated to intestinal injury in a rat ischemia/reperfusion model: Influence of monoclonal antibody to tumor necrosis factor. (In press)
32. Murray MJ, Gonze MD, Nowak LR, Cobb CF (1994) Serum D(−)-lactate levels as an aid to diagnosing acute intestinal ischemia. Am J Surg 167:575–578
33. Brandt RB, Siegel SA, Waters MG, Bloch MH (1980) Spectrophotometric assay for D(−)-lactate in plasma. Anal Biochem 102:39–46
34. Karlstad MD, Patteson SK, Guszcza JA, Langdon R, Chesney JT (1993) Methylprednisolone does not influence endotoxin translocation during cardiopulmonary bypass. J Cardiothorac Vasc Anesth 7:23–27
35. Schlag G, Redl H, Bahrami S, Davies J, Smuts P, Marzi I (1993) Trauma and Cytokines. In: Schlag G, Redl H, Traber DL (eds) Shock, Sepsis, and Organ Failure. Springer-Verlag, Berlin Heidelberg pp 128–155

36. Rush BFJ, Sori AJ, Murphy TF, Smith S, Flanagan JJ, Machiedo GW (1988) Endotoxemia and bacteremia during hemorrhagic shock: The link between trauma and sepsis? Ann Surg 207:549–554
37. Moore F, Poggetti R, McAnena O, Peterson V, Abernathy C, Parsons P (1991) Gut bacterial translocation via the portal vein: A clinical perspective with major torso trauma. J Trauma 31:629–638
38. Endo S, Inada K, Yamada Y, et al (1994) Plasma endotoxin and cytokine concentrations in patients with hemorrhagic shock. Crit Care Med 22:949–955
39. Roumen RM, Frieling JT, van Tits HW, van der Vliet JA, Goris RJ (1993) Endotoxemia after major vascular operations. J Vasc Surg 18:853–857
40. Bahrami S, Redl H, Yu Y, Jiang JX, Leichtfried G, Schlag G (1993) Bactericidal/permeability-increasing protein (BPI) reduces lipopolysaccharide (LPS) – induced cytokine formation and mortality in rats. Circ Shock (Suppl) 1:52 (Abst)
41. Deitch EA (1989) Simple intestinal obstruction causes bacterial translocation in man. Arch Surg 124:699–701
42. Peitzman A, Udekwu A, Ochoa J, Smith S (1991) Bacterial translocation in trauma patients. J Trauma 31:1083–1087
43. Sedman PC, Macfie J, Sagar P, et al (1994) The prevalence of gut translocation in humans. Gastroenterology 107:643–649
44. van Goor H, Rosman C, Grond J, Kooi K, Wubbels GH, Bleichrodt RP (1994) Translocation of bacteria and endotoxin in organ donors. Arch Surg 129:1063–1066
45. Berger D, Beger HG (1991) Neue Aspekte zur Pathogenese und Behandlung der Sepsis und des septischen Schocks. Chirurg 62:4–8
46. Yao YM, Bahrami S, Leichtfried G, Redl H, Schlag G (1995) Effects of N^G-monomethyl-L-arginine (L-NMMA) on hemodynamics and mortality in rats following hemorrhagic shock. Shock 3 (Suppl):71 (Abst)
47. Dobke MK, Simoni J, Ninnemann JL, Garrett J, Harnar TJ (1989) Endotoxemia after burn injury: Effect of early excision on circulating endotoxin levels. J Burn Care Rehabil 10:107–111
48. Yao YM, Sheng ZY, Tian HM, et al (1995) The association of circulating endotoxemia with the development of multiple organ failure in burned patients. Burns 21:255–258
49. Ziegler TR, Smith RJ, O'Dwyer ST, Demling RH, Wilmore DW (1988) Increased intestinal permeability associated with infection in burn patients. Arch Surg 123:1313–1319
50. Deitch EA (1990) Intestinal permeabilities increased in burn patients shortly after injuries. Surgery 107:411–416
51. Ryan CM, Yarmush ML, Burke JF, Tompkins RG (1992) Increased gut permeability early after burns correlates with the extent of burn injury. Crit Care Med 20:1508–1512
52. Gathiram P, Wells MT, Raidoo D, Brock-Utne JG, Gaffin SL (1989) Changes in lipopolysaccharide concentrations in hepatic portal and systemic arterial plasma during intestinal ischemia in monkeys. Circ Shock 27:103–109
53. Jacob A, Goldberg P, Bloom N, Degenshein A, Kozinn P (1977) Endotoxin and bacteria in portal blood. Gastroenterology 72:1268–1270
54. Yao YM, Sheng ZY, Yu Y, et al (1995) The potential etiologic role of tumor necrosis factor in mediating multiple organ dysfunction in rats following intestinal ischemia-reperfusion injury. Resuscitation 29:157–168
55. Haglund U, Jodal M, Lundgren O (1984) The small bowel in arterial hypotension and shock. In: Shepard AP, Granger DN (eds) Physiology of the Intestinal Circulation. Raven Press, New York, pp 305–319
56. Lundgren O, Svanvik J (1973) Mucosal hemodynamics in the small intestine of the cat during reduced perfusion pressure. Acta Physiol Scand 88:551–563
57. Herman CM, Kraft AR, Smith KR, et al (1974) The relationship of circulating endogenous endotoxin to hemorrhagic shock in the baboon. Ann Surg 179:910–916
58. Bahrami S, Schlag G, Yao YM, Redl H (1995) Significance of translocation/endotoxin in the development of systemic sepsis following trauma and/or hemorrhage. Prog Clin Biol Res 392:197–208
59. Deitch EA, Berg RD (1987) Bacterial translocation from the gut: A mechanism of infection. J Burn Care Rehabil 8:475–482

60. Alexander JW, Boyce ST, Babcock GF, et al (1990) The process of microbial translocation. Ann Surg 212:496–510
61. Jones WG2, Minei JP, Barber AE, et al (1990) Bacterial translocation and intestinal atrophy after thermal injury and burn wound sepsis. Ann Surg 211:399–405
62. Morris SE, Navaratnam N, Townsend CM, Herndon DN (1989) Decreased mesenteric blood flow independently promotes bacterial translocation in chronically instrumented sheep. Surg Forum 40:88 (Abst)
63. Marra MN, Graig G, Griffith JE, Snable J, Scott W (1990) Bactericidal/permeability-increasing protein has endotoxin-neutralizing activity. J Immunol 144:662–666
64. Gaffin SL, Grinberg Z, Abraham C, et al (1981) Protection against hemorrhagic shock in the cat by human plasma containing endotoxin specific antibodies. J Surg Res 31:18–21
65. Redl H, Bahrami S, Schlag G (1995) Possible therapeutic approaches to deal with bacterial/ endotoxin translocation. In: Vincent JL (ed) Yearbook of Intensive Care and Emergency Medicine. Springer-Verlag, Berlin Heidelberg, pp 693–702
66. Munster AM, Smith Meek M, Dickerson C, Winchurch RA (1993) Translocation. Incidental phenomenon or true pathology? Ann Surg 218:321–326
67. Hadfield RJ, Sinclair DG, Houldsworth PE, Evans TW (1995) Effects of enteral and parenteral nutrition on gut mucosal permeability in the critically ill. Am J Respir Crit Care Med 152:1545–1548
68. Lipman TO (1995) Bacterial translocation and enteral nutrition in humans: An outsider looks in. J Parent Enteral Nutr 19:156–165
69. Rush BFJ, Redan JA, Flanagan JJ, et al (1989) Does the bacteremia observed in hemorrhagic shock have clinical significance? A study in germfree animals. Ann Surg 210:342–347
70. Donohoe MK, Rush BFJ, Koziol JM, Machiedo GW (1986) Role of antibiotics in late survival from hemorrhagic shock. Surg Forum 27:62–64
71. Cruz N, Alvarez X, Specian RD, Berg RD, Deitch EA (1994) Role of mucin, mannose and β-1 integrin receptors in E. coli translocation across CaCO$_2$ cell monolayers. Shock 2: 121–126
72. Yao YM, Tian HM, Wang YP, Sheng ZY, Shi ZG, Xu SH (1992) Protective effect of re-LPS antiserum on experimental multiple system organ failure. Chin Med J 105:833–838
73. Bahrami S, Yao YM, Leichtfried G, Redl H, Schlag G, Di Padova FE (1996) Possible role of Enterobacteriaceae-derived endotoxin in hemorrhage-induced multiple organ injury and mortality in rats. Am Rev Respir Crit Care Med (in Press)
74. Pasquale MD, Cipolle MD, Cerra FB (1994) Bacterial translocation: Myth versus reality. In: Reinhart K, Eyrich K, Sprung C (eds) Sepsis. Springer-Verlag, Berlin Heidelberg New York, pp 86–106
75. Cruz N, Lu Q, Berg R, Deitch EA (1994) The Caco-2 cell monolayer system as an in vitro model for studying bacterial-enterocyte interactions and bacterial translocation. J Burn Care Rehabil 15:207–212
76. Foulkes R, Hughes B, Kingaby R, Woodger R, Vetterlein O (1994) Anti-TNF treatment reduces severity of organ damage in a concious rabbit model of hemorrhagic/traumatic shock. Intensive Care Med 20:72 (Abst)
77. Dentener MA, von Asmuth EJU, Francot GJM, Marra MN, Buurman WA (1993) Antagonists effects of lipopolysaccharide binding protein and bacterial/permeability-increasing protein on lipopolysaccharide-induced cytokine release by mononuclear phagocytes. J Immunol 151:4258–4263
78. Marra MN, Graig GW, Collins MS, Snable JL, Thornton MB, Scott RW (1992) The role of bactericidal/permeability-increasing protein as a natural inhibitor of bacterial endotoxin. J Immunol 148:532–537
79. Yao YM, Bahrami S, Leichtfried G, Redl H, Schlag G (1995) Pathogenesis of hemorrhage-induced bacteria-endotoxin translocation in rats: Effects of recombinant bactericidal-increasing protein (rBPI$_{21}$). Ann Surg 221:398–405
80. Smiddy FG, Fine J (1957) Host resistance to hemorrhagic shock. X. Induction of resistance by shock plasma and by endotoxins. Proc Soc Exp Biol Med 96:558–562
81. Baker CH, Sutton ET, Price JM (1995) Arteriolar reactivity of endotoxin-tolerant rats after hemorrhage and reinfusion. Shock 4:455–460

82. Van Leeuwen PA, Boermeester MA, Houdijk AP, et al (1994) Clinical significance of translocation. Gut 35:S28–S34
83. Tran DD, Cuesta MA, Van Leeuwen PA, Nauta JJ, Wesdorp RI (1993) Risk factors for multiple organ system failure and death in critically injured patients. Surgery 114:21–30
84. Fink MP (1994) Effect of critical illness on microbial translocation and gastrointestinal mucosa permeability. Semin Respir Infect 9:256–260

Experimental Multiple Organ Failure and Gut Dysfunction

R. J. A. Goris, G. A. P. Nieuwenhuijzen, and M. M. J. Jansen

Introduction

Sepsis associated with the sequential and progressive failure of multiple organs (MOF) presently is the major cause of death in surgical and ICU patients. The mortality from MOF still is around the 60%, despite optimal treatment and administration of a variety of antibiotic regimens. While by definition sepsis requires the causal involvement of bacteria, a clear, causal, exclusive, correlation between bacterial and/or (endo)toxin data and clinical data in patients with apparent sepsis/MOF has never been demonstrated [1, 2].

The impossibility to reliably and consistently correlate clinical signs and symptoms of "sepsis" with bacteriological data has led to the hypothesis that the gut, i.e. bacteria and endotoxins within the gut, may play an important role in generating MOF. Already in 1950, Fine et al. [3] demonstrated that transmural migration of *E. coli* into the peritoneal cavity occurs when chemical irritation of the intestinal serosa is maintained for a sufficiently long period, as with peritoneal dialysis in uremic patients. They noted that "the bacterial invasion of the peritoneal cavity in these circumstances is not dependent on bacterial motility, since dead and living bacteria gain entrance with equal facility". In 1972, Cuevas and Fine [4] demonstrated that in peritonitis live bacteria may pass from the intestinal lumen to the peritoneal cavity, and hypothesized that also the systemic appearance of endotoxin from the gut may contribute to irreversible shock.

Fueling this concept, experimental data demonstrated that intestinal permeability is increased in situations leading to MOF, such as in severe burns, mesenteric ischemia, hemorrhagic shock, sterile peritonitis, and endotoxin administration. In these conditions, gut bacteria were found to translocate to the peritoneal cavity, mesenterial lymph nodes (MLN), liver and spleen, eventually causing septicemia (for review see chapter by CL Wells) [5]. The gut therefore has been called the "motor" of MOF and "the undrained abscess".

However, the question still is unresolved whether this dysfunction of the gut barrier in life-threatening conditions plays a major causal role in increasing morbidity and mortality, or merely is one of the signs of severe illness without much clinical significance.

This chapter addresses experimental data regarding gut dysfunction in MOF, especially the role of gut dysfunction in generating MOF.

Animal Models of Gut Dysfunction in Sepsis

A number of principles have to be outlined before entering into the topic of gut dysfunction in experimental MOF:

1. The clinical problem of severely ill or traumatized patients is not (altered) gut permeability *per se*, and/or bacterial translocation *per se*, but sepsis, systemic inflammatory response syndrome (SIRS) and MOF. It therefore should be realized that studying gut permeability and/or bacterial translocation (BT) is relevant only in so far as a relationship can be established with subsequent infection, sepsis, SIRS and MOF.

2. Clinically as well as experimentally, it requires 5 to 7 days to fully develop MOF (see chapter by FA Moore) [1, 6–18]. Clinically, most episodes of septic shock (an acute event) can be treated well. Only in a limited number of patients with septic shock progresses to the more chronic clinical problem of sepsis, SIRS and MOF.

3. Most experimental models studying sepsis, SIRS, MOF, and gut dysfunction due to hypovolemic shock, ischemia or endotoxin administration are acute models, with an end-point of minutes, hours or maximally 2–5 days. Most phenomena encountered in this early phase may be, but are not necessarily, linked to the development of sepsis, SIRS or MOF.

4. While bacteria and their toxins are ubiquitously present, and are frequent initiators of the clinical problem of MOF, MOF is not the result of bacterial overgrowth but of an overwhelming reponse of the host's inflammatory cells. Thus, two factors are involved: live bacteria including their (endo)toxins, and the inflammatory response. A clean analysis of the pathophysiological processes involved requires that both factors should be studied separately, before studying them together.

This line of reasoning results in the conclusion that MOF is best studied in long-term (7–14 days) animal models, preferentially using a non-bacterial stimulus. Also studying germ-free or decontaminated animals should be considered. In these long-term models, it should be possible to establish if, respectively which early phenomena (i.e. gut dysfunction, increased permeability and/or BT) is essential for late MOF to develop. At present only a few models approach the above requirements: the cecal ligation and puncture model (CLP) [19–22], and the zymosan-induced generalized inflammation model (ZIGI) [6–18].

Early events are commonly studied in animal studies of hemorrhagic shock [23–26] or endotoxin administration [27, 28]. Local and systemic effects of direct mesenteric ischemia can be studied in the superior mesenteric artery occlusion (SMAO) model [29–31]. As early phenomena may be precursors of late MOF, attention will therefore be given to findings in acute models as well as in chronic models.

Gut Dysfunction in Acute Models

Hypovolemic Shock

One of the characteristic signs of inflammation is the passage of large proteins, i.e. albumin and immunoglobulins, through the capillary wall into the interstitium. In rats subject to a 2-h episode of hemorrhagic shock, orally administered low and high molecular weight dextran appeared in the systemic circulation in concentrations up to 5 times higher than in sham-treated controls. Reperfusion reduced these differences, with values approximately threefold greater than those of controls after 2 h [24].

Hypovolemic shock in rats, followed by adequate resuscitation, results in consistently elevated portal blood endotoxin levels (90 pg/mL) up to 60 min after the end of the shock period. Plasma endotoxin levels increased at the beginning of resuscitation, and peaked at 60 min after shock (66 pg/mL) [25, 26]. In this model, plasma tumor necrosis factor (TNF) levels were maximal at the end of the shock period, and subsequently decreased [26]. Higher systemic lipopolysaccharide (LPS) and TNF concentrations were found in non-survivors, rather than in 48-h survivors [26].

Pre- and post-treatment with recombinant bactericidal/permeability increasing protein ($rBPI_{21}$) resulted in plasma endotoxin levels decreasing to 14 pg/mL [25]. However, plasma TNF levels were not significantly influenced by $rBPI_{21}$. Though the morphological changes were relatively minor in the $rBPI_{21}$ group, mortality was not different from controls. These experiments indicate that, in the early phase after hemorrhagic shock in rats, plasma endotoxin and TNF levels are elevated, while plasma endotoxin levels lag behind and are less elevated than portal blood endotoxin, suggesting endotoxin absorption from the gut in the liver. Effectively neutralizing this endotoxin did not seem to improve short-term outcome [25].

Endotoxin Administration

24 h after endotoxin administration, BT was similar in small series of normal outbred (88%), complement deficient (67%), and macrophage-hyporesponsive (55%) mice, indicating that neither complement nor macrophage activation is necessary for endotoxin-induced BT to occur [28]. Ileal, not jejunal, permeability for ^{51}Cr-EDTA was increased twofold as early as 2 h after endotoxin challenge. Both the ileal increased permeability and BT were largely prevented by allopurinol, suggesting that the early changes found after endotoxin administration are mediated by activation of xanthine oxidase, not through complement activation or the liberation of macrophage products [28].

SMAO

Chiu et al. [23] found characteristic morphological alterations of the gut mucosa, resulting from reduced flow or SMAO. Within a 4-h observation period, these changes increased in severity and correlated with the severity of the ischemic insult.

The light microscopic changes were graded as follows:
Grade 0: normal villi
Grade 1: development of subepithelial Grünhagen's space, usually at the apex of the villus, often with capillary congestion
Grade 2: extension of the subepithelial space with moderate lifting of the epithelial layer from the lamina propria
Grade 3: massive epithelial lifting down the sides of the villi. A few villi may be denuded
Grade 4: denuded villi with lamina propria and dilated capillaries exposed. Increased cellularity of lamina propria may be noted
Grade 5: digestion and disintegration of the lamina propria; hemorrhage and ulceration.

These gradings of gut mucosal injury closely correlate with the severity of the original insult. Identical alterations have been identified as the result of various causes of shock (hypovolemic, septic), and could also be found dose-dependently in the ZIGI-model [10–12].

In the SMAO model in rats, mucosal permeability to ^{51}Cr-EDTA was increased fourfold as compared to sham-controls 30 min after reperfusion [32]. Pretreatment with inhibitors of free oxygen radicals or eicosanoids could not prevent this increased permeability. Indomethacin and PGE_2 significantly exacerbated the permeability changes. The authors concluded that the early increase in mucosal permeability in the SMAO model is not mediated by oxygen radicals or eicosanoids. In another study with the SMAO model in rats [33], morphological damage was accompanied by and correlated with oxygen radical formation. However, effective inhibition of oxygen radical formation by the 21-aminosteroid U74389F did not result in a decrease in morphological damage.

In the SMAO model, it was demonstrated that after reperfusion, the ischemic gut primes circulating PMNs, which subsequently sequester in the pulmonary vascular bed. At this site, these PMNs are relatively harmless, unless stimulated by a second trigger such as low dose endotoxin, making them migrate across the endothelium and release reactive oxygen species [31].

Lung injury was assessed in the SMAO model in rats, previously sham-operated or subject to a portacaval transposition. Pulmonary vascular permeability was significantly increased, regardless of the presence of a hepatic bypass, indicating that gut-origin mediators are responsible for pulmonary vascular permeability changes, and that these mediators are not appreciably influenced by the liver [30]. Therefore in this model, Kuppfer cell activation seems to play a less important role.

Gut Dysfunction in Chronic Models

The CLP Model

In the CLP model, laparotomy is performed in rats and the cecum identified, ligated without interfering with the blood supply, and punctured once or twice with needles of various sizes to vary the severity of the insult. Depending on the number of punctures and the size of the needle, 4-day mortality may vary from 20 to 100% [19]. Longer observation periods have barely been utilized with the CLP model.

Intraperitoneal infection induced by CLP results within 24 h in substantial bacterial overgrowth of the proximal gastrointestinal (GI) tract, while concentrations of *E. coli* increasing from 10^3 colony-forming units (CFU)/mL to more than 10^9 CFU/mL [20]. Meanwhile, the delayed hypersensitivity response decreases significantly, indicating that altered proximal GI tract flora can mediate suppression of cell-mediated immunity, one component of ongoing sepsis [20].

CLP, followed 24 h later by a colon anastomosis, results in a significant decrease in anastomotic bursting pressure and colon hydroxyproline concentration as an index of collagen content [21]. Sepsis thus significantly impairs the healing of the colon. CLP within 24 h adversely affects the gut absorptive function for aminoacids. This reduction in absorptive capacity of the gut may limit the ability of enteral feeding during sepsis and may contribute to the associated morbidity and mortality [21]. Mortality 4 days after CLP is significantly lower in endotoxin-resistant C3H/HeJ mice than in endotoxin sensitive C3H/HeN mice, indicating that the response to the bacterial stimulus may be more important than the bacterial challenge itself [34].

Chou et al. [35] demonstrated that ET-1 gene expression post-CLP with a single puncture of the cecum with a 23 gauge needle shows a 3,6-fold increase at 8 h, and a return to sham levels by 24 h. An increase of mRNA levels 24 h post-CLP was observed with a double puncture with a 18 gauge needle accompanied by an increase in serum ET-1 levels and higher tissue ET levels. These data indicate a time-dependent response of ET-1 gene expression in the terminal ileum post-CLP which is related to the severity of infection.

The ZIGI Model

In the ZIGI model [6], zymosan (an extract of the cell wall of the yeast *Saccharomyces Cerevesiae*) suspended in mineral oil or saline, is inoculated intraperitoneally in rats or mice. The usual dosage is 1 mg/g body weight. Zymosan is a strong activator of the alternative pathway of the complement system. The zymosan particles are also phagocytosed by macrophages, and induce a severe and prolonged inflammatory response, because macrophages can not break down zymosan particles. Furthermore, phagocytosis of zymosan particles is delayed by the presence of mineral oil.

Table 1. The zymosan-induced generalized inflammation (ZIGI) model in rats and mice

Phases	Time	Characteristics	Mortality
Acute phase	0–2 days	Lethargy Diarrhea Weight loss	20%
Recovery phase	3–7 days	Recovery of weight Normal behavior	0%
'Late' phase	8–12 days	Lethargy Weight loss Tachypnea Hypothermia	20–30%

Intraperitoneal zymosan results in a triphasic illness (Table 1). The first 24–48 h, the experimental animals display a hyperdynamic response, are severely ill, become febrile, lethargic and anorectic. They hyperventilate and lose liquid stools. Furthermore, they show a hunched back, ruffled fur and loose weight. In this first phase, there is leukopenia and increased oxygen consumption. In this early phase, BT to the peritoneal cavity and MLN are common, especially in early deaths. Also during the first 48 h, endotoxemia is regularly present [36]. At this time, dose-dependent microscopic alterations are observed in the gut mucosa (Fig. 1). Early mortality is around 30% with the above zymosan dosage. After 2 days, all surviving animals improve, become active and gain weight. Body temperature and pulse rate normalise, but respiratory rate remains elevated. After 7 days, the third hypodynamic MOF phase sets in with hypothermia, weight loss, increasing heart and respiratory rates, decreased oxygen consumption, lactic acidemia, elevated leukocyte and platelet counts. During the second and third phase, peritoneal cultures as well as all blood cultures remain sterile, and no endotoxemia is found.

Also in germ-free ZIGI-rats, MOF develops within the same time-frame, without the presence of gut bacteria, and obviously without BT [6]. However in germ-free rats, the first phase of illness is much less severe, and early mortality is barely seen.

Increased Permeability for Fluids in ZIGI: Increased permeability for fluids may be assessed by measuring wet to dry weight ratios. In the ZIGI-model in mice, a progressive and synchronous increase of the wet/dry ratio was found over the 12-day experimental period in various organs including the lung, liver, ileum and colon [17]. Similar findings were obtained during a 5-day observation period by Shayevitz et al. [18]. In another experiment with the ZIGI-model, the intestinal weight to body weight ratio on day 15 was highly significantly increased as compared to controls (11.4 ± 1.75 versus 8.8 ± 1.52) [13].

Permeability for Macromolecules in ZIGI: Microvascular permeability was assessed in the ZIGI-model by intravenous administration of ^{111}Indium labelled non-spe-

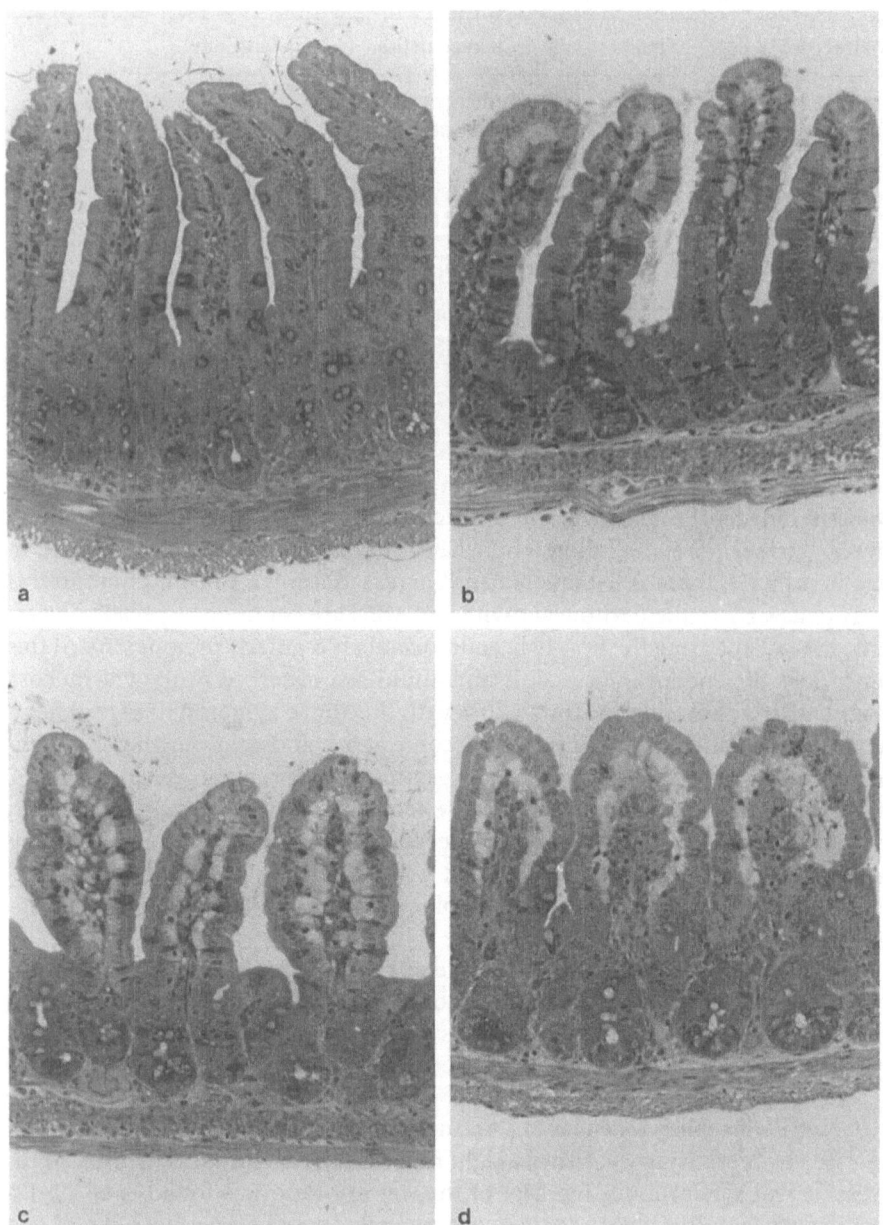

Fig. 1. Plastic sections of distal ileum 24 h after zymosan administration stained with toluidine blue (X220).

a Normal mucosa from a control mouse. **b** After 0.1 mg/g zymosan. Lifting of villus tip epithelium. **c** After 0.5 mg/g. More pronounced edema of villus. **d** After 1.0 mg/g. Complete dysruption of normal architecture of the mucosa. Scale bar = 100 µm

cific immunoglobulin G (^{111}In-IgG) 24 h before sacrifice, followed by scintigraphy of dissected organs [17]. Mice were sacrificed at various intervals after zymosan inoculation, up to day 12. The permeability index (PI) of each organ was calculated from the measured activity (percentage of the injected dose per gram dry weight) divided by the measured blood activity. On all days, PI was significantly elevated in the lungs, liver, ileum, colon and MLNs, while unchanged in the kidneys. In the MLNs, PI was constantly elevated. In the liver, ileum and colon, PI demonstrated the highest activity on day 2, with some improvement the next days. In the lungs, PI demonstrated a triphasic response, with an early increase, a temporary improvement and a late second peak, corresponding well with clinical illness (Fig. 2).

This experiment demonstrates that permeability changes show a different pattern and intensity in each organ, while permeability changes in the intestine occur simultaneously with, and are not preceded by permeability changes in other organs. As known in the ZIGI-model, functional organ damage is a late phenomenon, following maximal PI changes by several days. However a causal relationship between increased permeability and organ damage cannot be derived from this experiment.

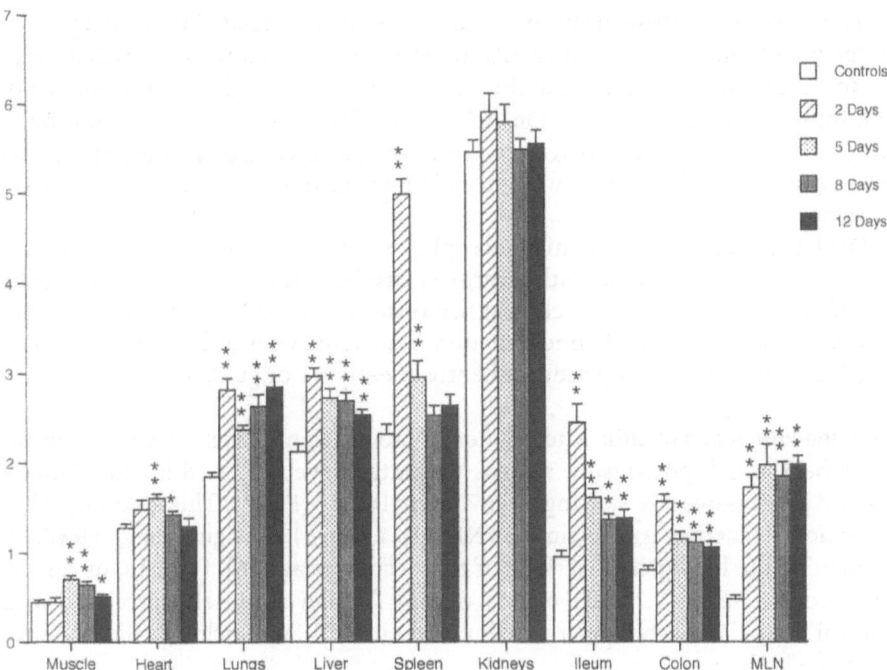

Fig. 2. Permeability index of various organs on different time points after zymosan challenge in mice. Tissue permeability index was calculated as follows: percentage of the injected dose Indium-111-immunoglobulin G per gram tissue dry weight divided by the percentage of the injected dose per gram blood weight. Data are expressed as mean ± SEM. Comparisons were made with the control group. * $p < 0.025$, ** $p < 0.01$. (From [17] with permission)

Bacterial Translocation and Selective Decontamination of the Gut in ZIGI: In the ZIGI-model, BT is a well documented early event, occurring during the first 24–48 h after zymosan inoculation, and related to early mortality [6, 7, 9–12]. However, in subsequent days, BT was only exceptionally observed, while MOF in this model develops after some 7 days. After inoculation of 0.1 mg/g zymosan, BT is limited to the MLN only. 0.5 mg/g zymosan promotes BT to MLN, blood and organs, while the magnitude of portal bacteremia is greater than systemic bacteremia [37].

Surprisingly, selective decontamination of the digestive tract (SDD) has been extensively studied in clinical trials, while barely any experimental work has been performed to study its effects in a model of sepsis and MOF. The ZIGI model is well suited to analyze the effects of SDD [7, 36]. SDD with trimethoprim in ZIGI-rats adequately eradicated all Enterobacteriaceae, preventing their translocation, but without any effect on early or late mortality, or MOF. On the other hand, SDD with streptomycin, in some experimental series, resulted in a 1000-fold overgrowth of the intestinal flora with Enterobacteriaceae before zymosan inoculation, while no BT occurred, and early mortality was almost absent [7, 9]. Late mortality and MOF, however, were as in undecontaminated controls. This surprising finding may be explained by the effects of streptomycin on macrophage function [9].

The correlation between survival and BT seems to be related to the magnitude of the inflammatory insult, since in another study [11] of low-dose ZIGI, mortality was reduced by cefoxitin, but this effect was lost when higher doses of zymosan were given. Rosman et al. [36] found that SDD with tobramycin and polymyxin E in ZIGI significantly reduced endotoxin levels and early mortality. However, experimental animals were terminated at day 4, a time before MOF develops in the ZIGI-model.

Depletion of liver and splenic macrophages prior to zymosan inoculation resulted in increased BT, but with improved survival [12], thus disconnecting the phenomenon of BT from the clinical response. These experiments indicate that in this model BT is an early phenomenon, associated with early death. However, late MOF seems to develop independently of early BT or gut bacteria.

Cytokine Production in ZIGI: After zymosan inoculation, plasma TNF concentrations peak at 2 h post-insult, returns to control levels after 18 h, and shows a second progressive rise starting after 7 days [16, 37] (Fig. 3). This second peak is biologically inactive. At this time, $sTNF_r$ (p_{55} and p_{75}) are significantly elevated, explaining the biological inactivity of this second peak [16]. Prior to, or during the second TNF-peak, no BT occurs. Serum TNF-levels closely correlated with clinical illness. However, pretreatment with anti-TNF monoclonals did not alter outcome [38].

Serum interleukin (IL)-6 plasma concentrations peak at 4 h post-zymosan challenge, decrease after 24 h, but remain above normal levels up to day 12 [16, 37]. Mainous et al. [37] extensively studied portal and systemic bioactivity of TNF and IL-1. This bioactivity was similar for either cytokine, and serum bioactivity did not correlate with zymosan dose. TNF bioactivity was increased in

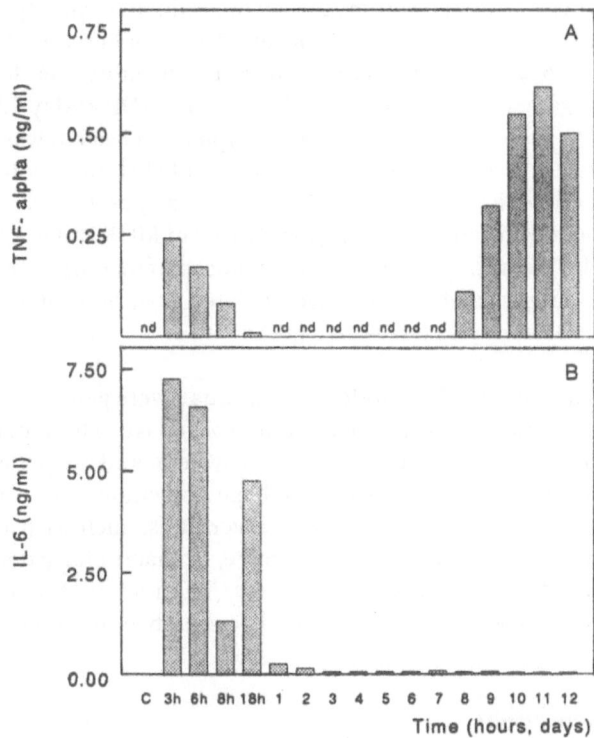

Fig. 3. Circulating TNF-α and IL-6 in ZIGI-mice. Plasma levels of immunoreactive TNF-α (**A**) and biologically active IL-6 (**B**) at various time points after intraperitoneal zymosan inoculation in mice. (nd = not detectable). (From [16] with permission)

the mesenteric lymph at 2 h post-challenge with 0.5 mg/g zymosan only. IL-6 bio-activity was increased in the mesenteric lymph at 4 through 10 h post-challenge, but was similar with either dosage of zymosan. The authors concluded that the gut may be capable of producing cytokines in response to an inflammatory stimulus, even in the absence of portal or systemic spread of bacteria. The magnitude of the cytokine response, however, did not correlate with the magnitude of BT.

Effects of Various Interventions in ZIGI: The ZIGI model is suitable for performing a variety of therapeutic interventions. Pre-treatment of rats with anti-TNF monoclonal antibody prevented the early TNF-peak [38] but failed to prevent late MOF and mortality [39]. Pretreatment with superoxide dismutase (SOD) and catalase [40], oxygen radical scavengers (mannitol, dimethylsulfoxide, dimethylthiourea, dihydrobenzoic acid, rosemarinic acid, U74006F) [39], fructose 1–6 diphosphate as a high-energy substrate [39], the protein-kinase-C activator 1-oleyl-2 acetyl-glycerol [39] did not alter early or late mortality or outcome. Pre-feeding with a fish oil enriched diet during 8 weeks decreased plasma TNF levels, but failed to alter outcome [15]. Early mortality was absent or decreased in germ free rats [6], streptomycin decontaminated rats [7], and elastase-deficient mice [39], but late MOF and mortality were unaltered in these series.

A significant decrease in early mortality was found in C5-deficient mice, together with significantly less severe MOF at day 12 [14]. Thus, in this model, the presence of a competent complement system was associated with early mortality, at a time when BT is also found [14]. In endotoxin resistant C3H/HeJ and endotoxin sensitive C3H/HeN mice, early as well as late mortality was almost absent, while animals were largely free of MOF at day 12 [2]. This effect is probably due to the hyposensitivity to zymosan of macrophages in both strains. Also in several series of macrophage depleted rats, mortality was significantly lower and MOF at day 12 less severe [12].

Thus, in the ZIGI model, continuous severe generalized inflammation is induced by intraperitoneal inoculation of zymosan. These particles activate the alternative pathway of the complement system, and are phagocytosed by macrophages, leading to continous macrophage activation and a triphasic illness resembling human MOF. Only a few interventions, such as using stimulus hyposensitive mice, complement-deficient mice, or macrophage depleted rats, were successful in decreasing severity of illness. The human corrolary for preventing and/or treating MOF probably should be searched for along the same lines.

Conclusion

While sepsis and various other stimuli have significant effects on the gut flora and function, the resulting alterations in gut barrier function and increased release of inflammatory mediators from the gut may contribute to the pathophysiologic processes leading to MOF. However, positive correlations between morphological alterations, gut mucosal permeability, bacterial and endotoxin translocation on one hand, and outcome on the other hand, have only been documented in short-term experiments. Such a relationship has hitherto not been demonstrated in 12 day experimental models. Therefore in severe illness, gut damage probably is an early event indicative of the severity of the condition, possibly not significantly related to outcome.

References

1. Goris RJA, te Boehorst TPA, Nuytinck JLM, Gimbrere JSF (1985) Multiple organ failure. Generalized autodestructive inflammation? Arch Surg 120:1109–1115
2. Goris RJA, van Bebber IPT, Hendriks TH (1991) Role of bacterial translocation and selective gut decontamination for the development of multiple organ failure. In: Schlag G, Redl H (eds) Second Wiggers-Bernard Symposium on Shock, Sepsis and Organ Failure. Springer-Verlag, Berlin Heidelberg New York, pp 133–144
3. Schweinburg FB, Seligman AM, Fine J (1950) Transmural migration of intestinal bacteria. A study on the use of radioactive Escherichia Coli. N Engl J Med 242:747–751
4. Cuevas P, Fine J (1972) Role of intestinal endotoxin in death from peritonitis. Surg Gynecol Obstet 134:953–957

5. Nieuwenhuijzen GAP, Deitch EA, Goris RJA (1996) The relationship between gut-derived bacteria and the development of the multiple organ dysfunction syndrome. Eur J Surg (In press)

6. Goris RJA, Boekholz WKF, van Bebber IPT, Nuytinck JLM, Schillings PHM (1986) Multiple organ failure and sepsis without bacteria. An experimental model. Arch Surg 121:897-901

7. Goris RJA, van Bebber IPT, Mollen RMH, Koopman JP (1991) Does selective decontamination of the gastrointestinal tract prevent multiple organ failure? An experimental study. Arch Surg 126:561-565

8. Mainous MR, Tso P, Berg RD, Deitch EA (1991) Studies of the route, magnitude, and time course of bacterial translocation in a model of systemic inflammation. Arch Surg 126:33-37

9. van Bebber IPT, Schillings PHM, Goris RJA (1992) Decontamination of the gastrointestinal tract by streptomycin in an experimental model of multiple organ failure reduces mortality by a mechanism independent of the presence of enterobacteriaceae. In: Thesis van Bebber IPT, Nijmegen, Netherlands

10. Deitch EA, Specian RD, Grisham MB, Berg RD (1992) Zymosan-induced bacterial translocation: A study of mechanisms. Crit Care Med 20:782-788

11. Deitch EA, Kemper AC, Specian RD, Berg RD (1992) A study of the relationships among survival, gut-origin sepsis, and bacterial translocation in a model of systemic inflammation. J Trauma 32:141-147

12. Nieuwenhuijzen GAP, Haskel Y, Lu Q, et al (1993) Macrophage elimination increases bacterial translocation and gut-origin septicemia but attenuates symptoms and mortality rate in a model of systemic inflammation. Ann Surg 218:791-799

13. Di Filippo A, Scardi S, Consalvo M, et al (1994) Valutazione di un modello sperimentale di disfuzione multipla di organo (MODS). Minerva Anesthesiol 60:157-164

14. Nieuwenhuijzen GAP, Meyer MPD, Hendriks Th, Goris RJA (1995) Deficiency of complement factor C5 reduces early mortality but does not prevent organ damage in an animal model of multiple organ failure. Crit Care Med 23:1686-1693

15. Gielen RCJM, van As AB, Goris RJA (1993) Do diets enriched with oil prevent MOF in mice? An experimental study. Eur J Surg 159:609-612

16. Jansen MJJ, Hendriks Th, Vogels MT, van der Meer JWM, Goris RJA (1996) Inflammatory cytokines in an experimental model for the multiple organ dysfunction syndrome. Crit Care Med (In press)

17. Nieuwenhuijzen GAP, Knapen MFC, Oyen WJG, Hendriks Th, Corstens FHM, Goris RJA (1996) Organ damage is preceded by changes in vascular permeability in an experimental model of the multiple organ dysfunction syndrome. Shock (In press)

18. Shayevitz JR, Miller C, Johnson KJ, Rodriguez JL (1995) Multiple organ dysfunction syndrome: End-organ and systemic inflammatory response in a mouse model of non-septic origin. Shock 4:389-396

19. Wichterman A, Baue AE, Chaudry IH (1980) Sepsis and septic shock: A review of laboratory models and a proposal. J Surg Res 29:189-201

20. Marshall JC, Christou NV, Meakins JL (1988) Small-bowel bacterial overgrowth and systemic immunosuppression in experimental peritonitis. Surgery 104:404-411

21. Ahrendt GM, Gardiner K, Barbul A (1994) Loss of colonic structural collagen impairs healing during intra-abdominal sepsis. Arch Surg 129:1179-1183

22. Sodeyama M, Gardiner K, Regan MC, Kirk SJ, Efron G, Barbul A (1993) Sepsis impairs gut amino acid absorption. Am J Surg 165:150-154

23. Chiu CJ, McArdle AH, Brown R, Scott HJ, Gurd FN (1970) Intestinal mucosal lesion in low-flow states. I. A morphological, hemodynamic and metabolic reappraisal. Arch Surg 101:478-483

24. Russell DH, Barreto JC, Klemm K, Miller TA (1995) Hemorrhagic shock increases gut macromolecular permeability in the rat. Shock 4:50-55

25. Yao Y-M, Bahrami S, Leichtfried G, Redl H, Schlag G (1995) Pathogenesis of hemorrhage-induced bacteria/endotoxin translocation in rats. Ann Surg 221:398-405

26. Jiang J, Bahrami S, Leichtfried G, Redl H, Ohlinger W, Schlag G (1995) Kinetics of endotoxin and tumor necrosis factor appearance in portal and systemic circulation after hemorrhagic shock in rats. Ann Surg 221:100-106

27. Deitch EA, Berg RD, Specian RD (1987) Endotoxin promotes the translocation of bacteria from the gut. Arch Surg 122:185–190
28. Deitch EA, Specian RD, Berg RD (1991) Endotoxin-induced bacterial translocation and mucosal permeability: Role of xanthine oxydase, complement activation, and macrophage products. Crit Care Med 19:785–791
29. Granger DN (1988) Role of xanthine oxidase and granulocytes in ischemia/reperfusion injury. Am J Physiol 255:H1260–H1275
30. Johnston TD, Fischer R, Chen Y, Reed RL (1993) Lung injury from gut ischemia: Insensitivity to portal blood flow diversion. J Trauma 35:508–511
31. Moore EE, Moore FA, Franciose RJ, Kim FJ, Biffi WL, Banerjee A (1994) The postischemic gut serves as a priming bed for circulating neutrophils that provoke multiple organ failure. J Trauma 37:881–887
32. Langer JC, Sohal SS, Blennerhassett (1995) Mucosal permeability after subclinical intestinal ischemia-reperfusion injury: An exploration of possible mechanisms. J Pediatr Surg 30:568–572
33. Van Ye TM, Roza AM, Pieper GM, Henderson J, Johnson CP, Adams MB (1993) Inhibition of intestinal lipid peroxidation does not minimize morphologic damage. J Surg Res 55:553–558
34. Baker CC, Kupper TS (1985) Clarification of the role of endotoxin in intra-abdominal and systemic sepsis. Surg Forum 36:68–70
35. Chou MC, Wilson MA, Spain DA, et al (1995) Endothelin-1 expression in the small intestine during chronic peritonitis. Shock 4:411–414
36. Rosman C, Wübbels GH, Manson WL, Bleichrodt RP (1992) Selective decontamination of the digestive tract prevents secondary infection of the abdominal cavity, and endotoxemia and mortality in sterile peritonitis in laboratory rats. Crit Care Med 20:1699–1704
37. Mainous MR, Ertel W, Chaudry IH, Deitch EA (1995) The gut: A cytokin-generating organ in systemic inflammation. Shock 4:193–199
38. von Asmuth EJV, Maessen JG, van der Linden CJ, Buurman WA (1990) TNF and IL-6 in a zymosan-induced shock model. Scand J Immunol 32:313–319
39. van Bebber IPT (1992) Zymosan induced MODS. An experimental model. Thesis, Nijmegen, Netherlands
40. van Bebber IPT, Lieners CFJ, Koldewijn EL, Redl H, Goris RJA (1992) Superoxide dismutase and catalase in an experimental model of multiple organ failure. J Surg Res 52:265–270

Intestinal Cytokines

J. Carlet, F. Tamion, and A. Cabie

Introduction

The past two decades have witnessed the emergence of a new syndrome, named multiple organ failure (MOF), which today continues to represent the very first cause of death in critical care patients. In contrast to the spectacular advances made in the therapy of end-stage single organ failure patients, our inability to treat successfully acutely ill patients with MOF and to prevent the syndrome will be the major challenge for the end of this century [1–6]. Increasing numbers of investigators [1, 5, 7–16] have focused on the role of the gastrointestinal (GI) tract in the pathogenesis of this syndrome. The gut is now very often described as "the undrained abscess" or the "motor of MOF" [7]. Because it contains such a huge amount of bacteria and bacterial products, the gut has been very logically suspected to be the major source for the bacteremia that are often detected during the course of MOF [4, 7, 8]. Endotoxin translocation is also suspected to occur frequently during severe insults to the body, and it is an attractive concept to imagine that endotoxin coming from the digestive tract could play an important role in this setting. However, bacterial or even endotoxin translocation has not been demonstrated in humans and is far from being constant in all animal models of gut ischemia [17, 18]. Moreover, it is still possible to create a severe MOF in germ free animals [19]. Thus, the concept of "bacterial translocation (BT)" remains highly controversial. On the other hand, high levels of a variety of cytokines have been described, not only in the systemic blood which is a very common finding in both animal models [20, 21] and in humans [22–24], but also in portal blood [23, 25, 26]. Moreover, the role of locally produced cytokines is widely accepted during inflammatory diseases of the bowel [27]. Thus the ability of the gut to produce cytokines, induced or not, and amplified or not by endotoxin release during both severe sepsis and MOF, and so the responsibility of this event in the pathophysiology of the syndrome is an important question to be solved.

This chapter focuses on the relationships between gut injury, bacterial or endotoxin translocation in severely injured patients and cytokine release with possible implication of those events in the pathophysiology of MOF.

Intestinal Cytokines In Acutely Ill Beings

Although the release in the systemic circulation of a variety of cytokines has been extensively demonstrated in both animal models of shock [9, 21, 22] (mainly septic) [28], and in acutely ill patients [22, 24], the site of production of those cytokines is far less well understood. The gut could indeed be the ideal candidate for this production. Those cytokines, especially tumor necrosis factor (TNF) α could be critical to damaging the liver and activating Kupffer cells [29, 30]. The activated Kupffer cells in the process of clearing these agents from portal venous blood plus the associated damaged hepatic tissue would then prime the liver for releasing its own destructive products which can amplify the inflammatory cascade and damage the lung. In this respect, it is worth recalling the work by Kahky et al. [31] which demonstrated in a rat model that the administration of TNF α via the venous portal route was significantly more toxic and led to higher mortality than via the systemic one. A vicious circle can very well be imagined remembering that both endotoxin and TNF are able, at high concentrations, to induce a significant ischemia of the gut leading sometimes to a total infarction of the small bowel [32]. High levels of TNF α have been shown not only in systemic but also in portal circulation in rat models of gut ischemia-reperfusion (I/R) (mesenteric arteries clamping and release) [20, 22]. In those models, a severe lung injury usually follows gut ischemia, which supports the concept of the "gut, liver, lung axis" [20, 21, 33, 34]. During abdominal aortic surgery with aortic cross-clamping, which creates an "experimental" model of gut I/R, Cabie et al. [25] have observed that both systemic and portal plasma levels of both lipopolysaccharide (LPS) and TNF α were elevated (Figs. 1–3). TNF production experienced a biphasic pattern, high levels being demonstrated in all patients even before aortic clamping, then returned to subnormal levels and peaked again after reperfusion (Fig. 2). Sustained levels of TNF were demonstrated after 90 min of reperfusion, and this up to the third day after surgery (end of the protocol), unrelated however to any clinical sign of systemic inflammatory response syndrome (SIRS) (Fig. 2). LPS levels were significant in one third of the patients even before aortic clamping (Fig. 1). They peaked after reperfusion (20 min) in 61% of the patients and returned to normal within a few hours in most (but not all) of them. The portal LPS levels were slightly higher than the systemic ones but this difference was not significant (Fig. 3). Interestingly enough, in contrast, the TNF portal levels were significantly higher than systemic ones over all the study period, suggesting a local production of this cytokine (Fig. 3). This production could be induced by both the ischemia of the gut with translocation of endotoxin or also with the manipulation of the intestine itself. Interleukin-6 (IL-6) levels, which were normal before clamping, peaked 20 min after reperfusion, thus after TNF, and remained moderately elevated up to the end of the protocol. They were similar in portal and systemic blood.

In contrast to IL-6, TNF is usually not detected in significant amounts after minor surgical stress [35]. Either bacterial products or ischemia seem mandatory to induce an important release of this cytokine. However, 2 out of the 7 control patients in the study from Cabie et al. [25], who were undergoing a carotid

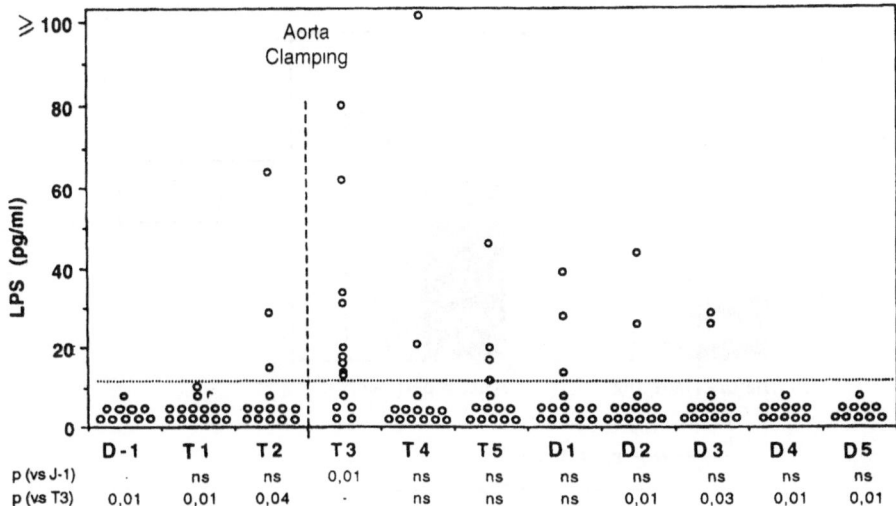

Fig. 1. Systemic endotoxin (LPS) levels before and after aortic cross-clamping for abdominal active surgery. Each point represents a patient. T1: induction of anesthesia, T2: before aortic clamping, T3: after reperfusion (mean 22 min), T4: after reperfusion (mean 90 min), T5: after reperfusion (mean 180 min). D-1, 2, 3, 4, 5: one ... five days after surgery. Detection limit 12 pg/mL

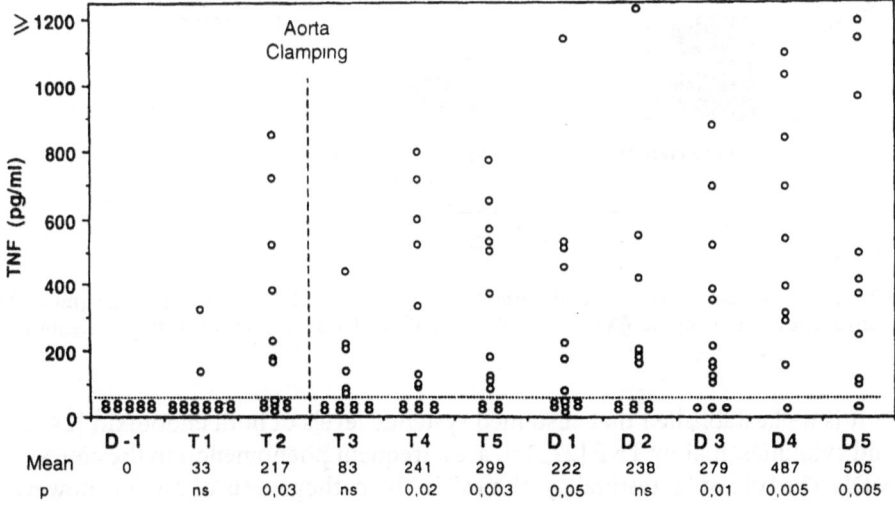

Fig. 2. TNF levels in systemic blood before and after aortic clamping (see legend of Fig. 1 for sampling schedule)

endarteriectomy, experienced significative TNF levels in the systemic circulation. In another study [36], the same authors demonstrated that monocytes of patients undergoing a routine laparotomy were primed to produce a far higher amount of TNF than the controls when stimulated with endotoxin.

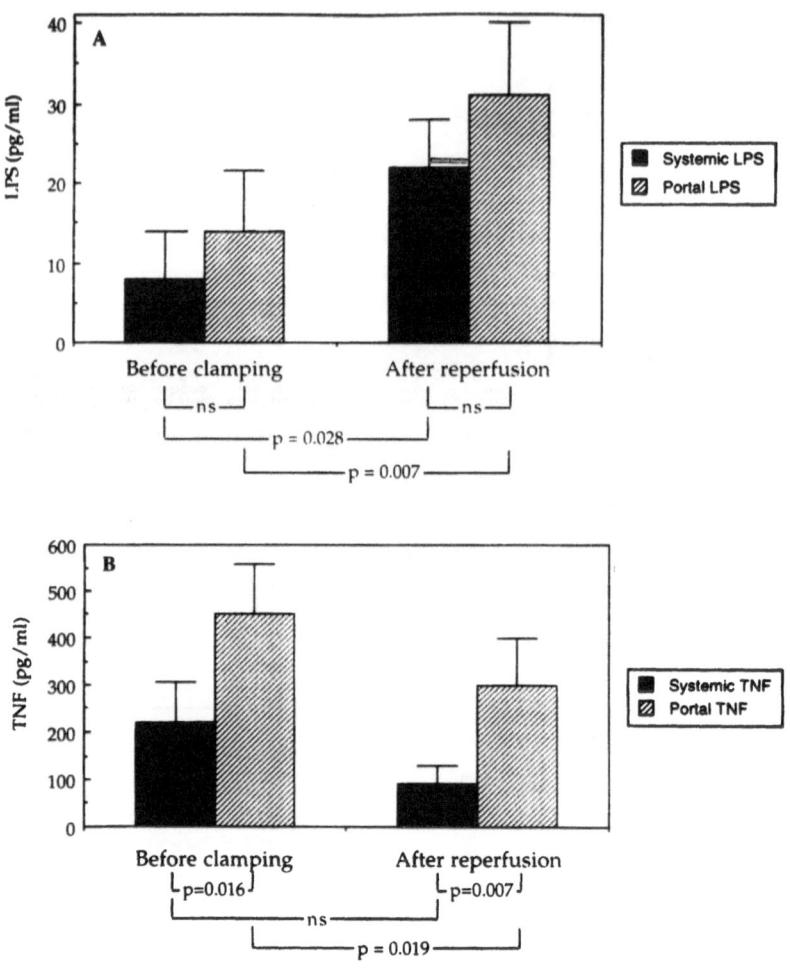

Fig. 3. Comparison of systemic and portal levels of LPS and TNFα before and after (mean 22 min) aortic cross clamping. ■ systemic blood; ▨ portal blood. (From [25] with permission)

It is well established that sustained systemic levels of both endotoxin [24, 37] and cytokines, mainly TNF [22, 27], are a frequent phenomenon in the course of MOF. The role of "intestinal cytokines" in the pathogenesis of MOF is however far more difficult to ascertain and has never been definitely settled. Indeed, there are very few models of "prolonged" MOF in animals and studies are difficult to perform in man. In 10 patients with MOF who underwent an exploratory laparotomy to rule out an intra-abdominal septic focus (and who indeed had none), we performed simultaneous samples in the portal vein and in a peripheral vein (unpublished data). We looked for LPS (chromogenic Limulus assay), for TNFα (radio-immunoassay), and for IL-1α (Elisa assay). Portal LPS was not detectable in all patients and the levels in the patients in whom it was detected were moder-

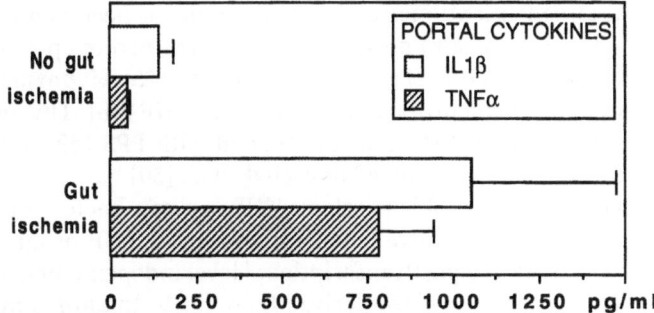

Fig. 4. TNFα and IL-1β levels in portal vein in 10 patients with multiple organ failure with (n = 6) or without (n = 4) gut ischemia

ate (15 to 40 pg/mL). There was no correlation between the presence or absence of gut ischemia (either morphologic or histologic) found in half of the patients, and portal LPS levels. In contrast, a very strong association was observed between IL-1 and TNFα portal levels and the presence of gut ischemia (Fig. 4). No correlation was found between either TNFα, or IL-1 and LPS levels.

Mechanism of Cytokine Production

Bacterial and Endotoxin Translocation

Among the numerous mechanisms which have been proposed to explain the activation of the cytokine network, which is considered to be a key factor in the pathophysiology of MOF, translocation of either alive or dead bacteria [1, 7, 9, 38–41], and/or realease of free endotoxin from the injured digestive tract [14, 16, 26, 41] has been extensively proposed as a mechanism. Indeed, the leakage of bacteria and/or bacterial toxins through the gut mucosa in unusually large amounts could very well produce an activation of the inflammatory cascade. Bacteria and bacterial toxins can reach systemic circulation via the portal route, but also, even more likely, through the lymphatic system [15, 42–46]. As an example, Glofsson et al. [47] using a partial gut ischemia model in rats, demonstrated that the development of systemic endotoxemia paralleled the appearance of endoxotin in the thoracic duct lymph and was identified before any significant portal endotoxemia. This lymphatic route has been demonstrated in both models of I/R [43] and experimental peritonitis [42]. The reticulo-endothelial system, usually able to deal with reasonnable amounts of bacteria or bacterial products could very well, during the phases of excessive leakage from the gut, be overwhelmed by this "high inoculum". If the lymphatic route is involved, then the liver is not in front line any more to clean this high inoculum. Moreover, it has been speculated that small but continuous amounts of endotoxin and bacterial products could be released in the most severe patients and then activate and perpetuate the inflammatory process.

As already mentioned above, endotoxin has been demonstrated to be present in both systemic and portal samples during severe episodes of gut I/R in some animal models [20, 21] as well as in humans [25]. Hypoxia followed by reoxygenation induces the production of IL-1 and TNF [48]. This production is far more important when these cells are treated with LPS [49]. However, this point remains controversial, since Matuschak et al. [50] have recently demonstrated that a transient I/R was able to release TNF in a non-bacteremic condition but downregulates gram-negative bacteremia-induced TNF production. This phenomenon occurred at a posttranscriptional level independent of cyclooxygenase products or xanthine oxydase-derived O_2 radicals. In animal models, BT to the mesenteric lymph nodes (MLN) can also be induced by simply altering normal gut flora. When *E. coli* counts exceeds 109/g of feces, MLN cultures become consistently positive [39]. Finally, the gut is strongly suspected to be responsible for the endotoxin release often present in the circulation of patients with severe grampositive infections [28]. The type of bacteria present in the portal circulation is probably of importance in the intensity of the cytokine production. Matuschak et al. [30] have demonstrated that TNF and IL-6 production by perfused rat liver was far higher with *E. coli* than with *S. aureus* or *Candida spp*. Finally, the way endotoxin translocates through the gut barrier (trans-cellular versus para-cellular) is of probable importance to activate or not the local cytokine production but this point requires further investigation. In summary, there are a rather high number of arguments in the literature supporting the role of endotoxin in the most critically ill patients.

Endotoxin-Independent Activation of Cytokines

Many contra-arguments can also be gathered to challenge the role of endotoxin and favor a direct activation of the cytokines network by ischemia itself during shock states and severe trauma (see also chapter by Moore et al.). First, although cytokines are usually found in the systemic blood of animals and patients with severe shock and I/R, endotoxinemia is far from being constant. Moore et al. [18], for example, showed that endotoxin was not found in portal or systemic samples up to 5 days after laparotomy performed for severe trauma. In this study, cytokines were not detected either. In contrast with high IL-6 and IL-8 levels, neither endotoxin nor TNF were found in the blood of severe trauma patients. In addition, in the study by Cabie et al. [25], endotoxin, in contrast to TNF, was not found in all patients after cross-clamping of the aorta, neither in portal nor in systemic blood, and LPS levels were not correlated with TNF ones. Similarly, in patients with MOF, endotoxin levels were either normal or not very high. However, we must point out that the presence, in most patients of high levels of bilirubin made the detection threshold for endotoxin difficult to define. An additional argument is provided by the study of Koike et al. [21]. In this study, the authors studied whether gut I/R, sufficient to produce lung injury, was associated with endotoxemia. Peak endotoxin concentrations occurred during early gut ischemia but further release was not obvious during reperfusion (Fig. 4). More-

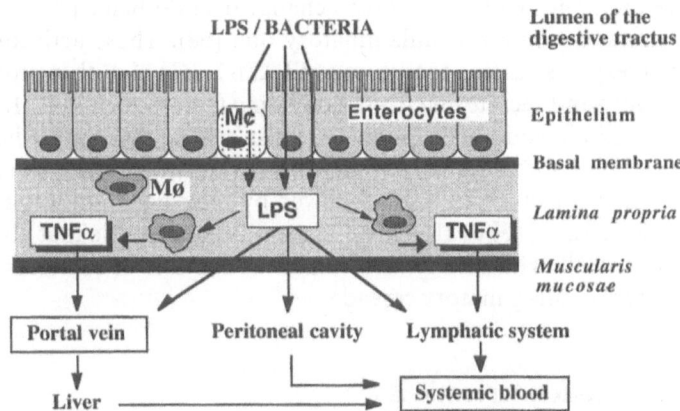

Fig. 5. Proposed mechanism for cytokine activation within lamina propria in relation with endotoxin (LPS) or bacterial translocation. TNF = tumor necrosis factor; LPS = lipopolysaccharide; Mo = monocytes; Mc = macrophages. (Modified from [64])

over, these concentrations were not significantly different from the levels in the sham-laparotomy animals. Moreover, the neutralization of endotoxin with an anti-endotoxin antibody (E 5 from Miles-Cutter), was unable to prevent the lung injury. This study however does not rule out an immediate action of endotoxin in the lamina propria of the gut which is known to be the production site of cytokines in the gut [51]. Very small amounts of endotoxin are probably sufficient during hypoxic situations to activate lamina propria to produce cytokines. In addition, E5 monoclonal antibody may not be efficient to neutralize completely endotoxin.

In contrast to anti-endotoxin antibodies, anti-TNF ones seem to be effective. Squadrito et al. [52] showed for example that passive immunization with anti-TNF in animal models of bowel ischemia injury attenuates the increase of pulmonary microvascular permeability and protects the animals from lethal effects. Although lung hyperpermeability was indeed prevented, the activation and sequestration of granulocytes in the lung, however, was not prevented by anti TNF pre-treatment in a study by Caty et al. [21]. This suggests that the neutrophils activation might result from the activation of TNF-independent pathways, namely gut ischemia itself.

Intestinal Cytokines and Splanchnic Ischemia

As pointed out in other chapters in this book, the gut is more susceptible to ischemia than the rest of the body [52]. Internal diary metabolism and energy production have an absolute dependence on oxygen. Inadequate oxygen rapidly leads to cellular dysfunction and injury [53]. One of the consequences is the production of oxygen radicals [55, 56]. These oxygen radicals have been shown to induce production of cytokines, especially TNF α by activating the promotor NF-

KB [57]. The cytokines induce a change in endothelial phenotype from a non-in-flammatory to a pro-inflammatory one [58]. These activated endothelial cells then express surface receptors as ELAM-1, ICAM-1, that promote leukocyte adherence and secrete leukocyte-activating factors such as IL-1, IL-8, and GM-CSF. This shift in endothelial phenotype results in leukocyte-mediated endothelial injury. Some studies have indeed demonstrated that during *in vitro* model of endothelial cell culture, hypoxia followed by reoxygenation was able to release cytokines as IL-1 [48] or IL-6 [59]. Thus, it is conceivable that gut micro-circulatory injury itself, without any involvement of bacteria or bacterial products, could activate the inflammatory cascade.

Therapeutic Interventions

A couple of therapeutic interventions could be used in the future to decrease cytokine production from the gut. They could be used either preventively, for example before surgical procedures known to induce cytokine release, or in a curative way. They include anti-endotoxins, anti-cytokines or soluble cytokine receptors (as soluble TNF receptors), or strategies able to decrease the amount of bacteria or endotoxin in the gut as the so-called selective digestive decontamination (SDD). It is far too early to know if the effects of those strategies, which for most of them remain controversial, could be due to any effect upon intestinal cytokines.

During experimental models, as mentionned above, anti-endotoxin monoclonal antibodies failed to prevent the pulmonary consequences of an experimental gut I/R [21]. However, additional data would be helpful in this area. Anti-cytokines could represent promizing drugs [21,52], provided they are used prophylactically, during situations known to induce acute I/R of the gut, as cardiopul-

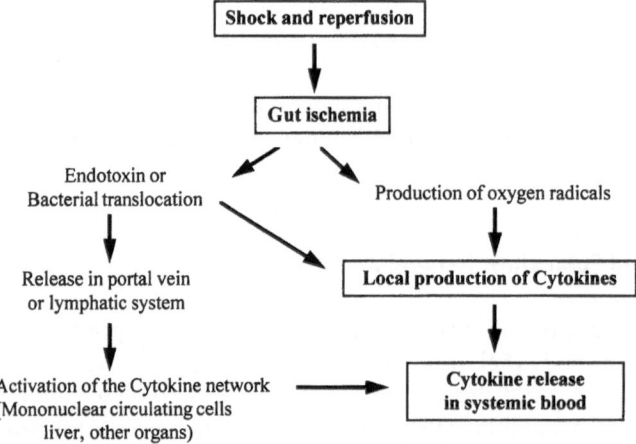

Fig. 6. Possible pathways for cytokine release during gut ischemia

monary bypass or vascular surgery. A recent experimental study shows that the lung injury induced by a model of intestinal I/R was efficiently prevented by soluble TNF receptors and anti-cytokine monoclonal antibodies [60]. The prerequisite for their usage should be our ability to detect, before surgery, the patients at risk to develop a profound gut ischemia. It could be useful to implement appropriate and well designed clinical studies in this setting.

The effect of SDD with non-absorbable antibiotics is treated elsewhere in this book. Some studies looked at endotoxin or cytokine release as endpoints. Martinez-Pelluz et al. [61] showed that TNF and IL-6 levels, as well as endotoxin ones were far lower than controls in patients experiencing a cardiopulmonary bypass and who were efficiently decontaminated with a combination of tobramicin and polymixin B. In contrast, Bion et al. [62] failed to demonstrate a significant decrease in endotoxin levels in patients with hepatic transplant performed for acute hepatic failure using the same strategy. Finally, Tetteroo et al. [63] showed a reduction in mortality and length of stay in patients experiencing very high risk surgical procedures. Additional informations are needed before being able to use this technique in patients at high risk to develop gut ischemia after trauma or surgery. Moreover, the respective role of the antimicrobial and of the anti-endotoxin effect of the strategy (polymixin) remain to be studied.

Conclusion

A substantial amount of evidence supports the implication of cytokines during episodes of gut ischemia. The mechanism by which they are activated remains controversial and the different pathways are in no way exclusive to each other. The translocation of either dead or alive bacteria, or of bacterial products mainly, but maybe not exclusively, endotoxin, is likely to occur at least in some cases. Those products could then very well activate the production of cytokines, in particular by the liver. They could also reach the systemic circulation via the lymphatic route or in the situations where the liver is significantly altered. On the other hand, small amounts of endotoxin can probably be able to activate a local production of cytokines in the lamina propria of the gut and this even into a higher extent if the gut is ischemic. The ischemia of the digestive cells by itself is probably able to activate the cytokines production via the production of oxygen free radicals. Those various mechanisms are likely to be associated and to be involved in the amplification of the inflammatory cascade. The respective responsibility of each phenomenon as well as the exact sequence of events remain to be fully understood before being able to propose preventive therapeutic strategies.

Acknowledgement: We thank J. M. Cavaillon, from Institut Pasteur, for his inestimable input in several of the studies mentionned in this chapter.

References

1. Deitch EA, Berg R (1987) Bacterial translocation from the gut: A mechanism of infection. J Burn Care Rehabil 8:475–482
2. Faist E, Baue AE, Dittmer H, et al (1983) Multiple organ failure in polytrauma patients. J Trauma 23:775–786
3. Fry DE, Pearlstein L, Fulton RL, et al (1980) Multiple system organ failure. Arch Surg 115:136–140
4. Goris R, Beokhorst P, Nuytinck K, et al (1985) Multiple organ failure: Generalized auto-destructive inflammation. Arch Surg 120:1109–1115
5. Border JR (1992) Multiple system organ failure. Ann Surg 216:111–116
6. Goodwin C (1990) Multiple organ failure: A clinical overview. J Trauma 30:5163–5165
7. Steinmetz O, Meakins J (1992) Translocation of bacteria from the gut: Clinically relevant? In: Fry D (ed) Multiple System Organ Failure. Mosby CV, Saint-Louis, pp 373–382
8. Wells C, Rotstein O, Pruett TL, et al (1986) Intestinal bacterial translocation into experimental intra-abdominal abscesses. Arch Surg 121:102–107
9. Fiddian Green R (1991) Role of the gut in shock and resuscitation. In: Ballière Trindall (ed) Ballière Clinical Anaesthesiology. London pp 75–99
10. Wilmore DN, Smith RJ, O'Duyer ST, et al (1988) The gut: A control organ after surgical stress. Surgery 104:917–923
11. Border JR, Manell S, La Ducca J (1987) The gut origin septic states in blunt multiple trauma (ISS=40) in the ICU. Ann Surg 206:427–448
12. Baker JW, Deitch EA, Li M, et al (1988) Hemorrhagic shock induces bacterial translocation from the gut. J Trauma 28:896–906
13. Deitch EF, Winterton J, Li M, Berg R (1987) The gut as a portal of entry of bacteremia. Role of protein malnutrition. Ann Surg 205:681–692
14. Deitch EA, Ma L, Ma WJ, et al (1989) Inhibition of endotoxin induced bacterial translocation in mice. J Clin Invest 84:36–42
15. Alexander JW, Boyce SJ, Babcock GF, et al (1990) The process of microbial translocation. Ann Surg 212:496–512
16. Rush BF, Sori AJ, Murphy TF, et al (1988) Endotoxin and bacteremia during hemorrhagic shock: The link between trauma and sepsis? Ann Surg 207:549–552
17. Ayala A, Perrin MM, Meldrum DR, et al (1990) Hemmorrhage induces an increase in serum TNF which is not associated with elevated levels of endotoxin. Cytokine 2:170–174
18. Moore FA, Moore EE, Poggetti R, et al (1991) Gut bacterial translocation via the portal vein: A clinical perspective with major torso trauma. J Trauma 31:629–639
19. Goris RJA, Boekholtz WKF, Van Bebber IPJ, et al (1986) Multiple organ failure and sepsis without bacteria. An experimental model. Arch Surg 121:897–901
20. Caty M, Guice K, Oldham K, Remick D, Kuntel S (1989) Evidence for TNF-induced pulmonary microvascular injury after intestinal ischemia-reperfusion injury. Ann Surg 212:694–700
21. Koike K, Moore E, Moore F, Read R, Carl V, Banerjee A (1994) Gut ischemia reperfusion produces lung injury independent of endotoxin. Crit Care Med 22:1438–1444
22. Marty C, Misset B, Tamion F, et al (1994) Circulating interleukin-8 concentrations in patients with multiple organ failure of septic and non-septic origin. Crit Care Med 22:673–679
23. Gathiram P, Wells MJ, Raidoo D, et al (1989) Changes in lipopolysaccharide concentrations in hepatic portal and systemic arterial plasma during intestinal ischemia in monkeys. Circ Shock 27:103–109
24. Pinsky MR, Vincent JL, Deviere J, et al (1993) Serum cytokine levels in human septic shock. Relationship to multiple-system organ failure and mortality. Chest 103:565–575
25. Cabie A, Farkas JC, Fitting C, et al (1993) High levels of portal TNF during abdominal aortic surgery in man. Cytokine 5:448–453
26. Jacob AI, Goldberg PK, Bloom N, et al (1977) Endotoxin and bacteria in portal blood. Gastroenterology 72:1268–1272
27. Panja A, Siden E, Mayer L, et al (1995) Synthesis and regulation of accessory-proinflammatory cytokines by intestinal epithelial cells. Clin Exp Immunol 100:298–305

28. Ramsay G, Newman PM, McCartney AC, et al (1988) Endotoxaemia in multiple organ failure due to sepsis. Prog Clin Biol Res 272:237–246
29. Marshall JC, Lee C, Meakins JL, et al (1987) Kupffer cell modulation of the systemic immune response. Arch Surg 122:191–196
30. Matuschak GM, Munoz C, Epperly NA, et al (1994) TNF alpha and IL-6 expression in perfused rat liver after intra portal candidemia vs E. coli vs S. aureus bacteremia. Am J Physiol 267:R446–R454
31. Kahky MP, Daniel CO, Cruz AB, et al (1990) Portal infusion of TNF increases mortality in rats. J Surg Res 49:138–145
32. Vanlanschot JJB, Mealy K, Wilmore DW, et al (1990) The effect of TNF on intestinal structure and metabolism. Ann Surg 212:663–670
33. Coletti LM, Burch GD, Remick DG, et al (1990) The production of TNF and the development of a pulmonary injury following hepatic ischemia-reperfusion. Transplantation 49:268–272
34. Coletti LM, Remick DG, Burtch GD, et al (1990) Role of TNF in the pathophysiologic alterations after hepatic ischemia-reperfusion injury in rat. J Clin Invest 85:1936–1943
35. Pulliccino EA, Carli F, Poole S, et al (1990) The relationship between the circulating concentration of interleukin-6 (IL-6), TNF, and the acute phase response to elective surgery and accidental injury. Lymphokine Res 9:231–238
36. Cabie A, Fitting C, Farkas JF, et al (1992) Influence of surgery on in vitro cytokine production by human monocytes. Cytokine 4:476–480
37. Casey LC, Balk RA, Bone RC, et al (1993) Plasmatic cytokine and endotoxin levels correlate with survival in patients with the sepsis syndrome. Ann Intern Med 119:771–778
38. Schwenberg FB, Seligman AM, Fine J (1950) Transmural migration of intestinal bacteria. N Engl J Med 242:747–751
39. Deitch EA, Ma Cjima K, Berg RD (1985) Effect of oral antibodies and bacterial overgrowth on the translocation of the GI-tract microflore in burned mice. J Trauma 25:385–392
40. Inoue S, Wirman JA, Alexander JW, et al (1988) Candida albicans translocation across the gut mucosa following burn injury. J Surg Res 44:479–492
41. Cueva SP, Fine J (1971) Demonstration of a lethal endotoxemia in experimental occlusion of superior mesenteric artery. Surg Gynecol Obstet 133:81–83
42. Olofson P, Nylander G, Olsson P, et al (1986) Endotoxin route of transport in experimental peritonitis. Am J Surg 151:443–447
43. Nozichova M, Bartos V, Sedlak J, et al (1977) Effect of transintestinal ischemia on the thoracic duct lymph absorption of endotoxin. Lymphology 10:161–165
44. Daniele R, Singh H, Appert HE, et al (1970) Lymphatic absorption of intraperitoneal endotoxin in dog. Surgery 67:484–487
45. Gans HG, Matsumoto K (1974) The escape of endotoxin from the intestine. Surg Gynecol Obstet 139:395–402
46. Mainous MR, Tso P, Berg RD, et al (1991) Studies of the route, magnitude, and time course of bacterial translocation in a model of systemic inflammation. Arch Surg 126:33–37
47. Olofsson P, Nylander G, Olsson P (1985) Endotoxin transport route and kinetics in intestinal ischemia. Acta Chir Scand 151:635–639
48. Koga S, Ogawa S, Kuwabara K, et al (1992) Synthesis and release of interleukin-1 by reoxygenated mononuclear phagocytes. J Clin Invest 90:1007–1015
49. Ghezzi P, Dinarello CA, Bianchi M, Rosandich M, Repine JE, White CW (1991) Hypoxia increases production of IL-1 and TNF by human mononuclear cells. Cytokine 3:189–194
50. Wibbenmeyer LA, Lechner AJ, Munoz CF, et al (1995) Downregulation of E. coli-induced TNF alpha expression in perfused liver by hypoxia-reoxygenation. Am J Physiol 268:G311–G319
51. Fiocchi C (1991) Production of inflammatory cytokines in the intestinal lamina propria. Immunol Res 10:1986–1995
52. Squadrito F, Altavilla D, Loculano M, et al (1992) Passive immunization with antibodies against TNF protects from lethality of splanchnic artery occlusion shock. Circ Shock 37:236–244
53. Nelson DP, King CE, Dodd SL, Schumaker PJ, Cain SM (1987) Systemic and intestinal limits of O_2 extraction in the dog. J Appl Physiol 63:387–394

54. Baneso-Aranda J, Schmid-Schonbein GW, Zweifach BW, Engler RL (1988) Granulocytes and NO reflexe phenomenon in irreversible hemorrhagic shock. Circ Res 63:437–447
55. Reilly PM, Schiller HJ, Bulkley GB (1991) Pharmacologic approach to tissue injury mediated by free radicals and other oxygen metabolites. Am J Surg 161:488–503
56. Granger DN (1988) Role of xanthine oxydase and granulocytes in ischemia-reperfusion injury. Am J Physiol 24:M1269–M1275
57. Pober JS, Cotran RS (1990) Cytokines and endothelial cell biology. Physiol Rev 70:427–451
58. Roebuck KA, Rahman A, Lakshminaray Avan V, Janakidevi K, Malik AB (1995) H_2O_2 and tumor necrosis factor activate intracellular adhesion molecule-1 (ICAM-1). Gene transcription through distinct regulatory elements within the ICAM promotor. J Biol Chem 270:18966–18974
59. Yan SF, Tritto I, Pinsky D, et al (1995) Induction of interleukin-6 (IL-6) by hypoxia in vascular cells. J Biol Chem 270:11463–11471
60. Sorkine P, Setton A, Halpern P, et al (1995) Soluble tumor necrosis factor receptors reduce bowel ischemia-induced lung permeability and neutrophil sequestration. Crit Care Med 23:1377–1381
61. Martinez-Pellus AE, Merino P, Bru M, et al (1993) Can selective digestive decontamination avoid the endotoxinemia and cytokine activation promoted by cardiopulmonary bypass? Crit Care Med 21:1684–1691
62. Bion JF, Badger I, Crosby HA, et al (1994) Selective decontamination of the digestive tract reduces gram-negative pulmonary colonization but not systemic endotoxinemia in patients undergoing elective liver transplantation. Crit Care Med 22:40–49
63. Tetteroo GW, Wagenvort HT, Mulder PG, et al (1993) Decreased mortality and length of hospital stay in surgical intensive care unit patients with successful selective decontamination of the digestive tract. Crit Care Med 21:1692–1698
64. Cavaillon JM, Tamion F, Marty C, et al (1994) Multiorgan dysfunction syndrome and the implication of cytokines. In: Mutz NJ, Koller W, Benzer H (eds) 7th European Congress on Intensive Care Medicine (Proceedings), pp 23–32

Selective Decontamination of the Digestive Tract

C. P. Stoutenbeek and H. K. F. van Saene

Introduction

Selective decontamination of the digestive tract (SDD) is an infection prevention technique used in granulocytopenic patients, transplantation surgery and in critically ill intensive care patients. It is based on the observation that many infections are caused by aerobic gram-negative bacteria (Enterobacteriaceae and Pseudomonadaceae), *Staphylococcus aureus* and yeast spp. carried in the oropharyngeal or intestinal flora (i.e. endogenous infections). It is called selective because the topical antibiotics used for SDD have little effect on the indigenous flora. The indigenous mostly anaerobic flora should be preserved as much as possible because it has important physiological functions and is seldom the cause of infection. More than 10 years after the introduction of SDD in intensive care [1] it is still controversial. In this chapter, the rationale for SDD in intensive care patients and the controversial issues will be discussed.

Rationale

Infections can be divided into endogenous and exogenous infections. Endogenous infections are defined as infections caused by potentially pathogenic microorganisms (PPM) carried in the throat and gastrointestinal (GI) tract, whereas exogenous infections are caused by PPM that have multiplied outside the body and that are introduced by an intervention (eg a contaminated nebulizer). Endogenous infections can be further subdivided into primary and secondary endogenous infections. Primary endogenous infections are caused by PPM that the patient is already carrying in throat or GI tract on admission to the ICU, whereas secondary endogenous infections are caused by PPM that have colonized the throat and GI tract during ICU stay. Although both exogenous infections and secondary endogenous infections are caused by hospital-acquired micro-organisms, the difference is that the multiplication phase of PPM in exogenous infections is outside the body, and in secondary endogenous infections it is inside the oropharynx or GI tract. This difference is important from the point of view of prophylaxis, because the multiplication of pathogens inside the body can be prevented by SDD.

Normal Flora

The normal flora is a very stable ecosystem. Exogenous micro-organisms ingested with food and beverages have little chance of survival in the body. After a transient presence in throat, stomach and gut, these are cleared by the defense mechanisms of the oropharynx and GI tract. This carriage defense is the first line of defense to control the microbial pressure from the outside world and comprises several factors including

1) the integrity of anatomy and physiology of the mucosal surfaces, which are covered by a protective blanket of mucus, preventing the adherence of micro-organisms;
2) motility: swallowing, chewing, deglutition, gastric emptying and peristalsis promote the clearance of micro-organisms present in the daily food intake;
3) mucosal cell renewal contributes to the removal of micro-organisms adhering to the mucosal surfaces;
4) gastric acidity;
5) secretions such as saliva, gastric and pancreatic juice, bile and mucus containing bactericidal products such as lysozyme, peroxidase and enzymes;
6) secretory immunoglobulin A preventing bacterial adherence to the mucosa; and
7) the indigenous flora inhibiting exogenous bacteria via competition for food, and production of bacterial toxins and volatile fatty acids (i.e. colonization resistance) [2, 3].

Impaired Carriage Defense

The carriage defense is the first line of defense to fail during illness. During illness the adherence of gram-negative bacilli (GNB) to mucosal cells is greatly increased due to the loss of fibronectin on the surface of mucosal cells exposing the receptors. Stasis in the GI tract due to paralytic ileus or mechanical obstruction leads to overgrowth of aerobic GNB. In critically ill patients gastric exocrine failure is common [4], showing a gastric pH of more than 4, even without the use of H_2-blockers or antacids. Starvation and lack of enteral feeding may impair the mucosal cell turnover and lead to mucosal atrophy. In critically ill patients, the quality of the mucous membrane as a "feeder layer" may change, and therewith its quality as a 'hopper' for the indigenous microflora. A starving indigenous flora appears to become easily replaced by GNB [5].

The endotracheal tube, nasogastric tube, sedatives and morphinomimetic drugs and dopamine all further contribute to the impairment of the carriage defense [6]. The presence of a nasogastric tube impairs the function of the gastro-oesophageal sphincter, leading to migration of gastric flora into the oesophagus and oropharynx. The salivary excretion may be reduced by atropin-like drugs. Administration of intravenous broad spectrum β-lactam antibiotics, which are excreted into the oropharynx and the GI canal via saliva, bile and mucus, may eradicate both the indigenous flora and the sensitive "community" PPM. As a consequence, resistant GNB, *S. aureus* and *Candida* spp are selected, followed by overgrowth in the oropharynx and GI tract.

Abnormal Carrier State

From a microbiological point of view, the impairment of carriage defense is associated with an abnormal carrier state. The incidence of abnormal carriage in mechanically ventilated patients is 60–90%. High concentrations of mostly gram-negative bacilli ($> 10^9$/mL), but also *S. aureus* and *Candida* spp can be found in saliva, stomach and gut [7] as soon as 48 h after admission to the ICU.

The clinical consequences of this rapid overgrowth by PPM are not yet fully understood. Is it a symptom of severe illness or a disease by itself? However, it is generally accepted that it predisposes to (secondary endogenous) infections and to emergence of resistance. It is also associated with multiple organ failure (MOF) [8]. The pathophysiological mechanisms by which infections and MOF may develop are (micro)aspiration, continuous spreading of PPM to neighboring organ systems, translocation and absorption of endotoxin. SDD is a technique to prevent and to treat abnormal carriage.

SDD

SDD includes three essential elements:
1. the application of topical non-absorbable antibiotics to the oropharyngeal cavity and GI tract;
2. a short period of systemic antibiotic prophylaxis in the first few days; and
3. intensive bacteriological monitoring of the oropharynx and GI tract.

Topical Non-Absorbable Antibiotics

The aim of the topical antibiotics is to selectively eliminate the aerobic PPM from the oropharyngeal cavity and GI tract, thereby preventing endogenous infections and emergence of resistance. The classical SDD regimen includes Polymyxin, Tobramycin and Amphotericine B (PTA-regimen). It covers all aerobic gram-negative PPM, *S. aureus* and yeast but has relatively little effect on the indigenous flora. Polymyxin is the cornerstone of SDD, because of its broad gram-negative spectrum and because there is no acquired resistance to polymyxin. However, the gap in the spectrum of polymyxin includes *Proteus* and *Providencia* spp. and therefore it should be combined with another agent (eg an aminoglycoside or a fluoro-quinolon). Tobramycin is the drug of choice because it has a potentiating bactericidal effect on *Pseudomonas* and *Acinetobacter* spp.

The correct choice and dosage of the topical antibiotics is crucial for the success of SDD, because many antibiotics are inactivated by feces [9] or by concomitant medication such as antacids or sucralfate [10] which makes them less suitable for decontamination. Agents like neomycin, nalidixic acid and erythromycin which were used in the preoperative preparation for colorectal surgery or in granulocytopenic patients are unsuitable for decontamination, because they are inactivated almost completely by feces.

The oropharynx is the most important reservoir of PPM causing respiratory tract infections and infections in the upper part of the body (eg mediastinitis, line infections), whereas the GI tract is more important for infections of the urinary tract, abdominal cavity, wounds etc. It is therefore of the utmost importance to decontaminate *both* the oropharynx *and* the GI tract.

In an effectively decontaminated patient only anaerobes, enterococci, viridans streptococci and coagulase negative staphylococci should be found in throat or rectal culture. It is obvious that these micro-organisms are not sensitive to the topical antibiotics used. This should not be regarded as overgrowth, because the absolute numbers do not increase. Most controlled clinical trials show that the isolation of enterococci and *Staphylococcus epidermidis* in the oropharynx and rectum has no clinical sequelae.

Systemic Antibiotic Prophylaxis

In mechanically ventilated intensive care patients, early onset infections are invariably caused by PPM carried by the patient in throat or GI tract upon admission to the ICU (i.e. primary endogenous infections). A typical example is a respiratory tract infection with *Streptococcus pneumoniae* developing on the second day in a multiple trauma patient admitted with a lung contusion. Primary endogenous infections, occurring within the first four days of intensive care stay, constitute about 50% of all respiratory infections developing in intensive care patients when no systemic antibiotic prophylaxis is given [11].

SDD should be combined with a short-term systemic antibiotic prophylaxis in the first 3–4 days of ICU stay in order to

1) eliminate gram-positive PPM from the oropharynx (eg pneumococci, hemolytic streptococci) which are insensitive to the topical antibiotics; and
2) prevent primary endogenous infections in the first few days when the decontamination is not yet complete.

Microbiological Surveillance

The bacteriological monitoring is another essential element of SDD:
1) to control the effectiveness of the decontamination procedure;
2) to adjust the antibiotic regimen in case of colonization by resistant strains eg methicillin-resistant *S. aureus* (MRSA); and
3) to recognize exogenous infections and to take the appropriate measures.

Systematic Reviews of SDD Trials

To date there are 46 trials on SDD and 4 meta-analyses. The first meta-analysis included only 1489 patients from 11 trials of which 6 randomized, controlled trials [12]. Recently three more meta-analyses of randomized, controlled trials of SDD have been published [13–15]. These meta-analyses differ not only in the number of trials and patients analyzed, but also in the methodology. Kollef analyzed only published trials including 2270 patients in 21 trials [15]. Heyland et al. [14] analyzed 3395 patients in 25 randomized published and unpublished trials. The SDD trialists' Collaborative Group analyzed 4142 patients from 22 randomized trials, both published and unpublished. They collected all patient data through direct contact with the investigators so that they could do an analysis on an intention-to-treat basis [13].

All meta-analyses show a significant reduction in the relative risk of respiratory infections in patients receiving intensive care. Kollef found a highly significant reduction in pneumonia rate but a small non-significant reduction in overall mortality (268 deaths out of 1105 for SDD-treated patients and 305 of 1165 control patients; $p = 0.291$) [15]. The SDD trialists' Collaborative Group found that SDD significantly reduced respiratory tract infections (odds ratio 0.37; 95% confidence interval 0.31–0.43). The value of the common odds ratio for total mortality (0.90; 0.79–1.04) suggested a moderate treatment effect, reaching statistical significance only when the subgroup of trials of topical and systemic treatment combined was considered separately (OR 0.80; CI 0.67–0.97) [13]. Heyland et al. [14] also found that the incidence of pneumonia was significantly lower in patients receiving SDD (Relative Risk (RR) 0.46; 95% CI 0.39–0.56) but they found a significant reduction in overall mortality (RR 0.87; 95% CI 0.79–0.97). In a subgroup analysis, the largest absolute difference was found in the comparison of studies using regimens including intravenous antibiotics (RR = 0.80; CI 0.68–0.95) and those that excluded systemic antibiotics (RR = 0.99; CI 0.83–1.19) [14].

Effectiveness of Decontamination

The fact that a mortality benefit was found only in the subgroup of 14 studies using topical antibiotics in combination with intravenous prophylaxis suggests that the systemic component is very important. However, this subgroup differs from the studies without systemic component also in the decontamination regimen used: in 9/14 studies oral and intestinal decontamination with the PTA-regimen has been used, whereas in only 2/14 studies no decontamination was achieved due to improper choice of topical antibiotics and these two studies were negative (Table 1).

On the other hand, in the subgroup of 9 studies that excluded intravenous antibiotic prophylaxis and in which no reduction of mortality was found; decontamination of *both* throat and gut was performed in only two studies (Table 1). The remaining 7 studies applied topical antibiotics either in the GI tract or only

Table 1. Trials using topical antibiotics and parenteral prophylaxis

Authors	Ref.	No. patients	Topical regimen	Topical application	Systemic prophylaxis
Verhaegen II et al.	[41]	268	Oflaxacine	oral + intestin	Ofloxa
Cockerill et al.	[42]	150	P, Gen, Nys	oral + intestin	Ctx
Aerdts et al.	[431]	88	P, Nor, A + Ctx	oral + intestin	Ctx
Ullrich et al.	[44]	112	P, Nor, A	oral + intestin	Tmp
Verhaegen et al.	[41]	385	PTA	oral + intestin	Ctx
Rocha et al.	[36]	101	PTA	oral + intestin	Ctx
Palomar et al.	[45]	97	PTA	oral + intestin	Ctx
Blair et al.	[46]	231	PTA	oral + intestin	Ctx
Kerver et al.	[47]	96	PTA	oral + intestin	Ctx
Hammond et al.	[19]	322	PTA	oral + intestin	Ctx
Ferrer et al.	[18]	80	PTA	oral + intestin	Ctx
Jacobs et al.	[48]	91	PTA	oral + intestin	Ctx
Sanchez et al.	[49]	271	PTA	oral + intestin	Ctx
Winter et al.	[50]	183	PTA	oral + intestin	Czd
Korinek et al.	[51]	191	PTA	oral + intestin	None
Gastinne et al.	[22]	445	PTA	oral + intestin	None
Cerra et al.	[52]	48	Nor, Nys	oral + intestin	None
Godard et al.	[53]	185	PT	intestin	None
Unertl et al.	[54]	39	P, Gen, A	intestin	None
Gaussorgues et al.	[55]	118	½ P, Gen, Van, A	intestin	None
Brun-Buisson et al.	[17]	133	½ P, Neo, Nali	intestin	None
Pugin et al.	[21]	79	P, Neo, Van	oral	None
Rodriguez et al.	[56]	31	PTA	oral	None

P: polymyxine/colistin; Gen: gentamicin; Nys: nystatin; Ctx: cefotaxime; N: norfloxacin; A: amphotericin B; Tmp: trimetoprim; ½ P: half dosis of polymyxin; Neo: neomycin; Van: vancomycin; Nali: nalidixic acid

in the oral cavity. Furthermore, many different antibiotic regimens were used without presenting any evidence of their effectiveness with regard to decontamination. Thus the difference in mortality in the two groups may not only be explained by the use of the systemic component but also by the effectiveness of the topical regimen.

The fact that the effectiveness of decontamination is a crucial factor has been demonstrated in a recent study by Tetteroo et al. [16]. Patients treated with SDD were divided into two groups: those who were effectively decontaminated within three days and those who were not. The actual death rate in patients who were effectively decontaminated within 3 days (n = 72) was significantly lower than the predicted death rate (as calculated by the APACHE II score) (18 versus 40%, p = 0.006), whereas no difference was found in those patients who were not effectively decontaminated despite the treatment with topical antibiotics (n = 25, death rate 44%). The unsuccessful decontaminated patients had a significantly longer hospital (52 versus 34 days) and length of ICU stay (23 versus 9 days; p = 0.002) and higher mortality rates (44 versus 18%, p = 0.20) when compared with the successfully decontaminated patients. This study is confounded by the fact that patients who are effectively decontaminated within 3 days probably have a functioning GI tract in contrast to those who cannot be decontaminated within that period, and this may reflect the severity on the underlying disease. However, the APACHE scores were similar in both groups. Furthermore, this study shows that as long as the patient is not effectively decontaminated, the infection rate remains high.

Diagnostic Criteria for Pneumonia

There is a strikingly wide range in the incidence of respiratory tract infections (18 to 80%) in the control groups of SDD-studies although apparently the criteria for diagnosis were very similar. This may be explained by differences in patient populations and in underlying diseases but it has also been argued that, due to aspecific criteria used for diagnosis of pneumonia in unblinded studies, the true pneumonia rate has been overestimated in SDD studies [17]. In fact, part of the respiratory tract infections in these studies might represent broncho-pneumonia, bronchitis or tracheitis rather than pneumonia. However, these infections cannot be disregarded as trivial and without clinical importance and their prevention is worthwhile.

There is little doubt that in studies in which pneumonia is diagnosed by the "protected brush technique" using a cut-off point of 10^3 CFU or by broncho-alveolar lavage with a cut-off point of 10^5 CFU/mL, the infection rate is much lower than in studies using clinical criteria. However, the SDD trialists' Collaborative Group demonstrated that the reduction of the relative pneumonia risk by SDD is independent of the criteria used for diagnosing pneumonia, and independent of the blinding of the study. In the subgroup of studies using the "protected brush" or broncho-alveolar lavage to diagnose pneumonia, the odds ratio was 0.38 (CI 0.29–0.49) versus 0.36 (0.29–0.44) in the subgroup of studies not using the protected brush.

Negative SDD Trials

A few trials using the full SDD-scheme, including oral and intestinal decontamination with the PTA-regimen and systemic antibiotic prophylaxis, did not find a significant reduction of the infection rate [18, 19]. There are several explanations for these negative results:
1. The impact of SDD on the ecology of the ICU by elimination of the patient sources. It has recently been shown that in a randomized, controlled trial the control group inside the same ICU as the SDD-treated group, had a significantly lower acquisition, colonization and infection rate than a concurrent control outside the ICU, or than a control group in the same ICU after discon-

tinuation of SDD [20]. Thus it should be realized that a randomized, controlled study inside one ICU may (partially) mask the effect of decontamination;

2. A number of double-blind studies have been conducted in an environment where methicillin-resistant *Staphylococcus aureus* (MRSA) was endemic. It is obvious that MRSA, which is also resistant to the tobramycin in the PTA-regimen, may be selected by SDD if no appropriate measures are taken, eg adding vancomycin to the regimen [21]. In these studies, the omission of the surveillance cultures or the blinding to its results has negatively influenced the results of the study due to colonization and infection with MRSA [18, 19, 22]; and

3. In some studies, the problem of exogenous infections appears not to be solved given the high incidence of exogenous gram-negative pulmonary infections in both treated and untreated patients [19].

Preoperative SDD High Risk Surgery

The meta-analyses have included only randomized trials in a general ICU population. Other trials with preoperative SDD have shown that it is highly effective in reducing the peri-operative infection risk in high risk surgery such as esophageal resections [23] and liver transplantation [24–26]. The advantage of preoperative SDD is that intestinal decontamination can be achieved within 48 h before the operation because the bowels are still functioning, whereas when it is started postoperatively it may take 7–10 days before complete decontamination is achieved.

SDD not only reduces the postoperative infection risk, but may also reduce the risk of serious surgical complications. Not only the risk of intestinal anastomotic leakage seems to be reduced but also the clinical consequences of leakage are less serious when there are no PPM in the intestinal contents. In an experimental study, anastomotic insufficiency following gastrectomy in rats could be increased by a high intraluminal concentration of PPM and could be significantly reduced by SDD [27].

SDD in Acute Pancreatitis

It is generally accepted that the initially sterile pancreatic necrosis secondarily infects with micro-organisms translocating from the gut. In experimental pancreatitis in rats, SDD is very effective in preventing translocation and infection of pancreatic necrosis [28, 29]. In a recent clinical study [30], it has been shown that SDD reduced the infection-related morbidity and mortality (35–22%) in severe acute pancreatitis. There was no difference in the early mortality from MOF associated with the acute pancreatitis, but late infection-related MOF and death were reduced by SDD. The number of patients with infected necrosis and the number of laparotomies per patient was significantly lower in the SDD-treated

group than in the control group [30].This study is one of the first studies showing the clinical importance of translocation in humans and the prevention by
SDD.

SDD in Fulminant Liver Failure and Burns

A few studies have shown that SDD reduces infections and mortality in patients
with acute fulminant liver failure waiting for transplantation [31, 32]. Also in
burn patients, SDD has been shown to be very effective in preventing infectious
complications by intestinal Enterobacteriaceae and Pseudomonadaceae [33, 34].
No controlled clinical SDD trials with mortality as endpoint have been performed in burn patients so far.

Emergence of Resistance

In most controlled SDD trials no evidence for emergence of resistance was
found. However, a few studies reported an increase in cefotaxime and tobramycin resistant strains in SDD-treated patient [35, 36]. In both studies, the copy-
strains (i.e. the same micro-organism from the same site from the same patient)
were not excluded. Moreover, although there was a relative increase in the percentage of tobramycin and cefotaxime-resistant strains, by effective elimination
of the sensitive ones, the absolute number of resistant strains decreased rather
than increased: eg tobramycin resistant *Acinetobacter* was found in 47/143 (33%)
isolates in the control group and in 14/23 (61%) of the treated group [35]. Recently, a 2-year surveillance showed that the prevalence of resistance did not increase during SDD [37]. In many ICUs using the same antibiotic regimen for
selective decontamination for more than 10 years, there is still no evidence of
emergence of resistance.

Selection of Gram-Positive Cocci

It has been suggested that SDD may lead to a gram-positive problem [38]. It is
obvious that enterococci and *S. epidermidis*, which belong to the normal indigenous flora, are the only micro-organisms isolated during successful decontamination. This does not represent overgrowth. Controlled trials that specifically
studied enterococci and *S. epidermidis* did *not* show an increased colonization or
infection with these micro-organisms during SDD [19, 39].

    As pointed out above, MRSA is an inherent limitation of the PTA-regimen,
and therefore, in an endemic MRSA environment, SDD may select this micro-organism [19, 22]. To avoid this, it should be considered to add vancomycin to the
PTA-regimen [40]. However, routine surveillance cultures to check the effectiveness of the decontamination remain the hallmark of SDD.

Conclusion

SDD is an infection prevention technique aiming to act against primary and secondary endogenous infections by aerobic gram-negative bacteria and yeast. The technique includes three elements: 1) oral and intestinal decontamination with topical non-absorbable antibiotics; 2) a short-term systemic antibiotic prophylaxis; and 3) microbiological surveillance. The meta-analyses have shown that SDD is highly effective in preventing respiratory tract infections in high risk patients. Exogenous infections are still important but can only be prevented with conventional hygienic measures. In an environment where MRSA is endemic, the PTA-regimen should be adjusted, to avoid selection of MRSA. Even in the most successful SDD trials, there seems to be a discrepancy between the dramatic reduction in infection rate and the modest reduction in mortality. This clearly demonstrates that the underlying disease is a more important determinant of mortality than acquired infections. However, when SDD is fully implemented (i.e. both oral and intestinal decontamination with the PTA-regimen in combination with a short-term antibiotic prophylaxis and microbiological surveillance), a 20% reduction in mortality can be achieved (Table 2). The clinical relevance of the observed reduction in mortality is clear when it is compared with the few other interventions that have a proven effect on mortality. The effect of thrombolytic agents in acute myocardial infarction on mortality could only be demonstrated after more than 14 000 patients treated with thrombolytic agents were included in a cumulative meta-analysis. In none of the available studies did SDD lead to emergence of resistance. However, bacteriological surveillance during SDD remains an essential part of the infection prevention technique. SDD is one of the best investigated and most effective infection prevention maneuvers in intensive care and should be considered in high risk patients.

Table 2. Indications for SDD

Indication	Topical antibiotics (PTA)	Systemic antibiotic prophylaxis
Oesophageal resection	Preoperatively	Perioperative (24 h)
Liver transplantation	Preoperatively	Perioperative (24 h)
Acute pancreatitis	Admission ICU	Day 1–4
Multiple trauma ISS > 16	Admission ICU	Day 1–4
Burns > 30% BSA	Admission ICU	Day 1–4
Medical or surgical patients with expected ventilatory support > 5 days	Admission ICU	Day 1–4 or systemic antibiotic therapy

ISS: injury severity score; BSA: body surface area

References

1. Stoutenbeek CP, Saene van HKF, Miranda DR, Zandstra DF (1984) The effect of selective decontamination of the digestive tract on colonization and infection rate in multiple trauma patients. Intensive Care Med 10:185–192
2. Wells CL, Maddaus MA, Jechorek RP, et al (1988) Role of intestinal anaerobic bacteria in colonisation resistance. Eur J Clin Microbiol Infect Dis 7:107–113
3. van der Waaij D (1982) Colonisation resistance of the digestive tract: Clinical consequences and implications. J Antimicrob Chemother 10:263–267
4. Stannard VA, Hutchinson A, Morris DL, et al (1988) Gastric exocrine "failure" in critically ill patients: Incidence and associated features. Br Med J 296:155–156
5. van der Waaij D (1988) Selective decontamination of the digestive tract: General principles. Eur J Cancer Clin Oncology 24S:1–4
6. Thülig B, van Saene HKF (1991) Impact of anaesthetic procedures on the oropharyngeal and gastrointestinal defence against carriage. In: Stoutenbeek CP, van Saene HKF (eds) Infection and the Anaesthetist. Bailliere's Clinical Anaesthesiology, Bailliere Tindall, London, pp 39–59
7. van Saene HKF, Stoutenbeek CP, Torres A (1992) The abnormal oropharyngeal carrier state: Symptom or disease? Respir Med 86:183– 186
8. Marshall JC, Christou NV, Meakins JL (1993) The gastrointestinal tract. The "undrained abscess" of multiple organ failure. Ann Surgery 218:111–119
9. van Saene JJM, van Saene HKF, Stoutenbeek CP, Lerk CF (1985) Influence of faeces on the activity of antimicrobial agents used for decontamination of the alimentary canal. Scand J Infect Dis 17:295–300
10. Feron B, Adair C, Gorman SP, McClurg B (1993) Interaction of sucralfate with antibiotics used for selective decontamination of the gastrointestinal tract. Am J Hosp Pharm 50: 2550–2553
11. Langer M, Cigada M, Mandelli M, et al (1987) Early onset pneumonia: A multicenter study in intensive care units. Intensive Care Med 13:342–346
12. Van den Broucke-Grauls CMJE, Van den Broucke JP (1991) Effect of selective decontamination of the digestive tract on respiratory tract infections and mortality in the intensive care units. Lancet 338:859–862
13. Selective Decontamination of the Digestive Tract Trialists' Collaborative group (1993) Meta-analysis of randomised controlled trials of selective decontamination of the digestive tract. Br Med J 307:525–532
14. Heyland DK, Cook DJ, Jaeschke R, Griffith L, Lee HN, Guyatt GH (1994) Selective decontamination of the digestive tract: An overview. Chest 105:1221–1229
15. Koleff MH (1994) The role of selective digestive tract decontamination on mortality and respiratory tract infections. A meta-analysis. Chest 105:1101–1108
16. Tetteroo GWM, Wagenvoort JHT, Mulder PGH, Ince C, Bruining HA (1993) Decreased mortality rate and length of stay in surgical intensive care unit patients with successful selective decontamination of the gut. Crit Care Med 21:1692–1698
17. Brun-Buisson C (1994) Selective decontamination in critical care. Interpreting the synthesized evidence. Chest 105:978–980
18. Ferrer M, Torres A, Gonzàlez J, et al (1994) Utility of selective digestive decontamination in a general population of mechanically ventilated patients. Ann Intern Med 120: 389–395
19. Hammond JMJ, Potgieter PD, Saunders GL, et al (1992) Double-blind study of selective decontamination of the digestive tract in intensive care. Lancet 340:5–9
20. Bonten MJM (1994) Colonization in patients receiving and not-receiving topical antimicrobial prophylaxis. Thesis, Maastrich, Netherlands, pp 99–118
21. Pugin J, Auckenthaler R, Lew DP, Suter PM (1991) Oropharyngeal decontamination decreases incidence of ventilator-associated pneumonia. JAMA 265:2704–2710
22. Gastinne H, Wolff M, Delatour F, et al (1992) A controlled trial in intensive care units of selective decontamination of the digestive tract with nonabsorbable antibiotics. N Engl J Med 326:594–599

23. Tetteroo GWM, Wagenvoort JHT, Castelein AL, Tilanus HW, Ince C, Bruining HA (1990) Selective decontamination to reduce gram-negative colonization and infection after oeso-phageal resection. Lancet 335:704–707

24. Wiesner RH, Krom RAF, Hermans P (1988) Selective bowel decontamination to decrease gram-negative aerobic bacterial and candida colonization and prevent infection after ortho-topic liver transplantation. Transplantation 45:570–574

25. Bion JF, Badger I, Crosby HA, et al (1994) Selective decontamination of the digestive tract reduces gram-negative pulmonary colonization but not systemic endotoxemia in patients undergoing elective liver transplantation. Crit Care Med 22:40–49

26. Smith SD, Jackson RJ, Hannakan CJ, Wadowsky RM, Tzakis AG, Rowe MI (1993) Selective decontamination in pediatric liver transplants. Transplantation 55:1306–1309

27. Schardey M, Kamps T, Rau HG, Gaterman S, Baretton G, Schildberg FW (1994) Bacteria: A major pathogenic factor for anastomotic insufficiency. Antimicrob Agents Chemother 38:2564–2567

28. Foitzik T, Fernandez del Castillo C, Ferraro MJ, Mithofer K, Rattner DW, Warshaw AL (1995) Pathogenesis and prevention of early pancreatic infection in experimental acute necrotizing pancreatitis. Ann Surg 222:179–185

29. Gianotti L, Munda R, Gennari R, Pyles R, Alexander JW (1995) Effect of different regimens of gut decontamination on bacterial translocation and mortality in experimental acute pancreatitis. Eur J Surg 161:85–92

30. Luiten EJ, Hop WC, Lange JF, Bruining HA (1995) Controlled clinical trial of selective decontamination for the treatment of severe acute pancreatitis. Ann Surg 222:57–65

31. Rolando N, Gimson A, Wade J, Philpott-Howard J, Casewell M, Williams R (1993) Prospec-tive controlled trial of selective parenteral and enteral antimicrobial regimen in fulminant liver failure. Hepatol 17:196–201

32. Salmeron JM, Titó I, Rimola A, et al (1992) Selective decontamination of the digestive tract in the prevention of bacterial infection in patients with acute liver failure. J Hepatol 14:280–285

33. Mackie DP, Hertum van WAJ, Schumburg T, Kuijper EC, Knape P (1992) Prevention of in-fection in burns: Preliminary experience with selective decontamination of the digestive tract in patients with extensive injuries. J Trauma 32:570–575

34. Manson WL, Pernod PGJ, Fidler V, Sauer EW, Klasen HJ (1992) Colonization of burns and the duration of hospital stay of severely burned patients. J Hosp Infect 22:55–63

35. Nardi G, Valentis U, Proietti A, et al (1993) Epidemiological impact of prolonged syste-matic use of topical SDD on bacterial colonization of the tracheobronchial tree and antibio-tic resistance. Intensive Care Med 19:273–278

36. Rocha L A, Martin MJ, Pita S, et al (1992) Prevention of nosocomial infection in critically ill patients by selective decontamination of the digestive tract. A randomized double blind, placebo controlled study. Intensive Care Med 18:398–404

37. Hammond JMJ, Potgieter PD (1995) Long-term effects of selective decontamination on anti-microbial resistance. Crit Care Med 23:637–645

38. Daschner F (1992) Emergence of resistance during selective decontamination of the diges-tive tract. Eur J Clin Microbiol Infect Dis 11:1–3

39. Humphreys H, Winter R, Pick A (1992) The effect of selective decontamination of the diges-tive tract on gastrointestinal enterococcal colonization in ITU patients. Intensive Care Med 18:459–463

40. Pugin J, Auckenthaler R, Lew DP, Suter PM (1991) Oropharyngeal decontamination de-creases incidence of ventilator-associated pneumonia. JAMA 265:2704–2710

41. Verhaegen J (1992) Randomized study of selective digestive decontamination on colonisa-tion and prevention of infections in mechanically ventilated patients in the ICU. Thesis, Leuven, Belgium

42. Cockerill FR, Muller SM, Anhalt JP, et al (1992) Prevention of infection in critically ill pa-tients by selective decontamination of the digestive tract. Ann Intern Med 117:545–553

43. Aerdts SJ, van Dalen R, Clasener HAL, Festen J, van Lier HJJ, Vollaard EJ (1991) Antibiotic prophylaxis of respiratory tract infections in mechanically ventilated patients. A prospec-tive, blinded, randomized trial of the effect of a novel regimen. Chest 100:783–791

44. Ulrich C, Harinck-de Weerd JE, Bakker NC, Jacz K, Doornbos L, de Ridder VA (1990) Selective decontamination of the digestive tract with norfloxacin in the prevention of ICU-acquired infections: A prospective randomized study. Intensive Care Med 15:424–431

45. Palomar M (1991) Prevention of nosocomial pneumonia in ventilated patients using cefotaxim (CTX) and SDD. 17th International Congress on Chemotherapy, Berlin

46. Blair P, Rowlands BJ, Lowry K, Webb H, Armstrong P, Smilie J (1991) Selective decontamination of the digestive tract: A stratified, randomized, prospective study in a mixed intensive care unit. Surgery 110:303–310

47. Kerver AJH, Rommes JH, Verhage EAE (1988) Prevention of colonization and subsequent infection in surgical intensive care patients. A prospective randomized study. Critical Care Med 16:1087–1093

48. Jacobs S, Foweraker JE, Roberts SE (1992) Effectiveness of selective decontamination of the digestive tract (SDD) in an ICU with a policy encouraging a low gastric pH. Clin Intensive Care 3:52–58

49. Sanchez M, Lopez J, Galvan B, et al (1990) Selective digestive tract decontamination (SDD) and sucralfate (S) in intubated patients. Intensive Care Med 16:S32 (Abst)

50. Winter R, Humphreys H, Pick A, MacGowan AP, Willatts SM, Speller DCE (1992) A controlled trial of selective decontamination of the digestive tract in intensive care and its effect on nosocomial infection. J Antimicrob Chemother 30:73–87

51. Korinek AM, Laisne MJ, Nicolas MH, et al (1993) Selective decontamination of the digestive tract in neurosurgical intensive care unit patients: A double blind, randomized, placebo-controlled study. Crit Care Med 21:1466–1473

52. Cerra FB, Maddaus MA, Dunn DL, et al (1992) Selective gut decontamination reduces nosocomial infections and length of stay but not mortality or organ failure in surgical intensive care unit patients. Arch Surg 127:163–169

53. Godard J, Guillaume C, Reverdy ME, et al (1990) Intestinal decontamination in a polyvalent ICU: A double-blind study. Intensive Care Med 16:307–311

54. Unertl K, Ruckdeschel G, Selbmann HK, et al (1987) Prevention of colonization and respiratory infections in long-term ventilated patients by local antimicrobial prophylaxis. Intensive Care Med 13:106–113

55. Gaussorgues Ph, Salord F, Sirodot M, et al (1991) Efficacité de la décontamination digestive sur la survenue des bactérémies nosocomiales chez les patients sous ventilation mécanique et recevant des bêta-mimétiques. Réan Soins Intens Méd Urg 7:169–174

56. Rodriguez-Roldan JM, Altuna-Cuesta A, Lopez A, et al (1990) Prevention of nosocomial lung infection in ventilated patients: Use of an antimicrobial pharyngeal nonabsorbable paste. Crit Care Med 18:1239–1242

Increased Gastrointestinal Permeability

D. G. Sinclair and T. W. Evans

Introduction

Advances in the application of supportive techniques to the critically ill have failed to influence significantly the high mortality associated with the development of multiple organ failure (MOF), to which the majority of such patients succumb. Sepsis and the associated systemic inflammatory response syndrome (SIRS) are together thought to account for the endothelial cell injury and loss of microvascular control that together lead to organ dysfunction [1]. Although an infective organism is identified in less than 50% of cases, in early studies of MOF occult sepsis was identified as the most important clinical correlate. However, more recent investigations have also suggested that organ failure can develop in the absence of an untreated focus of infection. Further, MOF can be reproduced experimentally by the infusion of a diverse spectrum of endogenously-derived mediators of inflammation. Studies have emphasized the central role of circulatory failure induced by SIRS in the development of MOF, which seems to carry an especially poor prognosis [2]. It has recently become apparent that hypoperfusion of the mucosa of the gastrointestinal (GI) tract is of fundamental importance in the development of MOF. While intestinal ischemia has been identified traditionally only with profound GI tract impairment or even transmural intestinal necrosis, it now appears that lesser degrees of ischemia, sufficient to produce a loss of the epithelial barrier function, may lead to equally important systemic injury. Thus, the mucosa of the GI tract in conjunction with the gut-associated lymphoid tissues, provides an effective barrier to the entry of bacteria and endotoxin to the bloodstream. Multiple factors support this barrier function, including the tight junctions between epithelial cells, specific epithelial IgA antibody and local cell-mediated immune responses [3]. Loss of barrier function and immunosuppression have long been recognized as complications of critical illness. The GI tract is particularly sensitive to ischemia during circulatory shock, and even when cardiac output is supranormal, displays anaerobic metabolism at a level of oxygen delivery (DO_2) sufficient for other organ systems to maintain aerobic cellular function [4]. Secondly, the GI tract is a reservoir of bacteria and endotoxin. Finally, the association between diminished cardiac output and decreased splanchnic blood flow in cardiogenic shock is established. It therefore seems increasingly likely that GI ischemia leads to disruption of the intestinal mucosa and the systemic absorption of bacteria, endotoxin and digestive en-

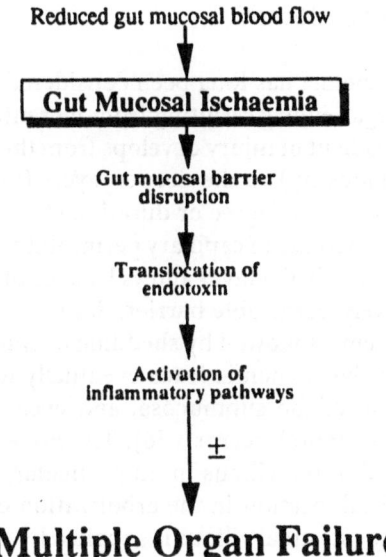

Fig. 1. The role of the gastrointestinal tract in modulating sepsis and multiple organ failure

zymes (Fig. 1). This may constitute an initiating or amplifying mechanism for the inflammatory cascades that are manifest as SIRS, or the establishing of a distant infective focus leading to the development of sepsis and septic shock.

Mechanism of Splanchnic Ischemia

Non-occlusive mesenteric hypoperfusion resulting in ischemia has long been considered to be the primary mechanism of GI injury. Low flow states may result from a number of pathological processes, including hypovolemia, and cardiogenic and septic shock. The physiological response to such states includes intense splanchnic vasoconstriction mediated by the renin-angiotensin axis. Surgery involving non-pulsatile cardiopulmonary bypass (CPB) is associated with this phenomenon and can be regarded as an iatrogenic form of hypovolemic or cardiogenic shock resulting in an ischemia/reperfusion injury.

Non-Pulsatile Perfusion

Non-pulsatile CPB leads to progressive, total systemic peripheral arterial vasoconstriction and reduced perfusion of peripheral organs. Numerous studies have documented a progressive increase in systemic vascular resistance (SVR) post-CPB, lasting from the onset of extracorporeal circulation, extending into the postoperative period. Decreased renal blood flow and a rise in angiotensin II (A-II) levels have been identified in these circumstances. A-II acts selectively on the hepatosplanchnic vascular bed to produce a disproportionate fall in perfusion [5].

Regional Sensitivity

Ischemia has long been considered to be the primary mechanism of splanchnic organ injury resulting from mesenteric hypoperfusion. Evidence suggests that a gradient of injury develops from the most superficial layers of the bowel wall (the villous tip) to the deeper layers (muscularis mucosa) as an ischemic insult increases in degree or duration (Fig. 2) [6]. The earliest manifestation of injury is an increase in capillary permeability to large molecules. Subsequently, the mucosal epithelial layer allows leakage of large molecules through the normally selectively-permeable barrier. Severe or prolonged ischemia produces subepithelial edema, followed by shedding of epithelial cells, initially from the villous tip. Still further ischemia leads eventually to full mucosal necrosis, followed by disruption of the submucosa, and eventually of the muscularis propria, producing transmural necrosis [6]. The preferential sensitivity of the mucosa in general, and of the villous tip in particular, to ischemic injury is probably related to its distal location in the arborization of the vascular tree. The microcirculation of the intestinal villous is supplied by a central arteriole which branches near the tip of the villous into a subepithelial network of capillaries and venules. Flow in the capillaries and venules is opposite in direction to the flow in the nutrient arteriole. Because the ascending and descending vessels are in close proximity, the countercurrent arrangement of the villous microvasculature permits arterial-venous diffusion of oxygen from the nutrient arteriole to the draining venules.

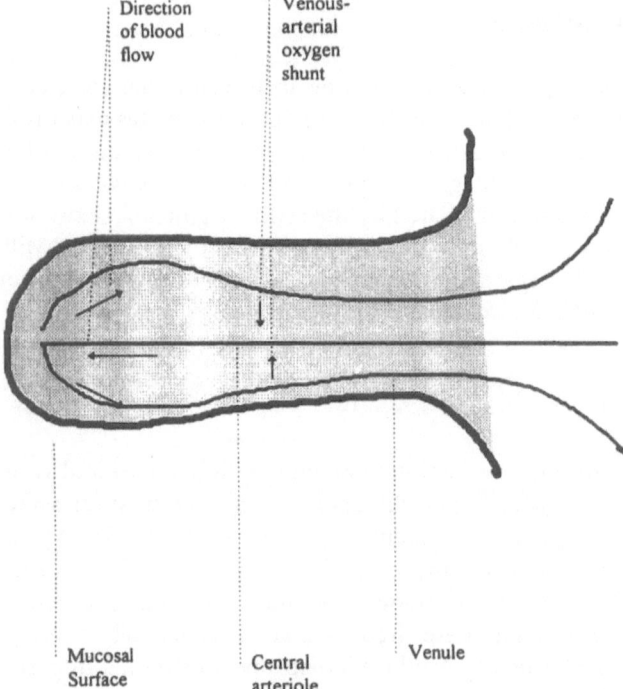

Fig. 2. Intestinal villous blood supply

As a result, oxygen tension is normally substantially lower at the tips of the villi than at the bases. Under certain pathological circumstances, such as systemic arterial hypotension or mediator-induced vasospasm of the splanchnic vessels, the linear velocity of red cells traversing the villous microvasculature is diminished and the countercurrent arterial-venous shunting of oxygen becomes exaggerated [7]. This phenomenon is probably important in the development of villous injury under ischemic conditions.

Reperfusion Injury

Whilst hypoxia plays a role in organ injury during hypoperfusion, much of the superficial injury incurred in the GI tract is thought to be sustained during reperfusion. Reactive oxygen species (ROS) generated by xanthine oxidase (high concentrations of which are found within the villous enterocyte) during reperfusion of ischemic bowel probably contribute significantly to the breakdown of mucosal integrity [8]. Work demonstrating that allopurinol, a specific inhibitor of xanthine oxidase, has a protective effect on gut permeability following experimental ischemia/reperfusion supports this hypothesis.

Toxic and Nutritional Factors

Numerous potent, corrosive factors are secreted into the lumen of the GI tract in health to facilitate normal function. These same agents, which include hydrochloric acid, bile salts, bacteria, bacterial toxins, protease's and other digestive enzymes have the potential to cause both local and systemic tissue injury when the gut epithelial barrier is breached. Further, an important requirement for the maintenance of normal GI integrity and function is the presence of appropriate nutrients within the gut lumen.

Measurement of GI Permeability

Tests used in the direct measurement of GI permeability in clinical practice can be divided into 3 groups: those that employ sugars, isotope-based tests, and those using polyethylene glycols (PEGS) as markers. Ideally, markers of intestinal permeability should be inert and cross the intestinal epithelium by non-mediated diffusion through defined pathways. Intestinal permeation is usually measured by renal excretion after oral ingestion, in which circumstance it is necessary to demonstrate that the test substance is qualitatively recoverable in urine after intravenous administration and can be reliably measured by a convenient technique. Secondly, the permeation of all substances is affected by a variety of non-mucosal factors including gastric emptying, intestinal transit, dilution by secretions, available surface area and altered renal clearance. The influence of these factors can be circumvented by the use of two markers that are affected equally by them but have different routes of permeation. Combining a large molecule with a smaller molecule allows a permeation ratio of large/small molecules to be calculated. This technique demonstrates greater clinical discrimination than the behavior of either type of marker alone [9].

Isotope Tests

Isotope probes are in general more easily measured than other markers of permeability, but suffer from the inherent disadvantages of single marker tests and the use of radioactivity. [51]Chromium-ethylenediaminetera-acetate (^{51}Cr-EDTA) has been employed for the estimation of intestinal permeability. The technique is disadvantaged by the wide variation in published control values and the relatively short half-life of ^{51}Cr which limits the shelf-life and length of time that samples can be kept prior to analysis.

Polyethylene Glycol (PEG) Test

Many different size PEGs have been used to assess intestinal permeability. Commercial formulations consist of polymers of different size: PEG-400, for example, is composed of 8 different sized molecules. The apparent advantage of differing molecular size is offset by substantial variation in the proportion of each individual polymer excreted after oral administration. There is also considerable disparity in the range of excretion after intravenous administration. Opinion differs as to whether PEG-400 excretion is increased or decreased in small intestinal disease and controversy about the route of PEG permeation persists.

Dual Saccharide Test

A number of dual saccharide tests (disaccharide/monosaccharide) have been developed for the assessment of intestinal permeability. There is little practical difference between them, although the tests and sources of error differ in detail. The cellobiose/mannitol and lactulose/mannitol combinations are the best documented; but there are potential sources of error arising from the metabolism and analysis of the sugars. Particular confusion exists about the route of mannitol permeation. *In vivo*, its behavior suggests transcellular permeation, whereas *in vitro* mannitol is used as a marker of paracellular permeability. It probably permeates by both routes. A further dual sugar technique employs lactulose and L-rhamnose (Fig. 3). Lactulose absorption is increased in celiac disease, whereas that of L-rhamnose is decreased, which leads to an increase in the lactulose/L-rhamnose (L/R) excretion ratio. This has shown complete discrimination between 13 patients with untreated celiac disease and healthy control subjects. Lactulose appears to be a reliable marker of paracellular permeation, but whilst urinary recovery of lactulose approaches 100% after intravenous injection, re-

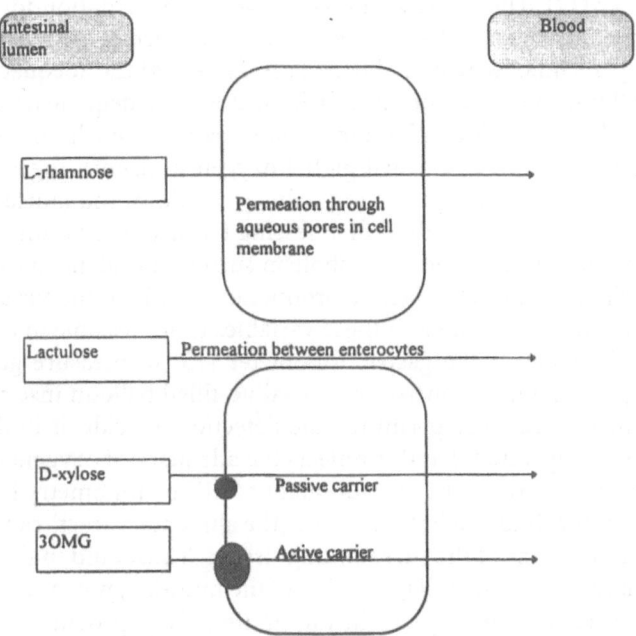

Fig. 3. Mechanisms and routes of absorption and permeation for 3-O-methyl-D-glucose (3-OMG), D-xylose, L-rhamnose and lactulose from the small intestinal lumen to the blood

covery of L-rhamnose is only about 75%. The fate of the missing fraction is unknown, but does not appear to vary widely between subjects. The route of L-rhamnose permeation is assumed to be transcellular *in vivo*, and the substance is transported 5 times more effectively across an artificial lipid barrier than mannitol [10].

Non-mediated permeation and mediated transport of carbohydrates can be measured simultaneously by combining lactulose and L-rhamnose with D-xylose and 3-O-methyl-D-glucose (3OMG), thus providing another measure of intestinal function with much better discrimination than a single marker test (Fig. 3) [11].

Assessment of Splanchnic Blood Flow

Conventional assessment of the adequacy of tissue oxygenation is by the measurement of various hemodynamic variables and the calculation of global arterial DO_2 and O_2 uptake (VO_2) together with metabolic markers of anaerobic metabolism (arterial pH, standard base excess, and blood lactate concentration). These measurements take no account of regional variations in DO_2. Blood flow to the splanchnic circulation may be disproportionately reduced in response to hypovolemia and in the critically ill, and both low flow rates and sepsis can lead to an ischemic mucosal injury that reduces the efficiency of the GI mucosal barrier [12]. These observations provide an explanation for the finding that global measurements of oxygenation can be normal in the presence of significant splanchnic ischemia. Thus, an assessment of the adequacy of oxygenation of the GI tract may provide an early indicator of inadequate tissue perfusion in the critically ill. The identification of those patients in whom there is gut ischemia, despite apparently normal global oxygen transport, together with its subsequent treatment may significantly reduce morbidity and mortality.

The optimal method of assessing tissue oxygenation is to measure metabolic markers of anaerobic metabolism such as the adenosine diphosphate/adenosine triphosphate ratio, lactate production, or pH in the tissue of interest. However, direct measurement of these variables is not feasible in clinical practice. The development of the gastric tonometer [13] to measure gastric intramucosal pH (pHi), a device consisting of a saline-filled balloon inserted nasogastrically into the stomach, has permitted the detection of acidosis in the stomach wall. It has been suggested that this reflects the adequacy of oxygenation of a segment of the upper GI tract. The measurement of pHi by tonometry is based on the principle that the fluid in a hollow viscus (the alimentary tract) can be used to estimate the gas tensions of the surrounding tissues. Thus, fluid in the lumen of the gut equilibrates with the PCO_2 and PO_2 of the intestinal mucosa, and an estimation of the tensions of these gases in the luminal fluid provides a valid measurement of intramucosal PCO_2 and PO_2. It is further based upon the assumption that the bicarbonate concentration in the tissue is the same as that delivered to it in arterial blood. Although this is a reasonable assumption in a well-perfused organ, it is likely that in an ischemic organ generating lactic acid, true intramucosal bicarbonate concentration is almost certainly lower than arterial bicarbonate concentration. Despite this potential source of error, there is still a very good correlation in animal studies between tonometric and microelectrode pHi measurements in different situations, including graded local GI ischemia and endotoxic shock [14].

Clinical Studies of GI Permeability

Cardiopulmonary Bypass

Patients undergoing surgery necessitating CPB have been studied extensively as they provide a homogeneous population and are readily accessible. Although the majority of patients recover uneventfully after cardiac surgery, MOF complicates the postoperative period in up to 2% of this population. This has a significant effect on the utilization of critical care resources given the large number of patients undergoing such procedures. It is therefore important to further understanding of the cause and pathophysiology of post-CPB organ dysfunction. Furthermore, CPB is associated with organ dysfunction similar to that occurring in critically ill patients. Gastric tonometry has been used to study prospectively changes in pHi. In parallel with observations made in critically ill patients, a perioperative fall in pHi is predictive of increased morbidity and mortality in patients undergoing

CPB [15]. Low pHi is thought to reflect GI ischemia, an important mechanism in the loss of GI mucosal integrity [16, 17]. Using the dual saccharide technique, an eight-fold rise in GI mucosal permeability has been demonstrated following CPB. This was attributed to splanchnic ischemia, as gastric mucosal blood flow, measured by laser Doppler flowmetry, was reduced by 50% and the magnitude of change in permeability was related to duration of bypass (i.e. the duration of ischemic insult) [18].

This finding has recently been confirmed using the same technique [19], and the relationship between such direct estimates of GI permeability and pHi examined. A total of 20 patients undergoing elective CPB surgery were studied. The L/R ratio rose significantly. In 12 patients (60%), a low pHi (<7.32) was recorded during and/or after surgery, whilst in the remainder pHi remained normal throughout. The L/R ratio in patients who developed an intramucosal acidosis was 0.59 ± 0.06 compared to 0.32 ± 0.07 in those whose pHi remained normal throughout ($p < 0.05$ (Fig. 4). No difference in L/R ratio was seen between patients with or without evidence of a metabolic acidosis. No significant correlation between bypass time and pHi or bypass time and L/R ratio could be demonstrated.

This study confirmed that GI injury is detectable following uncomplicated surgery involving CPB. Profound impairment of both active and passive carrier-mediated absorption of saccharides in the small bowel occurred, and a coincident increase in gut permeability was demonstrated by the rise in L/R permeability ratio. The reduction in absorption may be explained by a variety of factors other than GI mucosal injury, including gastric emptying and dilution, small intestinal peristalsis, blood flow, the volume of distribution of saccharides, and alterations in renal clearance. However, the rise in the L/R permeability index observed postoperatively cannot be explained by such phenomena, since these

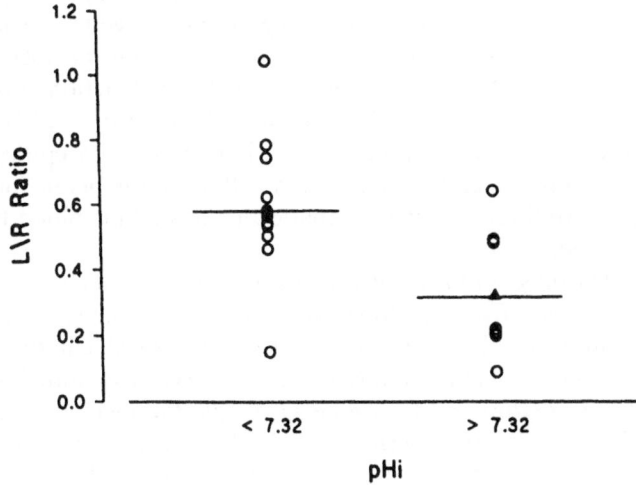

Fig. 4. Lactulose/rhamnose (L/R) ratio in patients with a gastric intramucosal pH (pHi) less than and greater than 7.32 ($p < 0.05$). (From [19] with permission)

factors should influence the clearance of both saccharides equally. The consequences of such impaired intestinal barrier function may be the initiation or perpetuation of inflammatory processes, although all the patients studied, with one exception, made an uncomplicated recovery post-operatively. It therefore seems that the splanchnic injury was probably transient and self-limiting.

Experimental studies have shown that a reduction in pHi measured tonometrically reflects gut ischemia. The increase in gut permeability seen in association with a low pHi seen in this study supports an ischemic etiology for this phenomenon post-CPB. The incidence of low pHi was similar to that reported elsewhere; other studies have reported abnormally low values for pHi in 50–60% of patients studied after CPB [13, 20, 21]. Although a sensitive but non-specific marker of postoperative complications, the nature and effect of any corrective therapy aimed at correcting a low pHi remains to be established. Although increased gut permeability in association with a low pHi was demonstrated, there is a degree of overlap between patients with a normal pHi and those with an abnormal pHi. This may be explained by the fact that gastric tonometry reflects blood flow specifically to the stomach via the celiac artery. Increased GI permeability is a reflection of small bowel absorption, the blood supply to which is the superior mesenteric artery. The presence of significant atheromatous disease from which this population might well suffer, might contribute to the disruption of blood flow in one or other of these arteries thereby creating local ischemia exacerbated by low systemic perfusion pressures during and after CPB. The result of such a process could be to create areas of localized ischemia which could effect either the pHi or L/R ratio in isolation.

Manipulation of GI Permeability following CPB

Significant reductions in mortality and morbidity for high risk surgical patients have been achieved by increasing perioperative DO_2 using dopexamine hydrochloride, an inodilator with specific effects on the splanchnic circulation [22]. Dopexamine is a novel dopamine analog with action at β_2-adrenoreceptors and DA_1-receptors, and only moderate activity at β_1- and DA_2-receptors. It has no direct α-adrenoreceptor activity, but inhibits norepinephrine re-uptake, producing peripheral vasodilatation with a simultaneous increase in cardiac index (CI). Additionally, renal, hepatic and splanchnic blood flow are specifically increased.

The effect of these regional hemodynamic changes on GI function were compared recently using dopexamine and dopamine [23]. Hemodynamic measurements were taken as soon as the patient was stable in the operating theatre, after which they were randomly allocated to receive an infusion of either dopexamine 2.0 mcg/kg/min or dopamine 2.5 mcg/kg/min which were continued until completion of the study period. Gastric pHi was measured after 90 min of CPB, or just as bypass was being terminated, whichever was the shorter; 2.5 h after the start, and at the end of the GI permeability study, which was performed once within 2 h of the patient's return to the ICU. Thirty patients were studied, 16 of whom re-

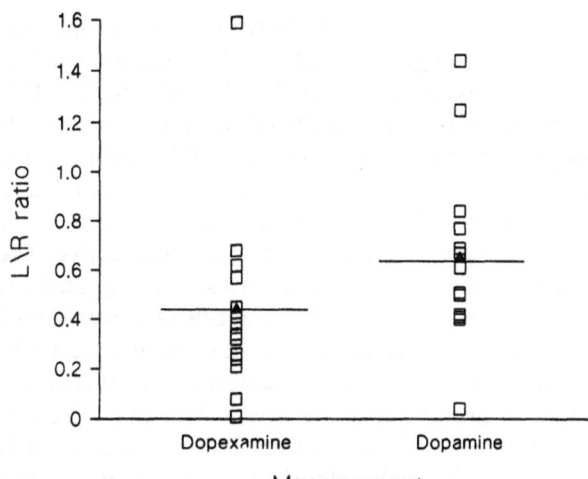

Fig. 5. Lactulose/rhamnose ratio in patients receiving dopexamine or dopamine ($p < 0.05$)

ceived dopamine and 14 dopexamine. There was a significant difference between the mean L/R ratio for the dopexamine and dopamine groups (Fig. 5). There were no significant changes in pHi observed within or between the two groups. Within the group as a whole, 18 patients developed an intramucosal acidosis (pHi < 7.32) during and/or after surgery. The L/R ratio in patients who developed an intramucosal acidosis was not significantly different from that measured in those who did not.

This randomized study demonstrated a reduction in gut permeability in patients treated with dopexamine compared with dopamine following CPB. For the study group as a whole, the urinary recovery of individual saccharides and the L/R ratio are similar to those previously reported following CPB. Although the mechanisms underlying a lower index of GI permeability in the patients treated with dopexamine remain unclear, a number of possibilities exists. Not surprisingly, there was a significant increase in DO_2 prior to commencement of CPB in the dopexamine group compared to the dopamine group, which was not maintained following termination of CPB. Increasing DO_2 perioperatively has been shown to reduce morbidity and mortality in high risk patients following non-CPB surgery [24, 25], a beneficial effect linked to increases in VO_2. Thus, a covert oxygen demand can be revealed if tissue perfusion is increased in the critically ill and VO_2 may depend on DO_2 in certain critical illnesses [26, 27]. Further, it has been suggested that post-operative increases in DO_2I are required to compensate for an intraoperative oxygen debt arising during surgery, which may exert a beneficial effect via this mechanism [28]. More recently, a marked reduction in mortality in high risk patients has been demonstrated when DO_2 was increased using dopexamine, independent of any effect on VO_2. The increase in DO_2 observed in the current study was not sustained following CPB, although an earlier rise in VO_2 was seen in those receiving dopexamine, suggesting that any oxygen debt occurring post-CPB would have been of shorter duration in the dopexamine group.

Dopexamine has been shown to increase splanchnic blood flow (SBF) in patients with congestive cardiac failure and to raise pHi in the critically ill, suggesting an increase in SBF in this population [29]. It is possible that dopexamine increased SBF in this study allowing regional VO_2 to rise. This lessening of the ischemic burden to the GI tract could permit the maintenance of improved mucosal integrity. Alterations in regional DO_2 and VO_2 are not detectable using global measures. Until such regional indices become available, the effects of dopexamine on gut permeability remain speculative. The relationship between pHi and GI mucosal permeability in a similar population of patients undergoing CPB described above, in which mean L/R ratio was significantly greater in those who developed an intramucosal acidosis compared to those in whom pHi remained normal, was not apparent and no significant changes in mean pHi were observed in either group during the study. This may be a reflection of the low operative risk of this population, in that all those patients studied made an uncomplicated recovery. Although splanchnic ischemia has long been considered to be the primary mechanism of GI mucosal injury, other factors may be relevant including the generation of reactive oxygen species by xanthine oxidase, high concentrations of which are found within the villous enterocyte during reperfusion of ischemic bowel [30, 31]. By maintaining SBF throughout the intra-operative period, dopexamine may have ameliorated this process. There is also evidence to suggest that endotoxin has a direct effect on GI mucosal integrity independent of changes in SBF [32]. Dopexamine may therefore have exerted this effect on GI permeability by means other than alterations in splanchnic oxygen transport and consumption. This study demonstrated that the mean L/R ratio was significantly lower in those patients who received dopexamine compared to dopamine. There were no significant differences between the two study groups in terms of hemodynamic measurements or pHi. These results suggest that dopexamine exerts a protective effect, at least compared to dopamine, on gut mucosal integrity during CPB.

Nutrition

Malnourished, critically ill patients tend to have poor wound healing and longer convalescence, with a high incidence of post-operative complications. Total parenteral nutrition (TPN) was introduced into ICU practice to provide nutritional support to catabolic patients if feeding via the enteral route (EN) was impossible. However, despite extensive use, there is little evidence to suggest that TPN affords any improvement in outcome in the critically ill, especially if feeding takes place for less than 10 days [33, 34] and may even be associated with a higher incidence of septic complications. The most important stimulus to mucosal viability is the presence of food in the GI lumen and sufficient nutrients, bulk and pancreatic enzymes. As the institution of TPN ensures the absence of these essentials, it is possible that non-enteral feeding also leads to increased GI mucosal permeability, translocation of bacteria into the portal circulation and the complications listed above. In an attempt to elucidate the relationship between mucosal viability and the use of TPN, a recent investigation measured GI permeability directly using the four sugar technique in normal individuals; and in a subsequent randomized trial assessed the effects of EN and TPN on this parameter in 24 critically ill subjects over a prolonged period [35]. Only patients admitted to the ICU for more than 3 days requiring nutritional support were eligible for study to permit a series of measurements of GI permeability to be made. Those with a history of malabsorption or who had undergone bowel surgery and those in renal failure, which precluded the acurate collection of urinary markers of GI permeability were also excluded. On the third day following admission to the ICU, APACHE II was calculated for all patients and baseline measurements of GI mucosal permeability performed, following which they were randomized to receive EN or TPN. On every third day, GI permeability was estimated to a maximum of three measurements. Ten normal volunteers, fasted for 10 h, also underwent a mucosal permeability study following an identical protocol. Baseline L/R ratio was markedly increased in both study groups compared to controls. During the study period, L/R ratio displayed a progressive and significant fall towards control values in the EN group, but in the TPN group fell initially before rising back to baseline levels (Fig. 6). Mortality in the enteral group was 15.4 compared with 54.6% in the TPN group. GI injury is therefore evident in critically ill patients at an early stage and is reversible with the institution of early EN, whilst reliance on TPN results in perpetuation of the injury. There is also a suggestion that this reversal of injury may be associated with improved outcome. The lack of a strong statistical correlation between type of feeding and outcome probably indicates that the factors dictating survival in this population are multi-factorial in origin and that the route of nutritional support is only one such contributory factor.

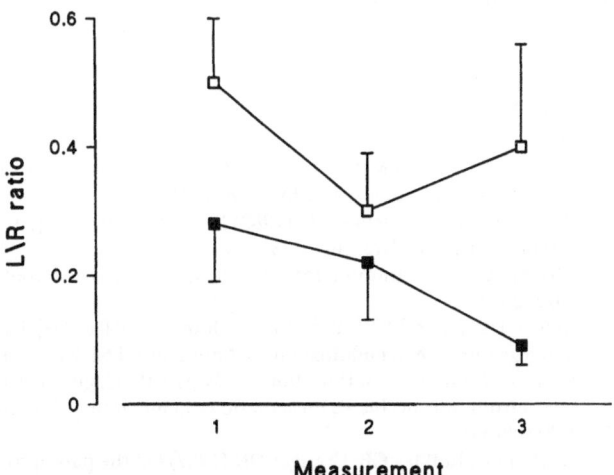

Fig. 6. Mean serial values for lactulose/rhamnose (L/R) ratio. Enteral nutrition group represented by solid squares, parenteral nutrition group represented by open squares. Significant difference from baseline p < 0.05; significant difference between patient groups p<0.05. (From [36] with permission)

EN, particularly if instituted early and supplemented with certain essential nutrients, may help to maintain mucosal integrity and enhance autoregulation of SBF, thereby preventing bacterial translocation [36]. Although histological studies have been performed and infection rates compared between patients receiving TPN and EN, this study represents the first attempt to make a functional assessment of GI absorption or permeability in these circumstances. TPN formulations lack glutamine, an amino acid which is unstable in solution, particularly during sterilisation, but which is now considered to be the main source of energy for the GI mucosa and in particular for the small bowel. In experimental studies in rats, it has been shown to contribute 46% of total jejunal CO_2 production [37, 38]. Studies have also demonstrated that during fever, endotoxemia and surgery, muscle free glutamine concentrations fall and muscle stores become depleted. TPN formulations also contain glucose, the presence of which suppresses ketone body formation, the latter now being recognized as an important fuel source for the gut [39]. This study has provided evidence that early administration of EN reverses GI mucosal injury where TPN fails to do so.

Conclusion

GI dysfunction in terms of increased permeability is a multifactorial phenomenon evident in a wide range of critically ill patients. It may be that differing mechanisms apply to differing populations of patients. Studies are now required to delineate these mechanisms in the relevant populations together with the effects of other pharmacological agents. Other investigations will be required to establish if the GI mucosa can be protected in the critically ill and the effect of such measures on outcome.

References

1. Curzen N, Griffiths MJD, Evans TW (1994) The role of the endothelium in modulating the vascular response to sepsis. Clin Sci 86:374–384
2. Pinsky MR, Matchuschak GM (1989) Multiple systems organ failure: Failure of host defense mechanisms. Crit Care Clin 5:199–200
3. Wright R (1982) Immunology of the gastrointestinal tract and liver. Practitioner 226: 2027–2032
4. Nelson DP, Samsel RW, Wood LD, Schumaker PT (1988) Pathological supply-dependency of oxygen uptake in endotoxemia. J Appl Physiol 64:2410–2419
5. Bailey RW, Bulkley GB, Hamilton SR, Morris JB, Haglund UH (1987) Protection of the small bowel from non-occlusive mesenteric ischemic injury due to cardiogenic shock. Am J Surg 153:108–116
6. Haglund U, Bulkley GB, Granger DN (1987) On the pathophysiology of intestinal ischaemic injury. Acta Chirg Scand 153:321–324
7. Lundgren O, Svanvik J (1973) Mucosal haemodynamics in the small intestine of the cat during reduced perfusion pressure. Acta Physiol Scand 88:551–553
8. Schiller HJ, Reilly PM, Bulkley GB (1993) Anti-oxidant therapy. Crit Care Med 21: S92–S103

9. Menzies IS (1974) Absorption of intact oligosaccharides in health and disease. Biochem Soc Trans 2:1042-1047
10. Crowther RS, Wen G (1991) Physiochemical properties of probe molecules used to assess intestinal permeability. Gastroenterol 100:A205 (Abst)
11. Cook GC, Menzies IS (1986) Intestinal absorption and unmediated permeation of sugars in post-infective tropical malabsorption (tropical sprue) Digestion 33:109-116
12. Fink MP, Antonsson JB, Wan H, Rothschild HR (1991) Increased intestinal permeability in endotoxic pigs: Mesenteric hypoperfusion as an etiologic factor. Arch Surg 126:211-218
13. Fiddian-Green RG, Baker S (1987) Predictive value of stomach wall pH for complications after operations: Comparison with other monitoring. Crit Care Med 15:153-156
14. Antonsson JB, Boyle CC, Kruitoff KL, et al (1990) Validation of tonometric measurement of gut intramural pH during endotoxemia and mesenteric hypoperfusion in pigs. Am J Physiol 259:G519-G523
15. Landow L, Phillips DA, Heard SO, Prevost D, Vandersalm TJ, Fink MP (1991) Gastric tonometry and venous oximetry in cardiac surgery patients. Crit Care Med 19:1226-1233
16. Meakins JL, Marshall JC (1986) The GI tract: The "motor" of MOF. Arch Surg 121:197-200
17. Border JR, Hasset J, LaDuca J, et al (1987) The gut origin of septic states in blunt multiple trauma (ISS = 40) in the ICU. Ann Surg 206:427-445
18. Ohri SK, Bjarnason I, Pathi V, et al (1993) Cardiopulmonary bypass impairs small intestinal transport and increases gut permeability. Ann Thorac Surg 55:1080-1086
19. Sinclair DG, Haslam PL, Houldsworth PE, Pepper JR, Evans TW (1995) The effect of cardiopulmonary bypass upon intestinal and pulmonary endothelial permeability. Chest 108:718-724
20. Landow L, Phillips DA, Heard SO, Prevost D, Vandersalm TJ, Fink MP (1991) Gastric tonometry and venous oximetry in cardiac surgery patients. Crit Care Med 19:1226-1233
21. Andersen LW, Landow L, Baek L, Jansen E, Baker S (1993) Association between gastric intramucosal pH and splanchnic endotoxin, antibody to endotoxin, and tumor necrosis factor-alpha concentrations in patients undergoing cardiopulmonary bypass. Crit Care Med 21:210-217
22. Boyd O, Grounds RM, Bennett ED (1993) A randomised clinical trial of the effect of deliberate perioperative increase of oxygen delivery on mortality in high risk surgical patients. JAMA 270:2699-2707
23. Hadfield R, Sinclair DG, Houldsworth PG, Morgan CJ, Evans TW (1995) Gut permeability following cardiopulmonary bypass surgery: A randomised study comparing the effects of dopexamine and dopamine. Am J Respir Crit Care Med 151:A770 (Abst)
24. Hunter DN, Gray H, Mudaliar Y, Morgan C, Evans TW (1989) The effects of dopexamine hydrochloride on cardiopulmonary haemodynamics following cardiopulmonary bypass surgery. Int J Cardiol 23:365-371
25. Shoemaker WC, Appel PL, Waxman K, Schwartz S, Chang P (1988) Prospective trial of supranormal values of survivors as therapeutic goals in high risk surgical patients. Chest 94:1176-1186
26. Shoemaker WC, Appel PL, Kram HB (1988) Tissue oxygen debt as a determinant of lethal and nonlethal postoperative failure. Crit Care Med 16:1117-1120
27. Clark C, Edwards JD, Nightingale P, Mortimer AJ, Morris J (1991) Persistence of supply dependence of oxygen uptake at high levels of delivery in the adult respiratory distress syndrome. Crit Care Med 19:497-502
28. Shoemaker WC, Appel PL, Kram HB (1992) Role of oxygen debt in the development of organ failure, sepsis and death in high risk surgical patients. Chest 102:208-215
29. Smithies M, Yee TH, Jackson L, Beale R, Bihari D (1992) Protecting the gut and the liver in the critically ill: Effects of dopexamine. Crit Care Med 22:789-795
30. Schiller HJ, Reilly PM, Bulkley GB (1993) Antioxidant therapy. Crit Care Med 21:S92-S102
31. Parks DA, Shah AK, Granger DN (1984) Oxygen radicals: Effects on intestinal vascular permeability. Am J Pathophysiol 247:167-170
32. Fink MP, Antonsson JB, Wang H, Rothschild HR (1991) Increased intestinal permeability in endotoxic pigs: Mesenteric hypoperfusion as an aetiologic factor. Arch Surg 126:211-218
33. Buzby TP (1990) Perioperative nutritional support. J Parent Enteral Nutr 14:197-198

34. Meguid MM, Campos AC, Hammond WG (1990) Nutritional support in surgical practice. Part 1. Am J Surg 159:345–348
35. Hadfield J, Sinclair DG, Evans TW (1995) Effects of enteral and parenteral nutrition on gut mucosal permeability in the critically ill. Am J Resp Crit Care Med 152:1545–1548
36. Alverdy TIC, Aoys E, Moss GS (1988) TPN promotes translocation from the gut. Surgery 104:185–190
37. Fiddian-Green RG (1989) Studies in splanchic ischaemia and multiple organ failure. In: Marston A, Bulkley G, Fiddian Green RG, Hagland U (eds) Splanchic ischaemia and multiple organ failure. Edward Arnold, London, Melbourne, Auckland, pp 339–348
38. Windmueller HG, Spaeth AE (1980) Respiratory fuels and nitrogen metabolism *in vivo* in small intestine of fed rats. J Biol Chem 255:107–112
39. Souba WW, Smith RJ, Wilmore DW(1985) Glutamine metabolism by the intestinal tract. J Parent Enteral Nutr 9:608–617

Gut Dysfunction in Trauma Patients

F. A. Moore and E. E. Moore

Introduction

With the development of regionalized trauma care, patients who were previously found dead in the field are now surviving to be admitted to regional trauma centers [1]. Early in-hospital deaths occur as a result of severe brain injury and irreversible shock while the leading cause of late deaths is multiple organ failure (MOF). Early risk factors for MOF include high injury severity score (ISS), advanced age, blood transfusions, and persistent shock [2, 3]. While it is difficult to implicate gut dysfunction in early brain death, it has recently been emphasized to be important in the pathogenesis of irreversible hemorrhagic shock and MOF [4–14]. The principle mechanism by which gut dysfunction is presumed to mediate these adverse outcomes is bacterial translocation (BT). In this chapter, we would like to discuss three gut-related questions that specifically differentiate time after injury into resuscitation, the early systemic inflammatory response syndrome (SIRS) and late organ failure.

Does Bacterial Translocation play a Decisive Role in the Pathogenesis of Irreversible Post-Injury Shock?

In a review article published 30 years ago based on a series of innovative laboratory models, Jacob Fine [15] hypothesized that the absorption of bacteria and endotoxin from the gut, in conjunction with shock-induced impairment of the hepatic reticuloendothelial system's ability to detoxify the portal venous effluent, potentiated the systemic spread of bacteria and endotoxin and that this was the fundamental basis for irreversible hemorrhagic shock. This theory faded from the literature because of a lack of corroborating experimental and clinical data. Recent experimental work has revived interest in this phenomenon. In the early 1980's, Berg and Deitch [16] popularized the term "bacterial translocation" which they initially defined "as the passage of viable indigenous bacteria from the GI tract through the intact epithelial mucosa to the mesenteric lymph nodes and other organs". Alexander et al. [17] in 1990 expanded this definition to "the passage of both viable and non-viable microbes and microbial products such as endotoxin across an anatomically intact intestinal barrier".

A variety of investigators have studied BT in hemorrhagic shock models. In Deitch and Berg's [4] model, rats were bled to a mean arterial pressure (MAP) of 30 mmHg for 30, 60, and 90 min. The rats were then sacrificed 24 h after shock and ileocolic mesenteric lymph nodes (MLN), spleens, and livers were harvested and then cultured quantitatively. 30 and 60 min of shock had roughly equivalent effects: half of the MLN cultures were positive, spread to the liver and spleen was less than 20%, and mortality was 15 and 20%, respectively. In contrast, after 90 min of shock, all MLNs had positive cultures and yielded significantly greater numbers of enteric bacteria, spread to systemic organs was 60%, and mortality increased to 40%. Of note, 35% of these rats had positive blood cultures. In a subsequent study, these authors performed histologic analysis of the ileum and cecum in rats subject to 30 min of shock (again bled to 30 mmHg). The mucosa was relatively intact 2 h after shock, but by 24 h there was frank mucosal damage in both the ileum and cecum [18]. In a similar model (rats bled to MAP of 30 to 35 mmHg for 90 min), Schlag, Redl and associates [19] noted that endotoxin levels in the portal vein increased significantly at the end of 90 min of shock and became evident in the systemic circulation during the first 60 min of resuscitation. These animals were also sacrificed for histologic examination after shock which revealed that the jejunum and ileum often had areas of mucosal necrosis, while the colon had relatively normal histology [7–9, 11, 12]. Rush et al. [6, 7, 8, 10] have also conducted a series of hemorrhagic shock studies (MAP 30 mmHg until 80% of shed blood returned) in rats. On average, this represents a shock period exceeding 4 h and thus is a much more severe model than above two models. Blood cultures became positive 30 min into the shock period, and bacteremia continued throughout the ensuing 48 h of observation [6]. In another study, rats were fed E. coli labelled with carbon 14 oleic acid [7]. After the same severe hemorrhagic shock insult, half were noted to have increased plasma C^{14} activity; all animals whose blood cultures were also positive were dead within 80 h. In contrast, 83% of the animals without plasma C^{14} activity survived. Moreover, Rush et al. [10] demonstrated that germ-free rats subject to their shock model had significantly better survival at 24, 48, and 72 h (62, 30, and 25 vs. 24, 11, and 5%).

Although these animal models are logical and consistent, clinical studies indicate that BT (as documented in laboratory models) is an infrequent event in humans after shock. In the Korean conflict, Lindberg et al. [20] found that among 30 soldiers who died, only 3 (10%) had positive blood cultures and only 3 cultures (8%) were positive in 38 other soldiers in shock for an average of 7.3 h. When their data were corrected for contamination, they estimated the incidence of early bacteremia would be less than 5% in combat casualties. More recently, as a correlate to their rat model, Rush et al. [12] sampled blood within 3 h of admission in acutely injured patients. Cultures were positive in 10 (45%) of the 18 patients who arrived in shock compared with 1 (4%) of the 25 patients without shock. 13 of the 18 patients with shock died within 24 h. Interestingly, 70% of the bacteria recovered from the blood were gram-positive, but the specific bacterial species were not reported. Additionally, they assayed blood for endotoxin in 10 patients. Of the 6 patients without shock, endotoxin was not detected. Of the 4 patients with shock, 2 had significant endotoxin levels. Subsequently, we performed [21] a similar blood culture study in 132 acutely injured patients requiring emergency laparotomy. Cultures were positive in 12 (32%) of the 38 patients who arrived in shock compared to 10 (12%) of the 94 patients who arrived not in shock. Breakdown of the culture results by injury mechanism and the presence or absence of shock in the emergency department is shown in Table 1. Like Rush et al., we had an exceptionally high incidence of gram-positive organisms. Most notably, coagulase-negative *Staphylococcus* was isolated in 5 (13%) of the patients with shock and in 6 (7%) of the patients without shock. This rate is too high to be dismissed as poor blood sampling technique. In general, the most common source of Staphylococcal bacteremia is direct injury to the skin, and, of course, many of our trauma patients did have disrupted skin. However, several laboratories have isolated *Staphylococcus* in their BT models. Irregardless of the source, in our experience these acute post-injury Staphylococcal bacteremia appeared to be of minimal clinical significance; none of our patients developed overt Staphylococcal infections nor did they die of hemorrhagic shock. In contrast, 7 patients with shock had more typical enteric bacteremias and 6 (86%) died within 24 h of irreversible shock. BT appeared to have occurred in 3 of these patients who did not have hollow viscus injuries. This is consistent with a more recent study by Raumen et al. [22] from the Netherlands. They measured serial endotoxin levels in 11 patients (5 with ruptured abdominal aortic aneurysms (AAA) and 6 trauma patients with ISS ≥ 25). 6 patients (5 (100%) with AAA and 1 (16%) with trauma) had endotoxemia at baseline and/or at 6 h, but endotoxemia was not demonstrated at 24 and 48 h in any of the patients. More recently, Endo et al.

Table 1. Blood culture results by mechanism and emergency department systolic blood pressure (SBP). (From [21] with permission)

	Blunt Trauma (n = 40)	Gunshot Wound (n = 42)	Stab Wound (n = 50)
SBP ≥ 90 mmHg			
No (%)	29 (72)	24 (57)	41 (82)
Positive culture, No (%)	3 (10)	4 (17)	3 (7)
Culture results	S, S, A	S, S, A, A	S, S, B
SBP < 90 mmHg			
No (%)	11 (28)	18 (43)	9 (18)
Positive culture, No (%)	3 (27)	5 (28)	4 (44)
Culture results	S, En, Et	S, S, S, En, E	S, E, A/C, B

S: coagulase-negative *Staphylococcus*; A: α-hemolytic *Streptococcus*; En: enterococcus; E: *Escherichia coli*; Et: *Enterobacter*; B: *Bacteroides fragilis*; A/C: combined α-hemolytic *Streptococcus* and *Clostridium* species. Each time a letter is used, it means one episode of bacteremia with that organism

[23] from Japan obtained serial early blood samples (0.5, 1, 2, 3, 6, 12, 24, 48, 72, 106, 120, 144, and 168 h after arrival) in 29 severely injured patients who arrived in shock. Elevated endotoxin levels were found in only 7 (2%) of 342 specimens. Finally, Hiki et al. [24] from Germany collected blood in 39 multiple injured patients at 0 to 3, and 6 to 12 h, and then at 1, 3, 5, and 10 days after admission. Again they noted that endotoxin levels were elevated early (i.e. 0 to 3 h, and 6 to 12 h), but not later.

In conclusion, the basic laboratory data supporting the notion that BT is responsible for irreversible postinjury shock are convincing, but of note, they are derived from severe shock models. Additionally, the clinical data indicate that BT can be documented in only a small number of injured patients who arrive in severe shock. Whether this contributes to early patient death or is just an epiphenomenon of severe shock is not clear. Answering this question will be challenging because the animal experiments do not represent human physiology. In many of these models, the shock insult causes small bowel mucosal necrosis which is uncommon clinically. Secondly, there is a tremendous variability among species. For example, even minor stress events in rats predictably result in endotoxemia and bacteremia. Moreover, there is a dramatic difference in the response to an endotoxin inoculation. Humans are extremely sensitive while rats are far relatively resistant. Finally, given the low frequency of early BT in patients at high risk for death secondary to hemorrhagic shock at a single regional trauma center (we had 7 such patients during 14 months), a multicenter trial would be required and a very large number of patients would be enrolled to control for confounding variables.

Is Bacterial Translocation a Pivotal Mechanism in Early Post-Injury SIRS?

MOF has traditionally been viewed to be "the fatal expression of uncontrolled infection" and consequently trauma research efforts in the 1980's were directed at determining how a traumatic insult creates an environment conducive for infection and how these infections then cause MOF [25–28]. However, in the mid 1980's, several reports from Europe (looking principally at blunt trauma), convincingly demonstrated that post-injury MOF could occur in the absence of an identifiable focus of infection [29, 30]. Jacob Fine's hypothesis was again revived, but now it was invoked to be the unifying mechanism in the post-injury SIRS (i.e. the "sepsis syndrome") that characterized MOF [5, 9, 11, 13, 14, 31, 32]. At the basic level, BT was demonstrated to occur by direct penetration of enterocytes, and translocation between the enterocytes was not observed [17]. In contrast, increased intestinal permeability to large water soluble molecules (eg lactulose) occurs via paracellular pores, the size of which are determined by the tight junctions of the enterocytes [33, 34]. Additionally, investigators convincingly documented that BT to MLNs can be induced in rodents by a variety of insults (eg hemorrhagic shock, thermal injury, and radiation) and that bacteria further spread into the liver, spleen, and systemic blood by altering a number of environmental cofactors (eg nutritional state, gut bacterial flora, immune status).

While these experimental models are consistent and logical, they are defining the mechanisms governing BT, but do not mechanistically link BT to remote organ failure. With this in mind, we developed a gut ischemia/reperfusion (I/R) acute lung injury (ALI) model [35]. To avoid excessive mucosal necrosis, we chose to use a limited period of gut ischemia (45 min of superior mesenteric artery occlusion) and documented relatively normal gut mucosal histology after 24 h [36, 37].

During the first 6 h of reperfusion, we observed the following pathogenic sequence leading to ALI:
1) gut phospholipase A_2 (PLA_2) activity is increased;
2) neutrophils (PMN) became sequestered in the gut;
3) circulating PMNs became primed (i.e. significantly increased superoxide generation when stimulated);
4) PMNs increased CD11b adhesion receptor expression and became sequestered in the lung; and
5) there is increased lung microvascular permeability.

Other investigators have observed the same type of ALI with longer periods of gut ischemia [38, 39]. In our model, we were surprised to find that plasma endotoxin levels were the same in the gut I/R and sham laparotomy animals, but the sham laparotomy animals had no evidence of ALI [40]. Additionally, the elimination of endotoxin by pretreatment with monoclonal antibodies did not alter gut I/R-induced ALI. Thus, in our model, gut I/R appears to provoke ALI via a mechanism independent of BT. Additionally, hind limb ischemia has been shown by other investigators to cause a similar PMN-mediated ALI, and this is presumed to be independent of endotoxin or bacteria [41].

Simultaneous with our basic laboratory studies, we began parallel studies in our trauma intensive care unit (ICU) [42]. Over a 9-month period in 1989, 20 high risk trauma patients (6 (30%) of whom later developed MOF) who required emergency laparotomy for their abdominal injuries had a portal vein catheter placed (patients with severe brain injury and those who were going to die early were excluded). Portal venous blood was obtained at laparotomy and then again at 6, 12, 24, 48 h, and at 5 days post-operatively. Simultaneous systemic blood samples were also obtained. The specific purpose of this study was to determine whether early gut translocation of bacteria and endotoxin via the portal vein occurred in patients at high risk for MOF. The blood samples were cultured for bacterial growth and to our surprise, they were virtually sterile (Table 2). 9 (2%) of 424 cultures were positive. In the portal blood, 5 grew coagulase-negative *Staphylococcus*, 2 grew *propionibacterium acnes*, and 1 grew an acinobacter species. The only positive systemic blood culture grew *Staph. aureus* in a patient who had a simultaneous *Staph. aureus* pneumonia. Additionally, the blood samples in the first 48 h were assayed for endotoxin, complement fragment C3a, tumor necrosis factor (TNF), and interleukin-6 (IL-6). As expected, C3a and IL-6 levels were elevated, but there was no difference between portal and systemic levels (Table 3). Of note, endotoxin was not detectable in the portal and systemic blood and TNF levels were not different from those in normal controls. Hoch et

Table 2. Portal and systemic culture results. (From [42] with permission)

Blood sample	Time					
	0 h	6 h	12 h	24 h	48 h	5 days
Portal positive cultures	1 (P)	1 (S)	1 (P)	0	3 (S, S, A)	2 (S, S)
Total cultures	40	40	36	34	32	30
Systemic positive cultures	0	0	0	0	0	1 (SA)
Total cultures	40	40	36	34	32	30

Portal and systemic cultures obtained in the operating room (0 h), at 6, 12, 24, 48 h, and 5 days postoperatively. P: *Propionibacterium acnes*; S: coagulase-negative *Staphylococcus*, A: *Acinobacter* species; SA: *Staphylococcus aureus*

Table 3. Portal and systemic culture results. (From [42] with permission)

Time	C3a (ng/mL)		TNF (pg/mL)		IL-6 (pg/mL)	
	Portal	Systemic	Portal	Systemic	Portal	Systemic
0 h	781 ± 107	802 ± 122	116 ± 17	118 ± 16	390 ± 85	414 ± 91
6 h	493 ± 76	434 ± 76	148 ± 17	141 ± 20	337 ± 49	373 ± 54
12 h	337 ± 47	370 ± 62	155 ± 23	149 ± 20	237 ± 46	269 ± 59
24 h	491 ± 67	412 ± 55	155 ± 20	166 ± 26	173 ± 40	180 ± 45
48 h	533 ± 64	503 ± 55	146 ± 24	139 ± 21	98 ± 38	94 ± 37

Portal and systemic levels (mean ± SEM) of complement fragment (C3a), tumor necrosis factor (TNF), and interleukin-6 (IL-6) obtained in the operating room (0 h), and 6, 12, 24, and 48 h postoperatively. Normal control values for C3a range from 184 to 376 ng/mL (mean ± SEM = 318 ± 34), for TNF range from 60 to 320 pg/mL (mean ± SEM = 169 ± 16) and IL-6 was not detected in normal controls

al. [43] have recently confirmed our findings. Despite marked elevations in IL-6 and IL-8, they could not identify endotoxin or TNF in the systemic circulation of high risk trauma patients admitted to their ICU. A criticism of our study was that we focused on the portal vein while ignoring that BT may preferentially spread via MLN to the thoracic duct. Our failure to detect systemic endotoxemia and the non-spiking nature of our TNF data suggest that this was not occurring. Additionally, several investigators (including ourselves) have subsequently cultured MLNs from patients requiring emergency trauma laparotomy. In Peitzman et al's [44] experience, 1 of 22 MLNs were cultured positive; in our experience, 4 of 49 MLNs were cultured positive; in Brathwaite et al's [45] experience, 1 of 22 MLNs were cultured positive, and in Reed et al's [46] experience, 4 of 16 MLNs were cultured positive [21]. Overall, 10 (9.2%) of the 109 MLNs cultured in these trauma studies were positive which is not different from the 10.3% culture positive rate recently documented in 267 patients undergoing elective general surgical procedures [47]. However, in the trauma studies, positive MLN cultures did not correlate with any adverse clinical outcome. Interestingtly, in Brathwaite et al's [45] study, indirect immunofluorescence analysis revealed *E. coli* β-galactosidase in the cytoplasm of macrophages in all 22 MLNs harvested, and in Reed et al's [46] study, electron microscopy demonstrated non-viable bacteria in 13 of 16 MLN harvested. One flaw in both of these studies is a lack of control patients. It is conceivable that the same results would be seen in normal healthy controls. Additionally, the key issue is not whether BT is occurring early post-injury, but whether it is a pathologic event. In fact, Wells et al. [48] have proposed that this is the normal response by which the gut-associated lymphoid tissue (GALT) sample foreign antigens following a stressful insult.

In conclusion, following severe injury patients are resuscitated into a state of systemic inflammation (i.e. SIRS) which in most cases is presumed to be beneficial. However, following a massive insult or sequential inflammatory insults, patients can develop intense SIRS that precipitate early MOF. While it is enticing to implicate BT as the driving mechanism of early MOF, there is very little supporting basic laboratory data. The majority of studies are defining the mechanisms of BT, but do not mechanistically link BT to remote organ failure. Additionally, the clinical investigators who have studied patients at risk for MOF (excluding those dying of irreversible hemorrhagic shock) have had difficulty demonstrating that BT is a pathologic event in early post-injury SIRS.

Is the Gut the Source of MOF-Associated Infections and are these Infections the Cause of Ongoing MOF?

It has long been recognized that MOF patients experience a high rate of major septic morbidity [25, 26]. The importance of infections as pathologic events in organ failure appears to be time dependent. This was first described in a 1976 report from Walker and Eiseman [49] from Denver who noted that the pattern of post-injury adult respiratory distress syndrome (ARDS) was changing. Of 78 trauma patients requiring mechanical ventilation, 13 (17%) developed ARDS. Of these, 9 had classic early onset ARDS (within 12 h) and all survived. The remaining 5 patients developed late ARDS (> 5 days). All were septic and all died of pulmonary failure or bacteremic hypotension. The presentation was so disparate that the authors concluded that they were dealing with different diseases. In 1983, Faist, Baue and associates [29], in an often quoted Bavarian study, similarly noted 2 patterns of MOF. Of the 433 blunt polytrauma patients studied, 34 (8%) developed MOF. In 15 (44%) the onset was rapid (12–36 h), apparently the result of combined severe tissue injury and shock. In the remaining 19 (56%), the onset was late (average 7.2 days) and uniformly associated with sepsis. Again, in 1992, Waydhas et al. [50] from Munich, in a prospective study of 100 severe multisystem injured patients (mean ISS = 37), noted that 45 developed organ failure within 2 days (primarily ARDS), and 14 evolved into MOF. A second peak of late MOF (predominated by liver failure) emerged in another 18 patients at 6–8 days. In 9 (50%) of these late MOF, patient infections immediately preceded or coincided with onset of MOF. These findings are quite similar to our recent study of post-injury ventilator-associated pneumonias [51]. In this prospective study of 123 high risk torso trauma patients (mean ISS $= 36 \pm 2$) who required > 24 h of mechanical ventilation, MOF was graded on a daily basis by our standard score and pneumonias were concurrently documented using a standard clinical defini- tion combined with bronchoalveolar lavage. 28 patients (23%) developed MOF. In 14 (50%), the onset was early (≤ 3 days). 11 of these patients developed pneu- monias; in 4 cases, the onset was temporally associated with worsening MOF, while the remaining 7 cases occurred late and had no significant impact on MOF scoring (i.e. they appeared to be "symptoms"). In the other 14 patients, the onset of MOF was late (> 3 days). 9 of these patients developed pneumonia, and in 8, the diagnosis of pneumonia was temporally associated with the onset of MOF (i.e. they appeared to be "triggers").

Finally, these findings were corroborated in a more recent comprehensive epi- demiology study of post-injury MOF. This was a prospective study of 457 trauma patients with an ISS > 15 who were admitted to our trauma ICU [3]. Again, MOF was scored on a daily basis and all infections were concurrently documented us- ing rigorous definitions. Overall, 70 (15%) developed MOF. In 27 (39%) the on- set was early, while in the remaining 43 (61%) MOF presented late. The classifi- cation of major infection in these early and late MOF patients is depicted in Table 4. 32 major infections occurred in 23 of the 27 early MOF patients (85%). By our classification, 2 (6%) were not related, 2 (6%) were potential "triggers", 5 (16%) worsened existing MOF, and 23 (72%) were symptoms. In contrast, 59 ma-

Table 4. Classification of major infection in early and late MOF. (From [3] with permission)

Early MOF (n = 27)	32 Major infections/23 patients (85%)			
	Not Related	Trigger	Worsen	Symptom
Pneumonia	2 (6%)	1 (3%)	3 (9%)	14 (44%)
Abdominal Abscess			2 (6%)	2 (6%)
Wound Infection		1 (3%)		4 (6%)
Other Infections				3 (9%)
Total	2 (6%)	2 (6%)*	5 (16%)	23 (72%)
Late MOF (n = 43)	59 Major infections/38 patients (88%)			
	Not Related	Trigger	Worsen	Symptom
Pneumonia	15 (25%)	11 (19%)	1 (2%)	13 (22%)
Empyema/abscess	1 (2%)			1 (2%)
Abdominal abscess	2 (3%)	3 (5%)	1 (2%)	3 (5%)
Wound infection		2 (2%)	1 (2%)	3 (7%)
Other	1 (2%)			1 (3%)
Total	19 (32%)	16 (27%)*	3 (5%)	21 (36%)

* $p = 0.025$ number of major infections serving as "triggers" for early MOF compared to late MOF

jor infections occurred in 38 of the 43 late MOF patients (88%). 19 (32%) were not related; 16 (27%) appeared to "trigger" late MOF; 3 (5%) significantly worsened late MOF; and the remaining 21 (36%) appeared to be late symptoms. Thus, early and late MOF patients experienced a similar high incidence of major infectious complications. However, in the late MOF patients, major infections appeared to trigger or worsen MOF in over a third of the patients.

The first part of the question is whether these MOF-associated infections originate from the gut. The data favoring this are strong. First, standard ICU therapy promotes gut dysfunction. In many trauma ICUs, the severely injured are maintained on total parenteral nutrition (TPN) and receive no enteral stimulation for weeks. These same patients receive narcotics that depress gut motility. Additionally, they may receive antacids or H_2-antagonists for stress gastritis prophylaxis as well as a variety of broad spectrum antibiotics. During prolonged ICU stays, these measures promote colonization of the upper gastrointestinal tract with drug-resistant organisms including enterococcus, *Staphylococcus epidermidis*, candida species, and numerous gram-negative organisms. In animal models, these are the organisms that translocate most easily. Additionally, the studies of Border et al. [13], Marshall et al. [52], and others provide convincing epidemiologic evidence that the gut is the reservoir for these pathogens in late MOF-associated infections [53]. Moreover, several gut specific interventions have been shown to reduce ICU infections. While sucralfate stress gastritis prophylaxis has not been extensively studied in trauma patients and the available data in non-trauma patients are not conclusive, it appears to reduce nosocomial pneumonias by maintaining normal gastric acidity. On the other hand, selective digestive decontamination (SDD) has been extensively tested in trauma and non-trauma populations and has been convincingly shown to reduce nosocomial infections (principally pneumonia) [54–56]. Whether the reduction in infections seen with SDD is due to reduced BT versus decreased aspiration of colonized secretions is not clear [57]. Finally, early enteral nutrition (EN) (most recently with immune-enhancing formulas) has primarily been tested in trauma patients and has consistently been shown to reduced delayed infections (both abdominal abscess and pneumonia) [58, 59]. While it is tempting to conclude that early EN reduces BT by maintaining normal gut flora, enhancing mucosal integrity and promoting local immunity; popular alternative explanations include that 1) the gut is an immunologic organ that can be modulated to enhance systemic immunity; or 2) by emphasizing the use of early EN, patients are not being exposed early to the immunosuppressive effects of TPN.

The second, more crucial part of the question is whether these late gut-associated infections are the cause of ongoing MOF and thus have attributable mortality. While the previously mentioned sucralfate stress gastritis trials and the early EN studies lack sufficient patient numbers to assess mortality as an outcome variable, there have been sufficiently large SDD trials to address this issue. Multiple studies have shown that SDD reduces major infections, but it does not reduce mortality. This has led some to conclude that infections are inconsequential symptoms of MOF. The trauma-related SDD trials, however, may be flawed because they enrolled a large portion of head injured patients. In a recent prospective trial in which we compared influence of pneumonia on outcome in ICU patients sustaining major head injuries compared to those with major torso trauma [60], we found that head injured patients die as a direct result of their brain injury while major torso trauma patients who survived to be admitted to the ICU primarily die of sepsis related to MOF.

In conclusion, we know that standard ICU care promotes colonization of the gut with hospital-acquired pathogens. Additionally, epidemiologic studies and interventional trials strongly implicate the gut as the reservoir for these pathogens in late MOF-associated infections. Unfortunately, the available data to date have failed to show that the prevention of these gut-associated infections improves survival.

Conclusion

Bacterial translocation is an enticing concept to explain how major trauma causes irreversible hemorrhagic shock and MOF. A high amount of resources have been expended studying this phenomenon at the basic level and the resulting laboratory data are good. However, there are several inherent flaws. The few studies that include gut histology demonstrate small bowel mucosal necrosis. This is uncommon clinically. Additionally, it is not consistent with the definition of BT as passage of viable and non-viable bacteria and their byproducts through an intact mucosa. A second issue is the tremendous variability among species. Rodents predictably translocate following even minor stress events and appear to tolerate endotoxemia quite well. In contrast, it is difficult to document translocation in humans and they appear extremely sensitive to endotoxemia. The third issue is that the vast majority of laboratory investigations are focused on studying the mechanisms governing BT, but do not mechanistically link BT to organ failure. Finally, and most importantly, clinical studies do not support that BT is an important pathogenic event following major trauma. It appears that a small number of patients who arrive in severe shock may experience BT. But these massively injured patients die early. For patients who survive and are resuscitated into SIRS, it has been difficult to document that early BT even occurs. On the other hand, BT may be a late MOF-associated event. However, the important issue here is not whether it occurs but whether it is the cause of ongoing MOF or just a symptom of a dying patient.

References

1. Sauaia A, Moore FA, Moore EE, et al (1995) Epidemiology of trauma deaths: A reassessment. J Trauma 38:185–193
2. Sauaia A, Moore FA, Moore EE, et al (1994) Early predictors of postinjury MOF. Arch Surg 129:39–45
3. Moore FA, Sauaia A, Moore EE, et al (1996) Postinjury multiple organ failure: A bimodal phenomenon. J Trauma 40:501–512
4. Baker J, Deitch EA, Berg RD, Li MA, Specian RD (1988) Hemorrhagic shock induces bacterial translocation from the gut. J Trauma 28:896–906

5. Deitch EA, Winterton J, Berg R (1987) The gut as a portal of entry for bacteremia. Ann Surg 205:681–692
6. Kozoil JM, Rush BF, Smith SM, Machiedo GW (1988) Occurrence of bacteremia during and after hemorrhagic shock. J Trauma 28:10–16
7. Redan JA, Rush BF, McCullough JN, et al (1990) Organ distribution of radiolabelled enteric *Escherichia coli* during and after hemorrhagic shock. Ann Surg 211:663–668
8. Sori AJ, Rush BF, Lysz TW, Smith S, Machiedo GW (1988) The gut as a source of sepsis after hemorrhagic shock. Am J Surg 155:187–192
9. Wilmore DW, Smith RJ, O'Dwyer ST, Jacobs DD, Zeigler TR, Wong XD (1988) The gut: A central organ after surgical stress. Surgery 104:917–923
10. Rush BF, Redan JA, Flanagan JJ, et al (1989) Does the bacteremia observed in hemorrhagic shock have clinical significance? Ann Surg 210:342–347
11. Fink MP (1991) Gastrointestinal mucosal injury in experimental models of shock, trauma, sepsis. Crit Care Med 19:627–641
12. Rush BF, Sori AJ, Murphy TF, Flanagan JJ, Machiedo G (1988) Endotoxemia and bacteremia during hemorrhagic shock. Ann Surg 207:549–554
13. Border JR, Hassett J, LaDuca J, et al (1987) The gut origin septic states in blunt multiple trauma (ISS = 40) in the ICU. Ann Surg 206:427–448
14. Marshall JC, Christou NV, Horn R, et al (1988) The microbiology of multiple organ failure. Arch Surg 123:309–315
15. Fine J (1965) Current status of the problem of traumatic shock. Surg Gynecol Obstet 120: 537–544
16. Deitch EA, Maejima K, Berg R (1985) Effect of oral antibiotics and bacterial overgrowth on the translocation of the GI tract micro-flora in burned rats. J Trauma 25:385–392
17. Alexander JW, Boyce ST, Babcock GF, et al (1990) The process of microbial translocation. Ann Surg 212:496–512
18. Deitch EA, Morrison J, Berg R, Specian RD (1990) Effect of hemorrhagic shock on bacterial translocation, intestinal morphology, and intestinal permeability in conventional and anti-biotic-decontaminated rats. Crit Care Med 18:529–536
19. Jiang J, Bahrami S, Leichfried G, Redi J, Ohlinger W, Schlag G (1995) Kinetics of endotoxin and tumor necrosis factor appearance in portal and systemic circulation after hemorrhagic shock in rats. Ann Surg 221:100–106
20. Lindberg RB, Wetzler TF, Newton A, et al (1954) The bacterial flora of the bloodstream in the Korean battle casualty. Ann Surg 141:366–368
21. Moore FA, Moore EE, Poggetti RS, Read RA (1992) Postinjury shock and early bacteremia: A lethal combination. Arch Surg 127:893–898
22. Roumen RM, Hendriks T, Wevers RA, Goris JA (1993) Intestinal permeability after severe trauma and hemorrhagic shock is increased without relation to septic complications. Arch Surg 128:453–457
23. Endo S, Inada K, Yamada Y, et al (1994) Plasma endotoxin and cytokine concentrations in patients with hemorrhagic shock. Crit Care Med 22:949–955
24. Hiki N, Berger D, Buttenschoen K, et al (1995) Endotoxemia and specific antibody behavior against different endotoxins following multiple injuries. J Trauma 38:794–801
25. Eisman B, Beart R, Norton L (1977) Multiple organ failure. Surg Gynecol Obstet 144: 323–326
26. Fry DE, Pearlstein L, Fulton RL, et al (1980) Multiple system organ failure. Arch Surg 115: 136–140
27. Moore FA, Moore EE (1995) Evolving concepts in the pathogenesis of postinjury multiple organ failure. Surg Clin N Am 75:257–277
28. Stillwell M, Caplan ES (1989) The septic multiple trauma patient. Infect Dis Clin N Am 3: 155–183
29. Faist E, Baue AE, Dittmer H, et al (1983) Multiple organ failure in polytrauma patients. J Trauma 23:775–786
30. Goris JA, Boekhoerst TP, Nuytinck JK, et al (1985) Multiple organ failure. Arch Surg 120: 1109–1115
31. AlexanderJW (1990) Nutrition and translocation. J Parent Enteral Nutr 14:170S–174S

32. Deitch EA, Kemper AC, Specian RD, Berg RD (1992) A study of the relationships among survival, gut-origin sepsis, and bacterial translocation in a model of systemic inflammation. J Trauma 32:141–147
33. Fink MP (1995) Intestinal mucosal hyperpermeability. Clin Intensive Care 6:13–18
34. Pape HC, Dwenger A, Gregel MA, et al (1994) Increased gut permeability after multiple trauma. Br J Surg 81:850–852
35. Moore EE, Moore FA, Franciose RJ, et al (1994) Postischemic gut serves as a priming bed for circulating neutrophils that provoke multiple organ failure. J Trauma 37:881–887
36. Poggetti RS, Moore FA, Moore EE, et al (1992) Simultaneous liver and lung following gut ischemia is mediated by xanthine oxidase. J Trauma 32:723–728
37. Koike K, Moore FA, Moore EE, et al (1993) Gut ischemia mediates lung injury by a xanthine oxidase-dependent neutrophil mechanism. J Surg Res 54:469–473
38. Hill J, Lindsay T, Rusche J, et al (1992) A Mac-1 antibody reduces liver and lung, but not neutrophil sequestration after intestinal ischemia-reperfusion. Surgery 112:166–174
39. Schmeling DJ, Caty MG, Oldham KT, et al (1989) Evidence for neutrophil-related acute lung injury after intestinal ischemia-reperfusion. Surgery 106:195–202
40. Koike K, Moore EE, Moore FA, et al (1994) Gut ischemia/reperfusion produces lung injury independent of endotoxin. Crit Care Med 22:1438–1444
41. Punch J, Ree R, Cashmer B, et al (1991) Acute lung injury following reperfusion after ischemia in the hind limbs of rats. J Trauma 31:760–777
42. Moore FA, Moore EE, Poggetti R, et al (1991) Gut bacterial translocation via the portal vein: A clinical perspective with major torso trauma. J Trauma 31:629–638
43. Hoch RC, Rodriguez R, Manning T, et al (1993) Effects of accidental trauma on cytokine and endotoxin production. Crit Care Med 21:839–845
44. Peitzman AB, Udekwu AO, Ochoa J, Smith S (1991) Bacterial translocation in trauma patients. J Trauma 31:1083–1087
45. Brathwaite CEM, Ross SE, Nagele R, Mure AJ, O'Malley KF, Garcia-Perez FA (1993) Bacterial translocation occurs in humans after traumatic injury: Evidence using immuno-fluorescence. J Trauma 34:586–589
46. Reed LL, Martin M, Manglano R, Newson B, Kocka F, Barrett J (1994) Bacterial translocation following abdominal trauma in humans. Circ Shock 42:1–6
47. Sedman PC, Macfie J, Sagar P, et al (1994) The prevalence of gut translocation in humans. Gastroenterology 107:643–649
48. Wells CL, Maddaus MA, Simmons RL (1988) Proposed mechanisms for the translocation of intestinal bacteria. Rev Infect Dis 10:958–979
49. Walker L, Eiseman B (1976) The changing pattern of post-traumatic respiratory distress syndrome. Ann Surg 181:693–696
50. Waydhas C, Nost-Kolb D, Jochum M, et al (1992) Inflammatory mediators, infection, sepsis, and multiple organ failure after severe trauma. Arch Surg 127:460–467
51. Sauaia A, Moore FA, Moore EE, et al (1993) Pneumonia: Cause or symptom of postinjury multiple organ failure? Am J Surg 166:607–611
52. Marshall JC, Christow NW, Horn R, et al (1988) The microbiology of multiple organ failure. Arch Surg 123:309–315
53. Garrison RN, Fry DE, Berberich S, Polk HC (1982) Enterococcal bacteremia: Clinical implications and determinants of death. Ann Surg 196:43–47
54. Van Saene HKF, Stoutenbeek CC, Stoller JK, et al (1992) Selective decontamination of the digestive tract in the intensive care unit: Current status and future prospects. Crit Care Med 20:691–698
55. Heyland DK, Cook DJ, Jaeschke A, et al (1994) Selective decontamination of the digestive tract: An overview. Chest 105:1221–1229
56. Cerra FB, Maddaus MA, Dunn DL, et al (1992) Selective gut decontamination reduces nosocomial infections and length of stay, but not mortality or organ failure in surgical intensive care unit patients. Arch Surg 127:163–169
57. Fiddian-Green RG, Baker S (1991) Nosocomial pneumonia in the critically ill: Product of aspiration or translocation? Crit Care Med 19:763–769

58. Moore FA, Feliciano DV, Andrassy RJ, et al (1992) Early enteral feeding, compared with parenteral, reduces postoperative septic complications. Ann Surg 216:62–69
59. Moore FA, Moore EE, Kudsk KA, et al (1994) Clinical benefits of an immune-enhancing diet for early postinjury enteral feeding. J Trauma 37:607–615
60. Sauaia A, Moore FA, Moore EE, et al (1992) Pneumonia-related multiple organ failure is not a primary cause of death in head trauma. Pan Am J Trauma 3:90–96

Gut Perfusion

Gastrointestinal Mucosal Ischemia

B. Vallet, R. Nevière, and J. L. Chagnon

Introduction

Beginning in the esophagus and continuing all the way to the anus, the wall of the digestive tube has the same basic arrangement of four layers. The four basic layers present are, from the lumen of the gut outward: the mucosa, the submucosa, the muscularis and the serosa. The mucosa is the mucous membrane that lines the digestive tract. It consists of three layers: an epithelial layer, the lamina propria, the muscularis mucosa. The submucosa contains blood vessels, lymphatics, nerves, and in some regions glands. The microcirculation of the alimentary tract is crucial not only for the nutritive maintenance of the alimentary tract itself, but also for its vital functions of secretion and absorption, since the circulation is the ultimate source of the secreted digestive juices and the recipient of absorbed digesta. Moreover, the integrity of mucosal barrier function is thought to play an important role in defending the host from translocation of intact micro-organisms or their breakdown products and toxins [1].

Mucosal blood flow in stomach as well as in intestine originates from the submucosal arterioles that arborise into a dense network of capillaries. These capillaries pass through, generally perpendicular to the plane of the mucosa, to reach the most luminal layer, just beneath the epithelial cells [2]. Blood from these most luminal capillaries drains into the mucosal venules at the most luminal level of the lamina propria. The arterioles which supply blood and the venules draining it conduct flow in the opposite direction. Arterioles and venules form "hairpin loop" arrangements which promote the development of a countercurrent exchange of oxygen (O_2) from the inflow vessels to the outflow vessels. As a consequence of this countercurrent exchange mechanism, there exists a base-to-tip gradient in the partial pressure of O_2, with lower O_2 tension at the apex of the hairpin loop [3]. This anatomical feature among others would make gastrointestinal (GI) mucosa highly susceptible to decreased O_2 delivery (DO_2). The countercurrent exchange mechanism is very likely to occur within small intestinal villi (at least in some species), but it is of importance to remind that there is a lack of data related to the existence of such a mechanism within the gastric mucosa. However, in spite of these potential discrepancies, it has been shown that gastric mucosal ischemia is indicative of intestinal mucosal ischemia in various hemodynamic disorders. This is of clinical importance since stomach is much easier to monitor than small intestine in critically ill patients.

Decreased mucosal perfusion will occur during two main circumstances:
1) global decrease in splanchnic flow as seen in low flow states; and
2) abnormal microvascular reactivity within GI mucosa as seen in septic states despite adequate global splanchnic flow.

Gastrointestinal Mucosal Ischemia in Low Flow States

Peripheral vasoconstriction is a major compensatory mechanism of hypovolemia. In the setting of both hypovolemic and cardiogenic shock, splanchnic ischemia occurs [4, 5] through normal vasoregulatory mechanisms, largely due to sympathetic and angiotensin II-induced reductions and/or redistribution in regional DO_2 [6, 7]. Redistribution of whole body DO_2 among organs promote macrovascular O_2 regulation by reducing perfusion of organs that are normally overperfused relative to need. Thus diversion of unnecessary flow from organs such as the kidneys and splanchnic viscera to the heart and brain during critically low whole body DO_2 would enhance O_2 uptake (VO_2) of the whole organism [8]. If this vasoconstriction is prolonged and/or severe, it may lead to ischemic insult of splanchnic organs which have been hypothesized to play a role in the pathogenesis of the multiple organ dysfunction syndrome (MODS). In 8 healthy male volunteers, Edouard et al. [9] clearly demonstrated that simulated hypovolemia (lower body negative pressure: LBNP) induced a parallel one-third decrease in cardiac output (bioimpedance), musculo-cutaneous (venous plethysmography) and splanchnic (indocyanine green clearance) blood flows. The major finding in this study was that during the recovery period, all the cardiovascular and biological variables returned to the pre-LBNP values, except for splanchnic blood flow which remained below control values 60 min after the return to atmospheric pressure. Evidently, the volunteers in this study did not suffer any MODS. In further experiments, the same group using LBNP in 7 volunteers [10] demonstrated that acute hypoperfusion in the splanchnic circulation was accompanied by a compensatory dilation of mucosal arterioles and an increase in gastric mucosal perfusion assessed by laser Doppler flowmetry. The authors speculated that a mechanism allowed redistribution of blood flow within gastric wall layers. If this is the case, one may consider that changes in GI mucosal perfusion do not fully predict changes in splanchnic perfusion. However, the authors demonstrated that for a -30 mmHg LBNP, gastric mucosal perfusion was significantly decreased. In contrast to splanchnic vascular resistances, gastric mucosal blood flow returned to control as soon as LBNP was interrupted.

Therefore, when hypovolemic shock is very severe, GI tissue dysoxia may appear. Indeed, in an animal model, Hartman et al. [11] demonstrated that intramucosal pH (pHi) in the stomach, small intestine and sigmoid colon rapidly decreases when blood pressure was lowered to 45 mmHg during hemorrhagic shock. pHi may be used as an indicator of tissue oxygenation. Grum et al. [12], and more recently Schlichtig and Bowles [13] showed that intestinal pHi remained constant as local DO_2 decreased to a point where VO_2 became supply dependent. The pHi fell precipitously when DO_2 to the tissue was reduced below critical levels. The current technique of clinical measurement of pHi is indirect. A tonometer is used that consists in a balloon filled with 0.9% NaCl solution incorporated near the distal end of a nasogastric tube. After a 30- to 90-min equilibration period, balloon CO_2 that is sampled merely represents gastric mucosal CO_2. pHi is estimated from PCO_2 measured on the fluid sampled and arterial bicarbonates, instead of mucosal bicarbonates, computed by the Henderson-Hasselbalch equation. Because gastric mucosal and arterial bicarbonates are not equal, it has been demonstrated that changes in gastric PCO_2 are more closely related to the hemodynamic state than changes in pHi [14]. Also, increases in mucosal PCO_2 are associated with the development of mucosal ischemia and correlate strongly with the histologic grade of injury.

The superficial mucosa rapidly demonstrates dysfunction and morphologic signs of injury during ischemia. But morphological and functional injury also can be exacerbated by events that occur following the re-establishment of tissue perfusion [15]. The relative contribution of ischemia-induced damage as compared to reperfusion-induced damage appears to depend on the duration, and perhaps the extent, of tissue hypoperfusion. In hemorrhagic shock, if tissue hypoperfusion duration is short enough, intestinal VO_2 [16] and intramucosal acidosis [14] recover when DO_2 is restituted with fluid. However, a severe denudation of apical villi after ischemia/reperfusion (I/R) injury, leaving exposed basement membrane, has been observed in experimental models with a 2-h period of mesenteric ischemia [17]. Salzman et al. [17] tested the hypothesis that intraluminal oxygenation could prevent mucosal injury caused by mesenteric I/R. They demonstrated that mucosal ATP levels normalized in oxygenated intestinal segments, whereas there was only partial recovery of ATP levels in nitrogenated segments. The authors considered that the amelioration of injury during reperfusion might have resulted from a protective effect of intraluminal oxygenation on cellular function during the period of ischemia. Considering the countercurrent exchange mechanism in the intestinal villus, they speculated that ischemia led to development of an O_2 debt at the level of the distal villus. By directly providing the distal villus of O_2 via an intraluminal route, it was possible to circumvent this O_2 "steal" by the proximal villus.

Likewise, an adequate blood flow is essential for gastric mucosal tissue to withstand the challenge of both endogenous and exogenous aggressors. Blood flow, by providing tissue oxygenation and nutrient delivery, acts to enhance the mucosal defense mechanisms, while reduction in blood flow leads to mucosal injury or make the tissue more susceptible to damage. An important factor in the relationship between mucosal blood flow, tissue integrity and mucosal defense is the maintenance of intramucosal acid-base neutrality [18]. Indeed, limitation of mucosal blood flow allows the intramucosal accumulation of hydrogen ions by reducing both their neutralization and their washout. It has been generally believed that gastric ulcers are caused by an imbalance between aggressive factors (such as gastric acid, pepsin, bile salts) and defensive factors (mucus, bicarbonate, mucosal blood flow, epithelial cell renewal, neuropeptides) [19].

Bleeding from acute stress ulcers or erosions occurs in 25 to 30% of all seriously ill patients in ICU, although in most patients this is minimal and not clinically

a problem [20, 21]. Stress-related mucosal damage refers to mucosal injury occurring in critically ill patients within 4 to 14 days of admission into ICU [19].
Subepithelial hemorrhages and erosions are common in these patients who
undergo endoscopy. These lesions usually lack clinical significance because they
do not cause bleeding, perforation or pain. Few data exist concerning the pathogenesis of inpatient ulceration and secondary bleeding regarding critically ill patients hospitalized for another problem. Gastric mucosal acidosis mainly results
from tissue ischemia. Clinically as well as experimentally, the frequency and severity of stress-induced gastric mucosal injury directly correlate with the severity of shock, while gastric acid secretion decreases in direct correlation with the
severity of shock [22, 23]. Recently, further studies have supported the hypothesis that shock and ischemia are the main factors promoting stress-induced gastric bleeding. However, the exact pathogenesis of stress-induced gastric mucosal
injury remains uncertain [24].

In support of the concept of a protective hyperemia is the finding that, when
the mucosa of rats is exposed to a mild irritant such as taurocholate, deep necrot-
ic damage occurs only with concurrent administration of a vasoconstrictor agent
such as vasopressin or norepinephrine [25]. A balance between the release of local vasoconstrictor (endothelin, neuropeptide Y) and vasodilator mediators
(prostacyclin (PGI_2), nitric oxide (NO)) in the microcirculation could be involved in the physiological control of mucosal blood flow, providing a mechanism for the rapid vascular response to the functional needs of the mucosa [18].
The systemic release of vasoactive factors may also influence the tone of the microvasculature. Pharmacological interventions to increase gastric mucosal levels
of NO or PGI_2 by augmenting their endogenous production or by providing an
exogenous source of NO or PGI_2 could prove effective in the prevention of acute
gastric mucosal injury in high risk settings.

Fiddian-Green et al. [26] examined the ability of pHi to predict the occurrence
of bleeding from stress ulcers and compared its ability with those of other measurements made in ICU patients. They found that the calculated measurements of
pHi were of predictive value for massive bleeding from stress ulceration in ICU
patient, and added significantly to the predictive ability of risk factors alone. The
occurrence of massive bleeding from stress ulceration in their patients, all of
whom were receiving antacids, was unrelated to the pH of gastric juice. The low-
est pH detected in the gastric juice of their patients who bled from stress ulcers
was 3.45. The target pH endpoint for titration of antisecretory therapy is considered to be higher than 3.5 [19]. There is increasing evidence from numerous
ICUs that stress ulcers can be effectively prevented without suppressing the
physiologic gastric acid barrier [24]. In Fiddian-Green's study, the finding of a
low pHi preceded the occurrence of bleeding from stress ulceration by one or
several days. The authors raised the possibility that the occurrence of bleeding
might have been prevented had it been possible to elevate pHi earlier. This study
antedated the discovery of *Helicobacter pylori* and its influence in gastroduodenal ulcer disease. The role of *H. pylori* in stress ulceration and secondary upper GI
bleeding has not been studied yet; nor has prophylactic treatment of *H. pylori* in
ICU patients been studied.

Gastrointestinal Mucosal Ischemia in Septic States

Risk factors associated with the development of stress ulceration appear to be multiorgan failure, prolonged mechanical ventilation, hypotension, sepsis (more often than hypotensive shock), major trauma, major surgery, and severe burns involving more than 35% of body surface area [27]. In a large heterogeneous cohort of critically ill patients (2252 patients)[28], main risk factors for clinically important bleeding were respiratory failure with mechanical ventilation for more than 48 h, coagulopathy, hypotension and sepsis. Interestingly, it has been demonstrated that thermal injury and/or sepsis are associated with disruption of GI homeostasis despite "adequate" indexes of resuscitation [29–31]. In these situations, decreased DO_2 due to reduced mesenteric blood flow cannot by itself explain the decreased intestinal pHi and increased mucosal damage: either GI mucosal DO_2 is increased, or VO_2 is abnormal.

Alterations of normal microcirculatory control mechanisms have been reported that may compromise further tissue nutrient blood flow. The presence of sustained tissue hypoxia as a consequence of septic microvascular injury has been proposed by a number of investigators. But still, there was no proof that a disruption in blood flow distribution occurs within organ during sepsis and that this disruption was linked to decreased O_2 extraction ability. We attempted to answer that question by generating surface tissue PO_2 ($PtiO_2$) measurements from skeletal muscle and gut mucosa and serosa during endotoxemia (lipopolysaccharide infusion, LPS), before and after volume resuscitation. Distribution of $PtiO_2$ histograms may be used to characterize the relationship between capillary DO_2 and cellular O_2 requirements and to reflect changes in microvascular control [32]. Under normal physiological conditions, relationship of capillary perfusion to cellular O_2 demand is well matched and the $PtiO_2$ histogram has a shape approximately Gaussian. When the microcirculation is disturbed, the histogram becomes irregular with a dispersion of values. In our study, skeletal muscle exhibited preserved O_2 extraction (O_2ER) ability. Its VO_2 remained unchanged and O_2ER reached 78% by the end of LPS infusion, suggesting that muscle microcirculation was probably not severely disturbed during LPS infusion. Consistent with this, $PtiO_2$ histograms in muscle maintained a near-Gaussian distribution supporting the finding of Gutierrez et al. [33], that skeletal muscle microcirculatory heterogeneity did not increase during endotoxin-induced sepsis. In the gut, VO_2 and pHi significantly decreased, and although intestinal DO_2 and serosal $PtiO_2$ returned to baseline with dextran infusion, intestinal VO_2, mucosal $PtiO_2$ and pHi never recovered (Fig. 1). The failure of gut VO_2 to rebound with resuscitation is consistent with earlier LPS dog studies [34], but is in sharp contrast to non-LPS models of gut ischemia, including studies of systemic hypoxic hypoxia [35] or ischemic hypoxia [16, 36] in which gut VO_2, as well as pHi, returned to baseline with resuscitation despite a more severe period of decreased DO_2 than in our study. This suggested that the physiology of shock associated with LPS has features such as inflammatory mediators that are not present in non-LPS hypoxia or ischemia that cause a sustained disturbance in gut VO_2. Therefore, after LPS infusion, blood flow-controlling sites in the gut microcirculation appeared to be

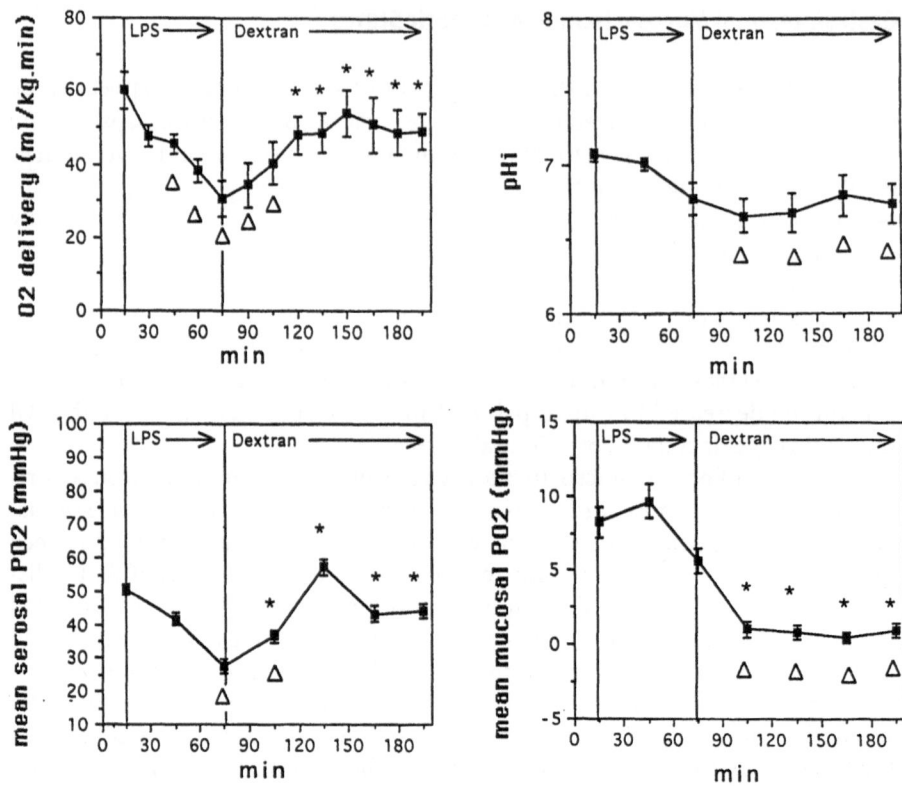

Fig. 1. Gut oyxgen delivery, intramucosal pH (pHi) and mean serosal and mucosal tissue PO_2 (mean $\pm$ SE) during endotoxin infusion (LPS) and resuscitation (dextran) Δ: different from baseline; *: different from end of LPS, $p < 0.05$. (Adapted from [30] with permission)

inadequate to maintain mucosal perfusion and oxygenation, and unable to prevent the preferential onset of supply dependency in the gut despite more than adequate blood flow following dextran infusion.

In support of changes in reactive properties of vascular tissue, Drazenovic et al. [37] recently showed that gut adjustments in perfused capillary surface density, in response to changes in DO_2, were impaired after LPS administration. Whithworth et al. [38] showed that vasoactive tone between intestinal little arterioles was imbalanced in a hyperdynamic model of sepsis in rats. Third-order arterioles, which terminate as central villous arterioles, were more constricted than first- or second-order arterioles, leading specifically to compromised mucosal blood flow. Gut mucosal blood flow decrease, using real time measurement of microvascular blood flow by laser Doppler flowmetry, has been described by several authors [39, 40]. Therefore, local tissue hypoperfusion during endotoxemia could result from a failure of vascular tissue to respond normally to metabolic vasodilatory stimuli and to match the local O_2 supply-to-demand. Even in the setting of systemic vasodilation, an inappropriate focal vasoconstriction could occur as a potential mechanism for focal tissue hypoxia.

Whether another kind of therapy than fluid could promote blood flow to the GI mucosa and improve its oxygenation must be explored. There is a number of ways by which blood flow to the gut might be promoted. These blood flow promoters include the early institution of enteral nutrition [41] and specific pharmacologic measures designed to influence mesenteric circulation. In endotoxic, live bacteria and cecal ligation puncture models [42–44], various potent adrenergic agents failed to redistribute total body volume and flow from non-vital organ system circulation, i.e. the gut, to vital organ system circulation such as the heart and the brain. At the opposite, inotropic and vasodilating agents in addition to fluid resuscitation are likely to increase mesenteric blood flow in endotoxic shock model.

Breslow et al. [42] evaluated the effects of norepinephrine, dopamine and phenylephrine on regional blood flow distribution in a porcine model of fluid-resuscitated endotoxic shock. Each vasopressor agent has a different spectrum of activity against the various adrenergic receptors, and theoretically each could affect regional blood flow distribution differently. The specific goal of the study was to determine whether elevation of systemic arterial blood pressure with vasopressors could improve blood flow to the brain and the heart at the expense of kidney and splanchnic blood flow in endotoxic shock. The results of this study suggest that blood pressure elevation with norepinephrine, dopamine and phenylephrine neither decreases blood flow to any organ nor increases blood flow to organs with reduced flow, and that norepinephrine, dopamine and phenylephrine affect regional blood flow to the same extent in this acute endotoxic shock model. Similarly, in a hyperdynamic model of sepsis secondary to cecal ligation and puncture in awake sheep, Bersten et al. [44] showed that sympathetic activation was not accompanied by redistribution of flow from non-vital organs to vital (heart and brain) circulations.

As stated above, evidence of gut mucosal hypoxia may be demonstrated in spite of normal or even increased total gut blood flow. Small intestinal mucosal damage was reported by Falk et al. [45] in 60% of cats subject to a standardized live *E. coli* septic shock with normal total intestinal blood flow. The authors concluded that even though regional DO_2 increased, compelling evidence suggested that this elevation was inadequate to satisfy tissue demand. In a hypodynamic model of septic shock, Fink et al. [46] demonstrated that mesenteric hypoperfusion was not by itself sufficient to cause a defect in the barrier function of the ileum as measured by clearance methods. The authors proposed that microvascular derangements in mucosal perfusion might be responsible for the observed changes in permeability and intramucosal acidosis. The effects of high dose dobutamine being titrated to maintain mesenteric blood flow in a porcine model of acute endotoxemia was published by the same laboratory [47]. The fluid-resuscitated group constituted a normodynamic model of acute endotoxemia. Additional resuscitation in form of either hetastarch or hetastarch plus dobutamine converted this into a hyperdynamic, hypotensive model. While mesenteric blood flow was reduced to about 50% of the baseline for the duration of the observation in control septic animals, the hetastarch plus dobutamine regimen succeeded in keeping mesenteric blood flow at or above the baseline value for the entire period of the experiment. Although hetastarch alone tended to support mesenteric blood flow, it also caused hemodilution and hence mesenteric DO_2 decrease. Adding dobutamine made it possible to maintain mesenteric DO_2 at baseline level. Permeability in this study was measured in the plasma-to-lumen direction which allowed a rigorous quantification of the degree of derangement in the permeability barrier. There was a sixfold increase in transmucosal permeability that hetastarch-dobutamine resuscitation regimen was able to prevent entirely. In this study, ileal pHi was also measured using tonometric techniques. Infusion of endotoxin into pigs caused a marked degree of mucosal acidosis. As the extent of resuscitation was increased first with hetastarch and then with hetastarch plus dobutamine, part of this mucosal acidosis could be ameliorated.

Whether a potent β-adrenergic agonist such as dobutamine could promote blood flow to the mucosa and improved its oxygenation has been explored. Shepherd et al. [48] using both radioactive microspheres and laser Doppler flowmetry demonstrated that $β_1$-$β_2$-adrenergic stimulation with isoproterenol was able to increase gut blood flow and to favor mucosal blood flow at the expense of flow to the muscularis layer in the gut wall in anesthetized animals. Cain and Curtis [49] recently showed in endotoxic dogs that dextran plus dopexamine, a potent $β_2$-adrenergic agonist, supported gut VO_2 at higher levels than did dextran alone. The authors postulated that the $β_2$-adrenergic agonist property of dopexamine could promote blood flow specially to the gut mucosa and prevent the rising output of lactate by the gut as a result of the correction of regional hypoxia within the gut wall. This was demonstrated by the observed effect of dopexamine that supported gut VO_2 at higher levels than in either dextran-treated or control animals. At the same time, lactate efflux from the gut in the dopexamine group remained lower than either in dextran-treated or control animals. The combined finding of lower lactate efflux and higher VO_2 in dopexamine-treated animals indicated that the treatment had a beneficial effect that was not achieved simply by maintaining high flow rate and DO_2 as the dextran infusion succeeded in doing so.

We recently reported the effects of low dose dobutamine on gastric and intestinal mucosal blood flow in a fluid-resuscitated porcine model of endotoxic shock [40]. Hemodynamics, O_2 transport and GI mucosal perfusion assessed by laser Doppler flowmetry and pHi were studied in saline-treated animals and saline plus dobutamine-treated animals. Despite the maintenance of systemic blood flow, endotoxin plus saline treatment produced both a decrease of gastric and intestinal microvascular blood flow and gastric and intestinal pHi. In contrast, gut microvascular blood flow returned to baseline values and gut pHi tended to normalize by the end of the saline plus dobutamine treatment (Fig. 2). The reason for these observations was assigned to the known effect of $β_2$-adrenergic stimulation to favor mucosal blood flow at the expense of flow to muscularis in the gut wall. Although the drop in pHi was not reversed entirely, the saline plus dobutamine resuscitative regimen limited gut pHi decrease. Since we did not measure gut VO_2, our data are insufficient to account for this incomplete gut acidosis amelioration. The effects of β-adrenergic stimulation on gut metabolism could participate in the persistent mucosal acidosis observed in this model.

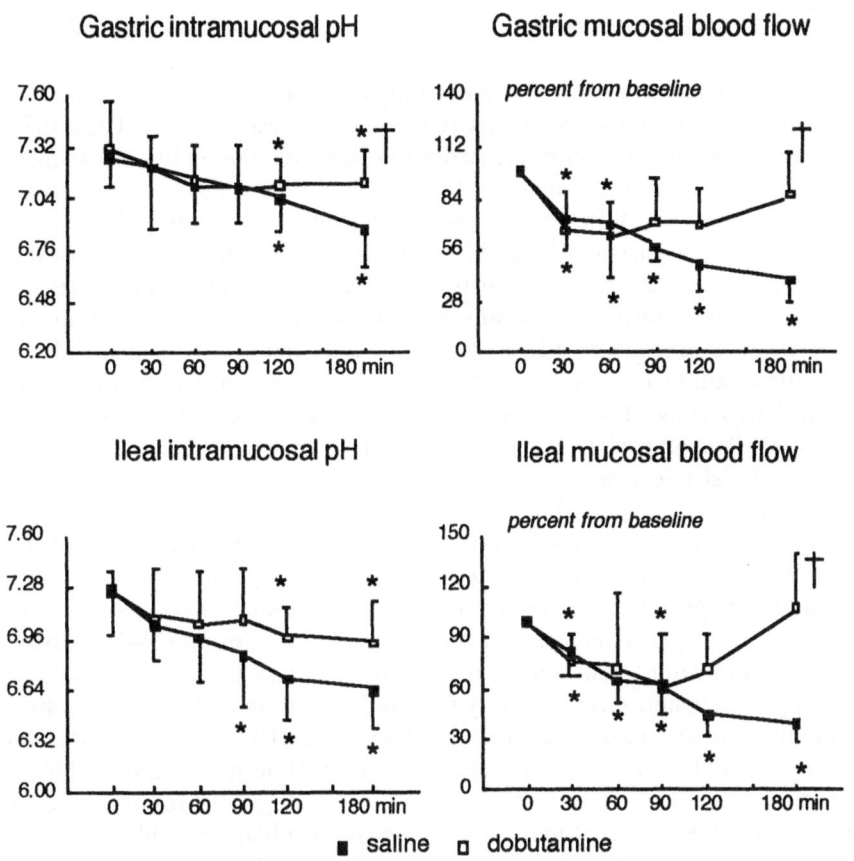

Fig. 2. Gastric and intestinal intramucosal pH and mucosal perfusion changes (mean ± SE) in endotoxic pigs resuscitated with either saline (closed square) or saline plus dobutamine (open square). Different from baseline: * $p < 0.05$; different from saline: † $p < 0.05$. (Adapted from [40] with permission)

Since experimental studies have shown that gut pHi is a good indicator of gut ischemia, clinical studies have demonstrated the potential utility of gut tonometry in identifying patients at risk for developing complications attributable to mucosal disruption in a variety of critical illness [50]. Also, experience with monitoring of pHi may help to identify alternative therapeutic options in patient with severe sepsis. Silverman et al. [51] demonstrated that dobutamine increases low gastric tonometric pHi values in septic patients, suggesting that this agent may improve splanchnic tissue oxygenation. In contrast, packed red blood cell transfusion in order to increase systemic DO_2 failed to improve gastric pHi. These findings have been confirmed by Marik and Sibbald [52]. These authors reported that the adverse effects of blood transfusion were related to the age of packed red blood cells, and assigned this observation to the loss of red cell pliability. Therefore, the failure of packed red blood cell transfusion to improve pHi was related to a decrease in mucosal blood flow caused by rheologic properties changes. Another explanation was an increased hematocrit level with enhanced blood viscosity.

In septic patients, a variety of pharmacological agents have been shown to reverse intramucosal acidosis refractory to increases in systemic DO_2. These drugs may reverse intramucosal acidosis in a dose-dependent manner by increasing regional DO_2 or redistributing regional DO_2 within different metabolic rate activity layers. Smithies et al. [53] demonstrated in septic patients that dopexamine was able to increase gastric pHi. In this study, splanchnic blood flow assessed by indocyanine green clearance was also measured. When gastric pHi increased with dopexamine infusion, indocyanine green clearance improved but not significantly. Changes in gastric pHi were unrelated to changes in splanchnic blood flow, cardiac output or systemic DO_2. The failure to observe any relationship between changes in gastric pHi and regional blood flow most likely represents a preferential effect on gastric mucosal perfusion.

The beneficial effect of dobutamine, a potent β_1-β_2-adrenergic agonist, on gastric intramucosal acidosis has been tested by Gutierrez et al. [54] in septic patients with and without elevated arterial lactate. The authors demonstrated that dobutamine when infused at 5 µg/kg·min and 10 µg/kg·min increased gastric pHi in both groups. It was speculated that dobutamine may reverse gastric intramucosal acidosis by increasing splanchnic blood flow and/or mucosal perfusion. The effects of low dose dobutamine on pHi and mucosal perfusion assessed by laser Doppler flowmetry were recently reported [55]. In the septic patients studied, dobutamine at 5 µg/kg·min increased systemic DO_2. This was associated with a significant increase of gastric pHi. At the same time, gastric mucosal blood flow measured by laser Doppler flowmetry increased out of proportion to the systemic DO_2. Likewise, treatment with a selective vasodilator in addition to conventional resuscitation (fluids and inoconstrictors) may help to increase GI mucosal flow when perfusion pressure is restored. In dopamine-resistant septic shock, Levy et al. [56] presented evidence that a low-dose dobutamine infusion in association with norepinephrine improved pHi much faster than did epinephrine alone. Radermacher et al. [57] demonstrated that infusing PGI_2 (10 ng/kg·min) in patients with septic shock further increased pHi even when conventional resuscitation goals had been achieved.

Therefore, improvements in blood flow to the gastric mucosa, and by implication to the intestinal mucosa, may become an appropriate goal for the treatment of critically ill patients with sepsis. Such therapeutics would be likely to prevent mucosal ischemia, bacterial translocation and the risk of MODS. Gutierrez et al. [58] showed in a large controlled, randomized study ($n = 260$) that patients monitored and treated for falls in pHi had lower mortality than those monitored only for conventional endpoints of resuscitation such as blood pressure and urine output. These findings have to be confirmed by other prospective controlled trials to determine whether such GI-directed therapies really improve the outcome of critically ill patients.

Conclusion

Gastrointestinal mucosal perfusion is the first to be affected in low flow states and the last to be restored to normality in resuscitation. In these states, mucosal perfusion remains within normal limits when DO_2 to the GI tract satisfies tissue metabolism requirements and when VO_2 is independent of DO_2. When the pathological processes that lead to inadequate tissue oxygenation overcome the resuscitative efforts, shock develops.

In covert compensated shock, there are no major hemodynamic derangements. The inadequacy of tissue oxygenation may be concentrated to the splanchnic organs, especially to the mucosal lining of the GI tract. A particularly important cause of covert compensated shock is an impaired ability of tissues to extract and utilize O_2. These abnormalities are commonly caused by sepsis and/or endotoxemia and might be often encountered in critical illness. Recent studies suggest that, even during hyperdynamic sepsis, the gut wall distribution of microvascular blood flow remains severely compromised with the presence of regional tissue hypoxia in the mucosal layer, despite more than adequate total gut blood flow following fluid infusion. Growing evidence suggests that β-adrenergic stimulation could promote blood flow to the GI mucosa and improve its oxygenation.

References

1. Wells C, Maddaus M, Simmons R (1988) Proposed mechanisms for the translocation of intestinal bacteria. Rev Infectious Dis 10:958–979
2. Gannon B, Browning J, O'Brien P, Rogers P (1984) Mucosal microvascular architecture of the fundus and body of human stomach. Gastroenterology 86:866–875
3. Landow L, Andersen LW (1994) Splanchnic ischemia and its role in multiple organ failure. Acta Anaesth Scand 38:626–639
4. Bailey RW, Bulkley GB, Levy KI, et al (1982) Pathogenesis of nonocclusive mesenteric ischemia: Study in a porcine model induced by pericardial tamponade. Surg Forum 33:194–197
5. Porter JM, Sussman MS, Bulkley GB (1989) Splanchnic vasospasm in circulatory shock. In: Marston A, Bulkley GB, Fiddian-Green RG, et al (eds) Splanchnic ischemia and multiple organ failure. E Arnold, London, pp 73–88
6. Bailey RW, Bulkley GB, Hamilton SR, et al (1987) Protection of the small intestine from non-occlusive mesenteric ischemic injury due to cardiogenic shock. Am J Surg 153:108–116
7. McNeil JR, Stark RD, Greenway CV (1970) Intestinal vasoconstriction after hemorrhage: Roles of vasopressin and angiotensin. Am J Physiol 219:1342–1347
8. Schlichtig R, Kramer DJ, Pinsky MR (1991) Flow redistribution during progressive hemorrhage is a determinant of critical O_2 delivery. J Appl Physiol 70:169–178
9. Edouard AR, Degrémont AC, Duranteau J, Pussard E, Berdeaux A, Samii K (1994) Heterogeneous regional vascular responses to simulated transient hypovolemia in man. Intensive Care Med 20:414–420
10. Duranteau J, Sitbon P, Vicaut E, Descorps-Declère A, Vigue B, Samii K (1996) Assessment of gastric mucosal perfusion during simulated hypovolemia in healthy volunteers. Am J Respir Crit Care Med (In press)
11. Hartmann M, Montgomery A, Jonsson K, et al (1991) Tissue oxygenation in hemorrhagic shock measured as transcutaneous oxygen tension, subcutaneous oxygen tension, and GI intramucosal pH in pigs. Crit Care Med 19:205–210

12. Grum CM, Fiddian-Green RG, Pittenger GL, et al (1984) Adequacy of tissue oxygenation in intact dog intestine. J Appl Physiol 56:1065–1069
13. Schlichtig R, Bowles SA (1994) Distinguishing between aerobic and anaerobic appearance of dissolved CO_2 in intestine during low flow. J Appl Physiol 76:2443–2451
14. Tang W, Weil MH, Sun S, Noc M, Gazmuri R, Bisera J (1994) Gastric intramural PCO_2 as monitor of perfusion failure during hemorrhagic and anaphylactic shock. J Appl Physiol 76:572–577
15. Haglund U, Bulkley G, Granger D (1987) On the pathophysiology of intestinal ischemic injury. Acta Chir Scand 153:321–324
16. Curtis SE, Cain SM (1992) Systemic and regional O_2 delivery and uptake in bled dogs given hypertonic saline, whole blood, or dextran. Am J Physiol 262:778–786
17. Salzman A, Wollert PS, Wang H, et al (1993) Intraluminal oxygenation ameliorates ischemia/reperfusion-induced gut mucosal hyperpermeability in pigs. Circ Shock 40:37–46
18. Whittle BJR (1993) Neuronal and endothelium-derived mediators in the modulation of gastric microcirculation: Integrity in the balance. Br J Pharmacol 110:3–17
19. Jutabha R, Poa L, Jensen DM (1995) Stress ulceration in the critically ill. Curr Opin Crit Care 1:125–129
20. Nash J, Lambert L, Deakin M (1994) Histamine H2-receptor antagonists in peptic ulcer disease. Evidence for a prophylactic use. Drugs 47:862–871
21. Chamberlain CE (1993) Acute hemorrhagic gastritis. Gastroenterol Clin N Am 22:843–873
22. Stannard VA, Hutchinson A, Morris DL, Byrne A (1988) Gastric exocrine failure in critically ill patients: Incidence and associated features. Br Med J 296:155–156
23. Urakawa T, Nagahata Y, Azumi Y, et al (1989) The mechanism of acute gastric ulcer after induced hemorrhagic shock. Scand J Gastroenterol 24:193–201
24. Tryba M, Kulka PJ (1993) Critical care pharmacology. A review. Drugs 45:338–352
25. Whittle BJR (1983) The potentiation of taurocholate-induced rat gastric erosions following parenteral administration of cyclooxygenase inhibitors. Br J Pharmacol 80:545–551
26. Fiddian-Green RG, McGough E, Pittenger G, Rothman E (1983) Predictive value of intramural pH and other risk factors for massive bleeding from stress ulceration. Gastroenterology 85:613–620
27. Fusamoto H, Hagiwara H, Meren H, et al (1991) A clinical study of acute gastrointestinal hemorrhage associated with various shock states. Am J Gastroenterol 86:429–433
28. Cook DJ, Fuller HD, Guyat GH, et al (1994) Risk factors for gastrointestinal bleeding in critically ill patients. N Engl J Med 330:377–381
29. Tokyay R, Zeigler S, Traber DL, et al (1993) Postburn gastrointestinal vasoconstriction increases bacterial and endotoxin translocation. J Appl Physiol 74:1521–1527
30. Vallet B, Lund N, Curtis SE, et al (1994) Gut and muscle tissue PO_2 in endotoxemic dogs during shock and resuscitation. J Appl Physiol 76:793–800
31. Payne JG, Bowen JC (1981) Hypoxia of canine gastric mucosa caused by E. coli sepsis and prevented with methylprednisolone therapy. Gastroenterology 80:84–93
32. Thorborg P, Malmqvist LA, Lund N (1988) Surface oxygen pressure distributions in rabbit skeletal muscle: Dependence on arterial PO_2. Microcirc Endothel Lymphatics 4:169–192
33. Gutierrez G, Lund N, Palizas F (1991) Rabbit skeletal muscle PO_2 during hypodynamic sepsis. Chest 99:224–229
34. Curtis SE, Cain SM (1992) Regional and systemic oxygen delivery/uptake relations and lactate flux in hyperdynamic, endotoxin-treated dogs. Am Rev Respir Dis 145:348–354
35. Dodd SL, King CE, Cain SM (1987) Responses of innervated and denervated gut to whole body hypoxia. J Appl Physiol 62:651–657
36. Montgomery A, Hartmann M, Jonsson K, Haglund UH (1989) Intramucosal pH measurement with tonometer for detecting gastrointestinal ischemia in porcine hemorrhagic shock. Circ Shock 29:319–327
37. Drazenovic R, Samsel RW, Wylam ME, Doerschuk CM, Schumacker PT (1999) Regulation of perfused capillary density in canine mucosa during endotoxemia. J Appl Physiol 72:259–265

38. Whitworth PW, Cryer HM, Garrisson RN, et al (1989) Hypoperfusion of the intestinal microcirculation without decreased cardiac output during live *Escherichia coli* in rats. Circ Shock 27:111-122
39. Theuer CJ, Wilson MA, Steeb GD, et al (1993) Microvascular vasoconstriction and mucosal hypoperfusion of the rat small intestine during bacteremia. Circ Shock 40:61-68
40. Nevière R, Chagnon LJ, Vallet B, et al (1995) Gut oxygenation in endotoxemic pigs during shock and resuscitation. Intensive Care Med 21:S18 (Abst)
41. Shepherd AP (1980) Intestinal blood flow autoregulation during foodstuff absorption. Am J Physiol 239:H156-H162
42. Breslow MJ, Miller CF, Parker SD, et al (1987) Effect of vasopressors on organ blood flow during endotoxin shock in pigs. Am J Physiol 252:H291-H300
43. Schneider AJ, Groeneveld AB, Teule GJ, et al (1991) Total body blood volume redistribution in porcine *E. coli* septic shock. Circ Shock 35:215-222
44. Bersten AD, Hersch M, Cheung H, et al (1992) The effect of various sympathomimetics on the regional circulations in hyperdynamic sepsis. Surgery 112:549-561
45. Falk A, Redfors S, Myrvold H, et al (1985) Small intestinal mucosal lesions in feline septic shock: A study on the pathogenesis. Circ Shock 17:327-337
46. Fink MP, Antonsson JB, Wang H, et al (1991) Increased intestinal permeability in endotoxic pigs . Arch Surg 126:211-218
47. Fink MP, Kaups KL, Wang H, et al (1991) Maintenance of superior mesenteric arterial perfusion prevents increased intestinal mucosal permeablity in endotoxic pigs. Surgery 110:154-161
48. Shepherd AP, Riedel GL, Maxwell LC, et al (1984) Selective vasodilators redistribute intestinal blood flow and depress oxygen uptake. Am J Physiol 247:G377-G384
49. Cain SM, Curtis SE (1992) Systemic and regional oxygen uptake and lactate flux in endotoxic dogs resuscitated with dextran and dopexamine or dextran alone. Circ Shock 38:173-181
50. Fiddian-Green RG (1995) Gastric intramucosal pH, tissue oxygenation and acid-base balance. Br J Anaesth 74:591-606
51. Silverman HJ, Tuma P (1992) Gastric tonometry in patients with sepsis: Effects of dobutamine infusion and packed red blood cell transfusions. Chest 102:184-188
52. Marik PE, Sibbald WJ (1993) The effect of stored blood transfusion on oxygen delivery in patients with sepsis. JAMA 269:3024-3029
53. Smithies M, Yee TH, Jackson L, et al (1994) Protecting the gut and the liver in the critically ill: Effects of dopexamine. Crit Care Med 22:789-795
54. Gutierrez G, Clark C, Brown SD, et al (1994) Effect of dobutamine on oxygen consumption and gastric mucosal pH in septic patients. Am J Respir Crit Care Med 150:324-329
55. Nevière R, Chagnon JL, Mathieu D, et al (1995) Effects of dobutamine and dopamine on gastric mucosal blood flow in septic patients. Am J Respir Crit Care Med 151:A446 (Abst)
56. Levy B, Bollaert PE, Nace L, Charpentier C, Bauer PH, Larcan A (1995) Epinephrine or norepinephrine-dobutamine for dopamine resistant septic shock. Am J Respir Crit Care Med 151:A447 (Abst)
57. Radermacher P, Buhl R, Santak B, et al (1995) The effects of prostacyclin on gastric intramucosal pH in patients with septic shock. Intensive Care Med 21:414-421
58. Gutierrez G, Palizas F, Doglio G, et al (1992) Gastric intramucosal pH as a therapeutic index of tissue oxygenation in critically ill patients. Lancet 339:195-199

Monitoring Gut Perfusion

M. Mythen and J. Faehnrich

Introduction

In pursuit of an ideal clinical monitor of tissue perfusion, attention has focused on the gastrointestinal (GI) tract. Its inner-most mucosal layer has a countercurrent system of arterioles and venules that improves absorptive function but makes it susceptible to reduced oxygen delivery (DO_2) states. Splanchnic vasoconstriction is an early response to a reduction in global DO_2 as blood is diverted to organs such as heart and brain. Whether due to myocardial failure and/or hypovolemia, the reduction in splanchnic blood volume is disproportionately greater than that seen in other beds [1]. There is also considerable evidence to suggest that splanchnic hypoperfusion may be a significant factor in the pathogenesis of the multiple organ dysfunction syndrome (MODS) [2].

There are many methods available to aid the clinician in monitoring gut perfusion but few are of practical use in the critically ill. A number of techniques will be discussed but the majority of this chapter will concentrate on the GI tonometer because, although it remains controversial, it is the only monitor of gut perfusion that is both commercially available and widely used.

Clinical Monitoring, Imaging Techniques and Endoscopy

Clinical examinations such as auscultation and palpation of the abdomen or measurement of residual gastric volume are part of the daily routine in the ICU. They are specific indicators that are suggestive of established GI tract dysfunction but are poor monitors of gut perfusion. Impairment of gut function, decreased bowel motility, paralysis and bowel distention are late signs of gut hypoperfusion which at this point may already be irreversible.

Abdominal ultrasound is a quick non-invasive method that is used frequently in the ICU, mainly to rule out edema of the intestinal wall, fluid retention, abscess or necrosis. The image quality is patient- and operator-dependent, and if bowel changes are seen they often represent late symptoms of intestinal ischemia.

The radiologic methods (X-ray and CT) expose patients to radioactivity and usually require them being moved to the facilities, which presents a considerable risk for critically ill patients. The use of contrast to enhance the bowel image may cause renal dysfunction. Angiography is limited by the resolution capability of the method, imaging only macrovascular, but not microvascular abnormalities. These techniques have their uses but are limited to the diagnosis of the manifestations of gut hypoperfusion rather than true monitoring.

Endoscopic visualization of the gut mucosa is a relatively safe and reliable method frequently used in the ICU. Examination is limited to the upper and lower portions of the GI tract and hypoperfusion can only be detected once mucosal injury has occurred.

Absorption and Clearance Tests

There are established methods for the determination of gut mucosal permeability that have been used in both animal models and clinical studies [3]. These methods indirectly provide some assessment of the adequacy of gut perfusion as it is assumed that a hypoperfused gut will leak. In animal models, the plasma-to-lumen clearance of two markers, such as chromium 51-labelled EDTA and urea, has been sucessfully used and correlated with other indices of gut perfusion [3]. Aside from the issues that surround the clinical use of radioactive substances, the technique is not practical in humans. The differential absorbtion of non-metabolizable sugars (eg lactulose and mannitol) can be used in clinical studies to determine gut permeability. The use of two inert markers expressed as a ratio (eg lactose/mannitol) reduces the confounding effects of irrelevant variables such as intestinal motility, surface absorption, renal clearance and accuracy of urine collection. These techniques are viable for clinical studies of gut permeability but not for routine clinical use. They are also not strictly monitors of gut perfusion as they can only aid in the diagnosis of an established abnormality.

Assessing Gut Blood Flow and Oxygen Delivery

ICG Clearance

Hepatic flow is estimated by the velocity of decrease in plasma indocyanine green (ICG) concentration after an IV bolus [4]. Assuming that ICG is cleared completely by the liver, hepatic flow is equal to systemic clearance of the dye. However in man, ICG is not eliminated completely by the liver. In fact variations in ICG extraction of 15 to 75%, depending on liver function, are common, so that this method is not viable for clinical determination of hepatic flow.

Doppler Flowmetry

The Doppler principle has found wide clinical application in diagnosis of blood flow abnormalities [5]. Laser light or ultrasound that is scattered by erythrocytes undergoes a frequency shift according to the Doppler principle, which allows an estimate of blood flow. Several flow meters are in use, measuring the blood flow in mesenteric vessels, or directly in the gut serosa or mucosa. A Doppler probe can be intraoperatively placed either on the external wall of the gut or around a blood vessel. Both these methods require a surgical approach, which makes them unsuitable for use in the ICU.

For several years, Doppler probes that can be advanced through the biopsy channel of an endoscope and placed under vision on the intestinal wall have been used for measuring the gastric mucosal blood flow operating either with ultrasound or with laser [6]. They are prone to artefacts as the flow measurements are influenced by breathing movements, peristalsis of the gut, the quality of contact between the probe and the intestinal wall (optical coupling) and the applied pressure to the wall. When using laser Doppler, wall thickness (gastric 5–7 mm, bowel 2.0–2.5 mm) influences the signal quality also, a fact that has to be regarded when calibrating a system. The degree of blood oxygenation influences the Doppler signal to a minor extent. Angulation of the probe does not affect the flowmeter signal. A linear relationship between flow and signal was seen in flow rates < 50 mL/min/kg, higher flow rates are underestimated by laser flow Doppler [6]. The method detects circumscript local changes in blood flow and can be used intraoperatively and during endoscopy. Validation studies versus hydrogen gas clearance in humans or versus measurement of the venous outflow of the stomach in rats showed a good correlation of both methods, respectively [6].

Reflectance Spectrophotometry

Reflectance spectrophotometry provides an index of mucosal hemoglobin concentration and an index of oxygen saturation of hemoglobin based on spectral analysis of light reflected from the mucosal surface [7]. Changes in these indices reflect changes in the mucosal perfusion of the bowel. The measuring probe consists of two coaxial light guides, one for emitted and one for reflected light, that couple the mucosal surface to the spectrophotometer. The spectrum of the reflected light is measured against a standard white surface, which is memorized by a microcomputer. The spectrum analyzer records the difference in absorption between a standard reference (almost zero) and a tissue sample. To obtain reproducible results, the measuring probe must be perpendicular to the mucosa touching it gently, without exercising pressure on the wall. In a validation study by Leung and coworkers [7], the index of oxygen saturation correlated very well with hydrogen gas clearance during hypoperfusion, whereas the index of mucosal hemoglobin correlated but fairly. In hyperemia, the hemoglobin index increased, but no significant change in the index of oxygen saturation was observed. They concluded that ischemia is well represented only by changes in index of oxygen saturation.

Oxygen Electrodes

Use of a transcutaneous O_2 electrode to measure visceral O_2 tension during colon surgery has been described [8]. A transcutaneous O_2 electrode can be either screwed into a suction ring and fixed to the organ transserously by applying a vacuum, or fixed to a gastric tonometer and placed subserously, measuring the PO_2 of an air calibrated isotonic saline solution, which flushes the intestines. If used discontinuously, a good correlation to PaO_2 was found.

Microspheres

Regional organ perfusion can be estimated with hematogenously delivered radioactive, fluorescent or color labelled microspheres. When an appropriate size is used, regional blood flow is proportional to the number of microspheres trapped in the region of interest. Methods for quantification of regional blood flow depend on the label attached to the microsphere. Microspheres are injected in a central vein or in the left ventricle and simultaneously a reference blood sample is withdrawn. Blood flow is assessed by measuring the amount of radioactivity or of the dye concentration in tissue biopsies. This method has been used frequently in animal studies, the need for tissue biopsies makes it unsuitable for routine clinical use [9].

Hydrogen Gas Clearance

This method is based on the clearance of hydrogen gas from mucosal tissue [10]. 3% hydrogen in air is inhaled and the washout of hydrogen by local gastric blood flow is detected by a needle-type platinum electrode that is inserted in or placed in contact with the gastric mucosa. The current produced by the hydrogen flux at the electrode corresponds to the hydrogen concentration in the tissue. The theory of blood flow measurement by the hydrogen clearance method is based on the assumption that the decrease of tissue hydrogen concentration is due solely to the washout by blood flow. It is possible, however, that a part of the gas diffuses into the gastric lumen, thus decreasing the concentration. To allow for this, the hydrogen concentration in the stomach is also registered. This method must be used intermittently and the placement of an electrode makes it unsuitable for routine clinical use.

Portal Vein Catheterization

Catheterization of the portal vein is invasive and allows measurements of portal venous blood flow, oxygen saturation and lactate concentration [11]. The method is practical in humans and allows on-line assessment of total splanchnic perfusion but subtle regional changes in perfusion may not be detected. Some animal and human studies have demonstrated a poor correlation between portal venous measurements and the adequacy of gut perfusion, particularly in sepsis [12]. There are no human studies that correlate changes in portal vein measurements with outcome.

Gut Oximetry

The use of a commercially available sterile pulse oximeter probe for intraoperative assessment of bowel viability has been investigated. Intraoperatively, the probe was attached on the antimesenteric border of the intestine and the oxygen saturation readings were compared to simultaneously obtained oxygen saturation readings from the tongue and showed a good correlation. There was also a good correlation between the intestinal oxygen saturation during ischemia and histological changes obtained from tissue biopsies [13].

It has also been reported that a pulse oximeter can be attached to a foley catheter and advanced into the colon or stomach. Once the foley balloon was inflated, if the pulse oximeter was in contact with the mucosa, a continuous signal was obtained analogous to the recordings on finger. This method was validated by Gardner and coworkers [14] in a porcine model against flow in the caudal mesenterial artery in decreasing perfusion states and showed a good correlation. During hypoperfusion, the signal decreased, but a curve and an oxygen reading still could be obtained. The method seems to work in elective operations; in cases where the stomach or the colon cannot be prepped, the method may not be practicable.

Assessing Gut Perfusion and Metabolism

The majority of techniques described above are restricted to research use only. The techniques that have some potential for clinical usage, such as portal vein catheterization or direct pulse oximetry, have very little human outcome data to support them. The above techniques are also focused on blood flow to the gut and, as we now recognize, DO_2 is no guarantee of adequate oxygen utilization (VO_2). To gauge the adequacy of cellular oxygen utilization a metabolic marker can be used, such as the adenosine diphosphate/adenosine triphosphate (ADP/ATP) ratio, lactate or tissue pH. The only currently available clinical monitor that can provide such information, is practical for use in critically ill patients and is supported by a reasonable quantity of published human data is the GI tonometer.

Gastrointestinal Tonometry: A Brief History

As early as 1860, the measurement of CO_2 in the lumen of the GI tract was a controversial subject. The debate was centered around whether the mode of accumulation of gases in the intestinal lumen was active, as suggested by Schierbeck in 1892, or passive as suggested by Planer in 1860 and Edkins in 1922? [15]. In 1926, McIver [15] published an elegant set of feline experiments and concluded that "... the movement of this gas (CO_2) into and out of the stomach is not due to secretory factors but is governed by the physical laws of diffusion". He also noted that partial obstruction of the portal vein caused a marked rise in CO_2 in an intestinal loop but dismissed the potential value of this sign as he believed it involved "... too gross a disturbance of the circulation to afford a useful comparison with clinical conditions."

In 1964, Bergofsky [16] showed that the PCO_2 and PO_2 of tissues could be estimated by sampling saline that was instilled in the bladder until it reached equilibrium with the surrounding tissue (60 min for 25 mL of saline). He referred to the technique "hollow visceral tonometry". The following year, Dawson et al. [17] reported in *Nature* that the same principals could be applied to the small gut of both dog and man but with a much quicker equilibration time (5 min for 40 mL of saline). They suggested that the method might be used to examine "... the relevance of mucosal tissue oxygen tension to small bowel function". In 1973, Kivisaari and Niinikoski [18] refined the tonometric technique for the determination of the PO_2 and PCO_2 in subcutaneous tissues of the forearm by using a gas permeable, saline filled, silastic balloon.

The current level of interest in GI tonometry is primarily a result of the research and teaching efforts of Richard Fiddian-Green, a surgeon from the United States of America. In the early 80's, Fiddian-Green and co-workers [19] adopted the saline tonometric technique for assessing gut luminal PCO_2 and extended its use to the calculation of what they refered to as the GI intramucosal pH (pHi). This was done initially without the use of a silicone balloon catheter. They assumed that the arterial bicarbonate (determined by arterial blood gas analysis) is the same as intramucosal bicarbonate and calculated the pHi by inserting the arterial bicarbonate and intraluminal PCO_2 values into the Henderson-Hasselbalch equation. Subsequently, the sampling technique was modified to use a silicone balloon catheter from which small aliquots of unsoiled saline could be withdrawn and analyzed in a routine blood gas analyzer [20].

GI tonometers are now produced commercially (Tonometrics Division, Intrumentarium Corp., Helsinki, Finland) and licensed for use in the human stomach (incorporating a nasogastric sump tube) and sigmoid colon. The most recent development is a semi-automated gas based system (The Tonocap, Datex, Helsinki, Finland) that is undergoing laboratory and clinical evaluation (see below).

The Balloon/Saline GI Tonometer

The gastric and sigmoid tonometers essentially work the same way. For ease, the gastric tonometer will be discussed unless stated otherwise. The tonometer consists of a gas impermeable sampling tube with a gas permeable silicone balloon on one end and a three-way tap on the other end. If it is inserted into the lumen

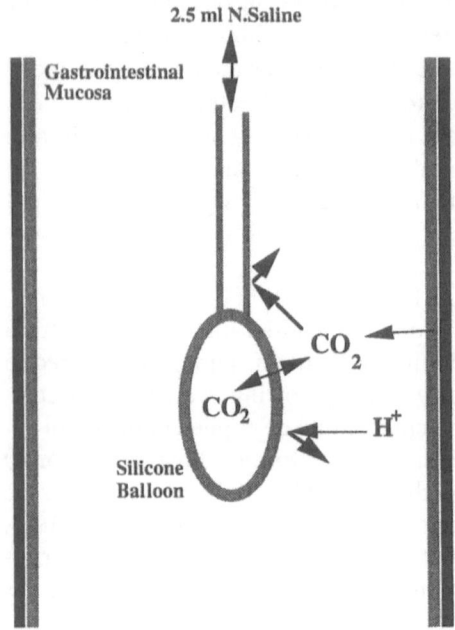

2.5 ml N.Saline

Gastrointestinal
Mucosa

CO_2

CO_2

H^+

Silicone
Balloon

Fig. 1. Diagrammatic representation of the gastrointestinal tonometer. Carbon dioxide is produced in the mucosal lining of the GI tract by both aerobic metabolism and the bicarbonate buffering of hydrogen ions produced during anaerobic metabolism

of the stomach, it allows the relatively non-invasive assessment of the carbon dioxide tension in the lumen of the stomach (Fig. 1). This is done by using a routine blood gas analyzer to measure the PCO_2 of a sample of saline aspirated from the tonometer balloon after time has been allowed for equilibration with the PCO_2 in the lumen of the gut. The pHi is calculated from a modified Henderson-Hasselbalch equation:

$$pHi = 6.1 + Log_{10}\left(\frac{arterial\ [HCO_3^-]}{PCO_2\,(tonometer) \times K}\right)$$

where K is a time-dependent equilibration constant provided by the manufacturer that corrects for the concentration gradient that exists across the tonometer membrane. It has been developed by the manufacturers *in vitro* using multiple readings over a wide range of equilibration periods and CO_2 tensions at 37°C (Boyle and Kent, Tonometrics Inc. – personal communication).

Full equilibration of luminal CO_2 with that in the balloon requires 90 min. Measurements can be made after as little as 10 min but the manufacturer recommend a minimum period of 30 min to reduce the errors associated with incomplete equilibration. With readings taken at 10 min after initial insertion of the tono-meter, there may be up to a 20% underestimation of the PCO_2 in the GI lumen. This is due to the first 1 mL of dead space saline in the tonometer tubing being non-carbonated whereas all subsequent dead space saline will contain CO_2 at the level of the immediate preceding sample. For first readings taken with an equilibration period of 15 min, the error is less than 5%, and for readings at 30 min less than 2% (Boyle and Kent, Tonometrics Inc. – personal communication).

The Tonometric Technique for Determining GI pHi

The tonometer is intended to be a monitor of tissue perfusion and relies on the assumption that reduced perfusion will result in anaerobic metabolism and in a fall in local pH. Increased lactic acid production is commonly thought to be the cause of tissue acidosis during hypoxia. If tissue hypoxia results in a local increase in hydrogen ions and these are buffered by bicarbonate, then additional CO_2 to that produced from aerobic metabolism will be generated. Carbon dioxide produced in the superficial layers of the mucosal surface of a viscus will rapidly equilibrate with the luminal contents. For the calculation of the pHi, it is assumed that the arterial bicarbonate (determined by arterial blood gas analysis) is the same as intramucosal bicarbonate. The pHi is calculated by inserting the arterial bicarbonate and intraluminal PCO_2 values into the Henderson-Hasselbalch equation. Using this technique, Fiddian-Green et al. [19] demonstrated a correlation between calculated pHi and pHi measured directly with a microprobe placed in the submucosa of the stomach, small bowel and colon of 16 dogs (114 paired readings, $r = 0.68$, $p < 0.001$).

Validation of the GI Tonometer

In animal models of septic and hemorrhagic shock, directly measured microprobe PCO_2 and tonometer measured PCO_2 in the GI tract have been shown to be the same [21, 22]. In anesthetized pigs in a steady state, Antonsson et al. [23] demonstrated that the indirect tonometric method of pH measurement was the same as that made with a microprobe placed in the interstitial layer of the gut mucosa. They also demonstrated a correlation between the two methods of gut mucosal pH measurement in pigs following the administration of endotoxin, partial vascular occlusion and total vascular occlusion [23]. In anesthetized dogs, Grum et al. [24] showed a linear relationship between splanchnic VO_2 and pHi whether DO_2 was reduced by limiting the flow of blood or oxygen content . Similarly, they showed that pHi was maintained until splanchnic DO_2 was equal to VO_2 when it fell precipitously [24]. Again in animal models, a persistently low pHi induced by vascular occlusion, endotoxemia or fecal peritonitis was associated with histological features of ischemia [25]. The direct infusion of oxygenated saline into the lumen of a section of hypoperfused gut corrected a low pHi and prevented histological damage [25]. In a study of patients undergoing cardiac surgery, Landow et al. [11] found that the gastric pHi was correlated with lactate concentration, pH and O_2 saturation measured directly from the hepatic vein. It seems therefore that a low calculated pHi is highly suggestive of inadequate gut mucosal and possibly splanchnic perfusion. However, a low pHi is not necessarily an absolute indicator of gut mucosal hypoxia.

Flaws in the Measurement of Luminal PCO_2 as an Indicator of GI Perfusion

A change in gut mucosal perfusion is not the only reason for a change in gut luminal PCO_2. The reflux of bicarbonate into acid in the stomach, for example, may liberate CO_2 independent of the gut mucosal redox state. Heard et al. [26] studied the effects of the administration of an H_2-blocker on pHi in healthy volunteers. They found that the administration of two oral doses of ranitidine 150 mg reduced the range of pHi measurements and increased reproducibility. They concluded that the H_2-blocker suppressed gastric acid production and thus CO_2 generation from refluxed duodenal bicarbonate. Kolkman et al. [27] confirmed and extended these findings. They studied the effects of an intravenous dose of 100 mg of ranitidine on gastric luminal PCO_2 and pH in 10 healthy volunteers before and after the oral ingestion of 100 mg of bicarbonate. Before receiving ranitidine, the volunteers had an elevated luminal PCO_2 in relation to arterial blood. The ingestion of bicarbonate produced a surge in gastric PCO_2 and fall in calculated pHi to levels that would suggest marked hypoperfusion. The ranitidine elevated gastric juice pH stabilized the basal readings such that gastric PCO_2 was identical to arterial and prevented any change occurring with a second dose of oral bicarbonate. The fact that their analyses of gastric juice pH data showed no correlation between alkaline shifts and gastric PCO_2 changes led them to conclude that a higher gastric luminal PCO_2 during normal versus suppressed acid secretion was due to buffering of gastric acid by gastric (rather than duodenal) bicarbonate.

The generation of GI luminal CO_2 from the mixing of bicarbonate with acid is probably less of a problem in critically ill patients as many have GI tract dysfunction resulting in a failure to produce gastric acid. In a study of 20 critically ill patients [28], we found that 13 had a gastric juice pH greater than 4 without preexisting H_2 blockade. Of the 13 patients with a gastric juice pH > 4, 6 had a calculated pH > 7.32 suggesting normal mucosal perfusion; all of these patients had a rapid decrease in their gastric juice pH in response to pentagastrin. Interestingly, this had no significant effect on the calculated pHi.

Pending the results of further investigations, it seems advisable to administer patients 100 mg of ranitidine intravenously at 8 hourly intervals and to check the gastric juice pH before trying to interpret the results from gastric tonometry.

Enteral feeding may also result in generation of GI luminal PCO_2 without modifying perfusion or interfere with diffusion of CO_2 into the tonometer balloon. These effects have not been formerly elucidated. However, we have examined the effects of the ingestion of a standard enteral feed formula on gastric pHi in 6 healthy volunteers who had taken 150 mg of ranitidine orally 1 h earlier. All subjects demonstrated a rise in luminal PCO_2 and thus a reduction in pHi to pathological values (Jacobsen et al. – unpublished observation). We assumed that, as they were healthy volunteers, these changes were unlikely to be indicative of gut mucosal hypoperfusion. The manufacturers recommend that enteral feed be stopped for 60 min prior to making a tonometer reading.

Gut luminal PCO_2 rises and falls in a linear fashion with arterial CO_2. Therefore, an abnormally high GI luminal PCO_2 and low calculated pHi in the face of a high $PaCO_2$ cannot be taken as evidence of gut mucosal hypoperfusion. Salzman et al. [29] have confirmed this finding in an animal model.

Flaws in the Measurement of Luminal PCO_2 as an Indicator of GI Hypoxia

Many publications have refered to the tonometer as an absolute indicator of tissue hypoxia. However, gut luminal PCO_2 may rise as a result of normal oxidative phosphorylation and impaired removal of CO_2. Consider, for example, where the flow is reduced to the gut mucosa but delivered O_2 exceeds a fixed requirement (Fig. 2). Venous O_2 saturation will fall (i.e. O_2 extraction ratio increases) and venous and tissue CO_2 will rise proportionally (the ratio dependent on the respiratory quotient). Only once O_2 supply falls below demand will anaerobic metabolism result in release of metabolic acid (such as lactate) and the liberation of CO_2 from bicarbonate. This sudden rise in tissue CO_2 will be disproportionate to the reduction in venous O_2 saturation (Fig. 2). The degree to which mucosal PCO_2 can be accounted for by aerobic or anaerobic metabolism has been determined by Schlichtig et al. [30] in a canine model of cardiac tamponade. They conclude from their measurements that GI tonometry can be a valid measure of tissue dysoxia, but calculated that the maximum human aerobic generation of CO_2 can exceed 70 mmHg (at an RQ of 1.0 and plasma pH of 7.26). Therefore, a high tonometer PCO_2 in relation to arterial blood should only be regarded as an index of tissue hypoperfusion and not as an absolute indicator of tissue hypoxia.

Flaws in the GI Tonometric Technique for the Determination of pHi

During periods of gut mucosal hypoxia, the assumption that arterial bicarbonate is the same as intramucosal bicarbonate or even that in local flowing capillary blood is flawed. The basic premise for the tonometric measurement depends on changes in gut luminal PCO_2 secondary to local bicarbonate buffering of H^+. If this is the case, then intramucosal bicarbonate concentration should be lower than arterial bicarbonate concentration and the pHi calculation should underestimate the magnitude of intramucosal acidosis. This hypothesis is borne out by the validation experiments of Antonsson et al. mentioned above [23]. When a mucosal acidosis was induced in pigs by total vascular occlusion, the tonometer

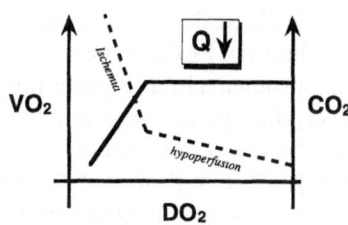

Fig. 2. If oxygen delivery (DO_2) is decreased to a tissue bed by decreasing blood flow (Q), then while DO_2 (shown with the *solid line*) exceeds consumption (VO_2), the rise in CO_2 (the *broken line*) is due to decreased removal of aerobically produced CO_2 (marked as *hypoperfusion*). Once VO_2 becomes flow dependent, anaerobic metabolism ensues and CO_2 is liberated more rapidly from the bicarbonate buffering of hydrogen ions (marked as *ischemia*)

pHi calculation underestimated the degree of acidosis measured directly with a microprobe. Desai et al. [21] have made direct measurements of GI PCO_2 and pH using microelectrodes placed into the ileal mucosa of rats. They calculated that the mucosal bicarbonate was actually higher than the arterial bicarbonate in normal but not hypotensive rats. However, the results are difficult to interpret as no indication is given in the methodology as to the calibration of the four different sets of electrodes (two pH and two PCO_2) used to calculate the different bicarbonate concentrations cited. In the same experiments, in spite of the proposed bicarbonate discrepancies, the directly measured pHi compared favorably with the calculated pHi using the Fiddian-Green technique.

Any change in the arterial bicarbonate concentration will modify the calculated pHi. For example, a low pHi in a patient with a metabolic acidosis due to renal failure does not necessarily imply gut mucosal hypoxia. Similarly, a normal pHi in a patient who has a metabolic alkalosis does not necessarily imply tissue normoxia. The administration of bicarbonate will raise arterial bicarbonate concentration and therefore can correct the calculated pHi despite the presence of mucosal ischemia. This was demonstrated by Benjamin et al. [31] who showed that the administration of bicarbonate to hypovolemic pigs apparently corrects the calculated gastric pHi. Closer scrutiny of the data shows that the administration of bicarbonate produces a metabolic alkalosis and a sharp increase in tonometer PCO_2 compared to arterial PCO_2. Therefore, the magnitude of the gap between the arterial pH and pHi remained abnormal until the hypovolemia was corrected.

In a study of 20 critically ill patients, Boyd et al. [32] demonstrated a close correlation between pHi and base deficit [28]. They found that a blood gas analyzer calculated base deficit of 4.65, predicted a gastric pHi < 7.32 with a specificity $> 95\%$. As stated above, patients with a low bicarbonate must have a low calculated pHi unless the gut lumenal PCO_2 is lower than arterial PCO_2, which is unlikely. Also base deficit and pHi must correlate as the same bicarbonate concentration is common to both calculations. However, as also demonstrated in the study of Boyd et al., not all patients with a low pHi have metabolic acidosis.

pHi, pH Gap or CO_2 Gap?

In order to solve many of the problems cited above, the difference between the arterial pH and the pHi or the arterial PCO_2 and tonometer PCO_2 have been proposed as more useful indices of gut mucosal perfusion. The pHi to arterial pH gap is illogical as pH is a logarithmic scale. The CO_2 gap is the most logical as the gut luminal PCO_2 is the true measure, and normalizing it to arterial CO_2 solves any problems in interpretation caused by respiratory acidosis or alkalosis. However, the vast majority of data available from clinical studies to date is reported as pHi, and it is difficult to retrospectively determine the CO_2 gaps. It may be that the predictive power of tonometry would be reduced if the studies were re-analyzed. One of the reasons for this being that calculating pHi combines a global index of tissue hypoperfusion (the arterial bicarbonate) with a regional one (the gut luminal PCO_2). Therefore, the calculated pHi may be abnormal when the components are both only mildly deranged. The pHi has been shown to be a very sensitive predictor of a poor outcome, the CO_2 gap will probably prove to be a more specific indicator of on-going, isolated, GI mucosal hypoperfusion.

The Measurement of PCO₂ in Saline

The balloon/saline tonometric technique relies on the measurement of PCO_2 in saline using routine blood gas analyzers. This presents two significant problems 1) saline contains no buffering system so CO_2 is very readily lost from solution; and 2) there may be considerable bias and imprecison when a routine blood gas analyzer is used for the determination of PCO_2 in saline samples.

The first problem makes the drawing and subsequent handling of saline samples of great importance. The same rules apply to the handling of blood gas samples (eg eliminate air, cap samples, keep on ice, don't delay) but the lack of stability of CO_2 in unbuffered saline greatly exaggerates the errors particularly at higher gas tensions. For example, if during the sampling process the three way tap on the end of the tonometer is opened to air while there is still negative pressure being generated in the syringe, some 25% of the CO_2 can be lost (JB Salmon – unpublished observations). Similarly, an uncaped sample at room temperature will de-gas rapidly whereas a caped sample on ice is stable for at least 20 min. Using the balloon/saline tonometric technique, there are at least five procedural steps where errors can occur. One study from Australia found a greater than 30% error in tonometric specimen collection/procedure despite a training process and awareness of being studied [33]. This could in part explain why tonometry enthusiasts, collecting their own data or using trained dedicated research staff, have published consistently encouraging results; yet some people report disappointing results from general clinical use.

Routine blood gas analyzers are calibrated for the determination of PCO_2 of blood, and for most machines there is a systematic error in the determination of PCO_2 in saline [34]. Most analyzers have no problem measuring saline samples *per se* but will often flash up an error warning as the pH is well outside the physiological range. For most commonly used analyzers, the manufacturers claim that the bias is small and comparable and the precision good (eg the Corning 178 and the Radiometer ABL 300). However, for other blood gas analyzers such as the Nova Stat Profile 7, the bias can be very large. Two studies have examined the measurement error of saline PCO_2 in blood gas analyzers using thin film tonometered saline as the reference [34, 35]. Both report a greater than 50% bias for the NOVA, and a greater than anticipated bias (up to 20%) for analyzers thought to be more suitable for the determination of CO_2 in saline such as the Radiometer ABL 300. The use of buffered solutions improved the reported bias. Most of the analyzers tested had good precision, and Takala et al. [34] concluded that a difference in calculated pHi of 0.06 pH units can be reliably detected by most analyzers in a clinically relevant PCO_2 range. One criticism of these papers is that they both assume that their gold standard (thin film tonometry) and sampling techniques are without error.

The systematic error does cast doubt on the validity of comparing absolute saline PCO_2 values or calculated pHi between centers, unless some form of bias correction has been used (see below). Tonometrics (Tonometrics Division, Instrumentarium Corp., Helsinki, Finland) can provide Tri-level Tonometered Saline for quality control and information about phosphate buffers that improve the bias and stability of PCO_2 measurement particularly for the NOVA blood gas machines.

Normal Range for Gastric pHi or Arterial-to-Mucosal CO$_2$ Gradient

In a group of 47 volunteers with known cardiac disease, Fiddian-Green et al. [20] found the group mean of triplicate recordings of gastric pHi to be 7.38 with a standard deviation of 0.03. Fiddian-Green's first peri-operative study took a gastric pHi of less than 7.32 as evidence of intramucosal acidosis, i.e. two standard deviations below the mean of the group reported above. However, most studies on ICU patients have used 7.35 as the lower limit of normality [36, 37]. No reasonable explanation is offered for these inconsistencies. As pointed out above, the bias in the measurement of CO_2 in saline probably invalidates comparison of absolute values between centers. However, the use of these previously reported values (7.32 or 7.35) have proven to be remarkably sensitive predictors of outcome. The current trend toward using the gap between GI tonometer saline PCO_2 and arterial CO_2 presents us with the question of what is a normal CO_2 gap. At least with pHi, we have some human outcome data to refer to. Available animal and human data suggest that under "normal" conditions there should be no gradient between arterial and mucosal CO_2. Therefore, accepting our measurement errors, a gradient of 8 mmHg would be abnormal (that allows for a 20% error on a blood gas analyzer assuming an arterial PCO_2 of 40 mmHg) [34]. This would give a lower limit of normal for the calculated pHi of 7.32 if the arterial bicarbonate was normal (24 mmol/L). According to the data presented in Schlichtig's study cited above, an arterial-to-mucosal CO_2 gradient of 25 to 35 mmHg can exist from aerobic metabolism and impaired blood flow alone [30]. This would mean that the calculated pHi would need to be below 7.19 to 7.13 before we could suggest that the gut mucosa was hypoxic (assuming a normal arterial CO_2 and bicarbonate). Therefore, pending further clarification in humans, it seems reasonable to suggest that an arterial-to-mucosal PCO_2 gradient > 8 mmHg is suggestive of gut mucosal hypoperfusion, but not necessarily ischemia or hypoxia.

Balloonless Saline and Air Tonometry

As mentioned above, the introduction of the silicone balloon was a fairly late development in the history of GI tonometry. The original saline techniques rely on sampling liquids that had been instilled into hollow viscera such as the bladder and gut [17]. The move to a balloon technique was primarily to prevent the soiling of blood gas analyzers. At least two fairly recent publications in humans have successfully used this technique, and a significant advantage is reported to be the rapid equilibration time [38, 39]. It is perfectly feasable just to sample gastric juice from an indwelling nasogastric tube and measure it in a blood gas analyzer, although we have found it to be logistically difficult particularly when trying to get the analyses carried out by a routine clinical laboratory. Mitch Fink's group have recently reported success with balloonless air tonometry in an animal model (the methodology is very similar to that reported by McIver in 1926 – see above) [14, 29]. By lavaging the lumen of the GI tract with 20–200 mL of air and then measuring the PCO_2 of the aspirated gas sample in a routine blood gas analyzer, they obtained results that correlated extremely well with standard saline tonometry. Like balloonless saline tonometry, air tonometry has the potential advantage of avoiding the expense of a specially designed catheter. However, its practical application in humans has yet to be reported and certainly in our institution, the laboratory charge for blood gas analyses is the major expense in performing any kind of blood gas analyzer-dependent tonometry.

Clinical Experiences with GI Tonometry

Despite all of the problems with GI tonometry discussed above, the technique has an impressive clinical research record. In all published studies of patients admitted to adult ICU, an abnormally low pHi has been found to be common and associated with a poor outcome [36]. In a prospective, randomized, multicenter trial of pHi-guided therapy, a $> 25\%$ improvement in survival was reported in patients admitted to the ICU with a normal pHi [36]. However, the same study failed to demonstrate any beneficial effects of pHi-guided therapy in the group of patients who had established splanchnic hypoperfusion on admission. This suggests that, if patients are to gain from the benefits of pHi measurement, it must be employed before GI ischemia is established. This may be an unreasonable aim for many patients admitted to the ICU, but not for those who have suffered accidental trauma or undergone elective major surgery. To date, all published studies that have examined the relationship between pHi and outcome following accidental trauma or major surgery have concluded that the presence of a low pHi is a predictor of a poor outcome [2]. In the studies that compared tonometry to other routinely used monitors of cardiorespiratory function, it was found to be a more sensitive predictor of morbidity than global measures such as blood pressure, cardiac output or urine flow measurement. Ivatury et al. [40] compared pHi and global O_2 variables (DO_2 and VO_2) as therapeutic indices in a prospective, randomized trial of patients in the first 24 h following major trauma. They found the mortality in the pHi group to be significantly lower (9.1 vs 31.3%). We have [41] recently reported the results of a prospective, randomized trial of the effects of fluid loading patients undergoing elective cardiac surgery with the aim of maintaining peri-operative gastric mucosal perfusion. We found that the incidence of a low pHi was significantly reduced in the protocol group when compared to controls as were the number of major complications and days spent in hospital. However in this study, pHi was used as an outcome variable and not a therapeutic goal.

Automated On-line Tonometry

One of the problems in using gastric tonometry clinically has been the slow response time with the balloon saline technique. This has made using it as a therapeutic index near impossible in settings such as major surgery where cardiorespiratory variables may change rapidly. The Tonocap (Datex, Helsinki, Finland) is a new device which can be used with the established Tonometric's catheters (Tonometrics Division, Instrumentarium Corp., Helsinki, Finland). The Tonocap fills the tonometer's balloon with air rather than saline. Following an equilibration period of 15 min, the gas is automatically sampled, measured with an infra-red sensor and the PCO_2 and calculated pHi are displayed. The air is then re-injected in an attempt to avoid CO_2 depletion.

The Tonocap is currently undergoing laboratory and human investigation. The first generation prototype revealed a new potential error in any form of GI tonometry. In hypoperfused states, although the level of CO_2 in the gut lumen is high, the production rate is limited and thus rapid repeated sampling of gut luminal contents seemed to deplete the CO_2 level. As mentioned above, the latest Tonocap re-injects the sampled air and this seems to have resolved the problem of depletion. Our own *in vitro* and *in vivo* experiments have so far been very encouraging. We have found that the Tonocap allows the reliable measurement of gut luminal PCO_2 and seems to be a far more stable technique than saline tonometry (Fig. 3) [42, 43].

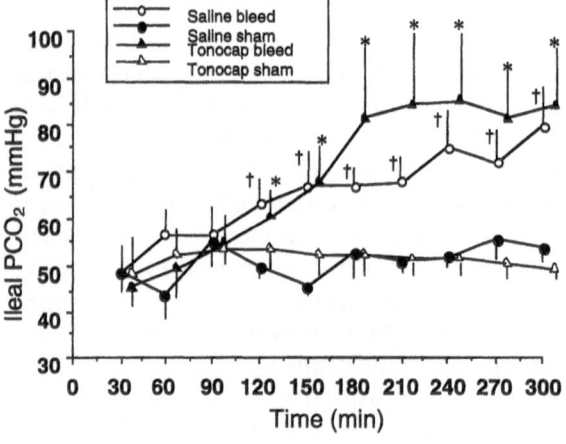

Fig. 3. Comparison of ileal PCO_2 measurements using the saline tonometer and the automated on-line tonometer (the Tonocap) in a canine sham controlled hemorrhage model. The bleed animals (n = 4) were hemorrhaged 30% of calculated blood volume at time 90 min. * $p < 0.05$ Tonocap PCO_2 compared to baseline and Tonocap sham, † saline PCO_2 compared to baseline and saline sham (ANOVA). (From [42] with permission)

Conclusion

The monitoring of gut perfusion is of established clinical interest. Despite all its faults, gastrointestinal tonometry is the most viable and widely used clinical monitor of gut perfusion. The research data published to date suggests that using the adequacy of gut perfusion as a therapeutic index may rationalize the treatment of critically ill patients and improve outcome. The appearence of a new automated on-line tonometer (Tonocap) is exciting and should accelerate the widespread assessment of the value of monitoring gut perfusion in the routine clinical setting. Hopefully, we can look forward to further developments in this field of monitoring because, although great progress has been made, there is plenty of room for improvement.

References

1. Lundgren O (1989) Physiology of the intestinal circulation. In: Marston A, Bulkley GB, Fiddian-Green RG, Haglund UH (eds) Splanchnic ischemia and multiple organ failure. Edward Arnold, London, pp 29–40
2. Mythen MG, Webb AR (1994) The role of gut mucosal hypoperfusion in the pathogenesis of post-operative organ dysfunction. Intensive Care Med 20:203–209
3. Fink MP (1991) Gastrointestinal mucosal injury in experimental models of shock, trauma, and sepsis. Crit Care Med 19:627–641
4. Uusaro A, Ruokonen E, Takala J (1995) Estimation of splanchnic blood flow by the Fick principle in man and problems in the use of indocyanine green. Cardiovasc Res 30:106–112
5. Nilson GE, Tenland T, Oberg PA (1980) Evaluation of laser Doppler flowmeter for measurement of tissue blood flow. IEE Trans Biomed Eng 27:597–604
6. Ahn H, Ivarsson LE, Johansson K, et al (1988) Assessment of gastric blood flow with laser Doppler flowmetry. Scand J Gastroenterol 23:1203–1210
7. Leung FW, Morishita T, Livingston EH (1987) Reflectance spectrophotometry for the assessment of gastroduodenal mucosal perfusion. Am J Physiol 252:G797–G804
8. Larsen PN, Moesgaard F, Naver L, et al (1991) Gastric and colonic oxygen tension measured with a vacuum-fixed oxygen electrode. Scand J Gastroenterol 26:409–418
9. Glenny RW, Bernard S, Brinkley M (1993) Validation of fluorescent labelled microspheres for measurement of regional organ perfusion. J Appl Physiol 74:2585–2597
10. Murakami M, Moriga M, Miyake T, et al (1982) Contact electrode method in hydrogen gas clearance technique: A new method for determination of regional gastric mucosal blood flow in animals and humans. Gastroenterology 82:457–467
11. Landow L, Phillips DA, Heard SO, Prevost D, Vandersalm TJ, Fink MP (1991) Gastric tonometry and venous oximetry in cardiac surgery patients. Crit Care Med 19:1226–1233
12. Rasmussen I, Haglund U (1992) Early ischemia in experimental fecal peritonitis. Circ Shock 38:22–28
13. De Nobile J, Guzzetta P, Patterson K (1990) Pulse oximetry as a means of assessing bowel viability. J Surg Res 48:21–23
14. Gardner GP, LaMorte WW, Obi-Tabot ET, et al (1994) Transanal intracolonic pulse oximetry as a means of monitoring the adequacy of colonic perfusion. J Surg Res 57:537–540
15. McIver MA, Redfield AC, Benedict EB (1926) Gaseous exchange between the blood and the lumen of the stomach and intestines. Am J Physiol 76:92–111
16. Bergofsky EH (1964) Determination of tissue O_2 tension by hollow visceral tonometers: Effect of breathing enriched O_2 mixtures. J Clin Invest 43:193–200
17. Dawson AM, Trenchard D, Guz A (1965) Small bowel tonometry: Assesment of small gut mucosal oxygen tension in dog and man. Nature (London) 206:943–944

18. Kivisaari J, Niinikoski J (1973) Use of silastic sampling tube and capillary sampling technic in the measurement of tissue PO_2 and PCO_2. Am J Surg 125:623–627
19. Fiddian-Green RG, Pittenger G, Whitehouse WM (1982) Back diffusion of CO_2 and its influence on the intramural pH in gastric mucosa. J Surg Res 33:39–48
20. Fiddian-Green RG, Baker S (1987) Predictive value of the stomach wall pH for complications after cardiac operations: Comparison with other monitoring. Crit Care Med 15: 153–156
21. Desai V, Weil MH, Tang W, Yang G, Bisera J (1993) Gastric intramural PCO_2 during peritonitis and shock. Chest 104:1254–1258
22. Nok M, Weil MH, Sun S, Gazmuri RJ, Tang W, Pakula JL (1993) Comparison of gastric wall PCO_2 during hemorrhagic shock. Circ Shock 40:194–199
23. Antonsson JB, Boyle CC, Kruithoff KL, et al (1990) Validity of tonometric measures of gut intramural pH during endotoxemia and mesenteric occlusion in pigs. Am J Physiol 259: G519–G523
24. Grum CM, Fiddian-Green RG, Pittenger GL, Grant BJB, Rothman D, Dantzker DR (1984) Adequacy of tissue oxygenation in intact dog intestine. J Appl Physiol 56:1065–1069
25. Fiddian-Green RG (1989) Studies in splanchnic ischemia and multiple organ failure. In: Marston A, Bulkely GB, Fiddian-Green RG, Haglund UH (eds) Splanchnic ischemia and multiple organ failure. Edward Arnold, London, pp 349–363
26. Heard SO, Helmsmoortel CM, Kent JC, Shahnarian A, Fink MP (1990) Gastric tonometry in healthy volunteers: Effect of ranitidine on calculated intramural pH. Crit Care Med 19: 271–274
27. Kolkman JJ, Groeneveld ABJ, Meuwissen SGM (1994) Effect of ranitidine on basal and bicarbonate enhanced intragastric PCO_2: A tonometric study. Gut 35:737–741
28. Higgins D, Mythen MG, Webb AR (1994) Low intramucosal pH is associated with failure to acidify the gastric lumen in response to pentagastrin. Intensive Care Med 20:105–108
29. Salzman AL, Strong KE, Wang H, Wollert PS, Vandermeer TJ, Fink MP (1994) Intraluminal "balloonless" air tonometry: A new method for determination of gastrointestinal mucosal carbon dioxide. Crit Care Med 22:126–134
30. Schlichtig R, Bowles SA (1994) Distinguishing between aerobic and anaerobic appearance of dissolved CO_2 in intestine during low flow. J Appl Physiol 76:2443–2451
31. Benjamin E, N-Fonayim JM, Hannon EM, et al (1992) Effects of systemic metabolic alkalosis on gastrointestinal tonometry. Crit Care Med 20 (Suppl):S65 (Abst)
32. Boyd O, Mackay CJ, Lamb G, Bland JM, Grounds RM, Bennett ED (1993) Comparison of clinical information gained from routine blood gas analysis and from gastric tonometry for intramural pH. Lancet 34:142–146
33. Crispin C, Jones W, Daffurn K (1995) How consistently do RNs perform the procedure of collecting specimens for measurement of gastric pHi and CO_2. Intensive Crit Care Nurs 11: 123–125
34. Takala J, Parviainen IMS, Ruokonen E, Hamalainen E (1994) Saline PCO_2 is an important source of error in the assessment of gastric intramucosal pH. Crit Care Med 22: 1877–1879
35. Riddington D, Venkatesh B, Clutton BT, Bion J (1994) Measuring carbon dioxide tension in saline and alternative solutions: Quantification of bias and precision in two blood gas analyzers. Crit Care Med 22:96–100
36. Doglio GR, Pusajo JF, Egurrola MA, et al (1991) Gastric mucosal pH as a prognostic index of mortality in critically ill patients. Crit Care Med 19:1037–1040
37. Maynard N, Biahari D, Beale R, et al (1993) Assessment of splanchnic oxygenation by gastric tonometry in patients with acute circulatory failure. JAMA 270:1203–1210
38. Gys T, Hubens A, Neels H, Ludo F, Lauwers F, Peeters R (1988) Prognostic value of gastric intramural pH in surgical intensive care patients. Crit Care Med 16:1222–1224
39. Mohsenifar Z, Goldbach P, Tashkin DP (1983) Relationship between oxygen delivery and oxygen consumption in the adult respiratory distress syndrome. Chest 84:267–271
40. Ivatury RR, Simon RJ, Havriliak D, Garcia G, Greenbarg J, Stahl WM (1995) Gastric mucosal pH and oxygen delivery and oxygen consumption indices in the assessment of adequacy of resuscitation after trauma: A prospective, randomized study. J Trauma 39:128–136

41. Mythen MG, Webb AR (1995) Per-operative plasma volume expansion reduces the incidence of gut mucosal hypoperfusion during cardiac surgery. Arch Surg 130:423–429
42. Noone RB, Yen MHN, Leone BJ, Mythen MG (1996) *In vitro* validation of an automated gastrointestinal tonometer (the Tonocap). Intensive Care Med 22:S65 (Abst)
43. Noone RB, Yen MHN, Leone BJ, Mythen MG (1996) *In vivo* validation of an automated gastrointestinal tonometer (the Tonocap) in a canine haemorrhage model. Intensive Care Med 22:S66 (Abst)

Effects of Pharmacologic Agents on Splanchnic Blood Flow

J. Takala

Introduction

The splanchnic circulation interacts closely with the systemic hemodynamics and participates in the control of blood pressure and volume. Acute reduction of splanchnic blood flow (SBF) and volume in acute hypovolemia helps to defend the perfusion of the brain and the heart [1, 2]. Inadequate splanchnic tissue perfusion may contribute to the development of multiple organ failure (MOF) and increase the risk of death in critically ill patients [3, 4]. In intensive care patients, there is a complex and poorly understood interaction between the splanchnic tissue perfusion, metabolic demands of the tissues, and the inflammatory response.

The splanchnic region is both an important source as well as target of inflammatory mediators, which can have a major impact on systemic and regional tissue perfusion and vasoregulation [5–7]. Changes in systemic hemodynamics and increased regional metabolic demands may both result in inadequate blood flow and tissue perfusion. Tissue hypoxia with consequent direct hypoxic tissue injury, increased intestinal mucosal permeability, and translocation of gut microbes and toxins may all occur, but their clinical relevance is not clear. All these factors and ischemia and reperfusion of splanchnic tissues may contribute to the activation of inflammatory mediator networks, and thereby further modify the circulatory and metabolic responses locally, within the splanchnic region, and in the extrasplanchnic organs [5–7].

Use of vasoactive drugs is often necessary to support tissue perfusion in circulatory failure. Drugs and therapeutic interventions aimed at improving systemic hemodynamics may have variable effects on splanchnic perfusion. In addition, the apparent link between inadequate splanchnic perfusion and MOF has prompted search for specific therapeutic interventions to improve the splanchnic perfusion.

Experimental studies have demonstrated that a wide variety of pharmacological agents can markedly influence SBF and metabolism. Changes in total SBF, redistribution of blood flow within the splanchnic region and within specific organs, changes in oxygen extraction, and alterations in the metabolic demands of tissues may occur [8, 9].

The effects of vasoactive drugs on splanchnic circulation and metabolism have not been well documented in humans. The available data, though limited, clearly demonstrate that the regional hemodynamic effects of various vasoactive drugs in intensive care patients can neither be predicted from their pharmacological characteristics alone nor extrapolated from experimental models or human studies done in healthy subjects or stable patients [10-17]. Altered vasoregulation and metabolic demands, endothelial injury, and the activation of inflammatory mediator networks are all likely to interact and modify the regional blood flow responses to vasoactive drugs. Due to these interactions, the effects of vasoactive drugs on SBF, oxygen transport, and substrate metabolism should be evaluated in intensive care patients.

This chapter discusses briefly some physiological aspects of SBF that are relevant for interpretation of the effects of vasoactive drugs on splanchnic perfusion. The most relevant effects of pharmacological agents in experimental models are discussed as well, but the focus is on the relatively limited available human data on the effects of vasoactive agents on SBF.

Physiological Aspects of Splanchnic Blood Flow

The regulation of gut perfusion has been discussed in detail in the chapter by Cholley and Payen. The arterial supply to the splanchnic region is via the celiac trunk and the superior and inferior mesenteric arteries. The venous return via the portal vein represents the sum of all arterial SBF, except the hepatic arterial flow. The venous efflux from the liver through the hepatic veins represents the total hepatosplanchnic blood flow, i.e. the sum of the hepatic arterial and portal venous blood flow.

Hepatic arterial and portal venous blood flow interact closely. Due to this hydrodynamic interaction (also called the hepatic arterial buffer response), an alteration of flow through one of the vascular beds leads to an opposite change in the other vascular system. The interaction helps to preserve total liver blood flow relatively constant during acute isolated perturbations of either hepatic arterial or portal venous blood flow [8, 18].

The blood flow of the small intestinal villus allows countercurrent exchange of O_2 from the artery to the vein along their course within the villus [19]. This and a higher metabolic activity of the absorptive cells at the tip of the villus result in a descending gradient of tissue PO_2 from the base to the tip of the villus. The gradient is inversely related to the blood flow. The tower PO_2 at the tip makes the villus susceptible to tissue hypoxia, if blood flow decreases for any reason.

Direct measurement of SBF in humans is practically impossible without surgery due to anatomical reasons: the multivessel blood inflow and outflow, and the mixing of the portal venous and hepatic arterial blood within the liver. Hence, the basic splanchnic circulatory physiology relies largely on extrapolation from experimental studies. Total hepatosplanchnic blood flow can be estimated using the Fick principle and hepatic venous catheterization. This technique and its application both in normal subjects and in intensive care patients has been described in detail [20]. All quantitative SBF studies in intensive care patients have measured the total hepatosplanchnic blood flow by the Fick principle [10–14, 20–31]. Gastrointestinal tonometry cannot be used as a surrogate measure of hepatosplanchnic blood flow, since there is no consistent relationship between SBF and measurements obtained by gastric tonometry [12, 14, 30, 31]. Rather, the assessment of intramucosal pH (pHi) or PCO_2 should be regarded as a measure of the adequacy of local tissue perfusion or the perfusion of the gastric mucosa.

Splanchnic Oxygen Transport

The total hepatosplanchnic blood flow at rest is normally 20–30% of cardiac output. Portal flow contributes approximately 80% of the total flow through the liver and the hepatic artery the remaining 20%. The splanchnic oxygen consumption (VO_2) at rest is approximately 20–35% of the whole body VO_2. The hepatosplanchnic oxygen extraction fraction (O_2ER) tends to be slightly higher than the systemic O_2ER at rest [4, 8]. If the blood flow is reduced, the O_2ER increases. When the tissue metabolic demands increase, blood flow to the relevant organs tends to increase in proportion and the splanchnic O_2ER remains relatively constant. Increased extraction may precede increases in blood flow, if O_2ER is initially very low [8]. During progressive reduction of flow, signs of gut ischemia appear, when the gut O_2ER approaches 70% [32]. On the other hand, the hepatosplanchnic O_2ER may briefly reach 90% until signs of deteriorating liver function appear during exercise and simultaneous hypoxia of inspired gases in normal subjects [33].

Gut Blood Flow

The total blood flow to the gut wall is unevenly distributed between the mucosa, the submucosa, the muscularis and the serosa. The mucosa and the submucosa receive most of the flow, up to 90%. Changes in the total gut blood flow may influence the flow to the different layers to varying extent. Intestinal blood pressure/flow autoregulation is much weaker than the autoregulation of e.g. renal blood flow [8].

   Catecholamines are the most important circulating endogenous vasoactive substances that influence the gut blood flow. α-adrenoceptor stimulation results in vasoconstriction and β-adrenoceptor stimulation in vasodilation. The net effects of circulating catecholamines on gut blood flow depend on the concomitant changes in cardiac output [8, 14]. Vasopressin and angiotensin are both potent intestinal vasoconstrictors, though their physiological role in the control of gut blood flow is not certain. They contribute to the intestinal vasoconstriction in acute hypovolemia, and modulate the response to sympathetic nerve stimulation and norepinephrine [2, 8].

Hepatic Blood Flow

There are three principal determinants of hepatic blood flow. The vascular resistance across the intestine determines the mesenteric influx and thereby the portal venous flow. The hepatic arterial resistance determines the hepatic arterial flow. The intrahepatic portal venous resistance is less important, since the portal venous flow is mainly determined by the outflow from the intestine, i.e. the resistance across the intestine. Finally, the hepatic arterial buffer response tends to compensate for any change in one of the inflows to the liver by a reciprocal change in the other [4, 18]. Autoregulation has little importance in the regulation of hepatic arterial pressure/volume relationship; the relationship between the arterial pressure and the flow is approximately linear. The hepatic portal venous bed clearly lacks autoregulation and has a linear pressure/flow relationship [4, 18].

Nitric Oxide and Splanchnic Blood Flow

Nitric oxide (NO) helps to maintain basal vasodilation in the mesenteric vasculature and the hepatic artery but not in the portal vein [34]. Endotoxin abolishes both the hepatic arterial buffer response and autoregulation, independent on NO. Inhibition of both the constitutive and inducible NO synthase after endotoxin increased the resistance of both hepatic artery and portal vein [34]. Accordingly, NO seems to be important in preserving the blood flow across the splanchnic bed in experimental endotoxin shock. Non-selective NO inhibition in septic shock may improve blood pressure at the expense of splanchnic perfusion.

Splanchnic Blood Flow in Intensive Care Patients

Only very few studies with quantitative measurements of SBF in intensive care patients have been published [10-14, 20-31]. The determinants, clinical relevance, and the time course of SBF abnormalities in patients at risk of MOF have not been well established. The patterns of changes in SBF and metabolic demand in low flow states [11, 12, 14] and in severe inflammation, infections and septic shock are substantially different [10, 21-28].

In low flow states (eg cardiogenic shock) and hypovolemia (without injury or sepsis), SBF decreases without major changes in splanchnic metabolic demand (Figs. 1, 2) [11, 12, 14]. Vasoregulation is usually well preserved and an increased O_2ER compensates for the reduction of blood flow. The limits of compensation and the time of tolerance for splanchnic hypoperfusion have not been well defined. Brief episodes of exposure to very low hepatic venous saturation (or increased splanchnic O_2ER) can be well tolerated during and immediately after cardiac surgery without any serious consequences [11, 14]. It is reasonable to assume that a slow reduction in SBF is better tolerated than an acute reduction.

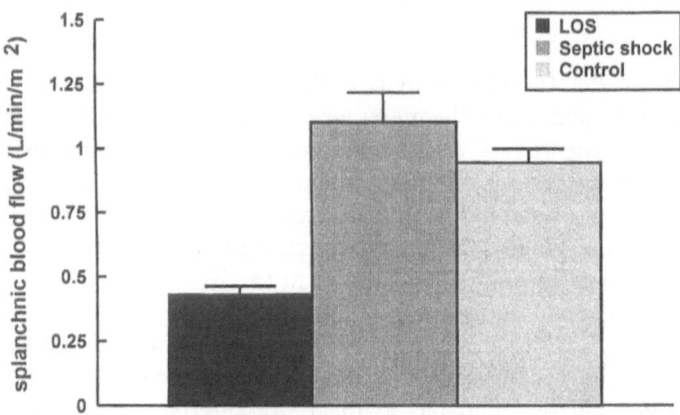

Fig. 1. Splanchnic blood flow in postoperative low cardiac output syndrome after cardiac surgery (LOS), in hyperdynamic septic shock treated with fluids and vasopressors, and in hemodynamically stable preoperative patients. (Data adapted from [3, 10, 14], J. Takala, unpublished)

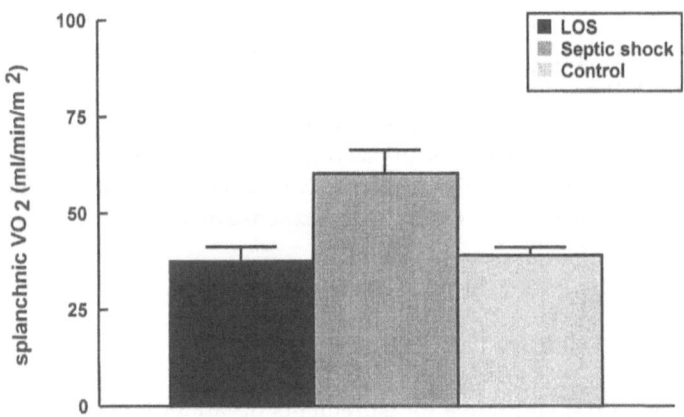

Fig. 2. Splanchnic oxygen consumption in postoperative low cardiac output syndrome after cardiac surgery (LOS), in hyperdynamic septic shock treated with fluids and vasopressors, and in hemodynamically stable preoperative patients. (Data adapted from [3, 10, 14], J. Takala, unpublished)

In severe inflammation (eg systemic inflammatory response syndrome (SIRS) septic infections, septic shock), the demand for O_2 in the splanchnic region is increased [10, 21–28]. The total splanchnic blood is increased as well, if the patient has adequate cardiovascular reserves to develop a hyperdynamic hemodynamic response (Figs. 1, 2). Despite the increased blood flow, the increase in VO_2 is even larger and the hepatosplanchnic O_2ER tends to be substantially increased.

Effect of Vasoactive Drugs on Splanchnic Blood Flow

Abnormal vascular tone, blood flow maldistribution, hypovolemia, and altered vasoregulation due to inflammatory mediators and endothelial injury is common in patients who need cardiovascular support with vasoactive drugs [3, 5, 7]. In addition, myocardial depression is relatively common in septic shock [35]. The blood volume has a major impact on SBF, and the volume status is likely to influence the response to vasoactive drugs [2, 36, 37].

Adrenergic Agents

The effects of adrenergic drugs on SBF in intensive care patients can neither be predicted from their pharmacological characteristics alone nor extrapolated from experimental models. The systemic hemodynamic response (both flow and pressure), volume status, adrenergic receptor downregulation, sympathetic nervous activity, and the metabolic demands in the splanchnic tissues may markedly modify the SBF response in individual patients and between patient groups [8–18].

Traditionally, the potential effects of adrenergic agents on regional perfusion have been interpreted in terms of their relative adrenergic receptor activity [4, 8, 18, 38]. α-adrenergic stimulation in general results in vasoconstriction in the splanchnic region. α-1 and α-2 receptors are both present in the splanchnic vasculature, and both participate in the vasoconstrictor response. β–adrenergic stimulation, especially β-2, results in splanchnic vasodilation. Dopaminergic receptors are present in the mesenteric and hepatic arterial vasculature. Their stimulation also produces vasodilation.

Experimental Studies: *Norepinephrine, epinephrine, α-adrenergic agonists.* α-adrenergic agonists, eg phenylephrine, metaraminol and methoxamine are intestinal vasoconstrictors in various experimental models [8, 9]. Norepinephrine acts as a vasoconstrictor under physiological conditions, but its α-adrenergic effects are markedly reduced in experimental endotoxin shock [8, 38, 39]. In volume-resuscitated endotoxin shock models, vasopressor doses of norepinephrine have no effect on the blood flow to the gut. In volume-resuscitated porcine endotoxin shock, restoration of blood pressure by norepinephrine, dopamine or phenylephrine have no effect on gut blood flow [39].

Epinephrine with its combined α- and β-receptor activity has variable effects on SBF [8, 9, 40]. Several studies have observed reduced intestinal blood flow in response to epinephrine, whereas others have observed increased blood flow. Most of the variability is probably related to the experimental models. In denervated preparations, a vasoconstrictor response is more likely due to the presence of vasodilatation before drug administration [8, 40]. In normally innervated models, the effects are dose-dependent: vasodilation at low doses shifts towards vasoconstriction at higher doses, where the α-mediated vasoconstrictor-response predominates.

Dobutamine, dopamine, dopexamine, β-adrenergic agonists. β-adrenergic agonists (eg isoproterenol) produce vasodilation in the splanchnic circulation
[8, 41]. Dobutamine has predominantly β-adrenergic effects (both β-1 and β-2),
although some α-adrenegic properties are also evident. Accordingly, dobutamine can be expected to induce vasodilation in the splanchnic vasculature,
although some authors suggest that the peripheral α- and β-2-agonist properties
of dobutamine may offset each other [42]. Resuscitation of experimental endotoxin shock with fluids and dobutamine is able to preserve mesenteric arterial
blood flow and prevent increase in gut mucosal permeability [43].

The effects of dopamine are dose-dependent and may be highly variable. At
low doses, the dopaminergic properties predominate and may result in splanchnic vasodilation and increased flow, whereas at higher doses, the α-agonist properties are more evident and result in splanchnic vasoconstriction [8, 40, 42, 44].
Dopexamine has both β-2 and dopaminergic properties. Both these characteristics favor splanchnic vasodilation, and dopexamine has been proposed as a tool
to improve the splanchnic tissue perfusion [45–47]. In a fluid-resuscitated fecal
peritonitis model, dopexamine resulted in reduced liver damage as compared to
dobutamine or fluids alone, despite similar SBF [46].

Adrenergic agents and SBF distribution. When isoproterenol or vasodilating
doses of epinephrine or dopamine are infused, gut mucosal blood flow distribution may change. In isolated, denervated intestinal loops, isoproterenol favors
gut mucosa at the expense of the muscularis [41]. Intra-arterial infusions of
vasodilating doses of epinephrine and dopamine in a normally innervated
canine model resulted in decreased gut mucosal blood flow despite an increase in
the total arterial inflow [40].

Human Studies in Healthy Subjects and Chronic Heart Failure: The effects of epinephrine and norepinephrine on hepatosplanchnic blood flow and metabolism in
healthy subjects were characterized already 45 years ago in the classic study by
Bearn et al. [13]. Epinephrine at pressor dose increased markedly, by roughly
100%, the hepatosplanchnic blood flow and VO_2 (Figs. 3, 4); concomitantly, the
hepatic glucose output increased by more than sixfold. Norepinephrine resulted
in slightly reduced hepatosplanchnic blood flow, although the reduction was
often transient. Pressor doses of norepinephrine increased splanchnic oxygen
VO_2 by 20–50% and the glucose output increased by 2–3-fold. Splanchnic O_2ER
remained relatively stable during epinephrine, whereas it increased during norepinephrine. Especially epinephrine increased the systemic blood lactate concentration.

The effects of dopamine on hepatosplanchnic blood flow in patients with
cardiac disease are somewhat controversial [17, 48, 49]. Dopamine increased
cardiac output but not the hepatosplanchnic blood flow in patients with chronic
congestive heart failure [49]. In patients without cardiac failure, cardiac output
and hepatosplanchnic blood flow increased in parallel; in addition, a tendency to
redistribution of blood flow to the hepatosplanchnic region was observed [48].
The different results despite similar increases in cardiac output may be explained

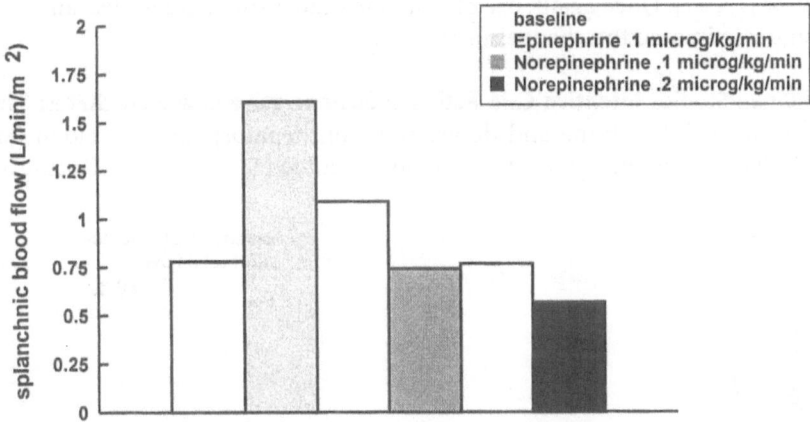

Fig. 3. Splanchnic blood flow in healthy subjects receiving epinephrine and norepinephrine. Separate group of subject was studied for each drug and dose. (Adapted from [13])

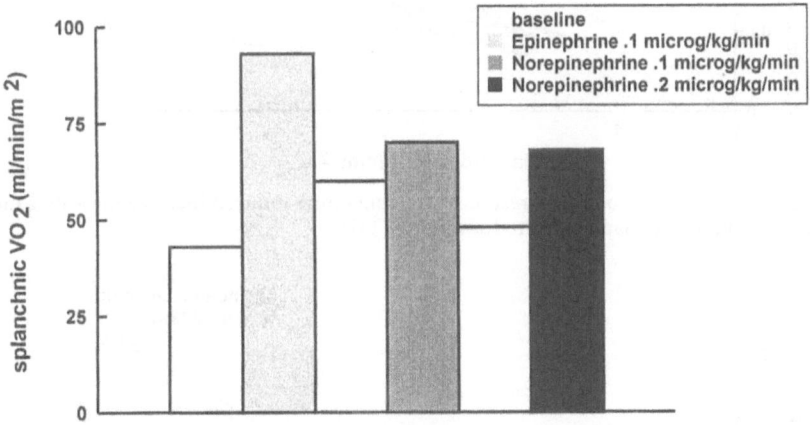

Fig. 4. Splanchnic oxygen consumption in healthy subjects receiving epinephrine and norepinephrine. Separate group of subject was studied for each drug and dose. (Adapted from [13])

at least in part by differences in methodology: the use of systemic indocyanine green clearance [49] underestimates the blood flow, if the hepatic dye extraction decreases concomitantly. The effects of adrenergic agents on the hepatic dye extraction are unpredictable: eg dobutamine may markedly decrease the dye extraction [20]. Other factors, such as splanchnic vasoconstriction due to activation of the renin-angiotensin system and the use of digitalis are likely to contribute as well.

Dobutamine had no consistent effect on the hepatosplanchnic blood flow in chronic heart failure despite substantial increase in cardiac output [17, 49], whereas dopexamine increased both cardiac output and hepatosplanchnic blood flow [17, 47]. Once again, use of systemic indocyanine green clearance may have underestimated the changes in SBF.

Human Studies Intensive Care Patients: Postoperative Low Flow States: The acute effects of dobutamine and dopexamine on hepatosplanchnic blood flow after cardiac surgery have recently been documented [11, 12, 14, 30]. During a 90-min

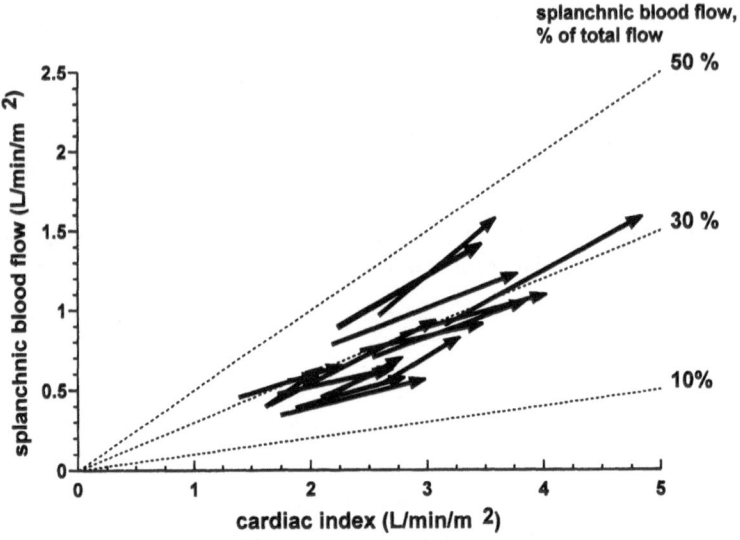

Fig. 5. Splanchnic blood flow response to dobutamine-induced increase in cardiac index after cardiac surgery. (Adapted and redrawn from [14])

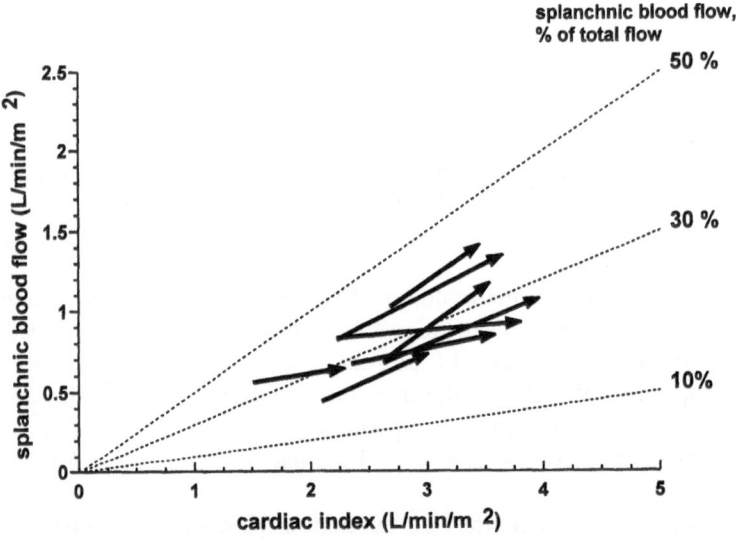

Fig. 6. Splanchnic blood flow response to dopexamine-induced increase in cardiac index after cardiac surgery. (Adapted and redrawn from [12])

infusion, both dobutamine and dopexamine induced parallel changes in cardiac output and hepatosplanchnic blood flow. The fraction of cardiac output that was distributed to the hepatosplanchnic region remained remarkably constant (Figs. 5, 6) [11, 12, 14, 30]. The response to these adrenergic agents was similar in patients with stable hemodynamics as compared to those with postoperative low cardiac output syndrome. Dobutamine in combination with sodium nitroprusside in severe low cardiac output syndrome had similar effects on regional blood

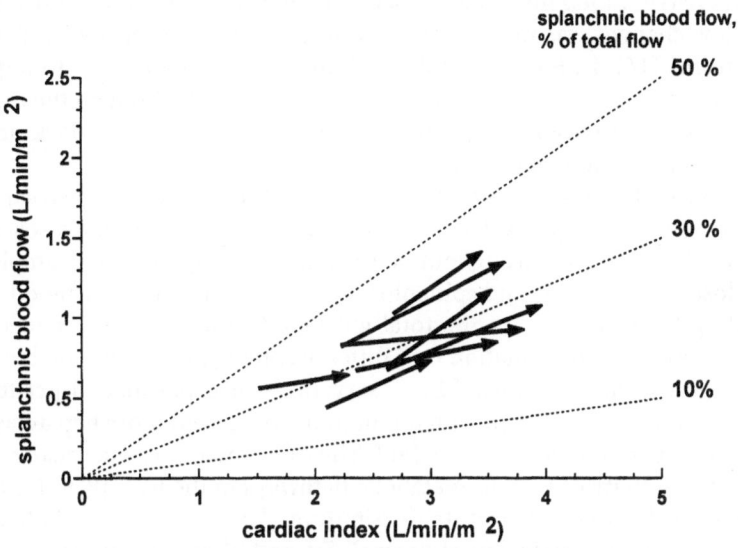

Fig. 7. Dissociation between gastric pHi and splanchnic blood flow following dobutamine-induced increase in cardiac output after cardiac surgery. (Redrawn from [14])

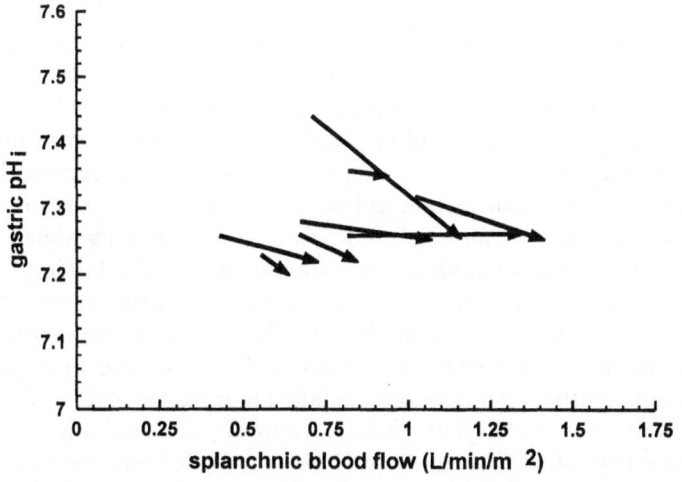

Fig. 8. Dissociation between gastric pHi and splanchnic blood flow following dopexamine-induced increase in cardiac output after cardiac surgery. (Redrawn from [12])

flow as dobutamine alone [11]. The effects of dopamine on regional blood flow after cardiac surgery resembled those of dobutamine: cardiac output and hepatosplanchnic blood flow both increased without evidence of redistribution (J. Takala, unpublished observations).

Simultaneous measurements of gastric pHi and hepatosplanchnic blood flow indicated a clear dissociation between changes in pHi and total SBF (Figs. 7, 8). Dopexamine induced a significant reduction of pHi despite marked increases in SBF [12]. Dobutamine also reduced pHi or failed to correct low pHi despite increased blood flow; the dissociation between pHi and hepatosplanchnic blood flow changes was more prominent in patients with the low cardiac output syndrome [14]. Failure of a prolonged infusion of dopexamine to improve low pHi after cardiac surgery has also been described [50], although the result is difficult to interpret because of problems of study design and the lack of systemic and regional hemodynamic data [50].

Several mechanisms may contribute to the decrease in gastric pHi despite increased total hepatosplanchnic blood flow. The effects of a vasoactive drug may not be uniform throughout the splanchnic region. For example, vasodilator doses of dopamine and epinephrine decreased the nutritive blood flow of the gut despite an increase in the total gut blood flow [40]. The effects of vasoactive drugs on microcirculation may differ despite similar effects on blood flow distribution in major vessels [9]. Observations in experimental peritonitis support this concept: treatment with dobutamine produced more hepatocellular damage as compared to dopexamine [46]. The catecholamines may also markedly modify the activity of various metabolic pathways in the liver [8, 9, 13, 17] and simultaneously alter SBF and its distribution. Accordingly, catecholamines may induce regional perfusion abnormalities and alter the balance between regional DO_2 and tissue metabolic demands.

Human studies in Intensive Care Patients: Sepsis and Septic Shock: Data on the effects of vasoactive drugs on SBF in clinical sepsis is very limited. Vasopressor doses of dopamine increased SBF in hyperdynamic septic shock, while norepinephrine had more variable effects (Fig. 9) [10].

Assessment of splanchnic tissue perfusion with tonometry has produced quite variable results. Improvement of gastric mucosal acidosis with norepinephrine and worsening with dopamine in septic shock has been observed, despite similar systemic hemodynamic responses [16]. In patients with sepsis and gastric mucosal acidosis, dobutamine improved pHi [15, 51]. Therapy aimed at improving pHi by volume resuscitation and dobutamine has resulted in improved outcome [52]. The effects of dobutamine on pHi or SBF in sepsis have not been prospectively evaluated in controlled trials. The effects of dopamine on pHi have also been variable. In one study, pHi increased in response to dopexamine [53], whereas in another trial dopamine failed to improve pHi [54].

Evidently, the underlying clinical condition, concomitant other therapeutic measures (eg volume management), the metabolic response to the disease and the drug, and alterations in vasoregulation all modify the individual responses to adrenergic agents. Since the regional blood flow changes cannot be predicted

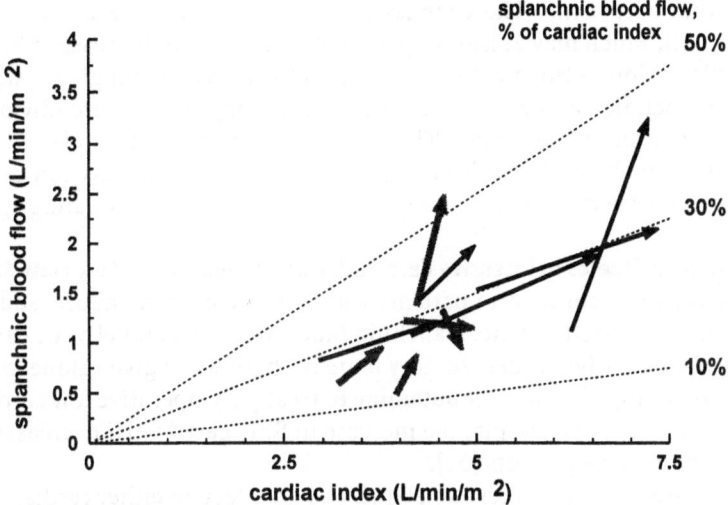

Fig. 9. Splanchnic blood flow response to correction of hypotension with vasopressor doses of dopamine and norepinephrine in hyperdynamic septic shock. Thick arrows dopamine, thin arrows norepinephrine. (Adapted and redrawn from [10])

from the pharmacological profile of the drug, the effects of these agents should be studied in more detail in those groups of patients they are used clinically.

Non-Adrenergic Vasodilators

Experimental Studies: The effects of vasodilators on SBF are controversial. As discussed earlier for vasodilating doses of epinephrine and dopamine, also adenosine may redistribute the blood flow away from the gut mucosa despite an overall increase in the intestinal blood flow [41]. Several studies have demonstrated that various direct vasodilators are able to increase SBF [8, 9, 18]. The overall effects in whole animal models are very likely to depend on the systemic hemodynamic responses and the blood volume management, although this has not been specifically addressed. Both sodium nitroprusside and nitroglycerin maintain the SBF in anesthetized animals during controlled hypotension, even if cardiac output is decreased [55, 56]. In conditions with increased activity of the renin-angiotensin axis, eg in hypovolemic and cardiogenic shock, inhibitors of the angiotensin converting enzyme (ACE) results in improved splanchnic tissue perfusion [57, 58].

Human Studies in Chronic Heart Failure: In patients with chronic congestive heart failure, nitrates and sodium nitroprusside had no effect on the hepatosplanchnic blood flow despite increased cardiac output, indicating blood flow redistribution [17, 59]. ACE inhibitors either had no effect or slightly reduced the hepatosplanchnic flow [17]. The lack of effect of all these vasodilators is somewhat surprising. The changes in cardiac output were in most cases relatively small, which may at least in part explain the lack of increase in hepatosplanchnic blood flow. Also, most of the patients were receiving digitalis, which is a known splanchnic vasoconstrictor. The vasodilatory effects were obviously more prominent in the periphery. These findings emphasize the role of the concomitant systemic hemodynamic changes and the interaction between different regional vascular beds in determining the SBF response to vasodilating agents.

Human Studies in Intensive Care Patients: Post-operative Low Flow States and Hypertension: In contrast to patients with chronic cardiac failure, sodium nitroprusside increased hepatosplanchnic blood flow in parallel with cardiac output in post-operative cardiac surgery patients, both when given alone to treat hypertension or together with dobutamine to treat post-operative low cardiac output syndrome [11, 31]. Despite the increase in SBF, gastric pHi decreased slightly in the hypertensive patients [31].

After cardiac surgery, enalapril had no effect on either cardiac output or hepatosplanchnic blood flow, but reduced the gastric pHi [29]. The lack of effect on SBF is particularly surprising, since the renin-angiotensin system is activated during cardiopulmonary bypass, and contributes to the reduction of hepatosplanchnic blood flow during bypass. This suggests that other factors contribute to the inadequate splanchnic perfusion after the operation. Post-operative transient endothelial damage could explain the lack of effect of the ACE-inhibitors.

The effects of sodium nitroprusside or ACE-inhibitors on hepatosplanchnic blood flow or gastric pHi have not been studied in other groups of intensive care patients. Nevertheless, the available data suggest that also the effects of these vasodilators are markedly modified by the underlying clinical condition. It seems likely that redistribution of blood flow may occur at the level of both macro- and microcirculation. This is supported by recent findings on the improvement of gastric mucosal acidosis in response to prostacyclin after conventional resuscitation with fluids and adrenergic agents had failed to correct the acidosis [60].

Metabolic Effects of Adrenergic Drugs

The effects of adrenergic agents on hepatosplanchnic blood flow should be considered together with their impact on metabolism. All adrenergic drugs have distinct metabolic effects, and tend to increase both systemic and hepatosplanchnic metabolic activity [61]. If improvement of tissue perfusion is attempted, the increase in metabolic demand may exceed the gain in perfusion. This will result in worsening of the perfusion/demand mismatch.

In sepsis, the hepatosplanchnic hypermetabolism [10, 21–28] increases the risk of inadequate tissue perfusion, and the effects of adrenergic agents on the metabolic demand or blood flow distribution may become critical. This may at least in part explain the controversial results that have been obtained with adrenergic agents in clinical sepsis.

Conclusion

The effects of vasoactive drugs on splanchnic circulation have not been well documented in humans. The regional hemodynamic effects of these drugs cannot be predicted from the pharmacological characteristics alone or extrapolated from experimental models or human studies done in healthy subjects or stabile patients. The underlined clinical condition of the patient is likely to remarkably modify both the effects of vasoactive drugs on tissue perfusion and their metabolic effects. These changes include a complex interaction between systemic, regional, and local tissue perfusion and metabolic demands. In order to optimize the treatment of the critically ill patient, better monitoring methods are necessary in order to evaluate the individual responses of regional tissue perfusion to vasoactive drugs.

References

1. Rowell LB, Detry JMR, Blackmon JR, Wyss C (1972) Importance of the splanchnic vascular bed in human blood pressure regulation. J Appl Physiol 32:213–220
2. Edouard AR, Degrémont AC, Duranteau J, Pussard E, Berdeaux A, Samii K (1994) Heterogenous regional vascular responses to simulated transient hypovolemia in man. Intensive Care Med 20:414–420
3. Carrico CJ, Meakins JL, Marshall JC, Fry D, Maier RV (1986) Multiple organ failure syndrome. Arch Surg 121:196–208
4. Bruns FJ, Fraley DS, Haigh J, et al (1987) Control of organ blood flow. In: Snyder JV, Pinsky MR (eds) Oxygen transport in the critically ill. Year Book Medical Publishers, Inc. Chicago, pp 87–124
5. Deitch EA (1992) Multiple organ failure. Pathophysiology and potential future therapy. Ann Surg 216:117–134
6. Matuschak GM (1994) Liver-lung interactions in critical illness. New Horizons 2:488–504
7. Matuschak GM (1995) Oxidative stress and oxygen-dependent cytokine production. In: Vincent JL (ed) Yearbook of intensive care medicine. Springer-Verlag, Germany, pp 413–421
8. Granger DN, Richardson PDI, Kvietys PR, Mortillaro NA (1980) Intestinal blood flow. Gastroenterology 78:837–863
9. Kvietys PR, Granger DN (1982) Vasoactive agents and splanchnic oxygen uptake. Am J Physiol 243:G1–G9
10. Ruokonen E, Takala J, Kari A, Saxén H, Mertsola J, Hansen EJ (1993) Regional blood flow and oxygen transport in septic shock. Crit Care Med 21:1296–1303
11. Ruokonen E, Takala J, Kari A (1993) Regional blood flow and oxygen transport in low cardiac output syndrome after cardiac surgery. Crit Care Med 21:1304–1311
12. Uusaro A, Ruokonen E, Takala J (1995) Gastric mucosal pH does not reflect change in splanchnic blood flow after cardiac surgery. Br J Anaesth 74:149–154
13. Bearn AG, Billing B, Sherlock S (1951) The effect of adrenaline and noradrenaline on hepatic blood flow and splanchnic carbohydrate metabolism in man. J Physiol 115:430–441
14. Parviainen I, Ruokonen E, Takala J (1995) Dobutamine-induced dissociation between changes in splanchnic blood flow and gastric intramucosal pH after cardiac surgery. Br J Anaesth 74:277–282
15. Gutierrez G, Clark C, Brown SD, Price K, Ortiz L, Nelson C (1994) Effect of dobutamine on oxygen consumption and gastric mucosal pH in septic patients. Am J Respir Crit Care Med 150:324–329
16. Marik PE, Mohedin M (1994) The contrasting effects of dopamine and norepinephrine on systemic and splanchnic oxygen utilization in hyperdynamic sepsis. JAMA 272:1354–1357

17. Leier CV (1988) Regional blood flow responses to vasodilators and inotropes in congestive heart failure. Am J Cardiol 62:86E–93E
18. Richardson PDI, Withrington PG (1981) Liver blood flow. Intrinsic and nervous control of liver blood flow. Gastroenterology 81:159–173
19. Lundgren O, Haglund U (1978) The pathophysiology of the intestinal countercurrent exchanger. Life Sci 23:1411–1422
20. Uusaro A, Ruokonen E, Takala J (1995) Estimation of splanchnic blood flow by the Fick principle in man and problems in the use of indocyanine green. Cardiovasc Res 30:106–112
21. Gump FE, Price JB Jr, Kinney JM (1970) Blood flow and oxygen consumption in patients with severe burns. Surg Gynecol Obstetr 130:23–28
22. Gump FE, Price JB Jr, Kinney JM (1970) Whole body and splanchnic blood flow and oxygen consumption measurements in patients with intraperitoneal infection. Ann Surg 171:321–328
23. Wilmore DW, Goodwin CW, Aulick LH, Powanda MC, Mason AD, Pruitt MD Jr (1980) Effect of injury and infection on visceral metabolism and circulation. Ann Surg 192:491–500
24. Aulick LH, Goodwin CW Jr, Becker RA, Wilmore DW (1981) Visceral blood flow following thermal injury. Ann Surg 193:112–116
25. Gottlieb ME, Sarfeh IJ, Stratton H, Goldman ML, Newell JC, Shah DM (1983) Hepatic perfusion and splanchnic oxygen consumption in patients postinjury. J Trauma 23:836–843
26. Dahn MS, Lange P, Lobdell K, Hans B, Jacobs LA, Mitchell RA (1987) Splanchnic and total body oxygen consumption differences in septic and injured patients. Surgery 101:69–80
27. Dahn MS, Lange P, Wilson RF, Jacobs LA, Mitchell RA (1990) Hepatic blood flow and splanchnic oxygen consumption measurements in clinical sepsis. Surgery 107:295–301
28. Steffes CP, Dahn MS, Lange MP (1994) Oxygen transport-dependent splanchnic metabolism in the sepsis syndrome. Arch Surg 129:46–52
29. Parviainen I, Rantala A, Ruokonen E, Takala J (1995) Failure of enalaprilat to reduce blood pressure in hypertensive cardiac surgery patients. Crit Care Med 23 (Suppl):A140 (Abst)
30. Uusaro A, Ruokonen E, Takala J (1995) Splanchnic oxygen transport after cardiac surgery: Evidence for inadequate tissue perfusion after stabilization of hemodynamics. Intensive Care Med 22:26–33
31. Parviainen I, Ruokonen E, Takala J (1996) Sodium nitroprusside after cardiac surgery: Central and regional hemodynamics. Acta Anaesth Scand (In press)
32. Nelson DP, Samsel RW, Wood LDH, Schumacker PT (1988) Pathological supply dependence of systemic and intestinal O_2 uptake during endotoxemia. J Appl Physiol 64:2410–2419
33. Rowell LB, Blackmon JR, Kenny MA, Escourrou P (1984) Splanchnic vasomotor and metabolic adjustments to hypoxia and exercise in humans. Am J Physiol 247:H251–H258
34. Ayuse T, Brienza J, Revelly P, Boitnott JK, Robotham JL (1995) Role of nitric oxide in porcine liver circulation under normal and endotoxemic conditions. J Appl Physiol 78:1319–1329
35. Parker MM, Shelhelmer JH, Bacharach SL, et al (1984) Profound but reversible myocardial depression in patients with septic shock. Ann Intern Med 100:483–490
36. Darle N, Lim RC Jr (1975) Hepatic arterial and portal venous flows during hemorrhage. Eur Surg Res 7:259–268
37. Dalton JM, Gore DC, Makhoul RG, Fisher MR, DeMaria EJ (1995) Decreased splanchnic perfusion measured by duplex ultrasound in humans undergoing small volume hemorrhage. Crit Care Med 23:491–497
38. Ruffolo RR Jr, Fondacaro JD, Levitt B, Edwards RM, Kinter LB (1987) Pharmacologic manipulation of regional blood flow. In: Snyder JV, Pinsky MR (eds) Oxygen transport in critically ill. Year Book Medical Publishers, Chicago, pp 450–474
39. Breslow MJ, Miller CF, Parker SD, Walman AT, Traystman RJ (1987) Effect of vasopressors on organ blood flow during endotoxin shock in pigs. Am J Physiol 252:H291–H300
40. Giraud GD, MacCannell KL (1984) Decreased nutrient blood flow during dopamine-and epinephrine-induced intestinal vasodilation. J Pharmacol Exp Ther 230:214–220
41. Shepherd AP, Riedel GL, Maxwell LC, Kiel JW (1984) Selective vasodilators redistribute intestinal blood flow and depress oxygen uptake. Am J Physiol 247:G377–G384

42. Löllgen H, Drexler H (1990) Use of inotropes in the critical care setting. Crit Care Med 18: S56–S60
43. Fink MP, Kaups KL, Wang H, Rothschild HR (1991) Maintenance of superior mesenteric arterial perfusion prevents increased intestinal permeability in endotoxic pigs. Surgery 110:154–161
44. Pawlik W, Mailman D, Shanbour LL, Jacobson ED (1976) Dopamine effects on the intestinal circulation. Am Heart J 91:325–331
45. Brown RA, Dixon J, Farmer JB, et al (1985) Dopexamine: A novel agonist at peripheral dopamine receptors and β2-adrenoreceptors. Br J Pharmacol 85:599–608
46. Webb AR, Moss RF, Tighe D, Al-Saady N, Bennett ED (1991) The effects of dobutamine, dopexamine and fluid on hepatic histological responses to porcine faecal peritonitis. Intensive Care Med 17:487–493
47. Leier CV, Binkley PF, Carpenter J, Randolph PH, Unverferth DV (1988) Cardiovascular pharmacology of dopexamine in low output congestive heart failure. Am J Cardiol 62:94–99
48. Angehrn W, Schmid E, Althaus F, Niedermann K, Rothlin M (1980) Effect of dopamine on hepatosplanchnic blood flow. J Cardiovasc Pharmacol 2:257–265
49. Leier CV, Heban PT, Huss P, Bush CA, Lewis RP (1978) Comparative systemic and regional hemodynamic effects of dopamine and dobutamine in patients with cardiomyopathic heart failure. Circulation 58:466–475
50. Gårdebäck M, Settergren G, Öhqvist G, Tirèn C (1995) Effect of dopexamine on calculated low gastric intramucosal pH following valve replacement. Acta Anaesth Scand 39:599–604
51. Gutierrez G, Palizas F, Doglio G, et al (1992) Gastric intramucosal pH as a therapeutic index of tissue oxygenation in critically ill patients. Lancet 339:195–199
52. Silverman HJ, Tuma P (1992) Gastric tonometry in patients with sepsis. Effects of dobutamine infusions and packed red blood cell transfusions. Chest 102:184–188
53. Smithies M, Yee TH, Jackson L, Beale R, Bihari D (1994) Protecting the gut and the liver in the critically ill: Effects of dopexamine. Crit Care Med 22:789–795
54. Trinder TJ, Lavery GG, Fee JPH, Lowry KG (1995) Correction of splanchnic oxygen deficit in the intensive care unit: Dopamine and colloid versus placebo. Anaesth Intensive Care 23: 178–182
55. Norlen K (1988) Central and regional haemodynamics during controlled hypotension produced by adenosine, sodium nitroprusside and nitroglycerin. Br J Anaesth 61:186–193
56. Colley PS, Sivarajan M (1984) Regional blood flow in dogs during halothane anesthesia and controlled hypotension produced by nitroprusside or nitroglycerin. Anesth Analg 63: 503–510
57. Bulkley GB, Oshima A, Bailey RW (1986) Pathophysiology of hepatic ischemia in cardiogenic shock. Am J Surg 151:87–97
58. Cullen JJ, Ephgrave KS, Broadhurst KA, Booth B (1994) Captopril decreases stress ulceration without affecting gastric perfusion during canine hemorrhagic shock. J Trauma 37:43–49
59. Leier CV, Bambach D, Thompson MJ, Gattaneo SM, Goldberg RJ, Unverferth DV (1981) Central and regional effects of intravenous isosorbide dinitrate, nitroglycerin and nitroprusside in patients with congestive heart failure. Am J Cardiol 48:1115–1123
60. Radermacher P, Buhl R, Santak B, et al (1995) The effects of prostacyclin on gastric intramucosal pH in patients with septic shock. Intensive Care Med 21:414–421
61. Ensinger H, Weichel T, Lindner KH, Grünert A, Georgieff M (1995) Are the effects of noradrenaline, adrenaline and dopamine infusions on VO_2 and metabolism transient? Intensive Care Med 21:50–56

Therapeutic Options to Increase Splanchnic Blood Flow

H. Zhang and J. L. Vincent

Introduction

The primary goal of the cardiorespiratory system is to deliver adequate amounts of oxygen to the tissues to meet their metabolic demands. If the cardiorespiratory system cannot meet the body's O_2 demands, organ system dysfunction occurs, as a result of tissue hypoxia or the resultant obligatory lactic acidosis. Gut hypoperfusion, in particular, has been implicated as initiating the sequence of events that leads to multiple organ failure (MOF). When blood flow is acutely reduced, splanchnic blood flow (SBF) may decrease more than in other regions, to allow maintenance of blood flow to vital organs, such as the heart and brain. Blood flow distribution to the organs is adjusted in response to changes in oxygen delivery (DO_2), through a balance between generalized vasoconstrictor tone, and local metabolic vasodilation, involving both the adrenergic and renin-angiotensin systems. The splanchnic circulation is very susceptible to damage from reduced blood flow and hypoxia. It is known that ischemia renders the splanchnic bed more permeable to bacteria and their products. These in turn may stimulate the immune system and hence the release of cytokines and other mediators resulting in an increase in O_2 demand, alterations in tissue O_2 extraction and myocardial depression. Among the mediators, oxygen free radicals (OFR) may play a key role in this pathophysiology of septic shock. The submucosal component of the gut itself contains many inflammatory cells and may, in fact, be the primary source of inflammatory mediators.

Alterations in gut barrier and function are the result of a combination of inadequate blood flow and the release of inflammatory mediators. Attempts to prevent, or limit, the cycle of events and the possible resultant MOF, must therefore aim to increase blood flow, but this alone may not be sufficient. A combination of improvement in blood flow and attenuation of mediators release may be the most effective strategy.

The present overview will focus on the effects of various therapeutic interventions to improve gut function, including established treatments using fluids and adrenergic agents, and more experimental methods affecting inflammatory mediators.

Fluid Resuscitation

In all forms of tissue hypoperfusion, fluids should be considered as a first priority. Fluids can often improve systemic blood flow, including to the gut. The quantity of fluids required to obtain adequate blood flow may amount to several liters per day. A reduction in SBF in some experimental models was clearly related to inadequate fluid repletion, and adequate fluid administration is essential to maintain splanchnic perfusion [1, 2]. The choice of fluids may be important. Colloids solution plasma expanders may be more effective than crystalloids. Nevertheless, colloids resuscitation with hydroxyethyl starch may fail to restore microvascular SBF, despite otherwise effective resuscitation [3]. Hypertonic saline solutions have demonstrated favorable circulatory effects in severe hemorrhagic and traumatic shock in animal models and in patients [4]. Small-volume resuscitation by adding a hyperoncotic colloid (i.e. 10% dextran-60) to the hypertonic saline solution has been shown to improve splanchnic microvascular perfusion in animal models of septic and hemorrhagic shock [5, 6]. In any case, fluid alone may be insufficient in some critically ill patients to restore adequate SBF so that vasoactive agents may be useful.

Adrenergic Agents

When fluid infusion fails to restore an acceptable arterial pressure or cardiac output, adrenergic agonists are the first line therapeutic intervention to increase DO_2. Studies on the effects of adrenergic agents on the distribution of blood flow generally showed increased mesenteric blood flow with β-, but not with α-adrenergic stimulation [7]. Shepherd et al. [8] showed that isoproterenol, a β1- and β2-adrenergic receptor agonist, redistributed intestinal blood flow, so that the mucosa was favored over muscularis in anesthetized animals. Another study [9] showed that isoproterenol induces increases in both blood flow and capillary filtration coefficient in the innervated small intestine of anesthetized cats. Because the vasodilator response was not blocked by practolol, the author concluded that β2-adrenoceptors were primarily responsible. Stimulation of dopaminergic receptors can selectively increase splanchnic perfusion. In control conditions, Johnson et al. [10] showed that dopamine improved blood flow and DO_2 to the gut in a positive end-expiratory pressure (PEEP)-induced low flow model in dog. Priebe et al. [11] recently showed that small intestinal and total hepatic blood flows could be increased by dopamine in anesthetized pigs. However, the physiological responses to dopamine are dose-dependent, wherein moderate doses may produce mesenteric vasodilation through β- and dopaminergic receptors activation, whereas higher doses may cause mesenteric vasoconstriction mediated by α-adrenoceptors.

Therapeutic interventions aiming at influencing blood flow distribution are less likely to be effective in septic conditions. Breslow et al. [12] found no major difference whether using dopamine, norepinephrine or phenylephrine in a porcine model of fluid resuscitated septic shock, and Bersten et al. [13] reached similar conclusions using dopamine, dobutamine, or norepinephrine in septic sheep. Van Lambalgen et al. [14] again found no significant differences between dopexamine and dobutamine in endotoxin-treated rats. However, different models and species used may result in different observations. We studied the effects of norepinephrine on systemic DO_2, oxygen uptake (VO_2), and regional blood flow in anesthetized dogs subject to stagnant hypoxia induced by cardiac tamponade following endotoxemia (unpublished data). At a dose of 1 µg/kg/min, norepinephrine increased arterial pressure but maintained cardiac index at least as high as in the endotoxin alone group for any given level of intrapericardial pressure. Norepinephrine administration did not significantly influence fractional blood flow to portal or mesenteric regions, and even increased fractional hepatic blood flow. On the other hand, norepinephrine decreased fractional blood flow to the renal bed. Norepinephrine infusion also decreased DO_{2crit} and increased critical oxygen extraction ratio (O_2ER_{crit}), indicating that the tissue O_2 extraction capabilities improved.

Several groups suggested that β-adrenergic stimulation can promote gastrointestinal mucosal blood flow and improve its oxygenation. Cain and Curtis [15] demonstrated that, in volume-expanded endotoxic dogs, dopexamine stimulates the dopaminergic receptors and has a potent β2-adrenergic receptor agonist effect, but no α-adrenergic properties, and may have caused gut mucosa to be preferentially perfused and thus to be kept better oxygenated and prevented the rise in lactate output. The better preserved SBF by β-adrenergic stimulation may also be associated with attenuation of cytotoxic mediators. Stimulation of β-adrenergic receptors inhibits endotoxin-induced tumor necrosis factor (TNF) production by mononuclear cells and whole blood *in vitro* [16, 17]. Furthermore, epinephrine and the β-receptor agonist salmeterol have been reported to attenuate the release of TNF after administration of endotoxin to mice and man [18, 19]. The inhibition of TNF production by β-adrenergic agents has been linked to their stimulating effect on adenylyl cyclase, leading to an increase in intracellular cAMP levels [16].

These observations have been reported in septic patients. Maynard et al. [20] recently compared the effect of dopexamine and dopamine on SBF in 25 critically ill patients. They demonstrated that dopexamine increases SBF as measured by gastric intramucosal pH (pHi), monoethylglycinexylidide (MEGX) formation from lidocaine, and indocyanine green clearance. However, dopamine had no effect on SBF, indicating that β-adrenergic stimulation may be more effective than dopaminergic stimulation in increasing SBF.

Dobutamine is such an adrenergic agent which has a more selective β-adrenergic effect, a slight α-adrenergic response, and no dopaminergic effect. Fink et al. [1] showed, in a porcine septic shock model, that fluid resuscitation with colloid and Ringer's lactate, in combination with dobutamine could preserve mesenteric blood flow, improve intramural pH and prevent endotoxin-induced intestinal mucosal permeability. In endotoxic dogs, De Backer et al. [21] showed that administration of 10 µg/kg/min of dobutamine could increase mesenteric blood flow and DO_2. Silverman et al. [22] and Gutierrez et al. [23] found dobutamine-increased pHi levels in critically ill patients. Thus, among the adrenergic agents available today, dobutamine is the most likely to effectively increase SBF. These effects are related to an increase in systemic flow to all regions (i.e. cardiac output) rather than to specific effects on regional blood flow. Thus, the combination of fluids with dobutamine may be particularly effective in limiting splanchnic hypoperfusion and its consequences.

Therapeutic Interventions on Mediators

Arachidonic Acid Metabolites

The metabolites of arachidonic acid, prostaglandins, thromboxanes and leukotrienes, may have both beneficial and deleterious consequences, and related therapies are therefore intended to enhance the favorable effects and/or reduce the harmful effects. Prostacyclin (PGI2), an endoperoxide derivative of arachidonic acid generated in the cyclooxygenase pathway, induces vasodilation and inhibition of platelet aggregation. The microcirculatory vasodilation induced by PGI2 seems to be particularly pronounced in the splanchnic region: PGI2 increased superior mesenteric artery blood flow in canine [24] and in porcine [25] shock models. PGI2 selectively enhanced blood flow to the gastric mucosa, the small bowel and the colon, even when cardiac output was nearly unaffected. In a porcine model of septic shock, iloprost, the stable PGI2 analog improved hepatic arterial blood flow and liver DO_2 after adequate volume expansion [26]. In patients with septic shock, Radermacher et al. [27] recently demonstrated that PGI2 enhanced DO_2 and pHi beyond the values obtained with conventional resuscitation suggesting an improvement in splanchnic oxygenation, probably by increasing regional perfusion.

Leukotrienes can decrease SBF. Etemadi et al. [28] showed that LY171883, a leukotriene inhibitor, substantially improved mesenteric blood flow in endotoxic animals which was not observed in normal controls.

Antioxidants

The pathogenesis of maldistribution of blood flow and impaired tissue O_2 extraction capabilities in septic states could be related to various factors including microvascular obstruction by activated cells, the release of vasoactive and toxic substances, and subsequent endothelial cell damage. Among other substances, OFR can have strong damaging effects on the endothelium, contributing to the maldistribution of blood flow and impaired O_2ER capabilities. They have also been implicated in the pathogenesis of sepsis-induced myocardial depression [29].

N-acetyl-L-cysteine: N-acetyl-L-cysteine (NAC) is a well-documented OFR scavenger. NAC can replenish intracellular glutathione, one of the pivots of cellular defense against oxidative stress [30]. NAC has been reported to block the acute toxicity of TNF [31]. According to recent studies, NAC may also stimulate endothelium-derived relaxing factor (EDRF), which exerts potent vasodilating and platelet inhibiting effects [32]. In a porcine model of endotoxin-induced pulmonary edema, NAC significantly increased cardiac output and DO_2, lowered pulmonary hypertension and intrapulmonary shunt, and decreased platelet aggregation [33]. NAC has been shown to increase DO_2, VO_2, and O_2ER in patients with fulminant hepatic failure [34]. We tested [35] the effects of NAC during endotoxic shock in anesthetized dogs. Interestingly, the alterations in O_2ER capabilities induced by endotoxin were markedly attenuated by prior administration of NAC. We demonstrated that NAC reduced DO_{2crit} from 10.8 to 8.1 mL/kg/min, and increased O_2ER_{crit} from 53 to 72%. NAC may exert these protective effects following endotoxemia by several intertwined mechanisms. An important one is the scavenging effect of NAC on OFR, since glutathione is one of the main intracellular defense mechanisms against oxidative stress, and cellular glutathione levels have been shown to be reduced during severe sepsis [36]. NAC can also exert important anti-inflammatory effects on neutrophils and monocytes. We found that a decreased inflammatory response was reflected by a complete inhibition of TNF release by NAC [37]. In a mouse endotoxic model, Peristeris et al. [31] recently demonstrated that pretreatment with NAC significantly inhibited TNF production both in the serum and in the spleen. This effect of NAC on TNF production is most likely due to a decreased release of OFR [37]. As a consequence, NAC may break a vicious circle, in that TNF can increase the production of OFR radicals, which in turn may activate inflammatory cells and induce further release of TNF [38].

An important question is whether NAC increases SBF. We studied the regional effects of NAC during endotoxic shock in the dog and found that NAC did increase absolute superior mesenteric blood flow but did not influence fractional blood flow to this region (Fig. 1) [39]. We therefore related the increase in O_2ER capabilities to an improvement in microcirculation within the tissues rather than among organs. A clinical study by Spies et al. [40] showed that NAC can increase pHi in septic patients, suggesting an improvement in the microcirculation of the gut. However, these observations applied only to a subgroup of responders.

Tirilazad mesylate (U74006F): The 21-aminosteroid, U74006F, exerts strong antioxidant effects through the inhibition of iron-dependent lipid peroxidation. U74006F has been reported to attenuate the accumulation of neutrophils [41], to protect endothelial structure [42], to diminish myocardial injury [43], to maintain a higher mean arterial pressure (MAP) and to increase survival [44] during ischemia/reperfusion. It has also been shown to suppress eicosanoid and TNF production [41], to prevent lactic acidosis [45], and to increase the survival rate [46] following endotoxemia in animals.

We explored the effects of U74006F on regional blood flow and O_2ER capabilities when blood flow was acutely reduced by cardiac tamponade in endotoxic dogs [2]. We found that U74006F administration significantly increased O_2ER_{crit} from 44 to 64% and reduced DO_{2crit} from 12 to 8 mL/kg/min, a value similar to the control without endotoxin levels [47]. The U74006F-treated dogs maintained

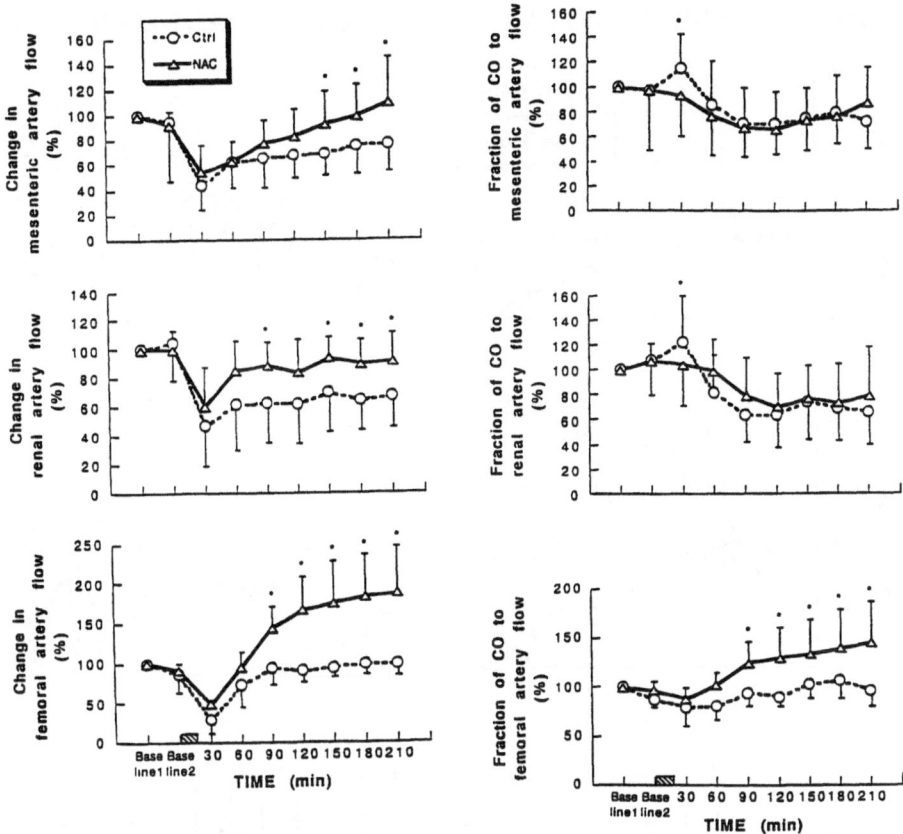

Fig. 1. Changes in absolute (*left panel*) and fractional (*right panel*) blood flow in mesenteric, renal and femoral vasculatures during time course in the endotoxin and NAC-treated groups. * $p < 0.05$ between the groups. (From [39] with permission)

a higher MAP than the dogs receiving placebo. U74006F administration increased stroke index and cardiac index, by an improvement in cardiac function. U74006F administration increased fractional blood flow to mesenteric and renal vasculatures but did not significantly influence femoral blood flow, indicating that U74006F may have beneficial effects on the distribution of blood flow in endotoxic shock (Fig. 2). Furthermore, U74006F significantly influenced individual organ O_2ER capabilities during endotoxic shock (Table 1). We explored the magnitude of changes in O_2ER in mesenteric beds, and observed that endotoxin significantly increased DO_{2crit} and decreased O_2ER_{crit} in mesenteric vasculatures. The administration of U74006F largely attenuated the endotoxin-induced alterations in O_2ER capabilities in mesenteric bed. These protective effects of U74006F after endotoxemia were associated with anti-inflammatory effects, reflected by significant lower serum TNF levels. Plasma nitrite levels were also reduced, suggesting a lower production of nitric oxide (NO). In contrast to the effects of specific NO inhibitors [47], this effect was not associated with any vasoconstriction, indicating that other important anti-inflammatory effects also took place.

CHANGE OF BLOOD FLOW (%)   FRACTIONAL BLOOD FLOW

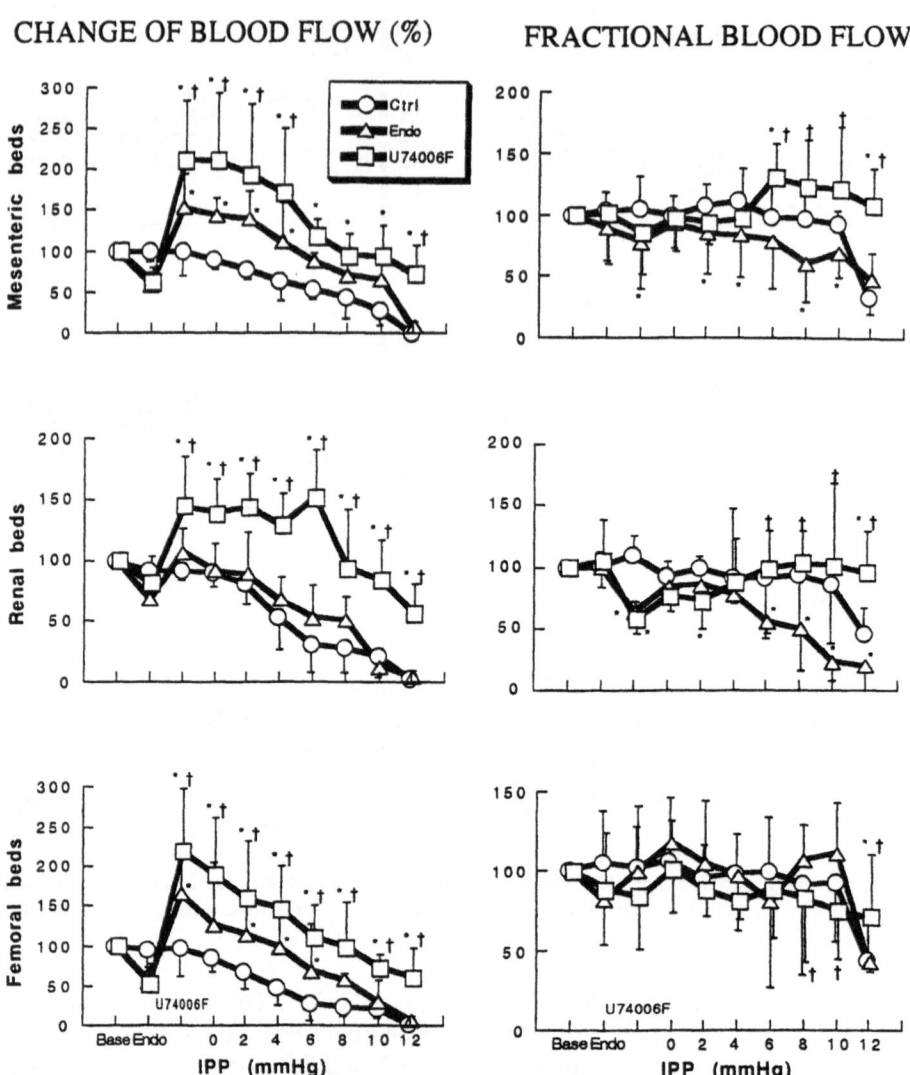

Fig. 2. Changes in absolute and fractional regional blood flow in three groups of dogs (controls; endotoxin; endotoxin plus U74006F) during acute blood flow reduction. * $p < 0.05$ vs ctrl, † $p < 0.05$ vs endo. (From [2] with permission)

Role of Nitric Oxide

NO, an EDRF, plays an important role in the regulation of blood pressure and organ blood flow distribution in normal conditions. This physiological role of NO is controlled by a constitutive, calcium-dependent NO synthase (NOS). Another NOS, inducible and calcium-independent, is expressed in various cells, including macrophages [49], endothelial cells [50] and vascular smooth muscle

Table 1. Systemic and regional VO_2, DO_2, and O_2ER values in endotoxic dogs after treatment with U74006F (From [2] with permission).

	Control	Endotoxin	U74006F
Whole body			
VO_2 (mL/kg/min)	5.6±1.2	5.2±0.9	4.8±0.7
DO_2 (mL/kg/min)	7.7±2.4	12.0±1.9*	7.8±2.0†
O_2ER (%)	75.0±12.7	44.3±8.7*	64.1±11.2†
Mesenteric vasculature			
VO_2 (mL/100 g tissue/min)	3.2±0.6	3.0±0.3	2.9±0.4
DO_2 (mL/100 g tissue/min)	4.3±0.6	9.1±2.9*	5.2±1.3†
O_2ER (%)	72.3±6.4	35.3±13.6*	61.0±10.0†
Renal vasculature			
VO_2 (mL/100 g tissue/min)	6.4±4.0	4.9±2.6	4.8±2.4
DO_2 (mL/100 g tissue/min)	12.4±4.7	15.0±3.3	10.7±4.5†
O_2ER (%)	53.9±25.9	33.0±13.1*	47.6±14.4†
Femoral vasculature			
VO_2 (mL/min)	3.6±0.7	4.0±0.6	3.0±1.0
DO_2 (mL/min)	4.7±1.0	8.6±2.1*	6.3±2.6
O_2ER (%)	77.4±10.7	48.0±7.9*	52.4±16.1*

* $p < 0.05$ vs Control, † $p < 0.05$ vs Endotoxin

cells [51], in response to endotoxin and several cytokines [49, 51]. A number of studies have incriminated an increased release of NO in the profound vasodilation characterizing septic shock.

NO Blockade

Inhibitors of NO synthesis such as N^G-monomethyl-L-arginine (L-NMMA) and N^G-nitro-L-arginine methyl ester (L-NAME) have been shown to reverse the fall in vascular tone induced by endotoxin or TNF [52], or to reverse the sepsis-induced myocardial depression [53]. However, an increased survival, or even an improvement in cardiovascular status, have not been consistently observed following these interventions [54]. Moreover, the administration of NOS inhibitors may decrease blood flow to organs including the gut. Billiar et al. [55] demonstrated that L-NMMA inhibited endotoxin-induced NOS, while promoting hepatic damage by reducing liver blood flow. Following endotoxic shock in rats and rabbits, Hutcheson [56] and Wright et al. [54] observed that L-NMMA pretreatment enhanced intestinal damage and increases in vascular permeability, and decreased hepatic blood flow. In sheep, NOS inhibitor has been shown to decrease blood flow to the splanchnic bed following endotoxemia [48]. More recently, Pastor et al. [57] demonstrated that N^W-nitro-L-arginine (L-NA) decreased aortic, portal vein and hepatic artery blood flow in a rabbit endotoxic shock model. Ayuse et al. [58] demonstrated that NOS inhibition in endotoxic shock could increase morbidity, due to a loss of local control of liver blood flow and marked increases in resistance to venous return across both the liver and the lungs in pigs.

Guanylate Cyclase Inhibition

NO activates a soluble guanylate cyclase which leads to increased levels of guanosine 3',5'-cyclic monophosphate (cGMP) in the endothelial and smooth muscle cells resulting in vasorelaxation. Methylene blue is an inhibitor of the soluble guanylate cyclase activity which counteracts the effects of NO and other nitrovasodilators in endothelium and vascular smooth muscle [59]. Methylene blue has been demonstrated to prevent the endotoxin- or interleukin-1-induced vasorelaxation by abolishing cGMP production [60], and to reverse endotoxin- or cytokine-induced hypotension and myocardial depression [53].

Differences in their mechanisms of action might lead to different effects being exhibited by methylene blue and NO inhibitors. We investigated [61] the effects of methylene blue at various doses during endotoxic shock in fluid-resuscitated dogs. Methylene blue markedly influenced regional blood flow: low to moderate doses of methylene blue selectively increased superior mesenteric blood flow following endotoxemia (Fig. 3). Importantly, methylene blue administration reduced mesenteric blood flow in the control group, so that the increase in mesenteric blood flow induced by methylene blue takes place only in the presence of endotoxin. These effects may be due to potentiating effects of methylene blue on the nitrovasodilator-induced endothelium-independent relaxation of the mesenteric vasculature [62]. Thus during endotoxic shock, methylene blue may have

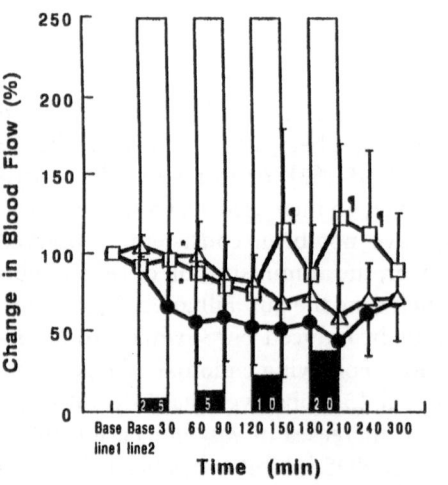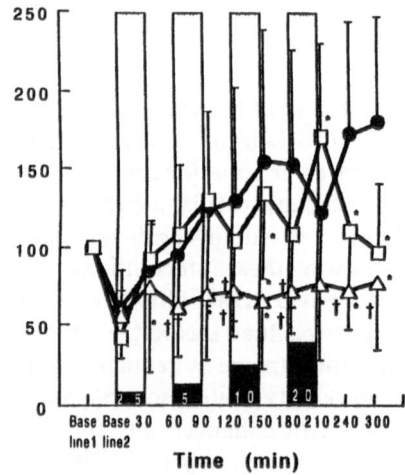

Fig. 3. Changes in blood flow in the superior mesenteric artery (*circles*), the left renal artery (*triangles*) and the left femoral artery (*squares*) after methylene blue administration in the control (*left panel*) and the endotoxic (*right panel*) groups, respectively. * p < 0.05 vs mesenteric, † p < 0.05 vs femoral, ¶ p < 0.05 vs mesenteric and renal beds. (From [61] with permission)

beneficial effects by diverting blood flow away from organs with a substantial oxygen extraction reserve (i.e. the femoral circulation), to organs that primarily depend on blood flow to maintain tissue oxygen availability (i.e. the splanchnic circulation) [63].

NO Donor

As mentioned above, NO blockade may decrease SBF, impair splanchnic organ function or increase mortality rates in septic shock [54]. Some recent studies have suggested that increased NO availability in septic shock may be more beneficial than harmful [35, 64]. It is intriguing, therefore, to test the hypothesis that NO-releasing compounds administered at judicious doses may have beneficial effects on the distribution of cardiac output in septic shock. We chose [65] to study the effectiveness of SIN-1, the vasoactive metabolite of molsidomide, as a NO donor. SIN-1 spontaneously decomposes into NO and the stable metabolite N-morpholinoiminoacetonitrile (SIN-1C). We tested the effects of SIN-1 at various doses on regional blood flow and tissue oxygen availability to the mesenteric, renal and femoral beds during endotoxic shock. Following SIN-1 infusion, we used methylene blue to partially block the effects of SIN-1 and thus to investigate the hemodynamic effects of methylene blue following SIN-1 administration during endotoxic shock. SIN-1 administration selectively increased mesenteric blood flow. Mulder et al. [66] demonstrated thats SBF is critically dependent on NO during the first hour of endotoxemia in rats. Boughton-Smith et al. [67] demonstrated that exogenous supplementation of NO by S-nitroso-N-acetyl-penicillamine administration, could preserve gut blood flow and attenuate endotoxin-induced macroscopic jejunal damage in the rat. Increased NO availability may improve tissue perfusion not only by a vasodilating effect but also by an inhibiting effect on platelet adhesion and aggregation, activation of leukocytes, mast cells, and other cellular elements involved in the inflammatory response [68, 69]. Payne and Kubes [70] recently demonstrated that exogenous administration of NO by NO donors can reduce reperfusion-induced mucosal barrier dysfunction, even independently of alterations in intestinal blood flow. Taken together, these studies suggest that NO has a protective effect against endotoxin-induced splanchnic injury. Thus, SIN-1 exerts some protective effects on splanchnic blood flow during endotoxic shock.

Conclusion

The splanchnic bed is a prime target in sepsis and frequently becomes hypoxic in the critically ill. Diverting splanchnic blood flow to vital organs may be incriminated in the release of mediators causing multiple organ failure, and resulting in increased mortality. Augmenting and maintaining splanchnic blood flow is therefore a fundamental, and effective therapy for acutely ill patients. To achieve this, fluid resuscitation is essential to maximize regional perfusion. Adrenergic agents are necessary to enhance vascular tone, improve blood flow distribution and possibly tissue oxygenation. Dobutamine is currently considered the most effective. Other therapeutic interventions affecting arachidonic acid metabolites, oxygen free radicals, and nitric oxide, require further study but may be relevant to clinical practice in the future.

References

1. Fink MP, Kaups KL, Wang H, Rothschild HR (1991) Maintenance of superior mesenteric arterial perfusion prevents increased intestinal mucosal permeability in endotoxic pigs. Surgery 110:154–161
2. Zhang H, Spapen H, Manikis P, Rogiers P, Vincent JL (1995) Tirilazad mesylate (U74006F) improves systemic and splanchnic oxygen extraction capabilities following endotoxic shock. Am J Physiol 268:H1847–H1855
3. Bauer M, Feucht K, Ziegenfuss T, Marzi I (1995) Attenuation of shock-induced hepatic microcirculatory disturbances by the use of a starch-deferoxamine conjugate for resuscitation. Crit Care Med 23:316–322
4. Kreimeier U, Frey L, Dentz J, Herbel T, Messmer K (1991) Hypertonic saline dextran resuscitation during the initial phase of acute endotoxemia: Effect on regional blood flow. Crit Care Med 19:801–809
5. Kreimeier U, Messmer K, Kox W, Gamble J (eds) (1988) Fluid resuscitation. Bailière Tindall, London. Small-volume resuscitation. pp 545–577
6. Vollmar B, Lang G, Menger MD, Messmer K (1994) Hypertonic hydroxyethyl starch restores hepatic microvascular perfusion in hemorrhagic shock. Am J Physiol 266:H1927–H1934
7. Schmartz D, Zhang H, Hoang C, et al (1995) Systemic and regional effects of adrenergic stimulation in septic shock. Effects of concurrent fluid administration. Am J Respir Crit Care Med 151:A446 (Abst)
8. Shepherd AP, Riedel GL, Maxwell LC, Kiel JW (1984) Selective vasodilators redistribute intestinal blood flow and depress oxygen uptake. Am J Physiol 247:G377–G384
9. Richardson PDI (1974) Drug-induced changes in capillary filtration coefficient and blood flow in the innerved small intestine of the anaesthetized cat. Br J Pharmacol 52:481–486
10. Johnson DJ, Johannigman JA, Branson RD, Davis KD, Hurst JM (1991) The effect of low dose dopamine on gut hemodynamics during PEEP ventilation for acute lung injury. J Surg Res 50:344–349
11. Priebe HJ, Nöldge GFE, Armbruster K, Geiger K (1995) Differential effects of dobutamine, dopamine, and noradrenaline on splanchnic haemodynamics and oxygenation in the pig. Acta Anaesthesiol Scand 39:1088–1096
12. Breslow MJ, Miller CF, Parker SD, Walman AT, Traystman RJ (1987) Effect of vasopressors on organ blood flow during endotoxin shock in pigs. Am J Physiol 252:H291–H300
13. Bersten AD, Hersch M, Cheung H, Rutledge FS, Sibbald WJ (1992) The effect of various sympathomimetics on the regional circulations in hyperdynamic sepsis. Surgery 112:549–561
14. Van Lambalgen AA, Van Kraats AA, Van de Vaart-Mulder MF, et al (1991) Systemic and renal actions of dopexamine and dobutamine during endotoxin shock in the rat. J Crit Care 6:61–70
15. Cain SM, Curtis SE (1992) Systemic and regional oxygen uptake and lactate flux in endotoxic dogs resuscitated with dextran and dopexamine or dextran alone. Circ Shock 38:173–181
16. Severn A, Rapson NT, Hunter CA, Liew FY (1992) Regulation of tumor necrosis factor production by adrenaline and beta-adrenergic agonists. J Immunol 148:3441–3445
17. Spengler RN, Chensue SW, Giachero DA, Blenk N, Kunkel SL (1994) Endogenous norepinephrine regulates tumor necrosis factor-α production from macrophages *in vitro*. J Immunol 152:3024–3031
18. Monastra G, Secchi EF (1993) β-adrenergic receptors mediate *in vivo* the adrenaline inhibition of lipopolysaccharide-induced tumor necrosis factor release. Immunology 38:127–130

19. Van der Poll T, Coyle SM, Barbosa K, Braxton CC, Lowry SF (1996) Epinephrine inhibits tumor necrosis factor-α and potentiates interleukin-10 production during human endotoxemia. J Clin Invest 97:713–719
20. Maynard ND, Bihari DJ, Dalton RN, Smithies MN, Mason RC (1995) Increasing splanchnic blood flow in the critically ill. Chest 108:1648–1654
21. De Backer D, Zhang H, Manikis P, et al (1994) Dobutamine can increase mesenteric blood flow during endotoxic shock in dogs. Am Rev Respir Dis 149:A19 (Abst)
22. Silverman HJ, Tuma P (1992) Gastric tonometry in patients with sepsis. Effects of dobutamine infusions and packed red blood cell transfusions. Chest 102:184–188
23. Gutierrez G, Clark C, Brown SD, Price K, Ortiz L, Nelson C (1994) Effects of dobutamine on oxygen consumption and gastric mucosal pH in septic patients. Am J Respir Crit Care Med 150:324–329
24. Seelig RF, Kerr JC, Hobson RW, Machiedo GW (1981) Prostacyclin (epopeostenol): Its effect on canine splanchnic blood flow during hemorrhagic shock. Arch Surg 116:428–430
25. Gaskill HV, Sirinek KR, Levine BA (1984) Prostacyclin selectively enhances blood flow in areas of the GI tract prone to stress ulceration. J Trauma 24:397–402
26. Rasmussen I, Arvidsson D, Zak A, Haglund U (1992) Splanchnic and total body oxygen consumption in experimental fecal peritonitis in pigs: Effects of dextran and iloprost. Circ Shock 36:299–306
27. Radermacher P, Buhl R, Klein M, Kniemeyer HW, Becker H, Tarnow J (1995) The effects of prostacyclin on gastric intramucosal pH in patients with septic shock. Intensive Care Med 21:414–421
28. Etemadi AR, Tempel GE, Farah BA, Wise WC, Halushka PV, Cook JA (1987) Beneficial effects of a leukotriene antagonist on endotoxin-induced acute hemodynamic alterations. Circ Shock 22:55–63
29. Prasad K, Kalra J, Chaudhary AK, Debnath D (1990) Effect of polymorphonuclear leukocyte-derived oxygen free radicals and hypochlorus acid on cardiac function and some biochemical parameters. Am Heart J 119:538–550
30. Bernard GR, Lucht WD, Niedermeyer ME, Snapper JR, Ogletree ML, Brigham KL (1984) Effect of N-acetylcysteine on the pulmonary response to endotoxin in the awake sheep and upon in vitro granulocyte function. J Clin Invest 73:1772–1784
31. Peristeris P, Clark BD, Gatti S, et al (1992) N-acetylcysteine and glutathione as inhibitors of tumor necrosis factor production. Cell Immunol 140:390–399
32. Stamler J, Mendelsohn ME, Amarante P, et al (1989) N-acetylcysteine potentiates platelet inhibition by endothelium-derived relaxing factor. Circ Res 65:789–795
33. Modig J, Sandin R (1987) Haematological, physiological and survival data in a porcine model of adult respiratory distress syndrome induced by endotoxaemia. Acta Chir Scand 154:169–177
34. Harrison PM, Wendon JA, Gimson AES, Alexander GJM, Williams R (1991) Improvement by acetylcysteine of hemodynamics and oxygen transport in fulminant hepatic failure. N Engl J Med 324:185–187
35. Zhang H, Spapen H, Nguyen DN, Benlabed M, Buurman WA, Vincent JL (1994) Protective effects of N-acetylcysteine in endotoxemia. Am J Physiol 266:H1746–H1754
36. Keller GA, Barke R, Harty JT, Humphrey E, Simmons RL (1985) Decreased hepatic glutathione levels in septic shock. Arch Surg 120:941–945
37. Pogrebniak HW, Merino MJ, Hahn SM, Mitchell JB, Pass HI (1992) Spin trap salvage from endotoxin: The role of cytokine down-regulation. Surgery 112:130–139
38. Jensen JC, Pogrebniak HW, Pass HI, et al (1992) Role of tumor necrosis factor in oxygen toxicity. J Appl Physiol 72:1902–1907
39. Zhang H, Spapen H, Nguyen DN, Rogiers P, Bakker J, Vincent JL (1995) Effects of N-acetyl-L-cysteine on regional blood flow during endotoxic shock. Eur Surg Res 27:292–300
40. Spies CD, Reinhart K, Witt I, Walensky C, Hannemann L, Specht M, Fohring U (1993) Influence of N-acetylcysteine on O_2 consumption and gastric intramucosal pH in septic patients. Crit Care Med 21:S183 (Abst)

41. Semrad SD, Rose ML, Adams JL (1993) Effect of tirilazad mesylate (U74006F) on eicosanoid and tumor necrosis factor generation in healthy and endotoxemic neonatal calves. Circ Shock 40:235–242
42. Eversole RR, Smith SL, Beuving LJ, Hall ED (1993) Protective effect of the 21-aminosteroid lipid peroxidation inhibitor tirilazad mesylate (U74006F) on hepatic endothelium in experimental hemorrhagic shock. Circ Shock 40:125–131
43. Carrea FP, Lesnefsky EJ, Kaiser DJ, Horwitz LD (1992) The lazaroid U74006F, a 21-aminosteroid inhibitor of lipid peroxidation, attenuates myocardial injury from ischemia and reperfusion. J Cardiovasc Pharmacol 20:230–235
44. Aoki N, Lefer AM (1990) Protective effects of a novel nonglucocorticoid 21-aminosteroid (U74006F) during traumatic shock in rats. J Cardiovasc Pharmacol 15:205–210
45. Rose ML, Semard SD (1992) Clinical efficacy of tirilazad mesylate for treatment of endotoxemia in neonatal calves. Am J Vet Res 53:2305–2310
46. Powell RJ, Machiedo GW, Rush BF, Dikdan GS (1991) Effects of oxygen-free radicals scavengers on survival in sepsis. Am Surg 57:86–88
47. Zhang H, Vincent JL (1993) Oxygen extraction is altered by endotoxin during tamponade-induced stagnant hypoxia in the dog. Circ Shock 40:168–176
48. Meyer J, Hinder F, Stothert J, et al (1994) Increased organ blood flow in chronic endotoxemia is reversed by nitric oxide synthesis inhibition. J Appl Physiol 76:2785–2793
49. Stuehr DJ, Marletta MA (1985) Mammalian nitrate biosynthesis: Mouse macrophages produce nitrite and nitrate in response to *Escherichia coli* lipopolysaccharide. Proc Natl Acad Sci USA 82:7738–7742
50. Radomski MW, Palmer RMJ, Moncada S (1990) Glucocorticoids inhibit the expression of an inducible, but not the constitutive, nitric oxide synthase in vascular endothelial cells. Proc Natl Acad Sci USA 87:10043–10047
51. Busse R, Mulsch A (1990) Induction of nitric oxide synthase by cytokines in vascular smooth muscle cells. FEBS Lett 275:87–90
52. Mayer B, Brunner F, Schmidt K (1993) Inhibition of nitric oxide synthesis by methylene blue. Biochem Pharmacol 45:367–374
53. Brady AJ, Poole-Wilson PA, Harding SZ, Warren JB (1992) Nitric oxide production within cardiac myocytes reduces their contractility in endotoxemia. Am J Physiol 32:H1963–H1966
54. Wright CH, Rees DD, Moncada S (1992) Protective and pathological roles of nitric oxide in endotoxin shock. Cardiovasc Res 26:48–57
55. Billiar TR, Curran RD, Harbrecht BG, Stuehr DJ, Demetris AJ, Simmons RL (1990) Modulation of nitrogen oxide synthesis *in vivo*: N^G-monomethyl-L-arginine inhibits endotoxin-induced nitrite/nitrate biosynthesis while promoting hepatic damage. J Leukoc Biol 48:565–569
56. Hutcheson IR, Whittle BJR, Boughton-Smith NK (1990) Role of nitric oxide in maintaining vascular integrity in endotoxin-induced acute intestinal damage in the rat. Br J Pharmacol 101:815–820
57. Pastor C, Teisseire B, Vicaut E, Payen D (1994) Effects of L-arginine and L-nitro-arginine treatment on blood pressure and cardiac output in rabbit endotoxin shock model. Crit Care Med 22:465–469
58. Ayuse T, Brienza N, Revelly JP, Boitnott JK, Robotham JL (1995) Role of nitric oxide in porcine liver circulation under normal and endotoxemic conditions. J Appl Physiol 78:1319–1329
59. Martin W, Villani GM, Jothianandan D, Furchgott RF (1985) Selective blockade of endothelium-dependent and glyceryl trinitrate-induced relaxation by hemoglobin and by methylene blue in the rabbit aorta. J Pharmacol Exp Ther 232:708–716
60. Beasley D (1990) Interleukin-1 and endotoxin activate soluble guanylate cyclase in vascular smooth muscle. Am J Physiol 259:R38–R44
61. Zhang H, Rogiers P, Preiser JC, Spapen H, Manikis P, Vincent JL (1995) Effects of methylene blue on oxygen availability and regional blood flow during endotoxic shock. Crit Care Med 23:1711–1721

62. Khan MT, Jothianandan D, Matsunaga K, Furchgott RF (1992) Vasodilation induced by acetylcholine and by glyceryl trinitrate in rat aortic and mesenteric vasculature. J Vasc Res 29:20–28
63. Samsel RW, Nelson DP, Sanders WM, Wood LDH, Schumacker PT (1988) Effect of endotoxin on systemic and skeletal muscle O_2 extraction. J Appl Physiol 65:1377–1382
64. Pastor CM, Billiar TR (1995) Nitric oxide causes hyporeactivity to phenylephrine in isolated perfused livers from endotoxin-treated rats. Am J Physiol 268:G177–G182
65. Zhang H, Rogiers P, Friedman G, et al (1996) Effects of nitric oxide donor SIN-1 on oxygen availability and regional blood flow during endotoxic shock. Arch. Surg (In press)
66. Mulder MF, Lambalgen AA, Huisman E, Visser JJ, Van den Bos GC, Thijs LG (1994) Protective role of NO in the regional hemodynamic changes during acute endotoxemia in rats. Am J Physiol 266:H1558–H1564
67. Boughton-Smith NK, Hucheson IR, Deaking AM (1994) Protective effect of S-nitroso-N-acetyl-penicillamine in endotoxin-induced acute intestinal damage in the rat. Eur J Pharmacol 191:485–488
68. Gauthier TW, Davenpeck KL, Lefer AM (1994) Nitric oxide attenuates leukocyte-endothelial interaction via P-selectin in splanchnic ischemia-reperfusion. Am J Physiol 267:G562–G568
69. Nishida J, McCuskey RS, McDonnell D, Fox E (1994) Protective role of NO in hepatic microcirculatory dysfunction during endotoxemia. Am J Physiol 267:G1135–G1141
70. Payne D, Kubes P (1993) Nitric oxide donors reduce the rise in reperfusion-induced intestinal mucosal permeability. Am J Physiol 265:G189–G195

Gut Metabolism

Gastrointestinal Exocrine Failure in Critical Illness

A. B. J. Groeneveld

Introduction

The main function of the gastrointestinal (GI) tract is to digest and absorb essential nutrients, including carbohydrates, lipids, amino acids, vitamins, minerals and water. This is critical for body homeostasis, at least when enteral feeding is applied.

During critical illness, GI complications may develop [1]. They may range from hemorrhagic gastritis with stress ulcer bleeding to gastric retention, absent bowel sounds and constipation following decreased gut motility [1–4]. After surgery, particularly stomach and colon motility is impaired, in extreme cases leading to pseudo-obstructive syndromes. This may relate to postoperative bowel paralysis, peritonitis and analgesic drugs [5]. In more than one-third of intensive care patients, however, GI dysfunction is primarily manifested by diarrhea, whether temporally related to tube-feeding or not [5–7]. This may be,

Table 1. GI exocrine failure in the critically ill

Organ	Potential dysfunction	Potential cause	Potential consequence
Stomach	Decreased acid production	Ischemia/reperfusion	– Stress ulcer and bleeding – Bacterial overgrowth
Small bowel	– Malabsorption of small carbohydrates, – Amino acids, – Fatty acids (?)	– Villous atrophy by ischemia/reperfusion and starvation, – Bacterial overgrowth, – Volume overload, – Hypoalbuminemia, – Defective brush border and transport proteins, – Reprioritization of intestinal protein synthesis	– Diarrhea, – Malabsorption, – Decreased motility, – Cardiac depression (?), – (Translocation) bacteremia owing to decreased barrier function, – Decreased immune function
Pancreas	Pancreatic injury	Ischemia	– Diarrhea – Malabsorption, – Ischemic pancreatitis, – Cardiac depression (?)

among others, associated with "intolerance to enteral nutrition (EN)" and may inhibit the uptake of enterally delivered nutrients [6, 7].

The causes and consequences of these complications are probably multifactorial (Table 1). It is therefore largely unclear what the major predisposing factors are as well as their impact on overall morbidity and mortality of critically ill patients [1], unless it is indeed true, as suggested by many animal studies, that the mucosa is injured and the gut mucosal barrier is broken down during various critical conditions, and that this plays a central role in translocation of bacteria and endotoxins from the gut lumen into the circulation, thereby contributing to the development of secondary sepsis, multiple organ failure (MOF) and ultimate death [8].

In this chapter, we will address if and how the function of the GI tract is deranged in critically ill patients.

Stomach

The major exocrine function of the stomach is production of acid and pepsin. The issue of gastric acid production during critical illness is controversial. In fact, gastric juice pH may spontaneously rise above 4 in critically ill patients, even in the absence of acid secretion inhibition, while it is usually below 4 in normal subjects [9, 10]. Also, administration of pentagastrin has been reported to fail to decrease gastric juice pH in some critically ill patients, as it would in normal subjects, and this was denoted as "exocrine" failure of the parietal cells of the gastric mucosa [10]. Whether this failure also extends to pepsin secretion by chief cells is currently unknown. On the other hand, authors have suggested that the gastric mucosa is able to secrete acid during sepsis in critically ill patients [11]. In fact, failure to control gastric juice pH above 4 by antacids and the H_2-blocker cimetidine was often associated with occult infection and development of sepsis [11].

Gut

The small gut produces the brush border enzymes disaccharidases and peptidases, and together with pancreatic proteolytic and lipolytic enzymes prepares enteral nutrients such as peptides, carbohydrates and lipids in small molecular forms amenable to absorption, together with fluids and electrolytes. The absorption of small molecular nutrients is an active, energy-consuming process and various carrier systems are involved. Furthermore, the gut produces some hormones, has an immunologic function and provides a barrier to luminal bacteria and endotoxins.

The mucosal epithelial permeability may be increased during critical illness, including trauma and hemorrhagic shock, as evidenced by an increased urinary lactulose to rhamnose or mannitol ratio after oral ingestion of these compounds, and this may be accompanied by, but relatively independent of diminished absorption capacity [12–14]. The consequences of this phenomenon remain unclear, since for instance no (temporal) relationship between increased permeability on the one hand and endotoxin translocation and development of septic complications on the other has been found in man [13]. Hence, the relation between increased permeability and (barrier) function of the GI mucosa in man is unknown.

The absorptive capacity of the small gut may be impaired during critical illness. Studies suggest that the ability to absorb sugars like D-xylose is decreased, during and early after trauma, hemorrhage, sepsis, shock and resuscitation in rodents, relatively independent of global hemodynamics [15–18]. The beneficial effect of a calcium antagonist or ATP on impaired D-xylose absorption after hemorraghic shock and sepsis suggests involvement of an energy deficit and cytosolic calcium overload in the mucosal injury [16, 17]. Alternatively, a decreased carrier (protein) activity and/or surface area of the absorptive epithelium, independently of blood flow, may underlie diminished absorptive capacity [5, 14, 16, 17]. In humans, the absorptive capacity of the gut may also be impaired, even early (within days) after trauma and onset of sepsis in critically ill patients, as shown by a fall in the D-xylose and 3-O-methyl-D-glucose urinary recovery, returning to normal 1–3 weeks after trauma or resolution of sepsis [5, 14]. Nevertheless, most patients tolerated EN, so that the clinical significance of these findings remained unclear. Also, the absorptive capacity for amino acids, including arginine, that plays a role in immune defense, and glutamine, that is considered as an essential gut nutrient, is impaired after induction of hemorrhagic shock, sepsis or endotoxemia in rodents, and even, in some studies, after resuscitation and amelioration of intestinal hypoperfusion [15, 18–21]. In other studies, impaired amino acid absorption normalized during recovery from sepsis [21]. Diminished glutamine uptake by the bowel wall during these conditions has been suggested to be associated with breakdown of the gut mucosal barrier and in the development of bacterial translocation [19, 20]. The impaired amino acid (glutamine) absorption during endotoxemia is likely to be mediated by interleukin-1 (IL-1) rather than by tumor necrosis factor (TNF) [20]. As in animal experiments, septic patients may also show diminished absorptive capacity for amino acids [18], but it is unknown if this also applies to lipids. In contrast, sepsis has been shown to increase the release of gut peptides in animals, including gastrin, secretin, vasoactive intestinal peptide, peptide YY, gastrin-releasing peptide and substance P, largely mediated by TNF rather than by IL-1 [22]. The implication of these latter findings for man remains unclear.

It is generally believed that relatively prolonged bowel rest (of more than about one week), particularly associated with total parenteral nutrition (TPN), leads to mucosal atrophy, diminished brush border enzyme activity, increased epithelial permeability and diminished absorptive capacity, and thereby contributes to diarrhea upon reinstitution of EN [8, 23–27]. TPN and bowel rest prior to a test dose of endotoxin in healthy volunteers may somewhat modify the inflammatory, circulatory and metabolic response to endotoxin as compared to EN [24]. Although on the one hand, EN may maintain gut structure and function by providing "gut nutrition" and may decrease translocation, morbidity and mortality in various animal models of shock and related conditions [8], EN may also have some drawback, even though it may increase GI blood flow. Indeed, EN and absorption of nutrients elevate the metabolic demands of the gut, so that, particularly in the absence of sufficient cardiac reserve as may occur in shock, EN may be harmful to the gut by diminishing the oxygen supply-to-demand ratio [28, 29]. This may even result in more severe mucosal damage than in the absence of EN, at least during bowel ischemia/reperfusion (I/R), following mesenteric clamping and declamping, in pigs [29].

Nevertheless, early start of EN has been widely recommended to replace TPN in critically ill patients, at least after initial resuscitation from shock [8]. The impact of this recommendation on the nutritional state of the patient remains unclear, however, particularly in case the absorptive capacity of the small bowel is diminished [14, 30]. In fact, the improvement in nutritional status may be similar during EN and TPN of similar nutritional value, in spite of more frequent occurrence of diarrhea during EN [30]. Glutamine, an amino acid considered as an essential nutrient for the bowel, can also be supplied, in modified and thus stable forms, via the parenteral route, so that, during critical conditions, small bowel histologic changes are prevented and gut protein synthesis and barrier function are improved, at least in animals [8, 19, 27, 31, 32]. In critically ill patients, glutamine dipeptide-containing TPN may improve D-xylose absorption [25] and nutritional status, and this may be associated with prevention of gut mucosal atrophy and increased permeability. However, modified EN, supplemented with arginine among others, may lessen morbidity in a variety of critical conditions as compared to standard EN, because of the arginine-induced improvement of immunologic function [33]. Other authors found that both during TPN and EN started early after admission of critically ill patients, absorption of sugars like D-xylose and 3-O-methyl-D-glucose were impaired but increased to a similar extent during both forms of nutrition [14]. In contrast, the urinary lactulose/rhamnose ratio, an index of gut epithelial permeability, was increased and returned to normal during EN but not TPN [14]. Enteral as opposed to parenteral feeding may thus improve gut mucosal barrier function, and may thereby diminish complications in the disease course of critically ill, mainly postoperative patients [8]. Other studies, however, failed to demonstrate such benefit, since EN as opposed to TPN did not decrease the frequency of MOF and mortality after sepsis [30].

Pancreas

The function of the pancreas is to secrete, among others, proteolytic (trypsin), carbohydrate-splitting (amylase) and lipolytic (lipase) enzymes. Animal studies in the seventies have suggested that circulatory shock is associated with release of lysosomal substances with negative inotropic properties in the blood stream, the so-called myocardial depressant factors, by the injured bowel mucosa, pancreas, or both [34]. The role of these factors and their precise nature remains a matter of debate. Nevertheless, there is evidence of pancreatic injury during critical illness such as trauma, burns, shock and the adult respiratory distress syndrome (ARDS) unrelated to acute pancreatitis; the serum concentration of pancreatic enzymes including lipase and trypsin may be elevated to levels seen during acute pancreatitis [35, 36]. The causes and consequences of these changes remain unclear however [35]. Nevertheless, there is experimental evidence that pancreatic enzymes are involved in the generation of mucosal injury of the small bowel during I/R [37]. In fact, pancreatic duct ligation prior to I/R of the porcine bowel, associated with hemorrhagic shock and resuscitation, ameliorated the development of mucosal damage [37]. Conversely, this must indicate somewhat preserved exocrine pancreas function during shock and resuscitation. Although above studies thus suggest some form of pancreatic injury during critical illness, the influence on luminal secretion and digestion of enteral nutrients remains unknown. However, it is likely, analogously to acute pancreatitis, that pancreatic injury is accompanied by some type and severity of exocrine failure. Although pancreatic function during acute pancreatitis has not been characterized well, some studies on residual pancreatic function after bouts of pancreatitis show impaired function in the majority of patients, as judged from subnormal contents of enzymes in duodenal contents after a test meal [38].

Causes of Potential Gastrointestinal Failure

The major etiologic factors associated with potential GI dysfunction in critically ill patients can be grouped as follows. The idea that prolonged bowel rest may contribute to mucosal atrophy and gut dysfunction has been alluded to above. Other factors involved in diminished absorptive capacity during critical illness (sepsis) independently from tissue oxygenation include defective transport proteins, for instance as a consequence of reprioritization of intestinal protein synthesis with increased production of acute phase proteins [18].

Ischemia

There is ample evidence that the oxygen supply-to-demand balance of the gut is compromised during shock, even if associated with a relatively high cardiac output as may occur during septic shock [39, 401. Although our knowledge largely stems from animals models, human data, using blood flow and oxygen balance parameters, also suggest relative underperfusion of the splanchnic area in hemorrhagic and septic shock [37, 39, 40]. Indeed, septic shock as opposed to hemorrhagic shock, may be accompanied by increased blood flow demands of stomach and intestines, so that (the rise in) blood flow may not fully compensate, rendering the GI tract susceptible to ischemia [40]. Increased demands may be associated with increased gluconeogenesis and protein synthesis in the bowel wall, while insufficient vasodilation or selective vasoconstriction may relate to an activated sympathetic nervous system and release of vasoconstricting angiotensin and vasopressin [41]. In fact, animal studies suggest a cytokine-induced increase in energy-consuming protein synthesis in the bowel wall during sepsis [42]. There are also other pieces of evidence for GI ischemia. Recently, tonometry has been introduced into clinical practice as a means to evaluate the adequacy of GI blood flow (description of principles and methodology in [43]). In fact, tonometry has allowed a major step forward in evaluating the frequency, causes and consequences of GI mucosal hypoperfusion in critical illness [10, 37, 43, 44]. Using this technique, evidence for mucosal hypoperfusion has been relatively frequently found in various clinical conditions [10, 13, 37, 40, 43, 44].

There are some data to suggest that bowel ischemia impairs bowel function in animals, and, conversely, that impaired GI function relates to hypoperfusion in critically ill patients. Animal studies have shown erosive lesions, with sloughing, hemorrhage, edema and necrosis, along the entire GI tract during various types of shock, and this may be accompanied by gastric "stress" ulcers and, particularly in dogs, by increased luminal fluid filtration, decreased fluid absorption and (bloody) diarrhea [1, 29, 31, 34, 37, 39, 41, 45–48]. It can be conceived that such lesions are associated with impairment of mucosal function and may, through release of toxic products or loss of barrier function and translocation, adversely affect remote organ function [8, 34]. Such lesions may also occur in man, and may remain clinically silent. Conversely, the clinical signs of GI dysfunction mentioned above may be caused by relative hypoperfusion of the GI tract.

As far as the stomach is concerned, it is known from animal experiments that gastric acid production, which is an active energy (and thus O_2 demanding process), is reduced during gastric mucosal ischemia [41, 47]. Although gastric stress ulcer bleeding is a relatively rare event in critically ill patients treated with some form of gastric mucosal protection and its pathogenesis is probably multifactorial, sepsis, hypotension and shock are major risk factors for these conditions suggesting that mucosal ischemia is involved [1–4, 11]. Although gastric acid may be a risk factor for stress ulcer bleeding, failure to produce acid may thus not be protective if associated with mucosal ischemia [9, 41, 47]. Indeed, a low intramucosal pH (pHi), as determined by tonometry and probably indicative of mucosal ischemia, may predict development of stress ulcer bleeding [43, 48]. Lack of gastric acid may also predispose critically ill patients to gastric colonization by mainly gram-negative enteric bacillae, since acid inhibiting or neutralizing drugs have been suggested to predispose to colonization and airway infections, although this is not beyond doubt.

Animal studies on hemorrhagic shock and sepsis in rats suggest that ischemic damage is an important factor in impaired gut absorptive capacity after resuscitation [15–18]. Very rarely, patients resuscitated from severe shock may develop non-occlusive ischemic bowel damage, as manifested by bowel paralysis, bloody diarrhea and, occasionally, perforation. Also, the development of acalculous cholecystitis might be caused by ischemia of the gall bladder wall and could be considered to contribute to "exocrine" failure of the GI tract during critical illness.

There is also some "direct" evidence for the role of hypoperfusion in GI mucosal dysfunction in critically ill patients. A relatively higher proportion of critically ill patients with, rather than without, hypotension and inotropic drugs had a gastric juice pH above 4, suggesting mucosal ischemia to be responsible for this defect in acid production [9]. A low gastric pHi (tonometry) predicted failure of pentagastrin to acidify gastric luminal contents in critically ill patients, suggesting that mucosal ischemia had impaired gastric acid secretion [10]. A high intra-gastric PCO_2 and a resultant low gastric pHi (tonometry), both indicators of inadequate mucosal perfusion, may sometimes coincide with increased small gut mucosal epithelial permeability, as reflected by an elevated lactulose/mannitol absorption ratio [43]. Although, in other studies, the causes of increased permeability in the absence of a relation with global circulatory abnormalities remained unclear [13]. The consequences of these phenomena remain largely unknown, at least in terms of associated morbidity and mortality, since, among others, there is no relation between epithelial permeability and potential endotoxin translocation [13]. Nevertheless, tonometric evidence for inadequate gastric mucosal perfusion is a prognostically bad sign. Conversely, authors have even suggested that therapy aimed at prevention or treatment of gastric mucosal hypoperfusion as shown by tonometric data, and generally consisting of improved cardiac output and tissue oxygen delivery by fluids and inotropes, may have beneficial effects on morbidity and mortality of critically ill (postoperative) patients [43, 44].

It is well known from most animal studies that blood flow to the pancreas falls during various types of circulatory failure, varying from low flow hemorrhagic and endotoxic to high flow septic shock. Since measurements in man are not available, there are no data on pancreatic perfusion and function during critical illness in man.

Volume Overload and Hypoalbuminemia

Plasma volume expansion with crystalloid infusions leads to increased transmucosal fluid filtration with losses of electrolytes and even plasma proteins into the intestinal lumen in the dog [49]. This diarrheogenic effect of volume expansion was accompanied by increased mucosal epithelial permeability to mannitol [49]. These effects largely related to the fall in plasma protein concentration and plasma colloid osmotic pressure [49]. In fact, hypoalbuminemia has been often implicated as a contributing factor to diarrhea in critically ill, tube-fed patients, although other factors may certainly be more important [6]. Hence, hypoalbuminemia may be a marker for malnutrition and mucosal atrophy rather than a cause of diarrhea [6]. Conversely, diarrhea may resolve during feeding whether or not supplemented with intravenous albumin, and this may be associated with improvement of nutritional state and serum albumin levels [6].

Conclusion

Critical illness may be accompanied by GI functional changes, which remain to be precisely characterized in man. They may range from impaired gastric acid secretion with susceptibility for stress ulcer formation, diarrhea and malabsorption of sugars and amino acids, as evidenced in animals and man with critical conditions, to impaired motility and constipation. This may hamper (efficacy of) EN, the preferred route for nutrition in the critically ill in the phase that mucosal ischemia is unlikely. The role of the pancreas is poorly defined, even though critical illness may be complicated by pancreatic injury. Future research should also better define potential causes that may include prolonged bowel rest, ischemia, volume overload and hypoalbuminemia, and management which may include measures to detect, prevent or treat the detrimental effects of ischemia, of GI failure in the critically ill.

References

1. Gottlieb JE, Menashe PI, Cruz E (1986) Gastrointestinal complications in critically ill patients: The intensivist's overview. Am J Gastroenterol 81:227–238
2. Fusamoto H, Hagiwara H, Meren H, et al (1991) A clinical study of acute gastrointestinal hemorrhage assiociated with various types of shock states. Am J Gastroenterol 86: 429–433
3. Cook DJ, Fuller HD, Guyatt GH, et al (1994) Risk factors for gastrointestinal bleeding in critically ill patients. N Engl J Med 330:377–381
4. Zandstra DF, Stoutenbeek CP (1994) The virtual absence of stress ulceration-related bleeding in ICU patients receiving prolonged mechanical ventilation without any prophylaxis. Intensive Care Med 20:335–340
5. Singh G, Harkema JM, Mayberry AJ, Chaudry IH (1994) Severe depression of gut absorptive capacity in patients following trauma or sepsis. J Trauma 36:803–809
6. Ringel AF, Jameson GL, Foster ES (1995) Diarrhea in the intensive care patient. Crit Care Clin 11:465–477
7. Edes TE, Walk BE, Austin JL (1990) Diarrhea in tube-fed patients: Feeding formula not necessarily the cause. Am J Med 88:91–93
8. Mainous MR, Block EFJ, Deitch EA (1994) Nutritional support of the gut: How and why. New Horizons 2:193–201
9. Stannard VA, Hutchinson A, Morris DL, Byrne A (1988) Gastric exocrine "failure" in critically ill patients: Incidence and associated features. Br Med J 296:155–156
10. Higgins D, Mythen MG, Webb AR (1994) Low intramucosal pH is associated with failure to acidify the gastric lumen in response to pentagastrin. Intensive Care Med 20:105–108
11. Martin LF, Max MH, Polk HC (1980) Failure of gastric pH control by antacids or cimetidine in the critically ill: A valid sign of sepsis. Surgery 88:59–68
12. Harris CE, Griffiths RD, Freestone N, Billington D, Atherton ST, Macmillan RR (1992) Intestinal permeability in the critically ill. Intensive Care Med 18:38–41
13. Roumen RMH, Hendrik T, Wevers RA, Goris RJA (1993) Intestinal permeability after severe trauma and hemorrhagic shock is increased without relation to septic complications. Arch Surg 128:453–457
14. Hadfield RJ, Sinclair DG, Houldsworth PE, Evans TW (1995) Effects of enteral and parenteral nutrition on gut mucosal permeability in the critically ill. Am J Respir Crit Care Med 152:1545–1548
15. Guthrie JE, Quastel JH (1956) Absorption of sugars and amino acids from isolated surviving intestine after experimental shock. Arch Biochem Biophys 62:485–496
16. Singh G, Chaudry KI, Chudler LC, Chaudry IH (1992) Sepsis produces early depression of gut absorptive capacity: Restoration with diltiazem treatment. Am J Physiol 263:R19–R23
17. Singh G, Chaudry KI, Chudler LC, Chaudry IH (1991) Depressed gut absorptive capacity early after trauma-hemorrhagic shock. Restoration with diltiazem treatment. Ann Surg 214:712–718

18. Gardiner K, Barbul A (1993) Intestinal amino acid absorption during sepsis. J Parent Enteral Nutr 17:277–283
19. Souba WW, Klimberg S, Plumley DA, et al (1990) The role of glutamine in maintaining a healthy gut and supporting the metabolic response to injury and infection. J Surg Res 48: 383–391
20. Austgen TR, Chen MK, Dudrick PS, Copeland EM, Souba WW (1992) Cytokine regulation of intestinal glutamine utilisation. Am J Surg 163:174–180
21. Gardiner KR, Gardiner RE, Barbul A (1995) Reduced intestinal absorption of arginine during sepsis. Crit Care Med 23:1227–1232
22. Zamir O, Hasselgren PO, Higashiguchi T, Frederick JA, Fisher JE (1992) Effect of sepsis or cytokine administration on release of gut peptides. Am J Surg 163:181–185
23. Hosoda N, Nishi M, Nakagawa M, Hiramatsu Y, Hioki K, Yamamoto M (1989) Structural and functional alterations in the gut of parenterally or enterally fed rats. J Surg Res 47: 129–133
24. Santos AA, Rodrick ML, Jacobs DO, et al (1994) Does the route of feeding modify the inflammatory response? Ann Surg 220:155–163
25. Tremel H, Kienle B, Weileman LS, Stehle P, Fürst P (1994) Glutamine dipeptide-supplemented parenteral nutrition maintains intestinal function in the critically ill. Gastroenterology 107:1595–1601
26. Guedon C, Schmitz E, Metayer J, Aurdan E, Hemet J, Colin R (1986) Decreased brush border hydrolase activities without gross morphologic changes in human intestinal mucosa after prolonged total parenteral nutrition in adults. Gastroenterology 90:373–378
27. Sarac TP, Souba WW, Miller JH, et al (1994) Starvation induces differential small bowel luminal amino acid transport. Surgery 146:679–686
28. Nowicki PT, Stonestreet BS, Hansen NB, Yao AC, Oh W (1983) Gastrointestinal blood flow and oxygen consumption in awake newborn piglets: Effect of feeding. Am J Physiol 245: G697–G702
29. Grootendorst AF, Van Leengoed LAMG, Nabuurs M, Bouman CSC, Groeneveld ABJ (1993) Enteral feeding increases bowel damage after ischemia/reperfusion in the pig. In: Grootendorst AF (ed) High volume hemofiltration in experimental shock. Thesis, Amsterdam, The Netherlands, pp 83–95
30. Cerra FB, McPherson JP, Konstantinides FN, Konstantinides NN, Tealey KM (1988) Enteral nutrition does not prevent multiple organ failure syndrome (MOFS) after sepsis. Surgery 104:727–733
31. Yoshida S, Leskiw MJ, Schluter MD, et al (1992) Effect of total parenteral nutrition, systemic sepsis, and glutamine on gut mucosa in rats. Am J Physiol 263:E368–E373
32. Okuma T, Kaneko H, Chen K, et al (1994) Total parenteral nutrition supplemented with L-alanyl-L-glutamine and gut structure and protein metabolism in septic rats. Nutrition 10:241–245
33. Bower RH, Cerra FB, Bershadsky B, et al (1995) Early enteral administration of a formula (Impact®) supplemented with arginine, nucleotides, and fish oil in intensive care unit patients: Results of a multicenter, prospective, randomized clinical trial. Crit Care Med 23:436–449
34. Haglund U, Lundgren O (1978) Intestinal ischemia and shock factors. Fed Proceed 37:2729–2733
35. Nicod L, Leuenberger P, Seydoux C, Rey F, Van Melle G, Perret Cl (1985) Evidence for pancreatic injury in adult respiratory distress syndrome. Am Rev Respir Dis 131:696–699
36. Uhl W, Büchler M, Nevalainen TJ, Deller A, Beger HG (1990) Serum phospholipase A_2 in patients with multiple injuries. J Trauma 30:1285–1290
37. Montgomery A, Borgström A, Haglund U (1992) Pancreatic proteases and intestinal mucosal injury after ischemia and reperfusion in the pig. Gastroenterology 102:216–222
38. Bozkurt T, Maroske D, Adler G (1995) Exocrine pancreatic function after recovery from necrotizing pancreatitis. Hepato-Gastroenterol 42:55–58
39. Fink MP (1991) Gastrointestinal mucosal injury in experimental models of shock, trauma, and sepsis. Crit Care Med 129:627–641

40. Groeneveld ABJ (1996) Redistribution of blood flow in hypovolemic and septic shock: Clinical and animal studies. Réanimation Urgences (in press)
41. Cullen JJ, Ephgrave KS, Broadhurst KA, Booth B (1994) Captopril decreases stress ulceration without affecting gastric perfusion during canine hemorrhagic shock. J Trauma 37:43-49
42. Breuille D, Rose F, Arnal M, Melin C, Obled C (1994) Sepsis modifies the contribution of different organs to whole-body protein synthesis in rats. Clin Sci 86:663-669
43. Groeneveld ABJ, Kolkman JJ (1994) Splanchnic tonometry: A review of physiology methodology and clinical applications. J Crit Care 9:198-210
44. Mythen MG, Webb AR (1995) Perioperative plasma volume expansion reduces the incidence of gut mucosal hypoperfusion during cardiac surgery. Arch Surg 130:423-429
45. Cook BH, Wilson ER, Taylor AE (1971) Intestinal fluid loss in hemorrhagic shock. Am J Physiol 221:1494-1498
46. Falk A, Redfors S, Myrvold H, Haglund U (1985) Small intestinal mucosal lesions in feline septic shock: A study of the pathogenesis. Circ Shock 17:327-337
47. Yasue N, Guth PH (1988) Role of exogenous acid and retransfusion in hemorrhagic shock-induced gastric lesions in the rat. Gastroenterology 94:1135-1143
48. Kiviluoto T, Voipio J, Kivilaakso E (1988) Subepithelial tissue pH of rat gastric mucosa exposed to luminal acid, barrier breaking agents and hemorrhagic shock. Gastroenterology 94:695-702
49. Duffy PA, Granger DN, Taylor AE (1978) Intestinal secretion induced by volume expansion in the dog. Gastroenterology 75:413-418

Early Enteral Nutrition in the Surgical Patient

M. Singer

Introduction

Malnutrition should clearly be avoided in both the high risk patient undergoing major surgery as well as the critically ill postoperative patient. Immune incompetence [1, 2], poor wound healing [3], increased postoperative complications [4], and prolonged hospital stay [5] have all been linked with malnutrition. Irrespective of the patient's nutritional status prior to ICU admission, a state of nutritional deficiency may occur through delayed and/or inadequate feeding.

This chapter will set out:
1) the proven and putative benefits of early and aggressive enteral feeding in the critically ill surgical patient;
2) its safety; and
3) evidence that early feeding equates with better tolerance.

Techniques of establishing early postoperative enteral nutrition (EN) will also be described.

Malnutrition

Deitch et al. [2, 6] used a rat model to demonstrate that protein malnutrition impaired systemic and gut-associated immunity; both intestinal permeability and the rate of bacterial translocation (BT) rate were increased. A good correlation has also been found in patients between impaired nutritional status, postoperative wound complications [1], and prolonged postoperative stay [5]. A large multicenter study in patients undergoing major elective surgery [4] showed improved outcome in the subgroup of severely malnourished patients receiving total parenteral nutrition (TPN).

Why Enteral?

Long-established convention has dictated that the gut be rested after abdominal surgery. The rationale for this unproven dogma is that the gut will not work after handling, and any bowel anastomosis would be at risk of bursting under the strain of intestinal contents. Passage of flatus and presence of bowel sounds are traditionally sought markers of a functioning bowel; absence of these signs may result in nutritional deprivation for days and, sometimes, weeks. Even the icono-clastic, dynamic intensivist will often wait for several days until cardiovascular stability is restored before attempting to feed the critically ill patient, surgical or not.

TPN is unnatural and unphysiological albeit a sometimes necessary route for the provision of adequate nutrition. Complications involving line placement, infection and metabolic abnormalities are well noted [7], though description of these tend to overshadow problems of lower profile but of potentially greater significance. Direct intestinal nutrition appears to confer specific protective effects not provided by TPN. Enterocytes receive nutrition directly from food within the bowel lumen. Depriving the cells of this immediate food source by provision of TPN alone leads to increased gut permeability and villous atrophy [8]. Bowel rest produces alterations in host resistance and metabolic response to injury independent of malnutrition [9]. Furthermore, it also promotes bacterial overgrowth in the intestinal lumen [10], a possible source of bacteremia and endotoxemia. Alverdy et al. [11, 12] demonstrated impairment of gut immunity and increased BT in TPN-fed rats. Resumption of EN resulted in a rapid return of secretory IgA to normal levels, suggesting that maintenance of secretory IgA depends on the intraluminal presence of food. Lower serum albumin and higher bilirubin levels were found after 70% hepatectomy in TPN-fed animals [13] while increased hepatocyte-associated tumor necrosis factor (TNF) levels have also been associated with a lack of direct intestinal nutrient provision [14]; the con-tribution of this towards the priming of any subsequent systemic inflammatory response syndrome (SIRS) must remain speculative at present. Both Kudsk et al. [15] and Zaloga et al. [16] found an increased mortality in their rat models with TPN following septic and hemorrhagic insults.

Another well-recognized benefit of EN is its prophylactic role against gastro-intestinal (GI) hemorrhage; Pingleton and Hadzima [17] claimed it to be sup-erior to either oral antacid or cimetidine. Whether this protective effect is brought about through direct substrate absorption by gastric mucosal cells [18] and/or by decreasing gastric acid secretion through changes in GI regulatory peptide levels [19] remains unknown.

Increased gut permeability has been found after major trauma [20], with SIRS [21] and with non-provision of EN [8]. Whether this association is causal or epi-phenomenonal requires further elucidation though an impaired gut barrier is probably not desirable, regardless of whether this indicates a generalized meta-bolic abnormality or hypoperfusion, or is a precursor of increased BT and endo-toxin across the bowel wall. If standard TPN and lack of direct intestinal nutri-tion contributes to the development of impaired gut integrity, the implication of covert harm can be drawn. It thus appears rational to feed the patient enterally whenever possible, even after bowel surgery where local metabolic demands may well be higher.

Does Ileus occur following Abdominal Surgery?

Small bowel peristalsis and absorptive capacity continues after surgery, even after bowel resection. Catchpole [22] found a control frequency of gastric activity of 3/min, 11–12/min in the duodenum, 6/min in the terminal ileum and of variable frequency in the colon. Following laparotomy, this motility was still present. While gastric activity remains disturbed for up to 36 h, the small bowel continues to empty. Traditionally, the reappearance of bowel sounds and passage of flatus are used to indicate that it is "safe" to recommence oral intake. However, bowel sounds mainly originate in the small intestine as a result of gas being passed from a contracting stomach. Small bowel motility may thus be normal in the absence of bowel sounds. The relationship of TPN to prolonged ileus is more likely a function of decreased gut usage than an effect of the TPN *per se*. This is possibly related to small bowel disuse atrophy. GI processing of nutrients produces trophic effects on rat intestinal histology, structure and function which do not occur with intravenous feeding [23, 24]. Weight gain, fat and nitrogen distribution differ depending on the route of delivery. Saito et al. [25] showed that intravenously fed burned guinea pigs had a reduced gut mucosal weight and thickness compared to an enterally fed group.

Is Early Enteral Feeding Better than a Delayed Start?

Early EN support has been shown to be clearly beneficial in terms of reduced complications and outcome to burns patients [26, 27]. Adams et al. [28] however found no difference in the incidence of major infection after surgery between patients fed enterally or parenterally, though delay in institution of enteral feed may have been a significant factor. Nevertheless, Moore et al. [29] did show a reduction through the use of total EN (20 to 3%) in trauma patients undergoing laparotomy as did Kudsk et al. [30] following laparotomy for blunt or penetrating abdominal trauma (38 vs 14%). This may be possibly related to earlier institution of feed. A prospective, randomized trial in trauma victims requiring surgery was performed by Moore and Jones [31]; early EN via a needle catheter jejunostomy was associated with a lower incidence of sepsis compared to EN delayed by 5 days. Moore et al. [32] performed a meta-analysis of 8 prospective, randomized trials comparing EN and TPN in high risk trauma and/or postoperative patients. 230 patients were assessed, of whom 118 had been randomized to receive EN. Though an improvement in mortality was not shown, significantly fewer septic complications (16 vs 35%, $p = 0.01$) occurred in patients receiving early EN started within a few days of surgery. Even when catheter-related sepsis was excluded, this remained significantly lower (16 vs 29%, $p = 0.03$). A recent study by Reissman et al. [33] of 161 patients undergoing elective colonic surgery randomized to receive either conventional management, with oral intake commencing after resolution of postoperative ileus, or starting a clear liquid diet on the first postoperative day followed by regular diet as tolerated thereafter, showed no difference in hospital stay or complications. 79% of patients tolerated early commencement of oral intake and advanced to normal intake within 24–48 h.

The only evidence for survival benefit from early EN in critically ill postoperative patients is indirect though does originate from the same investigators. Cerra et al. [34] studied 66 patients in whom either TPN or EN was commenced though not until 4–6 days from the onset of sepsis. No difference in subsequent mortality or morbidity was detected and EN in itself did not prevent multiple organ failure (MOF) from developing. However, a recent prospective, randomized, controlled trial of 296 patients [35] comparing early EN with a standard formula against an 'immuno-enhanced' formula containing supplemental arginine, dietary nucleotides and fish oil, where feeding was commenced within 48 h of the event necessitating ICU admission and at least 60 mL/h were administered within 96 h of the same event, showed no difference in mortality between the groups but *both* were significantly lower (p < 0.001) than that predicted by admission severity scores. The implication to be drawn is that early feeding is beneficial though this does require confirmation with a large prospective multicenter trial.

Immediate Postoperative Enteral Feeding?

Zaloga et al. [36] showed that immediate postoperative EN after abdominal surgery in rats resulted in decreased weight loss and improved wound strength compared to a group in which feeding was delayed by 72 h. Schroeder et al. [37] investigated immediate postoperative EN in patients after elective bowel resection delivered via a nasojejunal or nasoduodenal tube placed peroperatively. Successful immediate EN was achieved in 12 of the 16 patients and significantly improved wound healing was demonstrated. Though hospital stay was not significantly reduced, time to passage of flatus and first bowel motion, as well as complication rate all trended favorably compared to the control group managed in a conventional manner. We have recently undertaken a similar study in 28 patients undergoing elective small or large bowel surgery [38], the major difference between the two studies being the amount of EN delivered prior to commencement of oral intake. Our protocol used a regimen of 30 mL/h of full-strength standard formula feed commenced within 1 h of return to the ward and increases in volume of 30 mL/h at 4-hourly intervals until target calorie values were reached. We were able to achieve a mean daily calorie intake of 2086 ± 362 kcal compared to 1179 ± 388 kcal in the study by Schroeder et al. [37]. All our protocol patients tolerated immediate EN and showed a significant reduction in postoperative complications as well as a trend towards earlier hospital discharge compared to the control group (Table 1). Intestinal permeability, measured by the differential sugar (lactulose/mannitol) absorption test before and 5 days after surgery, showed a significant rise in the conventional 'starved' group but no change whatsoever in the group receiving immediate EN (Fig. 1). Another recent trial [39], albeit of just 9 patients undergoing laparoscopic colonic resection for neoplastic disease with epidural analgesia, demonstrated that immediate post-

Table 1. Clinical characteristics of patients undergoing gastrointestinal resection either given immediate EN or managed conventionally. (From [38] with permission)

Detail	Enteral feeding	Conventional feeding
n	14	14
Nausea/vomiting	1	7
Distension	2	4
Diarrhea	0	1
Bleeding duodenal ulcer	0	1
Infection (wound/urinary)	0	3
Deaths	0	1
Length of stay (days)	9.8 (6.6)	9.3 (2.8)
Days to oral intake	6	6
Days to passage at flatus	6	6
Days to defecation	4	5

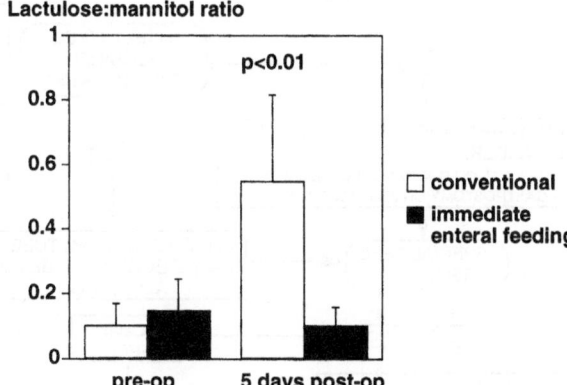

Fig. 1. Lactulose/mannitol ratio in patients receiving either immediate EN or conventional management after gastrointestinal resection

operative oral intake enhanced by 1 L of enteral protein solution was well tolerated and enabled the patients to be discharged on the 2nd–3rd postoperative day without complication.

How to feed Enterally after Surgery

EN is usually administered successfully via a nasogastric tube in the majority of intensive care patients. Figure 2 shows our intensive care unit protocol for EN. Nevertheless, a proportion, particularly after bowel surgery, will have high volumes of gastric residue secondary to gastric ileus and decreased gastric motility. Dive et al. [40] found severely impaired gastroduodenal motility in mechanically ventilated, critically ill patients compared to a control group of healthy volunteers. The stomach was markedly hypokinetic while the duodenum occasionally exhibited abnormal propagation (3 of 12 patients). As the small intestine usually continues to function immediately after surgery, it is nevertheless possible to

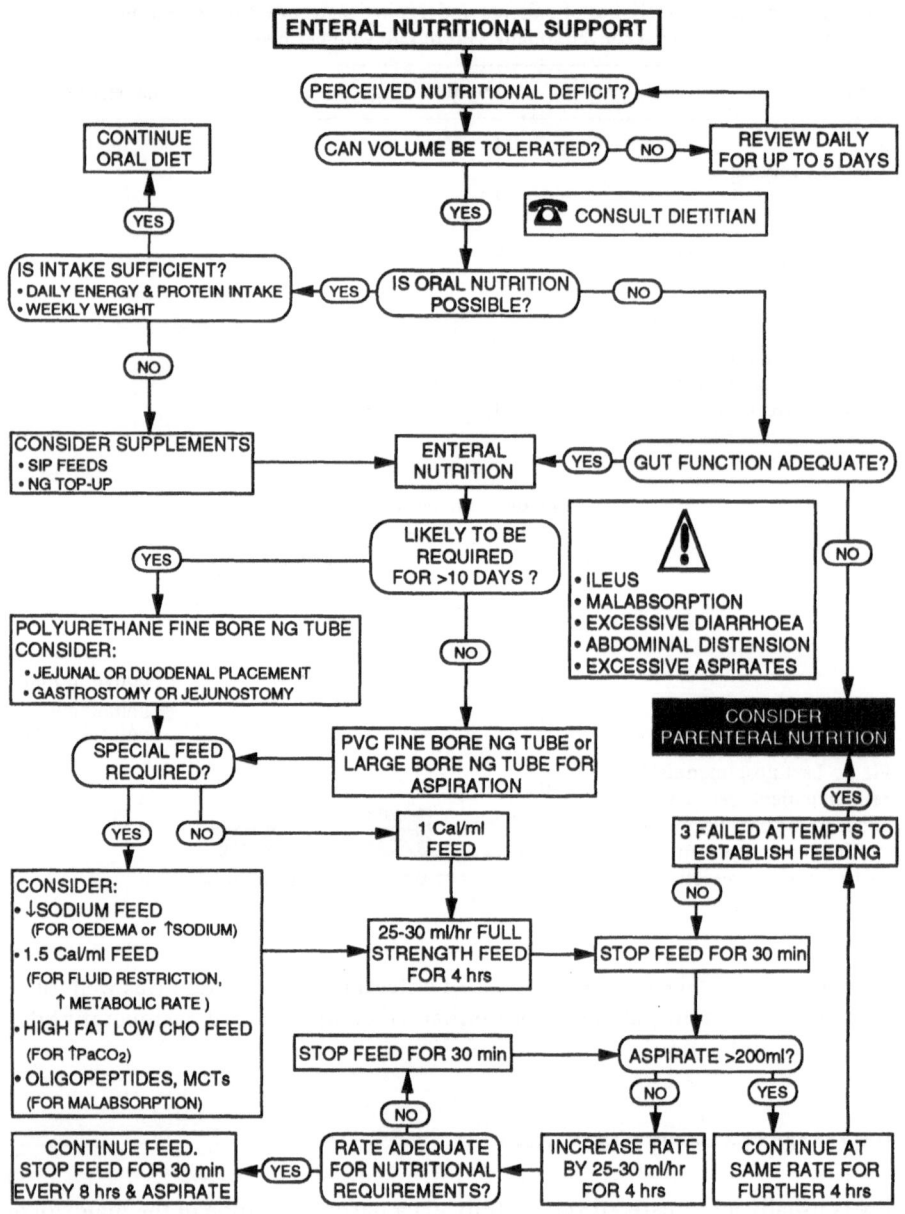

Fig. 2. University College London Hospitals Intensive Care Unit EN protocol: (MCT: medium chain triglyceride; CHO: carbohydrate; NG: nasogastric). (Reproduced with permission from Armstrong RF et al (eds) Critical Care Algorithms. (1991) Oxford University Press, Oxford)

feed most patients immediately by bypassing the stomach. The variable period of starvation traditionally endured or the need for TPN can thus be avoided. This can be achieved by insertion of a nasojejunal or nasoduodenal tube or via a jejunostomy. Adams et al. [28] showed that traumatized patients could be supported with jejunostomy feeding with equal efficacy, a similar complication rate, and with far less expense compared to TPN. Peroperative placement of a naso-duodenal or nasojejunal feeding tube in a patient undergoing abdominal surgery, with the surgeon 'milking' the tube through the pylorus, is generally successful and reasonably rapid [38]. Transpyloric placement of tubes can also be performed on the ICU either 'blind' [41], under direct vision using a fiber-optic endoscope [42] or under fluoroscopy [43]. Some newer tubes have double lumens which allow both small bowel feeding and gastric aspiration or decompression.

Fashioning of a jejunostomy, either peroperatively or percutaneously, is an alternative to transpyloric tube placement. Jones et al. [44] described successful use of a needle catheter jejunostomy placed at laparotomy for abdominal trauma victims. Early EN was commenced 12 h postoperatively. More patients complained of GI discomfort compared to a control group (83 versus 50%), but only 13% ultimately required supplementation with TPN. Another option is percutaneous endoscopic jejunostomy, though results with this technique have not proved overly encouraging with tube displacement, blockage and even aspiration pneumonia being reported [45].

Failure to feed by a nasogastric route may not infrequently be overcome by pharmacological stimulants. Metoclopramide, cisapride and erythromycin are often prescribed to intensive care patients though have been rarely examined formally in prospective controlled trials, either against placebo or each other. One recent study [46] fulfilling these criteria, albeit with only 21 patients in total, did show that cisapride significantly increased gastric emptying (mean time to 50% emptying of stomach was 18 ± 7 compared to 78 ± 40 min for patients given EN alone) and lowered gastric residue (17.7 ± 8.9 versus 94.5 ± 33.4 mL). Cisapride has also been shown to induce an earlier return of propagative colonic motility after surgery [47] and to reduce the morphine-induced delay in gastric emptying [48]. Erythromycin, which has motilin agonist and thus prokinetic properties, also increases gastric emptying [49, 50].

Medical and nursing staff should still be encouraged to persist with attempts to feed enterally. Our intensive care unit EN protocol requires three successive 200 mL gastric aspirates at 4-hourly intervals before failure to feed via the stomach is accepted and alternatives sought. Chang et al. [51] demonstrated that intensive care patients unable to tolerate EN had a higher mortality (51%) than those whose intestine remained functional (25%). Although this must be attributable to either the illness precipitating ICU admission or to GI dysfunction as a component of MOF, could the ability to feed enterally thereby providing protective and nutritive effects not otherwise achieved by TPN have some covert influence in determining outcome?

Immunonutrition?

A detailed assessment of the role of immunomodulation by specific feed supplementation is beyond the scope of this chapter and is discussed elsewhere in this book and in previous reviews [52]. However, some recent studies in postoperative patients do suggest that some additional benefit may be forthcoming. Daly et al. [53, 54] investigated the use of a standard formula supplemented with arginine, dietary nucleotides and fish oil given to patients following surgery for upper GI malignancy. Infectious complications and hospital stay were significantly reduced. A similar result was found by Bower et al. [35] in a heterogeneous group of critically ill surgical ICU patients given the same supplemented feed. Length of hospital stay was significantly shorter (8 days), and if the patient was septic on admission to the study, the hospital stay was shorter still (10 days) and the frequency of nosocomial infections was significantly reduced. However, no effect was seen on mortality.

Is EN safe in the Surgical Patient?

Apart from the rare mechanical and misplacement problems encountered during placement [55, 56] and the risk of bacterial contamination of the feed as a source of nosocomial infection [57, 58], the major concerns surround the possibility of aspiration and secondary nosocomial pneumonia [59–61], and of the threat to any bowel anastomosis present though evidence for this is lacking; if anything, direct nutrition appears to confer beneficial effects [37, 38]. Likewise, the reported occurrence of aspiration in enterally fed ICU patients is highly variable, from 0.8 to 77% [62].

Does postpyloric feeding reduce the complication rate? Strong et al. [63] showed that equal aspiration rates occurred from post-pylorus and intragastric-placed small-bore nasoenteric feeding tubes but, in contrast, Montecalvo et al. [64] found that patients fed by nasojejunal tube received a significantly higher proportion of their daily target calorie intake, had a significantly greater increase in serum prealbumin concentration and a lower rate of pneumonia than patients fed nasogastrically.

Another potential concern expressed but, as yet unproved, is that EN may cause an increased oxygen demand on a poorly perfused bowel, thereby exacerbating the degree of ischemia. A counter-argument is that the direct provision of fuel to the enterocyte may provide necessary substrate not being delivered by an inadequate blood supply. There is also a suggestion that oxygen may diffuse transluminally across the bowel wall.

Conclusion

All patients undergoing major surgery should be considered for nutritional support which, ideally, should be both enteral and early, if not immediate. Difficulties in establishing nasogastric feeding can be often overcome by the use of pharmacological stimulants or placement of distal tubes though early commencement of feed appears prokinetic in its own right. Preliminary data suggest that earlier enteral feeding is not only safe and well-tolerated but appears to reduce postoperative complications and improve outcome. Large prospective, randomized, controlled multicenter trials are required to confirm these findings.

References

1. Chandra RK (1983) Nutrition, infection and immunity: Present knowledge and future directions. Lancet 1:688–691
2. Deitch EA, Dazhong X, Qi L, Specian RD, Berg R (1992) Protein malnutrition alone and in combination with endotoxin impairs systemic and gut-associated immunity. J Parent Enteral Nutr 16:25–31
3. Shukla VK, Roy SK, Kumar J, et al (1985) Correlation of immune and nutritional status with wound complications in patients undergoing abdominal surgery. Ann Surg 51:442–445
4. Buzby GP and the VA Total Parenteral Nutrition Cooperative Study Group (1991) Perioperative total parenteral nutrition in surgical patients. A VA Cooperative study. N Engl J Med 325:525–532
5. Robinson G, Goldstein M, Levine GM (1987) Impact of nutritional status on DRG length of stay. J Parent Enteral Nutr 11:49–51
6. Deitch EA, Winterton J, Li M, Berg R (1987) The gut as a portal of entry for bacteremia. Role of protein malnutrition. Ann Surg 205:681–690
7. Clarke PJ, Ball MJ, Kettlewell MGW (1991) Liver function tests in patients receiving parenteral nutrition. J Parent Enteral Nutr 15:54–59
8. van der Hulst RR, van Kreel BK, von Meyenfeldt MF, et al (1993) Glutamine and the preservation of gut integrity. Lancet 341:1363–1365
9. Fong Y, Marano MA, Barber A, et al (1989) Total parenteral nutrition and bowel rest modify the metabolic response to endotoxin in humans. Ann Surg 210:449–456
10. Freund HR, Muggia-Sullam M, LaFrance R, et al (1985) A possible beneficial effect of metronidazole in reducing TPN-associated liver function derangements. J Surg Res 38:356–363
11. Alverdy JC, Chi HS, Sheldon GF (1985) The effect of parenteral nutrition on gastrointestinal immunity: The importance of enteral stimulation. Ann Surg 202:681–684
12. Alverdy JC, Aoys E, Moss GS (1988) Total parenteral nutrition promotes bacterial translocation from the gut. Surgery 104:185–190
13. Delany HM, John J, The EL, et al (1994) Contrasting effects of identical nutrients given parenterally or enterally after 70% hepatectomy. Am J Surg 167:135–144
14. Rock CS, Barber AE, Ng EH, et al (1990) TPN vs oral feeding: Bacterial translocation, cytokine response and mortality following E. coli LPS administration. Surg Forum 41:14–20
15. Kudsk KA, Stone JM, Carpenter G, Sheldon GF (1983) Enteral and parenteral feeding influences mortality after E. coli peritonitis in normal rats. J Trauma 23:605–609
16. Zaloga GP, Knowles R, Black KW, Prielipp R (1990) Total parenteral nutrition increases mortality after hemorrhage. Crit Care Med 19:54–59
17. Pingleton SK, Hadzima S (1983) Enteral alimentation and gastrointestinal bleeding in mechanically ventilated patients. Crit Care Med 11:13–16
18. Lally KP, Andrassy RJ, Foster JE, et al (1984) Evaluation of various nutritional supplements in the prevention of stress-induced gastric ulcers in the rat. Surg Gynecol Obstet 158:124–128
19. Layon A, Florete OG, Day AL, et al (1991) The effect of duodenojejunal alimentation on gastric pH and hormones in intensive care patients. Chest 99:695–702
20. Roumen RM, Hendriks T, Wevers RA, Goris JA (1993) Intestinal permeability after severe trauma and hemorrhagic shock is increased without relation to septic complications. Arch Surg 128:453–457
21. Pape HC, Dwenger A, Regel G, et al (1994) Increased gut permeability after multiple trauma. Br J Surg 81:850–852
22. Catchpole BN (1989) Smooth muscle and the surgeon. Austr NZ J Surg 59:199–208

23. McManus JPA, Isselbacher KJ (1970) Effects of fasting versus feeding on the rat small intestine. Morphological, biochemical and functional differences. Gastroenterology 49: 214–221
24. Johnson LR, Copeland EM, Dudrick SJ, Lichtenburger LM, Castro GA (1975) Structural and hormonal alterations in the gastrointestinal tract of parenterally fed rats. Gastroenterology 68:1177–1183
25. Saito H, Trocki O, Alexander JW, et al (1987) The effect of route of nutrient administration on the nutritional state, catabolic hormone secretion, and gut mucosal integrity after burn injury. J Parent Enteral Nutr 11:1–7
26. Chiarelli A, Enzi G, Casadei A, et al (1990) Very early nutrition supplementation in burned patients. Am J Clin Nutr 5:1035–1039
27. McDonald WS, Sharp CW, Deitch EA (1991) Immediate enteral feeding in burn patients is safe and effective. Ann Surg 213:177–183
28. Adams S, Dellinger EP, Wertz MJ, et al (1986) Enteral versus parenteral nutritional support following laparotomy for trauma: A randomized prospective trial. J Trauma 26:882–891
29. Moore FA, Moore EE, Jones TN, et al (1989) TEN versus TPN following major abdominal trauma reduced septic morbidity. J Trauma 29:916–921
30. Kudsk KA, Croce MA, Fabian TC, et al (1991) Enteral versus parenteral feeding: Effects on septic morbidity after blunt and penetrating abdominal trauma. Ann Surg 213:503–513
31. Moore EE, Jones TN (1986) Benefits of immediate jejunal feeding after major abdominal trauma: A prospective, randomized study. J Trauma 26:874–880
32. Moore FA, Feliciano DV, Andrassey RJ, et al (1992) Early enteral feeding, compared with parenteral, reduces postoperative septic complications: The results of a meta-analysis. Ann Surg 216:62–69
33. Reissman P, Teoh TA, Cohen SM, Weiss EG, Nogueras JJ, Wexner SD (1995) Is early oral feeding safe after elective colorectal surgery? Ann Surg 222:73–77
34. Cerra FB, McPherson JP, Konstantinides FN, Konstantinides NN, Teasley KM (1988) Enteral nutrition does not prevent multiple organ failure syndrome after sepsis. Surgery 104: 727–733
35. Bower RH, Cerra FB, Bershadsky B, et al (1995) Early enteral administration of a formula (Impact) supplemented with arginine, nucleotides, and fish oil in intensive care unit patients: Results of a multicenter, prospective, randomized clinical trial. Crit Care Med 23:436–449
36. Zaloga GP, Bortenschlager L, Ward Black K, Prielipp R (1992) Immediate postoperative enteral feeding decreases weight loss and improves wound healing after abdominal surgery in rats. Crit Care Med 20:115–118
37. Schroeder D, Gillanders L, Mahr K, Hill GL (1991) Effects of immediate postoperative enteral nutrition on body composition, muscle function and wound healing. J Parent Enteral Nutr 15:376–383
38. Carr C, Ling E, Boulos P, Singer M (1996) Immediate post-operative enteral feeding is safe and effective in patients who have had gastrointestinal resections. Br Med J 312:869–871
39. Bardram L, Funch-Jensen P, Jensen P, Crawford ME, Kehlet H (1995) Recovery after laparoscope colonic surgery with epidural analgesia, and early oral nutrition and mobilisation. Lancet 345:763–764
40. Dive A, Moulart M, Jonard P, Jamart J, Mahieu P (1994) Gastroduodenal motility in mechanically ventilated critically ill patients: A manometric study. Crit Care Med 22:441–447
41. Zaloga GP (1991) Bedside method for placing small bowel feeding tubes in critically ill patients. A prospective study. Chest 100:1643–1648
42. Hudspeth DA, Thorne MT, Meredith JW (1992) A prospective evaluation of a simplified endoscopic technique for nasoenteric feeding tube placement. Crit Care Med 20:58S (Abst)
43. Silk DBA, Rees RG, Keohane PP, Attrill H (1987) Clinical efficacy and design changes of 'fine-bore' nasogastric feeding tubes: A seven year experience involving 809 intubations in 403 patients. J Parent Enteral Nutr 11:378–383
44. Jones TN, Moore FA, Moore EE, McCroskey BL (1989) Gastrointestinal symptoms attributed to jejunostomy feeding after major abdominal trauma: A critical analysis. Crit Care Med 17:1146–1150

45. Henderson JM, Strodel WE, Gilinsky NH (1983) Limitations of percutaneous endoscopic jejunostomy. J Parent Enteral Nutr 17:546–550
46. Spaden HD, Duinslaeger L, Diltoer M, et al (1995) Gastric emptying in critically ill patients is accelerated by adding cisapride to a standard enteral feeding protocol: Results of a prospective, randomized, controlled trial. Crit Care Med 23:481–485
47. Tollesson PO, Cassuto J, Rimback G, et al (1991) Treatment of postoperative paralytic ileus with cisapride. Scand J Gastroenterol 26:477–482
48. Rowbotham DJ, Nimmo WS (1987) Effect of cisapride on morphine-induced delay in gastric emptying. Br J Anaesth 59:536–539
49. Keshavarzian A, Isaac RM (1993) Erythromycin accelerates gastric emptying of indigestible solids and transpyloric migration of the tip of an enteral feeding tube in fasting and fed states. Am J Gastroenterol 88:193–197
50. Weber FH Jr, Richards RD, McCallum RW (1993) Erythromycin: A motilin agonist and gastrointestinal prokinetic agent. Am J Gastroenterol 88:485–490
51. Chang RW, Jacobs S, Lee B (1987) Gastrointestinal dysfunction among intensive care unit patients. Crit Care Med 15:909–914
52. Heyland DK, Cook DJ, Guyatt GH (1994) Does the formulation of enteral feeding products influence infectious morbidity and mortality rates in the critically ill patient? A critical review of the evidence. Crit Care Med 22:1192–1202
53. Daly JM, Lieberman MD, Goldfine J, et al (1992) Enteral nutrition with supplemental arginine, RNA, and omega-3 fatty acids in patients after operation. Immunologic, metabolic, and clinical outcome. Surgery 112:56–67
54. Daly JM, Weintraub FM, Shou J, Rosato EF, Lucia M (1995) Enteral nutrition during multimodality therapy in upper gastrointestinal cancer patients. Ann Surg 221:327–338
55. Valentine SJ, Turner WW (1985) Pleural complications of nasoenteric feeding tubes. J Parent Enteral Nutr 9:605–607
56. Roubenoff R, Ravich WJ (1989) Pneumothorax due to nasogastric feeding tubes: Report of four cases, review of the literature and recommendations for prevention. Arch Intern Med 149:184–188
57. Anderson KR, Norris DJ, Godfrey LB, Avent CK, Butterworth CE (1984) Bacterial contamination of tube-feeding formulas. J Parent Enteral Nutr 8:673–678
58. Levy J, Van Laethem Y, Verhaegen G, et al (1989) Contaminated enteral nutrition solutions as a cause of nosocomial bloodstream infection: A study using plasmid fingerprinting. J Parent Enteral Nutr 13:228–234
59. Heyland DK, Cook DJ, Guyatt GH (1993) Enteral nutrition in the critically ill patient: A critical review of the literature. Intensive Care Med 19: 435–442
60. Cook DJ, Laine LA, Guyatt GH, Raffin T (1991) Nosocomial pneumonia and the role of gastric pH: A meta-analysis. Chest 100: 7–13
61. Pingleton SK, Hinthorn DR, Liu C (1986) Enteral nutrition in patients receiving mechanical ventilation. Am J Med 80: 827–832
62. Pingleton SK (1994) Aspiration of enteral feeding in mechanically ventilated patients. How do we monitor? Crit Care Med 22: 1524–1525
63. Strong RM, Condon SC, Solinger MR, et al (1992) Equal aspiration rates from postpylorus and intragastric-placed small-bore nasoenteric feeding tubes: A randomized prospective study. J Parent Enteral Nutr 16: 59–63
64. Montecalvo MA, Steger KA, Farber HW, et al (1992) Nutritional outcome and pneumonia in critical care patients randomized to gastric versus jejunal tube feeding. Crit Care Med 20: 1377–1387

Glutamine: A Gut Essential Amino Acid

R. R. W. J. van der Hulst, M. F. von Meyenfeldt, and P. B. Soeters

Introduction

The fact that nutritional support cannot completely abolish the increase in morbidity and mortality observed in nutritionally depleted patients [1] has resulted in the development of completely new "organ specific nutrients" with the purpose to increase host defense mechanisms. Each of these nutrients has its specific effect on a certain target organ [2]. In evaluating nutritional modulation, it is necessary to realize that the effect on overall clinical outcome is very difficult to assess and requires large numbers of patients. Therefore, the clinical relevance of a specific nutrient has to be assessed by studying effects in its target organ, eg the gut. This chapter discusses the effect of one of these "new" nutrients, glutamine, on the intestine.

Glutamine is a classically non-essential amino acid, implying that it is produced at a sufficient rate to adequately supply glutamine consuming tissues. Of all the amino acids incorporated into protein, glutamine is the most abundant amino acid in the human body. Its blood concentration varies between 0.4 and 0.9 mmol/L [3], which is the highest of all amino acids. Excluding taurine which is a non-proteinogenic amino acid, 50% of the total free amino acid pool consists of glutamine. In addition, glutamine has the most versatile function of all amino acids [4]. Glutamine has two nitrogen residues (an amino and an amide group), making it quantitatively the most important non-toxic nitrogen "transporter", accounting for 35% of all amino acid nitrogen transported in the blood. Glutamine also serves as a non-toxic carrier for ammonia. The first step in the degradation of glutamine is a deamination step, yielding ammonia. Degradation of glutamine mainly takes place in tissues that are anatomically situated in such a way that the subsequent release of ammonia is without risk because the ammonia is either excreted (kidney) or converted to urea (liver). Consequently, glutamine is the most important substrate for ammoniagenesis allowing it to play a role in the regulation of acid/base homeostasis in the kidney [5]. Glutamine may be involved in the regulation of protein synthesis and provides precursors for nucleotide and protein synthesis and the production of radical scavengers [4, 6]. Most importantly however, glutamine is the major fuel for rapidly replicating cells, such as immune cells and enterocytes [7, 8]. The main site of production of glutamine in the postabsorptive state is muscle tissue [9]. Because the extent of glutamine production capacity greatly exceeds the amount of glutamine incorporated in protein and present in the intracellular pool, glutamine must be largely derived from *de novo* synthesis. It has been shown that the most important nitrogen donors for this *de novo* synthesis are the branched chain amino acids released by protein breakdown [10]. Glutamine may also be released from the brain, heart, lungs and adipose tissue albeit these organs are probably quantitatively less important [11]. Uptake of glutamine largely takes place in the splanchnic area (gut, spleen, pancreas) [12], kidney [13] and by the immune system [14]. The liver is capable of both synthesizing and degrading glutamine, depending on several factors like ammonia concentration, pH and degree of metabolic stress. Under normal non-stressed physiological conditions, however, the breakdown and synthesis of glutamine in the liver are comparable resulting in a close-to-zero liver glutamine balance (Fig. 1).

From work carried out over the past two decades, it is now clear that glutamine is involved in multiple biochemical cell reactions, and has important roles in tissue-specific and inter-tissue physiology. It was recognized that muscle free glutamine concentrations are markedly declined during conditions involving metabolic stress [2, 4]. From these observations, the non-essential character of glutamine was questioned, and exogenous supply was considered of potential benefit during metabolic stress. A decline of the glutamine "pool" was thought to have especially consequences for tissues consuming glutamine at high rates such as the gut and the immune tissues. It is hypothesized that, in depleted patients and in patients suffering from severe metabolic stress, the intestinal glutamine supply becomes insufficient due to depleted free glutamine pools or due to decreased capacity to produce glutamine. In this chapter, the current knowledge concerning glutamine and the gut in nutritional depletion and critical illness is reviewed.

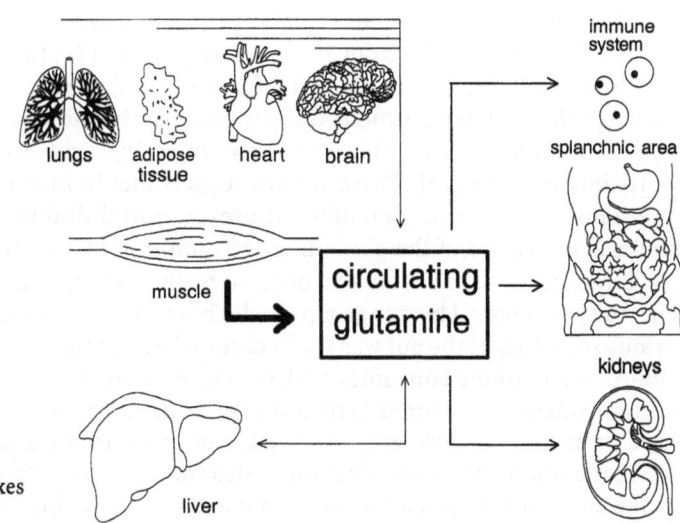

Fig. 1. Interorgan fluxes of glutamine

Glutamine Uptake by the Gut

Initial attention for glutamine as a metabolically important substrate came from the observation that glutamine is an essential nutrient for cells in culture [15]. First, fibroblasts were shown to be dependent of glutamine for their growth. The first reports suggesting consumption of glutamine by the gut were published in the 1960's. Neptune [16] discussed glutamine metabolism in the intestine observing the oxidation of ^{14}C glutamine to $^{14}CO_2$ *in vitro* in various animal species. Windmueller and Spaeth [8, 17] unequivocally demonstrated that glutamine was a major respiratory fuel for enterocytes *in vivo*. Enterocytes were shown to utilize glutamine to a greater extent than any other fuel source, even glucose. *In vivo* perfusion studies revealed that glutamine accounted for 55% of the respired CO_2, whereas acetoacetate and glucose together accounted for only 20% [8, 17]. Approximately 15% of the glutamine carbon is incorporated into protein [18]. Another 30% was discovered in lactate, citrate, citrulline, alanine, proline and several quantitatively less important amino acids. Glutamine nitrogen appears for 97% in ammonia, alanine, citrulline and proline. A small amount appears in glutamate and ornithine [8]. It is, however, important to realize that most of the *in vivo* studies concerned the metabolism of all portal drained viscera (including spleen and pancreas) rather than the gut alone. In addition, a substantial part of the gut (about 25%) consists of immune cells also consuming glutamine at a high rate. Thus, at least a part of the glutamine consumption by the gut may be caused by consumption of immune cells. A distinction can be made by the fact that *in vitro* studies showed that aspartate is a main product of glutamine metabolism in lymphocytes whereas almost no aspartate is produced by enterocytes. Aspartate not being an important end-product in the *in vivo* studies suggests that most of the glutamine is consumed by enterocytes.

Early *in vivo* human studies in which arterial and hepatic venous blood was sampled did not provide information concerning the relative contribution of the liver and the other splanchnic organs to amino acid metabolism [19, 20]. More recently, glutamine extraction by the portal drained viscera in humans was studied. Extraction varies from 3% in septic patients [21] to 14% in healthy individuals undergoing elective surgery for uncomplicated cholelithiasis [22]. In trauma patients, arterio-venous differences of amino acids were studied several days after surgery. Glutamine was the only amino acid extracted at a rate of approximately 15% [23]. These studies suggest that in man the gut is indeed an important consumer of glutamine. However, portal drained viscera glutamine uptake is indicative of the glutamine consumption by not only the small intestine, large intestine and stomach, but also by the pancreas and spleen [24]. A recent study performed by our group in which selective *in vivo* glutamine uptake at various segments of the gut was studied, revealed that the gut in man is indeed an important glutamine consumer [25]. Glutamine consumption was the highest in jejunum where a fractional extraction (percentage glutamine from the arterial blood extracted) of 30% was observed, compared to a fractional extraction of 10% in the colon and ileum. This study also showed a relation between glutamine uptake and arterial glutamine levels in the ileum. A decline in plasma glutamine may therefore result in decreased uptake of glutamine by the gut. In conclusion, there is convincing evidence that glutamine is extracted by the human gut.

Glutamine Supplementation

In the normal healthy man, glutamine is produced mainly by muscle tissue and in sufficient quantity to supply the gut and the immune system. There are, however, conditions in which the endogenous glutamine supply to the gut may become insufficient. In these conditions, exogenous glutamine supplementation may be beneficial by preventing a deterioration of gut function. Baskerville et al. [26] induced decreased circulating glutamine levels in various species using parenteral administration of glutaminase. This process was associated with edema and ulcerations of the intestinal mucosa. Conditions in which glutamine supply may become insufficient include the use of total parenteral nutrition (TPN), nutritional depletion and metabolic stress. Most commercial TPN solutions are lacking glutamine [4]. Due to decreased exogenous supply of glutamine, the prolonged use of TPN may therefore result in an insufficient supply of glutamine to tissues such as the gut. Nutritional depletion will result in decreased muscle mass on the one hand, and changes in intermediary metabolism on the other hand. Both may lead to decreased glutamine production capacity. During severe metabolic stress, glutamine utilization increases probably by an increased demand by the immune system [24]. Ongoing utilization of glutamine will eventually lead to a depletion of the glutamine pool. The risk of developing a glutamine deficiency depends on the combination and severity of each of these factors. For instance, it is unlikely that only the use of TPN will result in a glutamine deficiency, because there is sufficient supply of glutamine precursors to produce glutamine. However, in the clinical situation, TPN is often given to nutritionally depleted patients and/or patients with increased metabolic stress. These patients are more sensitive to develop a glutamine depletion (Fig. 2).

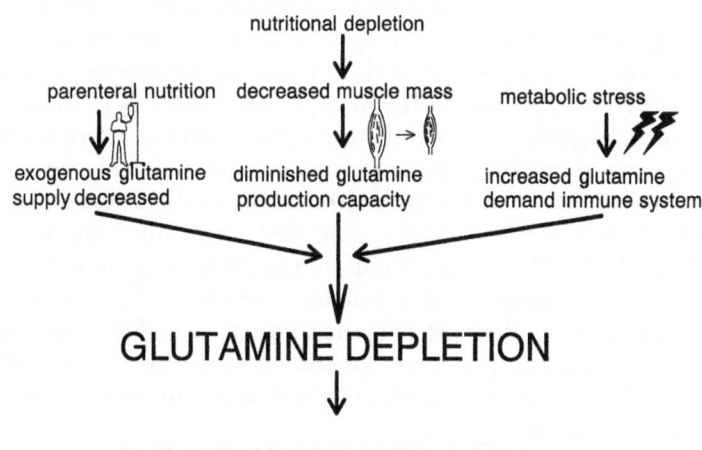

Fig. 2. Factors contributing to glutamine deficiency

In addition to the above mentioned factors, exogenous glutamine supply may also be beneficial in organ specific diseases like enterocolitis. The conditions in which glutamine supplementation is of interest will be discussed.

Parenteral Glutamine Supplementation in Animal Experiments

The villus atrophy frequently observed during TPN is ascribed to the absence of glutamine in commercially available amino acid solutions [4]. There are many animal studies investigating the effect of glutamine supplementation in TPN on gut function. Many studies performed in animals comparing the effect of standard TPN with glutamine-containing TPN on gut mucosa morphology demonstrate that glutamine supplementation attenuates mucosa atrophy [27–34]. The effect was comparable whether glutamine was given as a dipeptide or as a free amino acid [30]. Beyond a preserving effect on the intestinal mucosa, TPN supplemented with glutamine has also been shown to preserve smooth muscle morphology in the gut [32]. The effect of glutamine on gut immune status is demonstrated by the augmentation of IgA and IgM producing cells in the lamina propria, increased biliary s-IgA levels, and increased T-lymphocytes if glutamine is given [35, 36]. The combined effect of glutamine on the mucosal and immunological part of the intestine may explain the beneficial effects observed on gut integrity [37, 38] and bacterial translocation [36]. Although most studies have reported beneficial effects of glutamine supplementation on gut function and morphology, it is important to discuss the studies in which the effect of glutamine supplementation was not confirmed [39–41]. An important factor interfering with the observed effects of glutamine supplementation is the nutritional support given. In most animal experiments, nutritional solutions include only amino acids and dextrose. If a balanced "all in one" solution was given, including a fat emulsion, with adequate energy supply, the addition of glutamine had no effect on intestinal morphology. The effect of glutamine supplementation has been claimed to be reduced due to the trophic effect of intravenous lipid administration inducing stimulation of glucagon secretion [40]. Furthermore, intestinal protein synthesis was shown to be more activated by lipids compared to glutamine administration [42]. In addition, the degree of nutritional depletion may be an important factor in explaining differences in effect observed after parenteral glutamine administration; the beneficial effect of glutamine administration is more clearly demonstrated in starvation-induced atrophy of the small bowel [31, 34]. Finally, the degree of metabolic stress is an important determinant of the effect of exogenous glutamine administration. This is demonstrated by the effect of glutamine administration in endotoxemic rats. Rats given a continuous infusion of endotoxin have diminished endotoxin uptake by the gut and less morphological deterioration if parenteral glutamine is administered [38]. In addition, parenteral glutamine administration attenuates histological changes, and increases protein synthesis in intestinal mucosa in rats injected with *E. coli* [27].

Enteral Glutamine Supplementation in Animal Experiments

Compared to TPN, enteral nutrition (EN) has several advantages, one being the specific beneficial effect on gut function and morphology. EN is preferred because gut starvation, possibly inducing septic complications, is prevented. EN, already containing glutamine, supplemented with glutamine is therefore theoretically less likely to have the same effect compared to TPN supplemented with glutamine. Nevertheless, some studies report beneficial effects of enteral supplementation with glutamine. It is important to notice that these studies were performed in severely stressed animals. Bacterial translocation (BT) was lower in burned mice receiving a glutamine enriched diet compared to rats receiving an elemental diet. However, a chow diet was comparable or even better in preventing translocation [43, 44]. Endotoxin-induced changes in intestinal permeability can be prevented by luminal glutamine infusion [45]. In gut derived sepsis, enteral glutamine supplementation was shown to contribute to a decrease in BT and increased survival [46, 47]. No effect of glutamine supplementation was observed on BT after hemorrhage in rats [48], and on mucosal architecture after turpentine injections [49]. A question that should also be addressed if glutamine is given enterally is whether glutamine as a free amino acid added to the nutritional regimen remains stable in the stomach and is resorbed simultaneously with the amino acids derived from protein digestion. One study does not employ glutamine as a free amino acid or as a peptide but uses a combination of partially hydrolyzed wheat and casein proteins yielding 25% of glutamine of the protein given largely protected against gastric deamination inside the peptide chain. This study did not demonstrate an effect of feeding such a protein on the catabolic response to a zymosan challenge in rats [50]. The effect on gut mucosa, however, was not studied. In conclusion, the effect of glutamine supplementation in animal experiments depends on the degree of metabolic stress, the degree of nutritional depletion, and the way by which enteral glutamine is given.

Glutamine as a Mucosa Protectant

An interesting therapeutic area is the use of glutamine as a gut protectant during radiation therapy. The studies on glutamine as a mucosa protectant during radiotherapy are contradictory. Compared to a glutamine free diet, glutamine containing diets were shown to have a protective effect on BT and intestinal structure [51]. Later, it was found that the addition of glutamine to a chow diet was protective against radiation-induced damage [52]. McArdle [53] did not find an effect on BT if glutamine was added to a glutamine free diet. A potential explanation was given by the fact that the elemental diets used as control diets varied extensively between the different studies. In the last study mentioned, a decrease in radical scavengers was observed. McArdle therefore seriously questions the use of glutamine in radiation-induced enterocolitis because a decrease in scavengers may result in decreased protection of the intestine. Another explanation may be that the need of scavengers is decreased as a result of a decrease of oxygen radical formation resulting from less translocation. Parenteral gluta-mine administration has been shown to have no effect on morphology after radiation [54].

Several studies have examined the effect of glutamine-enriched diets on chemotherapeutic-induced enterocolitis. Glutamine enriched diets have been shown to have a protective effect on experimentally induced enterocolitis on intestinal structure, BT and survival [55, 56].

Glutamine Supplementation in Man

Clinical trials designed to investigate glutamine effects initially focused on safety of the intravenous administration of glutamine. On the one hand, studies were performed to investigate the safety of the administration of intravenous L-gluta-mine [57], whereas on the other hand, studies mainly described the alternative form of glutamine administration in the form of a dipeptide (glycyl-glutamine, alanyl-glutamine) [58]. The potential toxicity of glutamine administration re-sides in the fact that glutamine deaminates to form ammonia and potentially toxic L-pyrrolidone carboxylic acid (pyroglutamic acid) during prolonged sto-rage or heat sterilization [57]. In addition, it can be metabolized to ammonia and glutamic acid in the body.

The effect of storage on the stability of L-glutamine containing solutions is minimal. The breakdown of L-glutamine containing solutions stored at 4°C is less than 2% over a period of two weeks [59]. Studies investigating the safety of intravenous L-glutamine administration in control subjects and patients did not show any clinical or biochemical side effects if glutamine was given in a dosage of 0.57 g/kg/day [57]. From these studies, it was concluded that glutamine can be given in its free form. It is important, however, to notice that during shelf storage breakdown of glutamine may become relevant. In addition, even heating for short periods (sterilization) may cause a substantial breakdown of glutamine. Therefore, the preparation of L-glutamine containing solutions requires special care in the pharmacy. An alternative may be the use of glutamine containing stable dipeptides. These dipeptides (alanyl-glutamine and glycyl-glutamine) are hydrolyzed and cleared rapidly form plasma [58]. Metabolism is efficient in healthy controls as well as in critically ill and postoperative patients.

Because there are indications that glutamine pools may become depleted in man, glutamine supplementation may be beneficial. After surgery, there is ap-proximately a 50% fall of muscle glutamine concentration [60]. Glutamine plas-ma concentrations decrease with 10 to 30%, and only slowly return to normal values during convalescence. In severe metabolic stress such as sepsis, the chan-ges in muscle glutamine levels are even more pronounced: they may decrease with 95% of the normal concentration [61]. Plasma amino acids decrease with about 50% [61]. We observed a decrease in mucosal alanine and glutamine con-centration of respectively 30 and 10% in nutritionally depleted patients [62]. This was associated with a decline in plasma glutamine and alanine. Glutamine sup-plementation may therefore be indicated in these patients.

Data on the effect of glutamine supplementation on the gut in humans are scarce. A study in bone marrow transplanted patients showed a decrease of clinical infections and hospital stay in patients who received glutamine enriched TPN [63]. In another study in cancer patients hospital stay was reduced [64]. One study did not confirm these results. However, this study was performed in a small group of patients [65]. A possible explanation for the beneficial effects of glutamine may be its protecting effect on the mucosa.

If TPN is supplemented with glutamine, the mucosa and plasma glutamine levels increased significantly in patients with inflammatory bowel disease and cancer [66]. Interestingly, this increase in glutamine concentration was limited to the nutritionally depleted patients. Glutamine-enriched TPN also preserved intestinal morphology and integrity in this patient group [67]. The beneficial effects of glutamine supplementation in TPN were confirmed in a study in intensive care patients [68]. In six patients receiving glutamine-enriched TPN, the intestinal absorption capacity measured with the D-xylose method was significantly improved compared to six patients receiving standard TPN. The effect of glutamine on intestinal proliferation was investigated in an *ex vivo* study [69]. Human intestinal biopsies were shown to have increased proliferative activity when they were incubated with glutamine either as a free amino acid or as a dipeptide.

Another indication for the beneficial effect of glutamine on the intestine comes from two studies of the one group investigating the effect of administration of glutamine, growth hormone and a modified diet in patients with short bowel syndrome [70, 71]. Absorption of protein and carbohydrate was improved, resulting in a decreased stool output. In a follow up period of 1 year, 40% of the patients came off their TPN, in another 40% the amount of TPN could be reduced, and the remaining 20% required an unaltered TPN regimen.

These results are very promising. As these studies were uncontrolled, further confirmation is necessary, first to assess whether admission to a center specialized in the treatment of short bowel disease itself may reduce TPN requirement, and second to assess what is the contribution of the different aspects of the treatment on outcome.

One important question which should be solved is the amount of glutamine to be given. In the studies performed, dosages varied from 0.2 until 0.6 g glutamine/kg bodyweight. The beneficial effect on gut function and morphology was observed if 0.2 g was given. It is unclear whether the amount of 0.6 g used in bone marrow transplanted patients and short bowel patients is necessary to obtain a benefit.

In conclusion, there is increasing evidence that glutamine may become an essential nutrient for the gut in conditions were the endogenous glutamine production is insufficient. Due to a decrease of the plasma glutamine concentration, the uptake of glutamine by the gut will be reduced. A decline in the plasma glutamine concentration may be caused by nutritional depletion, increased metabolic stress and/or TPN. Nutritionally depleted patients undergoing surgery and in need of TPN should therefore receive glutamine-supplemented TPN. The increasing evidence of the beneficial effect of TPN supplemented with glutamine cannot automatically be applied to promote glutamine enrichment in EN. Because EN already includes glutamine, there may be no additional effect or only a minimal effect of glutamine supplementation. One should be careful in promoting the use of EN enriched with glutamine because at this moment there is no controlled trial published indicating a beneficial effect of glutamine in the enteral diet.

How does Glutamine work?

The physiological mechanism by which glutamine exerts its effect on the intestine is largely unknown. Several potential mechanisms may be involved. First, glutamine is used as a fuel and precursor for DNA synthesis in the rapidly dividing cells in the intestine. Decreased enterocyte formation could be the result of a lack of glutamine. Proliferation will decrease and villus atrophy will develop. The relation between villus atrophy and glutamine has already been discussed. In addition to decreased cell proliferation, the cell life span may also be decreased resulting in preterm cell death and or decreased quality of the enterocyte. Synthesis of important proteins, such as the proteins necessary for the formation of tight junctions may be diminished [72]. In addition, glutamine may serve as a regulator of the spontaneous life span of proteins [73].

A second pathway by which glutamine may have an effect is by the stimulation of immune cells. Glutamine has been shown to have several immunological functions [14]. The intestine is one of the most important immune cells containing organs. These immune cells are part of the intestinal barrier, protecting the host against translocation of bacteria and/or their products. The beneficial effect of glutamine on BT may be explained by the immune cell preserving effect of glutamine.

A third possible beneficial effect of glutamine may be the stimulatory effect of blood flow through the intestine. Flynn et al. [74] studied the effect of glutamine on intestinal blood flow after hemorrhage. Glutamine attenuated the flow impairment during hemorrhage by dilation of previllous arterioles, and overrided the effect of hemorrhage suggesting a mechanism for preserving mucosal energy supply.

Intestinal ischemia is associated with the generation of reactive oxygen intermediates (ROI). These ROI are thought to have an effect on the intestinal barrier. ROI are degraded by scavengers such as glutathione. Glutamine is essential for the production of glutathione. Harward et al. [75] observed a preservation of intestinal glutathione levels in glutamine-supplemented rats after ischemia/reperfusion.

Finally, glutamine could serve as a secretagogue, stimulating the elaboration of peptide hormones such as glucagon, exerting stimulatory effects on the mucosa. An indication for this mechanism is given by the observation that the glucagon concentration is increased in the portal circulation during glutamine administration [76].

Conclusion

In periods of severe metabolic stress, during nutritional depletion and/or insufficient nutritional support, the endogenous supply of the amino acid glutamine may become insufficient. This has consequences for glutamine consuming tissues such as the gut and the immune system. Uptake of glutamine by the gut has been shown in animals as well as in man. Glutamine supplementation of parenteral nutrition preserves gut morphology and function in man. A beneficial effect of enteral nutrition enriched with glutamine has still to be established in man.

References

1. Von Meyenfeldt MF, Meyerink WJ, Rouflart MM, Buil-Maassen MT, Soeters PB (1992) Perioperative nutritional support: A randomised clinical trial. Clin Nutr 11:180-186
2. Grimble KG (1993) Essential and conditionally-essential nutrients in clinical nutrition. Nutrition Res Rev 6:97-119
3. Van Eijk HM, Dejong CH, Deutz NE, Soeters PB (1994) Influence of storage conditions on normal plasma amino acid concentrations. Clin Nutr 13:374-380
4. Lacey JM, Wilmore DW (1990) Is glutamine a conditionally essential amino acid? Nutr Rev 48:297-309
5. Halperin ML, Ethier JH, Kamel KS (1990) The excretion of ammonium ions and acid base balance. Clin Biochem 23:185-188
6. Hong RW, Rounds JD, Helton WS, Robinson MK, Wilmore DW (1992) Glutamine preserves liver glutathione after lethal hepatic injury. Ann Surg 215:114-119
7. Ardawi MS, Newsholme EA (1983) Glutamine metabolism in lymphocytes of the rat. Biochem J 212:835-842
8. Windmueller HG (1982) Glutamine utilization by the small intestine. Adv Enzym 53: 201-237
9. Souba WW (1987) Interorgan ammonia metabolism in health and disease: A surgeon's view. J Parent Enteral Nutr 11:569-579
10. Darmaun D, Déchelotte P (1991) Role of leucine as a precursor of glutamine α-amino nitrogen *in vivo* in humans. Am J Phys 260:E326-E329
11. Elia M (1993) Glutamine metabolism in human adipose tissue *in vivo*. Clin Nutr 12:51-53
12. Dudrick PS, Souba WW (1991) The role of glutamine in nutrition. Curr Opin Gastro 7: 299-305
13. Welbourne TC, Joshi S (1990) Interorgan glutamine metabolism during acidosis. J Parent Enteral Nutr 14:77S-88S
14. Calder PC (1994) Glutamine and the immune system. Clin Nutr 13:2-8
15. Eagle H (1955) Nutrition needs of mammalian cells in tissue cultures. Science 122:501-504
16. Neptune EM Jr (1965) Respiration and oxidation of various substrates by ileum *in vitro*. Am J Phys 209:329-332
17. Windmueller HG, Spaeth AE (1980) Respiratory fuels and nitrogen metabolism *in vivo* in small intestine of fed rats. J Biol Chem 255:107-112
18. Windmueller HG, Spaeth AE (1974) Uptake and metabolism of plasma glutamine by the small intestine. J Biol Chem 249:5070-5079
19. Erikson LS, Olsson M, Björk O (1988) Splanchnic metabolism of amino acids in healthy subjects: Effect of 60 hours of fasting. Metabolism 37:1159-1162
20. Marliss EB, Aoki TT, Pozefsky T, Most AS, Cahill GF (1971) Muscle and splanchnic glutamine and glutamate metabolism in postabsorptive and starved man. J Clin Invest 50:814-817
21. Souba WW, Herskowitz K, Klimberg VS, et al (1990) The effects of sepsis and endotoxemia on gut glutamine metabolism. Ann Surg 211:543-551

22. Felig P, Wahren J, Karl I, Cerasi E, Luft R, Kipnis DM (1973) Glutamine and glutamate metabolism in normal and diabetic subjects. Diabetes 22:573–576
23. Mc Anena OJ, Moore FA, Moore EE, Jones TN, Parsons P (1991) Selective uptake of glutamine in the gastrointestinal tract: Confirmation in a human study. Br J Surg 78:480–482
24. Deutz NE, Reijven PL, Athanasas G, Soeters PB (1992) Post-operative changes in hepatic, intestinal, splenic and muscle fluxes of amino acids and ammonia in pigs. Clin Science 83:607–613
25. Van der Hulst RR, von Meyenfeldt MF, Deutz NE, Soeters PB (1996) Glutamine uptake by the gut is reduced in depleted gastrointestinal cancer patients. Ann Surg (In press)
26. Baskerville A, Hambleton P, Benbough JE (1980) Pathological features of glutaminase toxicity. Br J Exp Path 61:132–138
27. Yoshida S, Leskiwm MJ, Schluter MD, et al (1992) Effect of total parenteral nutrition, systemic sepsis, and glutamine on gut mucosa in rats. Am J Phys 263:E368–E373
28. O'Dwyer ST, Smith RJ, Hwang TL, Wilmore DW (1989) Maintenance of small bowel mucosa with glutamine-enriched parenteral nutrition. J Parent Enteral Nutr 13:579–585
29. Tamada H, Nezu R, Imamura I, et al (1992) The dipeptide alanyl-glutamine prevents intestinal mucosal atrophy in parenterally fed rats. J Parent Enteral Nutr 16:110–116
30. Jiang ZM, Wang LJ, Qi Y, et al (1993) Comparison of parenteral nutrition supplemented with L-glutamine or glutamine dipeptides. J Parent Enteral Nutr 17:134–141
31. Inoue Y, Grant JP, Snyder PJ (1993) Effect of glutamine-supplemented total parenteral nutrition recovery of the small intestine after starvation atrophy. J Parent Enteral Nutr 17:165–170
32. Meritt J, Witkowski TA, Nagele R, Norcross ED, Stein TP (1989) Glutamine and smooth muscle morphology of the gut in rats on total parenteral nutrition. J Am Coll Nutr 8:537–544
33. Burrin DG, Shulman RJ, Langston C, Storm MC (1994) Supplemental alanylglutamine, organ growth, and nitrogen metabolism in neonatal pigs fed by total parenteral nutrition. J Parent Enteral Nutr 18:313–319
34. Platell C, McCauley R, McCulloch R, Hall J (1993) The influence of parenteral glutamine and branched-chain amino acids on total parenteral nutrition-induced atrophy of the gut. J Parent Enteral Nutr 17:348–354
35. Alverdy JA, Aoys E, Weiss-Carrington P, Burke DA (1992) The effect of glutamine-enriched TPN on gut immune cellularity. J Surg Res 52:34–38
36. Burke DJ, Alberdy JC, Aoys E, Moss GS (1989) Glutamine-supplemented total parenteral nutrition improves gut immune function. Arch Surg 124:1396–1399
37. Li J, Langkamp-Henken B, Suzuki K, Stahlgren LH (1994) Glutamine prevents parenteral nutrition-induced increases in intestinal permeability. J Parent Enteral Nutr 18:303–307
38. Chen K, Okuma T, Okamura K, Torigoe Y, Miyauchi Y (1994) Glutamine-supplemented parenteral nutrition improves gut mucosa integrity and function in endotoxemic rats. J Parent Enteral Nutr 18:167–171
39. Spaeth G, Gottwald T, Haas W, Holmer M (1993) Glutamine does not improve gut barrier function and mucosal immunity in total parenteral nutrition. J Parent Enteral Nutr 17:317–323
40. Bark T, Svenberg T, Theodorsson E, Uribe A, Wennberg A (1994) Glutamine supplementation does not prevent small bowel mucosal atrophy after total parenteral nutrition in the rat. Clin Nutr 13:79–84
41. Babst R, Horig T, Stehle P, et al (1993) Glutamine peptide-supplemented long-term total parenteral nutrition: Effects on intracellular and extracellular amino acid patterns, nitrogen economy, and tissue morphology in growing rats. J Parent Enteral Nutr 17:566–574
42. Stein TP, Yoshida S, Schluter MD, Drews D, Assimon A, Leskiw MJ (1994) Comparison of intravenous nutrients on gut mucosal protein synthesis. J Parent Enteral Nutr 18:447–452
43. Zapata-Sirvent RL, Hansbrough JF, Ohara MM, Rice-Asaro M, Nyhan WL (1994) Bacterial translocation in burned mice after administration of various diets including fiber- and glutamine-enriched formulas. Crit Care Med 22:690–696
44. Tenenhaus M, Hansbrough JF, Zapata-Sirvent RL, Ohara M, Nyhan W (1994) Supplementation of an elemental diet with alanyl-glutamine decreases bacterial translocation in burned mice. Burns 20:220–225

45. Dugan ME, McBurney MI (1995) Luminal glutamine perfusion alters endotoxin-related changes in ileal permeability of the piglet. J Parent Enteral Nutr 19:83–87
46. Gianotti L, Alexander JW, Gennari RF, Pyles T, Babcock GF (1995) Oral glutamine decreases bacterial translocation and improves survival in experimental gut-origin sepsis. J Parent Enteral Nutr 19:69–74
47. Gennari R, Alexander JW, Eaves-Pyles T (1995) Effect of different combinations of dietary additives on bacterial translocation and survival in gut-derived sepsis. J Parent Enteral Nutr 19:319–325
48. Bark T, Katouli M, Ljungquist O, Mollby R, Svenberg T (1995) Glutamine supplementation does not prevent bacterial translocation after non-lethal haemorrhage in rats. Eur J Surg 161:3–8
49. Wusteman M, Tate H, Weaver L, Austin S, Neale G, Elia M (1995) The effect of enteral glutamine deprivation and supplementation on the structure of rat small-intestine mucosa during a systemic injury response. J Parent Enteral Nutr 19:22–27
50. Rooyackers OE, Soeters PB, Saris WH, Wagemakers AJ (1995) Effect of an enterally administered glutamine-rich protein on catabolic response to a zymosan challenge in rats. Clin Nutr 14:105–115
51. Klimberg VS, Souba WW, Dolson DJ, et al (1990) Prophylactic glutamine protects the intestinal mucosa from radiation injury. Cancer 66:62–68
52. Karatzas T, Scopa S, Tsoni I, et al (1991) Effect of glutamine on intestinal mucosal integrity and bacterial translocation after abdominal radiation. Clin Nutr 10:199–205
53. McArdle AH (1994) Protection form radiation injury by elemental diet: Does added glutamine change the effect? Gut 35 (Suppl):S60–S64
54. Scott TE, Moellman JR (1992) Intravenous glutamine fails to improve gut morphology after radiation injury. J Parent Enteral Nutr 16:440–444
55. Rombeau JL (1990) A review of the effects of glutamine-enriched diets on experimentally induced enterocolitis. J Parent Enteral Nutr 14 (Suppl):100S–105S
56. Zhang W, Frankel WL, Bain A, Choi D, Klurfeld DM, Rombeau JL (1995) Glutamine reduces bacterial translocation after small bowel translocation in cyclosporine-treated rats. J Surg Res 58:159–164
57. Ziegler TR, Benfell K, Smith RJ, et al (1990) Safety and metabolic effects of L-glutamine administration in humans. J Parent Enteral Nutr 14:137S–146S
58. Fürst P, Albers S, Stehle P (1990) Glutamine-containing dipeptides in parenteral nutrition. J Parent Enteral Nutr 14:118S–124S
59. Khan K, Hardy G, McElroy B, Elia M (1991) The stability of L-glutamine in total parenteral nutrition solutions. Clin Nutr 10:193–198
60. Askanazi J, Carpentier YA, Michelsen CB, et al (1980) Muscle and plasma amino acids following injury. Influence of intercurrent infection. Ann Surg 192:78–85
61. Roth E, Funovics J, Mühlbacher F, et al (1982) Metabolic disorders in severe abdominal sepsis: Glutamine deficiency in skeletal muscle. Clin Nutr 1:25–41
62. van der Hulst RR, Deutz NE, von Meyenfeldt MF, Elbers JM, Stockbrügger RW, Soeters PB (1994) Decrease of mucosal glutamine concentration in the nutritionally depleted patient. Clin Nutr 13:228–233
63. Ziegler TR, Young LS, Benfell K, et al (1992) Clinical and metabolic efficacy of glutamine-supplemented parenteral nutrition after bone marrow transplantation. Ann Intern Med 116:821–828
64. Schloerb PR, Amare M (1993) Total parenteral nutrition with glutamine in bone marrow transplantation and other clinical applications (a randomized, double blind study). J Parent Enteral Nutr 17:407–413
65. van Zaanen HC, van der Lelie H, Timmer JG, Fürst P, Sauerwein HP (1994) Parenteral glutamine dipeptide supplementation does not ameliorate chemotherapy-induced toxicity. Cancer 74:2879–2884
66. van der Hulst RR, von Meyenfeldt MF, Deutz NE, Stockbrügger RW, Soeters PB (1996) The effect of glutamine administration on intestinal glutamine content. J Surg Res 61:30–34
67. van der Hulst RR, van Kreel BK, von Meyenfeldt MF, et al (1993) Glutamine and the preservation of gut integrity. Lancet 334:1363–1365

68. Tremel H, Kienle B, Weilemann LS, Stehle P, Fürst P (1994) Glutamine dipeptide–supplemented parenteral nutrition maintains intestinal function in the critically ill. Gastroenterology 107:1595–1601

69. Scheppach W, Loges C, Bartram P, et al (1994) Effect of free glutamine and alanyl-glutamine dipeptide on mucosal proliferation of the human ileum and colon. Gastroenterology 107: 429–434

70. Byrne TA, Morrissey TB, Nattakom TV, Ziegler TR, Wilmore DW (1995) Growth hormone, glutamine, and a modified diet enhance nutrient absorption in patients with severe short bowel syndrome. J Parent Enteral Nutr 19:296–302

71. Byrne TA, Persinger RL, Young LS, Ziegler TR, Wilmore DW (1995) A new treatment for patients with short-bowel syndrome: Growth hormone, glutamine, and a modified diet. Ann Surg 222:243–255

72. Higashiguchi T, Hasselgren PO, Wagner K, Fischer JE (1993) Effect of glutamine on protein synthesis in isolated intestinal eptihelial cells. J Parent Enteral Nutr 17:307–314

73. Robinson AB, Robinson LR (1991) Distribution of glutamine and asparaginine residues and their near neighbors in peptides and proteins. Proc Natl Acad Sci USA 88:8880–8884

74. Flynn WJ, Gosche FR, Garrison N (1992) Intestinal blood flow is restored with glutamine or glucose suffusion after hemorrhage. J Surg Res 52:499–504

75. Harward TR, Coe D, Souba WW, Klingman N, Seeger JM (1994) Glutamine preserves gut glutathione levels during intestinal ischemia/reperfusion. J Surg Res 56:351–355

76. Li S, Nussbaum MS, McFadden DW, et al (1990) Addition of L-Glutamine to total parenteral nutrition and its effects on portal insulin and glucagon and the development of hepatic steatosis in rats. J Surg Res 48:421–426

Enteral Nutrition Support
in Surgical Intensive Care Patients

F. B. Cerra

Introduction

Nutrition support has become a standard of care in the management of intensive care unit (ICU) patients with the systemic inflammatory response syndrome (SIRS) with or without sepsis. Much of critical care therapy has been delivered on a physician preference basis. World-wide, there is a major effort to shift to evidenced-based medical decision-making. This effort requires the evaluation of medical literature that is based on objective methodologies for evaluating the quality of the data as well as the strength of the data in promoting evidence-based medical decision-making. This technology is available today.

This chapter applies an evidence-based approach to the medical literature regarding nutrition support in ICU patients with SIRS-sepsis [1].

Evidence-based Approach

The first step in the evidence-based approach was to define the minimum improvement(s) in clinical benefit (MICB) that would qualify to be used as an outcome that evidence could be gathered for. The second step was to gather the evidence through a review of the medical literature. The third step was to apply the standards of evidence to the data gathered.

The MICBs chosen for this analysis were the length of hospital stay and the incidence of acquired infectious complications. The considerations used in selecting the MICBs were the type, magnitude and clinical relevance of the medical benefit demonstrated, the risks and benefits of the therapy, and the cost of the therapy. Since little evaluable cost data for nutrition support was available in the literature, the definition of the MICBs occurred from the first two criteria.

The literature search was performed on Medline for the years 1970 to 1995, inclusive. The patient groups that the search was restricted to were: 1) adults; 2) received the therapy mainly in an ICU; 3) had a reason for ICU admission that included polytrauma, surgical intervention, surgical complication or infection; and 4) had data to support the presence of SIRS-sepsis during the ICU stay. With these constraints, the search was performed to seek either primary research (individual studies or multicenter trials), or overview studies of nutrition support (eg meta-analysis). Each of these studies identified was then evaluated for information pertaining to the MICBs. This evaluation included: 1) statement of hypothesis and primary and secondary outcome variables; 2) description of patients included in the study and whether or not they were accounted for in the results; 3) a description of the nutrition therapy provided; and 4) an analysis of study design and data collection (randomization, blinding, concurrent or prospective enrollment and data collection).

Each of the primary research studies (single center and multicenter trials) were evaluated by criteria and a judgment made as to the appropriate level of evidence [1]. Each of the scientific overviews (eg meta-analysis) was likewise evaluated. Two key aspects of the evaluations were quality and heterogeneity. The quality evaluation included an analysis of the methodology employed in the analysis and the appropriateness and design of the primary studies. Heterogeneity was assessed from the patient descriptions, presence and analysis of co-morbidities, and descriptions of the treatments employed. The relationship of the 95% confidence interval to the MICB was then assessed. Based on these variables, the level of review quality was assigned. For this chapter, only studies that were ranked as I or II are reported.

Three areas of efficacy of nutrition support were assessed:
1) The effect of perioperative total parenteral nutrition (TPN) on surgical complications (including infections);
2) The effect of enteral nutrition (EN) on infectious complications; and
3) The effect of enhanced EN (immunonutrition) on length of hospital stay or hospital-acquired infections.

The therapeutic impact of nutrition support was estimated by calculating the number of patients that would need to be treated to realize the effect in similar clinical circumstances.

The evidence was then used as a basis for recommendations for the use of nutritional support in the ICU in patients with SIRS-sepsis.

The results of the evidence analysis are presented for each of the defined MICBs. This is followed by the therapeutic impact analysis.

Perioperative TPN Affect on Complications

There were 6 studies that met evidence-level criteria for reporting (Table 1). Of these, one was a meta-analysis [2] and one was prospective, but not randomized [3]. Of the randomized trials, two stratified patients based on the degree of malnutrition present at entrance to the study [4, 5].

Four of 5 primary studies and the meta-analysis observed clinically relevant improvement in patient outcomes. However, in three studies, this benefit was only observed in the presence of moderate to severe malnutrition [3–7]. In one study in patients with a moderate level of malnutrition, the complication rate was increased with TPN use [6]. In the meta-analysis, the reduction in major complications associated with TPN was 7.1% (95% confidence; 2.1 to 12.4%). However, therapy-related complications (pneumothorax, line infection, vein

Table 1. Evidence summary for perioperative total parenteral nutrition

Patient type	Number		Days pre-operative	Complications			Mortality	Evidence level	Ref.
	C	T		Major	Infections				
UGI Cancer	59	66	10	p < 0.05	—		p < 0.05	I	[2]
General surgery: Abdominal	145 Patients all	50 Post-Op	> 7	p < 0.005 with PNI > 50%			p < 0.005 with PNI > 50%	III	[3]
General surgery: Abdominal	51	40	7		p < 0.005 with mod/severe MTN			II	[4]
General surgery: Abdominal and thoracic multicenter trial	228	231	7–15	p < 0.005 (decreased) with severe MTN	p < 0.005 (increased) with mild MTN			II	[5]
General surgery	149	151	Only Post-Op	No difference based on intent to treat				II	[6]
Meta-analysis	11 randomized trials 18 controlled trials			p < 0.05				II	[7]

C = control; T = treatment (TPN); UGI = Upper gastrointestinal; Post-Op = postoperative; MTN = malnutrition; PNI = prognostic nutrition index

thrombosis) occurred at 6.7% (95% confidence: 4 to 10%). No significant effect on mortality was observed [7].

Route of Nutrition Administration: Affect on Infectious Complications

There were 3 studies that met evidence-level criteria for reporting (Table 2). Two studies were randomized and prospective [8, 9]; one was a meta-analysis [10]. There were 8 prospective, randomized trials in the meta-analysis, 6 of which were unpublished data. Of the 2 published studies used, one is reported here [8], and one was judged to be of low quality and not included in this report.

All of the studies reported in Table 2 use infectious complications as the primary outcome variable. Nutrition was begun within 72 h of surgery; the patients were well-nourished. A reduction in infectious complications (pneumonia, wound, intra-abdominal abscess, central venous line) was observed in all 3 studies. In one study where the data is present [9], the central line sepsis incidence was increased in the patients receiving TPN (1.9 EN vs. 13.3% TPN). When the data in the meta-analysis was analyzed without line infections, the incidence of infectious complications was still reduced ($p < 0.05$). The study populations were more homogeneous than in most nutrition studies: younger, non-malnourished patients with high injury severity scores and abdominal trauma requiring laparotomy and subsequent ICU care. It is of note that the nutrition support was begun within 72 h of injury and that the MICB was observed in the absence of malnutrition at entrance to the study.

Enhanced EN

There were 7 studies suitable for analysis, 4 randomized, controlled trials and 3 multicenter, randomized, controlled trials [11–17]. Four studies were performed in patients undergoing upper gastrointestinal tract surgery for cancer of the

Table 2. Evidence summary for enteral nutrition

Patient type	Number		Initiation of feeding	Infectious complication	Evidence level	Ref.
	C	T				
Abdominal trauma with laparotomy	39	36	within 12 h after surgery	reduced in EN $p < 0.05$	I	[8]
Abdominal trauma with laparotomy	51	45	within 24 h after surgery	reduced in EN $p < 0.05$	I	[9]
Meta-analysis: abdominal trauma with laparotomy general surgery: 8 trials	118	112	within 72 h after surgery	reduced in EN $p < 0.05$	II	[10]

EN = enteral nutrition; C = control; T = treated

Table 3. Evidence summary for enhanced enteral nutrition

Patient type	Number		Formula		Outcome		Evidence level	Ref.
	C	T	C	T	Los	Inf.		
UGI cancer surgery RCT	44	41	Osm	Imp	↓ 4.4 days	↓ 36%	I	[11]
SIRS and sepsis trauma	143	153	Osm	Imp	I ↓ 8 days SIRS ↓ 5.5 days S ↓ 10 days SF ↓ 11.5 days	↓ 59% ↓ 60%	I	[12]
UGI cancer RCT	30	30	TrmCal	Imp	↓ 6 days	↓ 23%	II	[13]
Trauma RCT	18	19	Osm	Canola ARg HPro	NS	↓ 70%	II	[14]
UGI cancer RCT	24/TPN 27	26	Base Gly n-6	TPN/Imp	↓ 6 days to TPN	↓ 50%	II	[15]
Trauma MRCT	47	51	TEN	ImmAid	MOF ↓ 11%	↓ 11%	I	[16]
UGI cancer MRCT	77	77	Base n-6	Imp	↓ 4 days; cost 32%	↓ 62%	I	[17]

RCT = randomized controlled trial; MRCT = multicenter randomized controlled trial; Osm = osmolite; Imp = Impact; TrmCal = Trauma Cal; I = intent to treat and fed; SIRS = Systemic Inflammatory Response Syndrome; S = septic; SF = septic and fed; NS = not significant; TPN = total parenteral nutrition; MOF = multiple organ failure; Gly = Glycine

esophagus, stomach, pancreas, or ampulla [11–13, 15, 17]. Three studies were performed in multiple trauma patients [12, 14, 16]. Five studies used Impact as the experimental formula [11–13, 15, 17], a common use control was employed in 3 [11–13], and an unenhanced base formula the same as the Impact base in 2 [15, 17]. In one study, the control formula was isocaloric and isonitrogenous to Impact [17], in 2 studies canola oil was used as the source of n − 3 fat (Table 3) [14–16].

In 3 studies, the primary outcome variable was hospital length of stay [11–13], in one study it was the acquired infection rate [17], and in 3 studies the primary outcome variable was unspecified [14–16]. All studies prospectively analyzed the number of infectious complications acquired after inclusion in the study with similar definitions employed.

All the studies observed reductions in infectious complications that were clinically and statistically relevant. In those studies designed to evaluate hospital length of stay, significant and clinically relevant reductions were observed. A retrospective analysis of the cost of complications was performed in one study [17]. A 32% reduction in cost was observed in the group receiving the experimental formula.

Number-Needed-to-Treat (NNT) Analysis (Therapeutic Impact)

Three studies are of sufficient quality to permit NNT analysis (Table 4). Two of these are multicenter trials [5, 12], and one is a meta-analysis [8]. The relevant clinical outcomes are complications after surgical intervention, infectious complications, and length of hospital stay. In all of the clinical settings, the NNT would indicate significant potential clinical benefit when nutrition support is

Table 4. Therapeutic impact analysis based on number needed to treat

Clinical setting	Complication	Risk of developing complication, %	Reduction in risk from therapy, %	NNT	Ref.
Perioperative TPN in severe malnutrition	Major noninfectious complications	42.9	88	2.6	[5]
Enteral nutrition after abdominal trauma	Major infectious complications	35	54	6.2	[8]
Enhanced enteral nutrition in septic patients	Median length of stay of 28 days	100	36	1.6	[12]
Enhanced enteral nutrition in septic patients	Mean number of infections per patient of 0.88 or greater	100	59	2.4	[12]

NNT = Number needed to treat

provided in clinical situations the same or similar to those used in these clinical studies. In addition, it must be clarified that appropriate administration and monitoring techniques must be used. This is particularly so with TPN where complications related to the therapy have the potential of offsetting much of the benefit of the therapy itself (narrow therapeutic margin).

Conclusion

1) Perioperative nutrition support as TPN can be associated with a reduction in the incidence of postoperative surgical complications. Two qualifications must be added to this Grade B conclusion:
   a) The patient's need to be moderately to severely malnourished.
   b) The complications related to TPN must be kept low, preferably under 4-5%.
2) EN begun within 72 h of injury from trauma requiring surgical intervention and ICU admission is associated with a reduction in the incidence of major septic complications. The conclusion Grade is A^-/B^+.
3) EN formulas fortified with immune-enhancing nutrients and antioxidants is associated with a reduction in the length of hospital stay and acquired infectious complications when it is initiated within 96 h of an event necessitating ICU care and continued for at least 7 days. The conclusion Grade is A^-/B^+.

Recommendations

1) Perioperative TPN can be utilized to reduce surgical complications if:
   a) The patient is moderately to severely malnourished.
   b) Seven days of preoperative therapy are given and TPN is continued into the postoperative period.
   c) The therapy-related complications are kept under 4-5%.
   d) The enteral route of nutrition administration is not possible.
Grade B

2) EN should be initiated whenever possible within 72 h of polytrauma requiring surgical intervention, even in the absence of malnutrition.
Grade A^-/B^+

3) Enhanced EN should be given strong consideration when EN therapy is provided:
   a) in ICU settings of trauma, complications of major surgery and sepsis
   b) within 96 h of an event requiring ICU admission
   c) in the absence of malnutrition.
Grade A^-/B^+

References

1. Cook DJ (1994) Clinical trials in the treatment of sepsis: An evidence-based approach. In: Sibbald WJ, Vincent JL (eds) Update in Intensive Care and Emergency Medicine, Vol. 19. Springer, Berlin Heidelberg New York, pp XIX–XXXI
2. Muller JM, Brenner U, Dienst C, Pichlmaier H (1982) Preoperative parenteral feeding in patients with gastrointestinal carcinoma. Lancet 1:68–71
3. Mullen JL, Buzby GP, Matthews DC, Smale BF, Rosato EF (1980) Reduction of operative morbidity and mortality by combined preoperative and postoperative nutritional support. Ann Surg 192:604–613
4. Bellantone R, Doglietto GB, Bossola M, et al (1990) Preoperative parenteral nutrition in the high risk surgical patient. Am Soc Parent Enteral Nutr 12:195–197
5. The Veterans Affairs Total Parenteral Nutrition Cooperative Study Group (1991) Perioperative total parenteral nutrition in surgical patients. N Engl J Med 325:525–532
6. Sandstrom R, Drott C, Aforvidsson B, et al (1993) The effect of postoperative TPN on outcome following major surgery evaluated in a randomized study. Ann Surg 217:185–195
7. Detsky AS, Baker JP, O'Rourke K, Goel V (1987) Perioperative parenteral nutrition: A meta-analysis. Am Coll Phys 107:195–203
8. Moore FA, Moore EE, Jones TN, McCroskey BL, Peterson VM (1989) TEN versus TPN following major abdominal trauma-reduced septic morbidity. Trauma 29:916–923
9. Kudsk KA, Croce MA, Fabian TC, et al (1992) Enteral versus parenteral feeding. Ann Surg 215:503–513
10. Moore FA, Feliciano DV, Andrassy RJ, et al (1992) Early enteral feeding, compared with parenteral, reduces postoperative septic complications. Ann Surg 216:172–183
11. Daly JM, Lieberman MD, Goldfine J, et al (1992) Enteral nutrition with supplemental arginine, RNA and omega-3 fatty acids in patients after operation. Immunologic, metabolic, and clinical outcome. Surgery 112:56–67
12. Bower RH, Cerra FB, Bershadsky B, et al (1993) Early enteral administration of a formula supplemented with arginine, nucleotides and fish oils in ICU patients: Results of a prospective, randomized clinical trial. J Crit Care Med 23:436–449
13. Daly J, Weintraub FN, Shou J, Rosato EF, Lucia M (1995) Enteral nutrition during multimodality therapy in UGI cancer patients. Ann Surg 221:327–338
14. Brown R, Hunt H, Mowatt-Larson CA, Wajtsiah SL, Henningfield MF, Kudsh KA (1994) Comparison of specialized and standard enteral formulas in trauma patients. Pharmacotherapy 14:314–320
15. Braga M, Vignali A, Gianotti L, Cestari A, Profili M, DiCarlo V (1995) Benefits of early postoperative enteral feeding in cancer patients. Infusion Ther Transfusion Med 22:1–6
16. Moore FA, Moore EE, Kudsk KA, et al (1994) Clinical benefits of an immune-enhancing diet for early post–injury feeding. J Trauma 37:607–615
17. Senkal M, Kollig E, Mumme M, et al (1996) Early postoperative immunonutrition: Clinical outcome and cost benefit analysis in surgical patients. (In press)

Enteral Diets in Critically Ill Patients

H. L. Frankel and J. L. Rombeau

Introduction

The need to provide nutrition for critically ill or severely injured patients has become axiomatic throughout the world. Recognition of the gastrointestinal (GI) tract as a possible contributor to the septic inflammatory response syndrome has led to development of protocols whereby critically ill and severely injured patients are fed early in their disease course [1]. Moreover the use of specialized diets with gut specific nutrients have been advocated in an attempt to ameliorate GI dysfunction and possibly reduce gut-derived sepsis [2, 3].

The following indications have been proposed as guidelines for the initiation of nutritional support in the critically ill or severely injured patient:
1) The patient has been without nutrition for 5 to 7 days. (In a well-nourished individual, body stores are generally adequate to provide nutrients during shorter periods without compromising physiologic functions, altering resistance to infection, or impairing wound healing).
2) The duration of illness is anticipated to be > 10 days. Examples of these illnesses include patients with peritonitis, pancreatitis, severe injury or extensive burns.
3) The patient is malnourished (weight loss > 10% of usual body weight) [10].

The enteral route is the preferred method of nutrition if the GI tract can be used safely. Contraindications to enteral feeding include excessive GI output (> 600 mL/day), major GI tract hemorrhage, severe diarrhea, emesis, and pronounced abdominal distension (Table 1) [11].

As a result of rapidly escalating health care costs and possible morbidity from the administration of specialized feeding *per se*, there is an increasing need to select those patients who are most likely to benefit from administration of enteral feeding. Selection of these patients can be based, in part, on careful analysis of data from controlled clinical trials. Due to the heterogeneity of critically ill and injured patients, especially in multicenter trials, it is extremely difficult to perform such studies with comparable patient populations. Moreover, because nutritional support is now accepted as a mandatory component of the care of the critically ill, there is an ethical concern about the use of a minimally fed control group in these studies. Nonetheless, controlled clinical trials of high quality have been performed in this setting. The purpose of this chapter is to objectively

Table 1. Indications for enteral nutrition (partial listing)

Considered routine care in the following:
- Protein-calorie malnutrition with inadequate oral intake of nutrients for the previous 5–7 days
- Normal nutritional status but < 50% of required oral intake of nutrients for the previous 7–10 days
- Severe dysphagia
- Major full-thickness burns
- Low output enterocutaneous fistulas
- Major trauma

Usually helpful in the following:
- Radiation therapy
- Mild chemotherapy
- Liver failure and severe renal dysfunction
- Massive small bowel resection (> 50%) in combination with administration of total parenteral nutrition

Of limited or undetermined value in the following:
- Intensive chemotherapy
- Immediate postoperative period or poststress period
- Acute enteritis
- > 90% resection of small bowel

Contraindicated in the following:
- Complete, mechanical intestinal obstruction
- Moderate to severe abdominal distension
- Ileus or intestinal hypomotility
- Severe diarrhea
- Severe GI bleeding
- High-output external fistulas
- Severe, acute pancreatitis
- Shock
- Aggressive nutritional support not desired by the patient or legal guardian and respect of such wish being in accordance with hospital policy and existing law
- Prognosis not warranting aggressive nutritional support

evaluate several of these trials in order to identify recommendations for enteral feeding of the critically ill and severely injured patient. The 9 studies selected for this review are, for the most part, recent prospective, controlled clinical trials of standard or specialized enteral nutrition (EN) in critically ill, severely injured patients, or individuals undergoing major surgery [2–10]. We are very aware of the difficulty and expense of performing such studies. Additionally, it is not clinically feasible to control for every important outcome variable. Because of these realities, we have attempted to present our comments and evaluations within this context. The 9 studies to be reviewed address whether initiation of EN earlier than 5 to 7 days from the admission for severe illness and injury is indicated, and whether the use of special immune-enhancing formulas is efficacious.

Review of Controlled Clinical Trials

1. JR Border et al. [4] (1987) The gut origin septic states in blunt multiple trauma in the ICU

Study Design, Patients and Diets: This retrospective report included 66 multiple blunt trauma patients (age 16–60 years; mean 29 years ± 12) with an Injury Severity Score (ISS) > 22 (mean 40 ± 11). A standard enteral polymeric diet was compared to total parenteral nutrition (TPN). Some patients received both enteral and parenteral feedings. Clinical outcome variables included a multiple variable sepsis score, ventilator days, positive blood cultures and number of antibiotics per day.

Results: Pearson correlation coefficients (r) between enteral protein administration and the following variables were derived:

	(r)
– sepsis severity score	0.38
– ventilator days	0.48
– positive blood cultures	0.10
– antibiotics/day	0.25

In addition, subgroup analysis of patients who received no enteral protein versus minimal enteral protein versus control (standard enteral diet) revealed the following:

	N	Sepsis severity	Ventilator days	Positive blood culture
No enteral protein	10	73.6 ± 26.1	43.0 ± 32.0	0.27 ± 0.76
Minimal enteral protein	9	55.5 ± 12.9	26.0 ± 23.0	0.15 ± 0.52
Control	8	48.0 ± 11.5	13.0 ± 4.6	0.03 ± 0.23

Although these data reveal trends in favor of normal enteral protein delivery, there was no significant difference among groups.

Authors' Conclusions: Enteral protein administration reduces the magnitude and bacteriologic evidence of the septic state.

Critique: This study has often been cited to justify the use of EN to diminish septic complications in injured patients. Additionally, it has provided rationale for many of the prospective controlled trials to be reviewed in this chapter. Importantly, it is one of the few clinical trials to compare the amount of protein intake with ensuing sepsis.

There are numerous concerns about the relevance of this study to clinical decision-making for EN. The authors did not design their study with a clearly stated hypothesis, namely that enteral protein administration in the blunt-injured cohort will decrease septic complications. The variables studied are not assigned as *a priori* dependent or independent status, and multiple associations are entered into a database to derive a *post-hoc* hypothesis.

The patient population is small, not consecutive and is accrued over 12 years. During this time, major changes occurred in the management of the ICU and injured patient, all of which independently could affect clinical outcome. The authors do not provide their rationale or specific indications for administering either EN or TPN. Were patients not given EN because of intolerance to same or due to a concern that EN is contraindicated in certain types of injured ICU patients? Moreover, were the patients who were able to be fed enterally merely less ill than their parenterally fed counterparts? The authors attempt to ensure homogeneity of the patient population by providing data on age and Injury Severity Score for enterally and parenterally-fed groups. They do not provide equally cogent variables such as transfusion requirements and the presence or absence of torso injury among others which could impact on septic and overall outcome. Additionally, there is evidence suggesting that the groups are not homogeneous. The TPN patients received a greater overall protein intake than the EN group. This confounding finding makes it difficult to determine whether the higher sepsis score in TPN patients represents a consequence of overfeeding rather than of the route of administration.

There are additional methodologic concerns with the study. Correlation coefficients are expressed as r, rather than the more applicable r^2. No definitions are provided for "control" versus "minimal enteral protein" administration versus "no" enteral protein administration. In fact, because of small numbers and large standard deviations, there is not a statistically significant difference in the amount of protein administered enterally to patients in these groups. Furthermore, most patients in the study received both EN and TPN. Finally, when measurements were not available on a given day in the study, they were extrapolated by averaging results obtained the day prior and after. This is not a statistically valid method of analysis.

The correlations between EN and sepsis score, ventilator days, antibiotics/day and positive blood cultures are weak. Subgroup analyses of patients who received no enteral protein, minimal enteral protein or control is performed on groups too small to provide significant data.

Take-home Message: The importance of this study is to provide the rationale and preliminary data for prospective, well controlled investigations in this patient population. Meaningful data supporting a lower incidence of septic complications in enterally fed patients are not provided in this oft-quoted study. Its retrospective nature limits its usefulness for clinical recommendations.

2. W. Alexander et al. [5] (1980) Beneficial effects of aggressive protein feeding in severely burned children

Study Design, Patients and Diet: This prospective, randomized trial included 18 pediatric patients (mean age 9 ± 2 years) with major burns (mean burn size $60 \pm 5\%$). A balanced diet with normal protein content (16%) given either parenterally or enterally was compared to a protein supplemented (23% of calories) enteral diet. Study variables included several laboratory indices and measures of clinical outcome such as the number of bacteremic days and survival.

Results: The protein-supplemented group had significant improvements in opsonization (0.62 ± 0.05 vs. 0.42 ± 0.04), levels of C3 (1585 ± 44 vs. 1371 ± 55 mg/mL), IgG (975 ± 56 vs. 805 ± 52 mg/mL), transferrin (283 ± 18 vs. 200 ± 10 mg/dL), total protein (6.3 ± 0.2 vs 5.5 ± 0.1 g/dL) and amino acids over the standard fed group with fewer bacteremic days (8 vs. 11%) and higher survival (100 vs. 56%).

Authors' Conclusion: In severely burned children, protein supplementation results in improved immune function and survival.

Critique: This well-controlled clinical trial investigates a scientific hypothesis with readily measured outcome variables. Although the sample size is small, treatment can be expected to affect the outcome variables resulting in low standard deviations and meaningful data. The study was conducted in severely burned pediatric patients, an important group in need of EN. Extrapolation to an adult population of burn patients may not be valid.

The control and treatment groups are reasonably well-matched. Their average burn size, proportion of full-thickness burns, age, weight and concomitant smoke inhalation are nearly identical in both groups. The protein composition of the diet therefore appears to be the main variable affecting clinical outcome. However, several disparate variables existed between groups. The control group received a greater percentage of calories from parenteral alimentation than did the treatment group. Moreover, the control group received an increased proportion of intravenous lipid calories, known to be immunosuppressive, compared to the treatment group. Finally, the control group received greater total calories than did the treatment group. Therefore, the difference in immune function and overall outcome between the two groups could be ascribed to overfeeding, lipid administration or decreased use of EN instead of differences in dietary protein contents. Additionally, immune parameters were not measured in the two groups prior to treatment and, although unlikely, these variables could have differed for reasons other than those studied.

Take-home Message: Protein supplementation *might* benefit severely burned children. Extrapolation to adult burn patients is probably not warranted.

3. EE Moore et al. [6] (1986) Benefits of immediate jejunostomy feeding after major abdominal trauma: A prospective, randomized study

Study Design, Patients and Diet: This prospective, randomized trials included 63 adult injured patients with an Abdominal Trauma Index (ATI) of 15–40. Patients underwent emergency celiotomy at a Level I trauma center. An elemental diet delivered by needle catheter jejunostomy was compared to a control group who received 5% dextrose and water. Study variables included several standard laboratory indices in addition to minor and major septic complications.

Results: Serum protein markers and overall complication rate were not significantly different between the two groups. Septic complications were significantly reduced in the enterally fed group (4 vs. 26%).

Authors' Conclusion: Immediate postoperative EN via needle catheter jejunostomy reduces septic complications after major abdominal trauma.

Critique: This study is a well-controlled clinical trial which addresses the effect of early EN via needle catheter jejunostomy in injured patients at a single center. The relatively large number of patients studied appears to be well-matched in each group. The patients were analyzed for the development of septic complications, a very important outcome variable which, in turn, could be affected by many non-nutritional variables.

There are several questions about patient selection. Ideally, the control group should have consisted of patients who underwent insertion of the jejunostomy tube but were not fed. This would have enabled the investigators to control for jejunostomy-associated complications. This was not permitted by the authors' Human Research Committee, arguing that half of the patients enrolled could potentially be subjected to undue risk from the jejunostomy. Similar to other clinical trials of this nature, it was unclear as to whether the enterally administered diets were indeed absorbed. In 1996, it would be argued that a minimally fed control group of severely injured patients is not proper from an ethical standpoint, however, this is not a valid disagreement for a study designed in 1985. Finally, selection of patients for study with an ATI 15–40 might exclude those at highest risk for sepsis; however, it would be unethical to randomize this group to a non-nutrition control subgroup.

Both groups were well-matched for age, gender, injury mechanism, ATI, presence of shock, colon injury, need for splenectomy, and initial nutrition assessment. However, several factors not assessed might also have affected septic complications especially pneumonia. The control group did not achieve the target caloric rate for many days after initiation, thereby rendering many patients in this group profoundly malnourished.

Additionally, it is not clear how the data of treated patients who did not tolerate EN was assessed; two patients who received TPN appear in the enterally-fed group. Finally, the diminution of septic complications in the enterally fed group occurred without significant differences in the immune profile between groups.

Take-home Message: Many patients with major abdominal injury can safely tolerate immediate post-operative EN via needle catheter jejunostomy. Although no differences in immune profile or overall complications are realized, septic complications are diminished in patients receiving early EN compared to no nutrition. Because of the heterogeneous nature of injured patients requiring emergency celiotomy, it is difficult to determine whether early EN *per se* or other factors are responsible for this decrease in septic sequelae. Despite a few of the previously stated concerns, this study remains as a seminal investigation in support of the safety and reduction of sepsis in trauma patients who received early postoperative EN.

4. DV Feliciano et al. [7] (1991) Enteral versus parenteral nutrition in patients with severe penetrating trauma

Study Design, Patients and Diets: This prospective, randomized study included 22 adult trauma patients with penetrating trauma injuries and ATI 15–40. Early administration of an elemental diet, delivered by needle catheter jejunostomy, was compared to TPN. Important clinical outcome study variables included the cost of nutrient delivery, length of hospital stay and septic complications.

Results: Septic complications occurred in one of the EN patients and three of the TPN patients. This difference was not statistically significant. Length of hospital stay was reduced in the EN group (12.7 ± 5.2 vs. 26.9 ± 22.2 days). All but one of the EN patients tolerated the prescribed feedings. There was a mean cost savings of $ 870/patient for feeding when the enteral route was used.

Authors' Conclusion: Early EN in abdominally injured patients is a safe and effective alternative to TPN and it may decrease postoperative infection and reduce the cost of hospitalization.

Critique: The authors have conducted a controlled clinical trial to compare early EN to TPN in patients with penetrating abdominal injury at a single center. A small number of patients was studied. The patients were investigated for the development of septic complications and duration of hospital stay. These are important nutritionally related outcome measures, however, they are also affected by many non-nutritional variables.

The authors state that the enterally and parenterally fed groups are well-matched, with equivalent age, Injury Severity Score, metabolic status, and time to "goal" calories. However, data are not provided on equally cogent variables such as transfusion requirements, presence of colonic or splenic injuries or antibiotics prescribed. Of major concern is that the dietary intake between groups was neither isocaloric nor isonitrogenous. Additionally, the TPN group was given more calories than the EN group. Moreover, the EN group received more protein and glutamine which was not given to the TPN group. Therefore, observed outcome differences between the two groups could be due to the differences in the total amount of nutrients given rather than the route of nutrient administration. Finally, exclusion of patients with $ATI > 40$ might eliminate those patients at greatest risk for developing sepsis and not tolerating EN.

The modest, non-significant diminution in septic complications in EN patients attests to the fact that the sample size was probably too small to derive meaningful conclusions. Moreover, pneumonia is included among septic complications; however, additional information such as atelectasis, prolonged endotracheal intubation, and thoracic injury should be provided. Similarly, the data on hospital length of stay are difficult to interpret given the large standard deviations. If the author eliminated "outlyers" would the differences between the groups still be statistically significant? Important factors affecting prolonged length of hospital stay in addition to septic complications could include concomitant spinal cord injury, multiple extremity fractures and diffuse socioeconomic concerns. Moreover, in controlled clinical trials *a priori* discharge criteria must be established to correctly interpret data relating to length of stay. Finally, one would expect that a savings of greater than $ 870 should occur in EN over TPN patients regardless of the clinical outcome.

Take-home Message: Patients with major abdominal trauma can safely tolerate postoperative EN by needle catheter jejunostomy. Because of the small number and possibly heterogeneous nature of the patients studied and the differences in dietary intakes between groups, it is not possible to determine whether early postoperative EN improves outcome in this cohort.

5. KA Kudsk et al. [8] (1992) Enteral versus parenteral feeding: Effects on septic morbidity after blunt and penetrating abdominal trauma

Study Design, Patients and Diets: This prospective, randomized study included 96 adult patients with either penetrating or blunt trauma. Patients had ATI of 15 and required emergency laparotomy. A standard polymeric EN delivered by jejunostomy tube was compared to TPN. Study variables included measures of postoperative sepsis such as pneumonia and abdominal abscesses.

Results: The EN group sustained significantly fewer septic complications than did the TPN group: pneumonia (11.8 versus 31.0%), abscesses (1.7 versus 13.3%), sepsis (1.9 versus 13.3%) and overall infection rate (15.7 versus 40%), respectively.

Analysis of EN patients revealed a lower septic complication rate in the following subgroups compared to TPN patients: penetrating injury, ISS > 20 and ATI > 24. Patients with blunt injury or ISS < 20/ATI had a similar infectious complication rate despite the route of nutritional support.

Authors' Conclusions: There is a significantly lower incidence of septic morbidity in EN patients when compared to TPN after blunt and penetrating trauma, with most of the significant improvement occurring in the more severely injured patients. The surgeon should obtain enteral access at the time of initial celiotomy to provide an opportunity for delivery of nutrients, particularly in the most severely injured patients.

Critique: The study is a large controlled clinical trial addressing the effects of early EN (delivered via jejunostomy) in injured patients at a single center. All patients underwent placement of a jejunostomy tube, thereby providing a well-matched control group. Moreover, patients with $ATI > 40$ (a group that one would expect to have a high incidence of septic morbidity and inability to tolerate enteral feedings) were not excluded. Although the measurement of septic complications is dichotomous, it is still of great clinical importance and the authors attempted to elucidate all possible confounding variables.

The groups were well-matched in terms of age, ISS, ATI, mechanism of injury, transfusion requirements, ventilator and antibiotic usage and organs injured. However, the TPN group received more total non-protein calories, introducing a possible bias.

As mentioned, some of the outcome variables are similarly influenced by non-nutritional factors. Pneumonia is, perhaps, the most problematic. For example, the diagnosis of pneumonia is difficult to differentiate from pulmonary contusions and atelectasis in the acutely injured patient. Moreover, although it is intuitive that TPN patients should have a higher incidence of line sepsis, perhaps it is this complication that predisposes the patient to other infections sequelae. The authors' conclusion that severe injury necessitating emergency laparotomy should warrant placement of a surgical jejunostomy is not fully supported by the study because other methods of obtaining enteral access such as placement of a double lumen nasoenteric tube may be equally effective.

Nonetheless, the significant reduction in intra-abdominal infection rate in the EN group is impressive, especially in the most severely injured patients. Another important finding was the ability of most patients to tolerate EN.

Take-home Message: Patients with major abdominal trauma can tolerate early postoperative jejunal EN without major morbidity. Additionally, early administration of EN significantly decreases septic morbidity in severely injured patients.

6. FA Moore et al. [9] (1992) Early enteral feeding, compared with parenteral, reduces postoperative septic complications

Study Design, Patients and Diets: This report consisted of a meta-analysis of prospective, controlled trials of early EN with an elemental diet delivered into the jejunum compared to TPN. It included data from 2 published studies (including the aforementioned study by E. Moore and associates) and 6 additional trials. 230 patients from 8 centers were analyzed. The major study variables included sepsis and tolerance to feeding.

Results: When treatment failures were excluded from analysis, 17 EN versus 44 TPN patients had septic complications. Intention-to-treat analysis revealed 16 septic complications in the EN group and 35 in the TPN group. There were 29 septic complications in the TPN group if catheter-related infections were excluded. Subgroup analysis revealed differences in combined groups of trauma patients and blunt-trauma patients, but not in penetrating-injured, or non-trauma patients (Fig. 1).

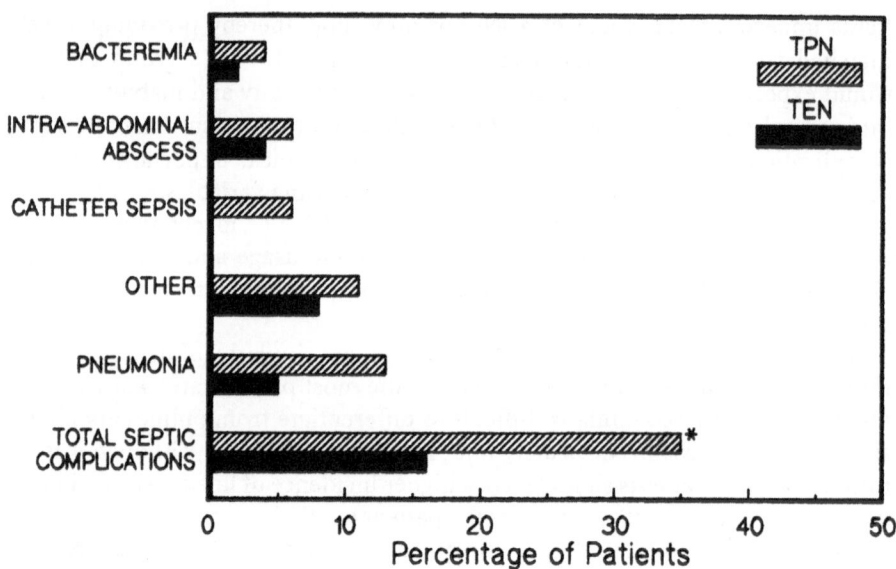

Fig. 1. Post-operative septic complications. (From [9] with permission). * $p < 0.05$

Authors' Conclusion: Early postoperative EN is well tolerated in high risk surgical patients. These patients have reduced septic morbidity when compared with those receiving TPN.

Critique: The patients in the two treatment arms were well-matched with respect to age, gender, ISS, ATI and metabolic profile at the time of hospital admission. However, the authors acknowledged that the TPN penetrating injured cohort had a higher mean ISS than the EN counterpart. Moreover, the method of EN differed among the centers as did the time to initiate nutrition, varying from 8–72 h. Similar to other meta-analysis of clinical outcome studies, this report includes patients of widely disparate demographics including 60 non-trauma patients who underwent oncologic and general surgical emergent and elective operations.

The report largely compared the use of standard TPN to Vivonex (Norwich NY), a commercial elemental formula. In most instances, the diets were not administered in an isocaloric, isonitrogenous manner. Despite these concerns, the reduction in sepsis with EN is impressive. Is this due to the efficacious components of the EN formula or the adverse effects of TPN?

Take-home Message: Early administration of EN is well-tolerated in most high risk surgical patients. Early EN decreases septic morbidity in these patient populations.

7. FB Cerra et al. [2] (1991) Improvement in immune function in ICU patients by enteral nutrition supplemented with arginine, RNA, and Menhaden oil is independent of nitrogen balance

Study Design, Patients and Diets: This prospective, randomized, blinded trial included 20 patients with polytrauma, major elective general surgery or a major surgical infection. Patients were in the ICU for at least 5 days with persistent hypermetabolism, mild malnutrition and they were able to tolerate EN. A special immune enhancing elemental diet (supplemented with arginine, nucleotides, and omega-3 fatty acids) was compared to a standard commercially available enteral diet. The diets were isocaloric and isonitrogenous. Study variables included several *in vitro* tests of immune function in addition to measures of clinical outcome.

Results: Both groups had significant pre-study depression of immune proliferative assays relative to normal. There were significant increases in the proliferative responses to all stimulants (concavalin A, tetanus antigen, phytohemagglutinin, and pokeweed mitogen) in the experimental group compared to no improvements or progressive suppression of the same tests in the control group. Nonetheless, both groups remained anergic with a depressed T_4/T_8 for the duration of the experiment. Six and twelve-month follow-up revealed no significant differences in mortality, number of infections, hospitalizations, physician visits or work status.

Authors' Conclusion: Nutrients targeted to effect disease-induced *in vitro* suppression of immune function appear to achieve that end.

Critique: The study is a multiple-blinded prospective, randomized clinical trial comparing the immune and overall consequences of a specialized immune-enhancing and a standard EN formula. Although the sample size is small, treatment should have a predictable effect with small standard deviations on the outcome variables, most of which are continuous. Importantly, the diets compared were administered in an isocaloric/isonitrogenous manner.

The age, admission, nutritional and immunological profiles, and degree of metabolic stress were similar in the treatment groups. Although not quite statistically significant, the control group received more calories prior to study initiation than did the treatment group. Because of the heterogeneity of diagnoses, it is difficult to determine how well-matched the groups are without additional data on numerous other non-nutritional variables which could affect immune status.

Finally, although treatment improved *in vitro* immune function, there were no significant differences in long-term clinical outcome between groups. Therefore, is this a difference that makes a difference? Perhaps if the authors had examined in-hospital septic complications, significant differences might have been noted.

Take-home Message: Administration of an immune-enhanced EN improves *in vitro* immune function in high risk surgical patients. This improvement is not associated with significant differences in morbidity and mortality.

8. RH Bower et al. [3] (1995) Early enteral administration of a formula (Impact) supplemented with arginine, nucleotides, and fish oil in intensive care unit patients: Results of a multicenter, prospective, randomized clinical trial

Study Design, Patients and Diets: This report was a prospective, randomized, double-blinded multicenter trial. 296 adult critically ill or injured patients were investigated. An immune enhanced diet (supplemented with arginine, nucleotides and fish oil) was compared to a standard elemental diet. Major study variables included measures of clinical outcome such as sepsis, length of hospital stay and mortality.

Results: Treatment with the immune diet was associated with an 8-day reduction in length of hospital stay compared to control patients. There were no significant differences in infectious morbidity or mortality between groups. Subgroup analysis of septic patients in the treatment arm revealed a 10-day reduction in hospital stay with decreased infectious morbidity.

Authors' Conclusion: Early administration of an immune-enhanced EN to critically ill and injured patients, particularly if they were septic at the time of hospital admission, resulted in reduced hospital stay and fewer infectious complications.

Critique: Based on conclusions that immune-enhanced diets improve *in vitro* immune function in the previously discussed study, the present authors investigated whether a significant difference in short-term complication rates might occur between the patients fed immune-enhanced versus standard diets. The authors did not replicate the *in vitro* data in this study which could have validated a mechanism for their findings. As previously discussed, hospital stay and infectious complication rate are outcome measures that are difficult to interpret in the absence of stringent *a priori* criteria. Moreover, confounding factors always present in a multicenter study with heterogeneous patients may have significantly influenced the data. Inasmuch as patients in the treatment arm had significantly decreased hospital stays without reduced infectious morbidity, it is unclear as to why the immune-enhanced diet reduced hospital stay. Only in the *post hoc* analyses of a septic subgroup could the authors demonstrate a concurrent diminished length of hospital stay and decreased infection rate. However, the standard deviations are large with respect to infectious morbidity. Finally, and most importantly, the diets administered were neither isocaloric nor isonitrogenous. The inequality of dietary intake between groups precludes a valid conclusion of nutritional-induced improvement in clinical outcome.

Take-home Message: Specialized immune-enhancing enteral diets have not yet been shown to decrease infections morbidity in critically ill or injured patients.

9. JM Daly et al. [10] (1995) Enteral nutrition during multimodality therapy in upper gastrointestinal cancer patients

Study Design, Patients and Diets: This prospective, randomized trial consisted of 60 patients who underwent surgery for esophageal, gastric or pancreatic cancer. The patients were followed in the hospital and outpatient setting. Clinical outcome measures included infectious complications and duration of hospital stay. Additionally, study variables included measured of plasma fatty acids and PGE_2. The study diet was a special immune-enhanced formula (Impact, Sandoz) supplemented with arginine, nucleotides and omega-3 fatty acids. The control diet was a polymeric formula. The composition of the diets were neither isocaloric nor isonitrogenous. The objective was to determine if early EN with the specialized diet could reduce infectious complications and hospital stay when compared to a standard diet.

Results: Patients fed the immune-supplemented diet had a 10% infectious complication rate and 16-day mean hospital length of stay compared to 43% and 22 days, respectively, in the standard diet group. Plasma omega-3 fatty acids were significantly higher and PGE_2 levels lower in the patients receiving the immune-enhanced diet.

Authors' Conclusion: Supplemental immune-enhanced EN decreases postoperative infectious/wound complications compared with standard EN in upper GI cancer patients.

Critique: This study is a prospective, randomized, controlled clinical trial comparing the immune and overall consequences of an immune-enhanced formula with a standard enteral diet in postoperative population conventionally thought to benefit from perioperative nutrition, but not presumed to be able to tolerate EN. The sample size is adequate and the outcome variables addressed are appropriate given the concerns discussed previously.

The authors undertook a formidable endeavor by following the patients both in hospital and upon discharge. However, they do analyze the data both via intention-to-treat and exclusionary methods, with little difference in results.

The diets administered are neither isonitrogenous nor isocaloric. The patients in the standard diet group received less protein and more calories overall, potentially affecting the results. In addition, patients receiving standard diets had more advanced cancers (mean pathological score of 3.8 versus 2.2), underwent a greater proportion of pancreatic operations (which may inherently have higher morbidity), and had lower preoperative transferrin levels than the standard diet group. The authors may have been better served to limit their study to the in-patient setting to minimize heterogeneity in the outpatient setting.

Take-home Message: The vast majority of patients with upper GI cancer can tolerate early postoperative EN given by jejunostomy tube. Administration of immune-enhanced formulas may be beneficial in improving clinical outcome.

Conclusions

Based on an in-depth review of the 9 described clinical trials in ICU patients, the following recommendations can be made:

Strong conclusions based on the studies:
1) A large proportion of patients can tolerate immediate postoperative EN following major abdominal surgery through a variety of access routes.
2) The diminished cost of EN compared to TPN as well as the elimination of line-related complications support the use of EN as the preferred route of nutrient administration.
3) Early post-operative administration EN decreases septic morbidity in selected severely injured patients.
4) Specialized enteral immune-enhanced formulas improve *in vitro* immune proliferative function in critically ill and injured patients.

Supportive though inconclusive data to date:
1) Immune-enhanced EN formulas decrease septic complications in critically ill and injured patients.

Take-home recommendations:
1) Establish enteral access early in severely ill or injured patients. Consider jejunostomy tube insertion at the time of laparotomy.
2) Use enteral access whenever possible when nutrition is initiated.
3) Standard EN formulas are tolerated well in most patients.
4) Avoid administration of excessive calories.

References

1. Deitch EA, Winterton J, Li M, Berg R, et al (1987) The gut as a portal for entry for bacteremia: Role of protein malnutrition. Ann Surg 205:681–692
2. Cerra FB, Lehmann S, Konstantinides N, et al (1991) Improvement in immune function in ICU patients by enteral nutrition supplemented with arginine, RNA and Menhaden oil is independent of nitrogen balance. Nutrition 7:193–199
3. Bower RH, Cerra FB, Bershadsny B, et al (1995) Early enteral administration of a formula (Impact) supplemented with arginine, nucleotides, and fish oil in intensive care unit patients: Results of a multicenter, prospective, randomized clinical trial. Crit Car Med 23:436–449
4. Border JF, Hassett J, LaDuca J, et al (1987) The gut origin septic states in blunt multiple trauma (ISS = 40) in the ICU. Ann Surg 206:427–448
5. Alexander W, Macmillan BG, Stinnett JD, et al (1980) Beneficial effects of aggressive protein feeding in severely burned children. Ann Surg 192:505–517
6. Moore EE, Jones TN (1986) Benefits of immediate jejunostomy feeding after major abdominal trauma. A prospective randomized study. J Trauma 26:874–881

7. Feliciano DV, Spjut-Patrinely V, Burch JM (1991) Enteral versus parenteral nutrition in patients with severe penetrating abdominal trauma. Contemp Surg 39:30–36
8. Kudsk KA, Croce MA, Fabian TC, et al (1992) Enteral versus parenteral feeding: Effects on septic morbidity after blunt and penetrating abdominal trauma. Ann Surg 215:503–505
9. Moore FA, Feliciano DV, Andrassy RJ, et al (1992) Early enteral feeding, compared with parenteral, reduces post-operative septic complications: The results of a meta-analysis. Ann Surg 216:172–183
10. Daly JM, Weintraub FN, Shou J, et al (1995) Enteral nutrition during multimodality therapy in upper gastrointestinal cancer patients. Ann Surg 221:327–338
11. Rombeau JL, Rolandelli RH, Wilmore DW (1994) Nutritional Support. In: Care in the ICU. Scientific American Vol II Chapter 10 pp 1–35

Future Directions

Experimental Advances in Intestinal Monitoring

P. Radermacher and M. Georgieff

Introduction

Assessment of splanchnic tissue perfusion, oxygenation and function has gained increased interest in intensive care research. Currently, no methods to directly measure splanchnic blood flow and oxygenation are routinely available. Indirect methods that have been introduced into clinical practice include the measurement of systemic indocyanine green clearance, the determination of the MEGX concentration, a metabolite of lignocaine, after a lignocaine bolus injection, and gastric tonometry [1]. This chapter will discuss two techniques which have recently been applied to assess gut and liver perfusion, oxygenation and metabolic performance. On the one hand, remission spectrophotometry using the *Erlanger Micro-lightguide Photometer* (EMPHO) allows to measure intracapillary hemoglobin O_2 saturation and relative hemoglobin content, the latter being a mirror of capillary blood flow [2, 3]. On the other hand, the use of stable, non-radioactive isotope-labelled substrates in tracer amounts permits to obtain information on global systemic as well as organ specific metabolic performance [4–6].

Technical and Physiological Basis of EMPHO

EMPHO measurements are technically based on tissue light remission spectrophotometry. Light emitted from a xenon lamp is radiated into the tissue and the remitted light collected via recipient light conductors. Both the illuminating fiber and the collecting micro-lightguides are encased in a flexible rubber tube. The remitted light passes through a rotating interference filter-disc, and extinction signals for a wavelength range between 502 and 628 nm are recorded allowing the construction of hemoglobin absorption spectra. Figure 1 shows a block diagram of the EMPHO setting as described recently by our group [3]. Oxygenated hemoglobin has two characteristic extinction maxima at 542 and 577 nm, while desoxygenated hemoglobin has only one single extinction maximum at 556 nm. Therefore, the hemoglobin O_2 saturation (HbO_2) can be precisely evaluated: light emitted into the tissue is both scattered and absorbed and subsequently remitted. The characteristics of the remitted light are determined by the basic tissue absorbtion and scattering, the respective concentrations of oxygenated (Hb_{oxy}) and desoxygenated (Hb_{desoxy}) hemoglobin and wavelength dependent scattering

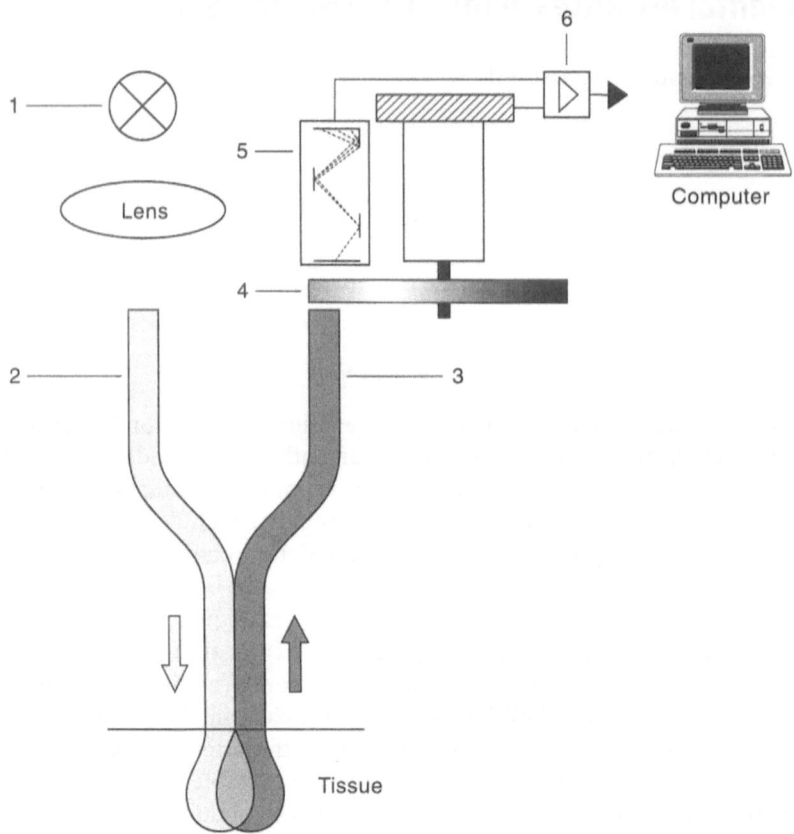

Fig. 1. Block diagram of the Erlanger Micro-lightguide Photometer (EMPHO). Light is radiated from a high-pressure xenon-lamp (1) into the tissue via a transmitting light conductor (2) with a diameter of 250 μm. The remitted light is conducted to a rotating interference bandpass filter-disc (4) via 6 recipient light conductors (3) arranged circularly around the transmitting conductor. The filter-disc rotates at 90 Hz, and 64-wavelength signals between 502 and 628 nm are recorded to construct a hemoglobin spectrum. The spectrum signal then passes through a photomultiplier (5) and an analog-digital converter (6), and is stored on a hard disc at a rate of 100 spectra per second. (Adapted from [3])

[7]. Since hemoglobin spectra are measured at 64 wavelenghts these parameters can be precisely determined via iterative techniques, and HbO_2 can be calculated as

$$\% HbO_2 = [Hb_{oxy}]/([Hb_{oxy}] + [Hb_{desoxy}]) \ [2].$$

Although the absolute concentrations cannot be determined because the exact volume of tissue picked up is unknown, the relative hemoglobin content in arbitratry units can be derived allowing to estimate capillary blood flow.

The physiological background of EMPHO is the fact that the capillary framework is formed by interacting supply units each consisting of one terminal arteriole and several capillaries supplied by that arteriole [8–11]. According to the Krogh-model, two different PO_2 gradients arise, one parallel to the capillary resulting from the tissue O_2 uptake [12], the other one perpendicular to the capillary representing the intercapillary tissue PO_2 [13]. Due to the hemoglobin O_2 dissociation curve the former, i.e. the intracapillary PO_2 gradient, is proportional to a HbO_2 gradient from the arterial beginning to the venous end of the capil-

a   Real intracapillary HbO_2-gradients of three individual units of supply

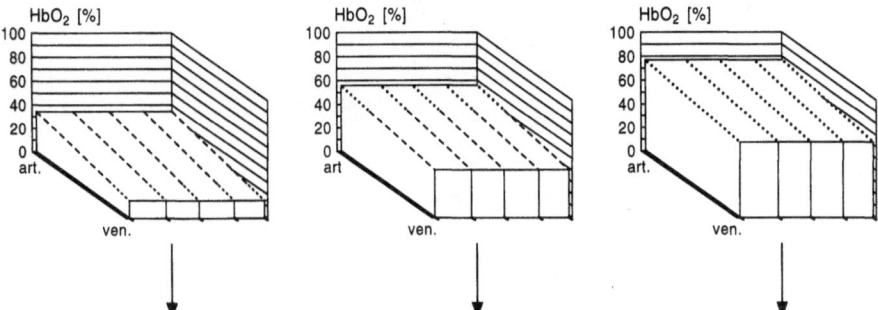

b   Pertinent integrated intracapillary HbO_2-gradients of these three individual units of supply

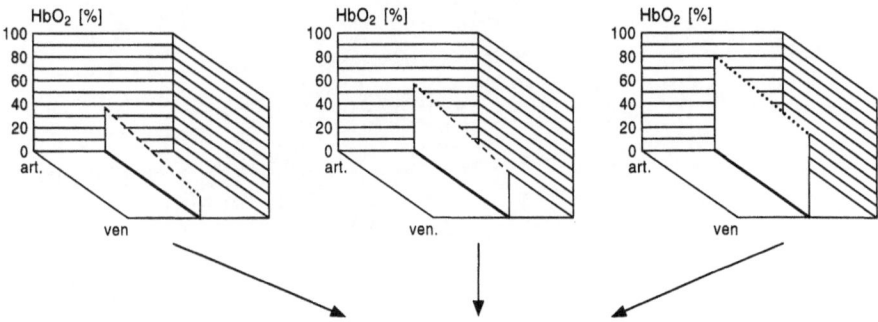

c   Integrated intracapillary HbO_2-gradient along a capillary representative for these three units of supply

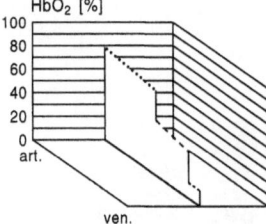

Fig. 2. Computation of an integrated hemoglobin O_2 saturation (HbO_2) gradient along theoretical capillary representing several interacting supply units. Within a single unit, the HbO_2 distribution is homogeneous (**a**), so that one single unit can be represented by one HbO_2 saturation gradient (**b**). Then an integrated gradient is constructed for a theoretical capillary representing these interacting units (**c**). (Adapted from [3])

lary. While the HbO$_2$ distribution is homogeneous within one single supply unit and, hence, can be represented by one integrated HbO$_2$ gradient for this unit (Fig. 2), there are substantial differences between interacting units due to the fact that "high" and "low flow" interacting capillary units exist [9, 10]. From the recorded spectra, a representative HbO$_2$ gradient can be calculated for a theoretical single capillary supplying these different interacting units (Fig. 2), and the combination of adjacent measurement points allows to construct an integrated spatial distribution of HbO$_2$ gradients (Fig. 3). Three intracapillary HbO$_2$ levels can be discriminated according to their functional importance: while a HbO$_2$ beyond 50% characterizes normal tissue O$_2$ availability, values below 20% corre-

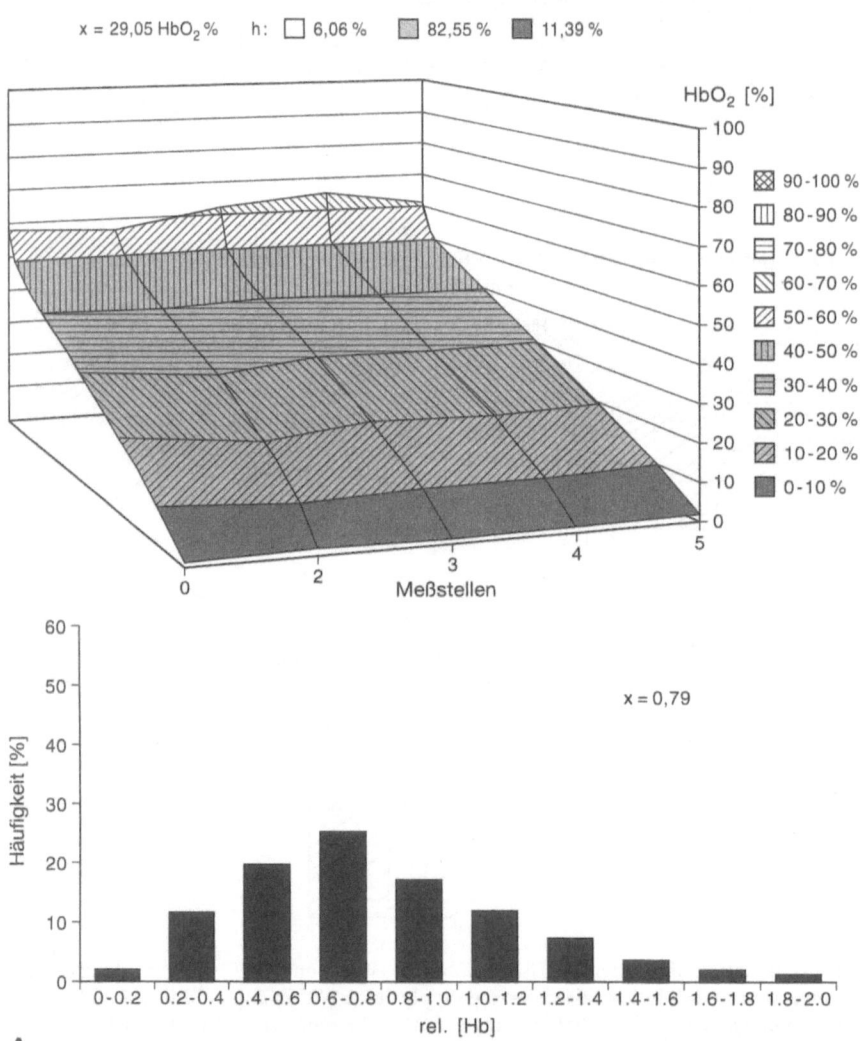

A

spond to intercapillary PO_2 resulting in impaired cellular oxidative capacities [14–16]. Levels between 20 and 50% constitute a reserve range corresponding to the potential of compensatory mechanisms such as redistribution of blood flow between different supply units [14].

Despite the promising preliminary results, limitations of EMPHO have to be taken into account. On the one hand, depending on the measurement site, the light remittance may be influenced by other biological pigments such as melanin and bilirubin. While the former is in particular important when remitted light is collected from the skin, bilirubin probably only assumes major importance at very high concentrations since the molar absorption is nearly negligible at wave-

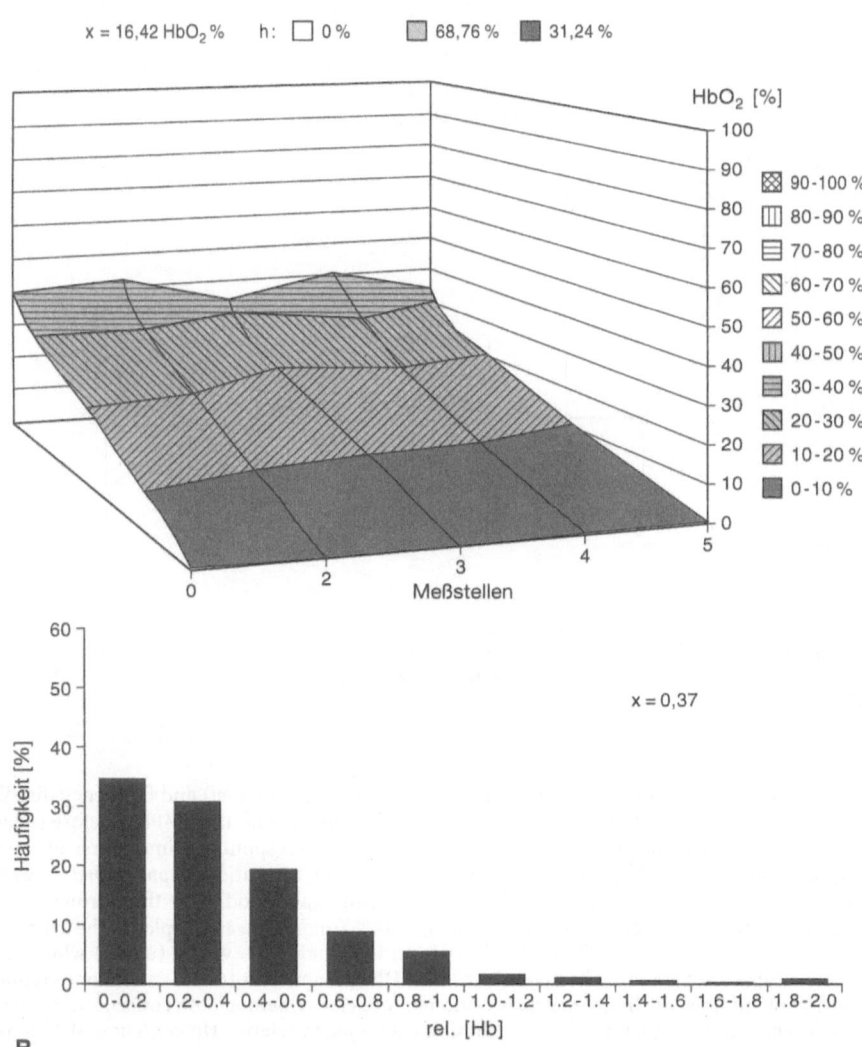

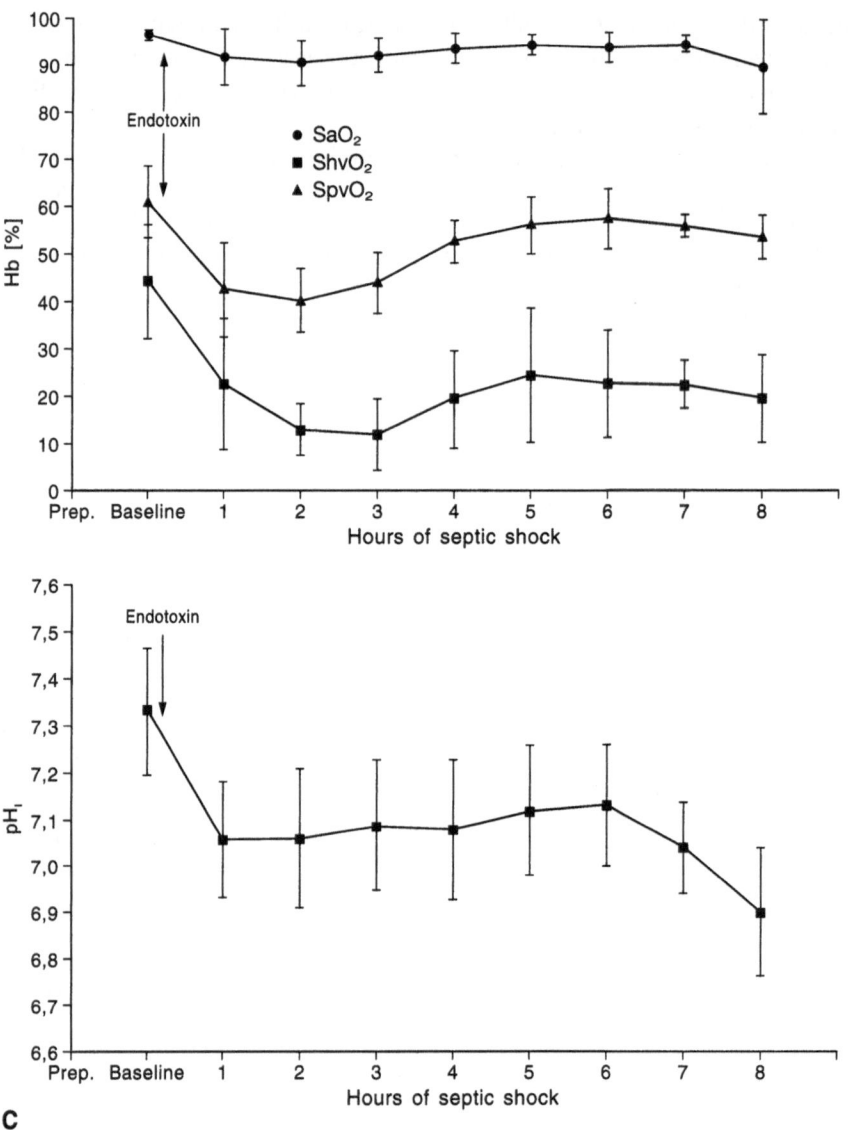

C

Fig. 3. Spatial distribution of hemoglobin O_2 saturation (*upper panel*) and frequency distribution of relative hemoglobin content (*lower panel*) as assessed with the EMPHO before (**A**) and 8 h after endotoxin infusion (**B**) in pigs. Fig. **C** shows the corresponding time course of arterial (*hyphen*), portal (*triangles*) and hepatic (*rhombi*) venous O_2 saturations (*upper panel*) as well as gastric pHi (*squares*) (*lower panel*) during the experimental period. Note that throughout the experiment, the fractional contribution of $HbO_2 < 10\%$ (middle) nearly tripled at the expense of the reserve range ($10\% < HbO_2 < 50\%$) (lower) and normal HbO_2 values (upper) which completely disappeared resulting in a fall of the mean HbO_2 from 29 to 16%. As a mirror of reduced mucosal blood flow, the frequency distribution of the relative hemoglobin concentrations fell in parallel changing from a Gaussian distribution with a mean relative Hb content of 0.79 to predominantly low Hb content values (mean relative [Hb] =0.37). (Adapted from [22])

lengths beyond 500 nm. On the other hand, movement artefacts may substantially influence the recorded signal: the pressure exerted on the measurement site when positioning the light guide may vary and thereby influence *per se* the capillary blood volume and/or oxygen content. Moreover, the light guide may slightly move when positioned onto the mucosa, and, hence, the signal recorded does not necessarily reflect the remittance from a single point but rather from an area of variable size. Finally, up to now, the EMPHO system does not provide a mathematically rigorous technique to eliminate artefactual spectra. This problem is attenuated to some extent by the large number and the high frequency of spectra recorded. Nevertheless, currently, the proportion of spectra which need to be discarded still largely depends on the skill and the experience of the individual investigator.

Experimental and Clinical Results obtained with EMPHO

Remission spectrophotometry has been applied in various investigations on the intestinal microcirculation. Sato et al. [17] as early as 1979 introduced the technique for calculating the amount and O_2 saturation of hemoglobin in gastric mucosal vessels. They were able to prove that indeed the volume caught by spectrophotometery is limited to mucosal and, to some extent, submucosal vessels. Leung et al. [18] could further demonstrate that microvascular HbO_2 and the relative Hb content, similar to tissue PO_2, depend on local oxygen uptake as well as supply, i.e. microhematocrit and blood flow. In a hemorrhagic shock model in rats, these authors found a positive correlation between gastric mucosal HbO_2 and Hb content indices and mucosal blood flow as measured using the hydrogen clearance technique. In addition, the reflectance spectrophotometry data also closely mirrored ischemia with congestion induced by portal vein occlusion as well as postischemic hyperemia after release of the celiac artery. Limitations of reflectance spectrophotometry however, were observed when global hematocrit changes occur or during artificial hyperoxia or hypoxic hypoxemia; under these circumstances, mucosal HbO_2 and relative Hb content do not always correctly reflect changes in mucosal blood flow [19].

Hasibeder et al. [20] studied the mucosal and serosal microcirculation of an *in vivo* perfused jejunal segment with intact autonomic innervation using the EMPHO device. In contrast to the serosa, mucosal HbO_2 and relative Hb content showed large slow (4–5 cycles/min) rhythmic fluctuations which were paralleled by tissue PO_2 variations. These fluctuations were unrelated to hemodynamic parameters, respiratory frequency, jejunal electromyographic activity or visible peristalsis. Since the results on relative Hb content represent strictly intravascular phenomena, the authors attributed the observed changes to variations in blood volume or microhematocrit within the villus microvessels. In fact, in a subsequent study [21], the authors found evidence that the fluctuations in the villus capillary blood flow are probably caused by vasomotion of the submucosal vessels: by infusing increasing doses of dopamine, the mucosal HbO_2 could be enhanced in a dose-dependent manner without changes in electromyographic activity. The amplitude of the HbO_2 and relative Hb content variations decreased in parallel and disappeared completely at high doses of dopamine.

In a hypodynamic endotoxin shock model, we compared gastric mucosal HbO_2 and relative Hb content recorded at 5 different measurement sites in the great curvature as well as the anterior gastric wall with intramucosal pH (pHi) tonometry, and portal as well as hepatic venous O_2 saturation [22]. Throughout the study, there was a continuous increase of the fractional contribution of critical ($< 20\%$) HbO_2 values at the expense of the reserve ($20\% < HbO_2\% < 50\%$). At the end of the experiment, normal HbO_2 levels ($> 50\%$) had completely vanished (Fig. 3). These findings were concomitant with a redistribution of the relative Hb content histograms towards levels predominantly below 0.5 indicating that the fall in capillary hemoglobin oxygenation was at least in part caused by a drop in capillary blood flow (Fig. 3). These findings were underscored by a pathologically low gastric pHi and substantially reduced portal and hepatic venous O_2 saturations (Fig. 3).

Although remission spectrophotometry has already been used for measuring liver hemodynamics in patients [23], until now clinical experience with EMPHO is only scarce. In hemodynamically stable, mechanically ventilated patients, Specht et al. [24] found substantial differences between HbO_2 levels in the gastric and duodenal mucosa, the latter being mostly lower. Ventilation with increased PEEP levels predominantly resulted in a fall of capillary hemoglobin oxygenation probably due to the decreased microcirculatory blood flow as assessed by laser Doppler flowmetry [25]. Consistently, lower gastric and duodenal mucosa HbO_2 as well as relative Hb content were found in patients with sepsis and patients after coronary artery bypass surgery (CABG) when compared to normals (mean HbO_2 76%) [26]) while mucosal capillary hemoglobin oxygenation (mean HbO_2 48 and 60% in the septic and CABG patients, respectively) as well as relative hemoglobin content were impaired upon admission to the ICU in both groups. Infusing dopexamine (2 µg/kg/min) allowed to achieve normal distributions only in the patients after cardiac surgery (mean HbO_2 60–70 vs. 59% in the patients with septic shock).

Biochemical and Physiological Aspects of Stable Isotope Approaches

The currently available monitoring techniques such as the measurement of splanchnic blood flow and O_2 kinetics and gastric pHi tonometry yield information about regional perfusion, oxygen transport and uptake [1]. Interpretation of these data, however, has two major restrictions. On the one hand, there is no discrimination between gut and hepatic circulation, a distinction which may assume clinical importance [27]. On the other hand, blood flow and oxygen kinetics are not necessarily in parallel with the metabolic responses, be they global or regional [28]. Therefore, we advocate the use of stable, non-radioactive isotope-labelled substrates for the analysis of metabolic pathways.

Several aspects discriminate the stable isotope approach from conventional assessment of metabolic pathways [4]. Routine measurement of substrate concentrations and organ blood flow can only provide information on net balances rather than absolute rates of uptake and release, a drawback which is particularly important in the splanchnic region where results represent a weighted average from the intestine, pancreas and liver. Moreover, routine assessment of metabolic rates crucially depends on correct flow measurement and is highly sensitive to errors in arterio-venous content differences, in particular when the differences are small when compared to the absolute concentrations, eg in the case of glucose. Finally, different oxygen or substrate consuming processes cannot be differentiated.

The theoretical basis of the stable isotope approach conjects that the metabolism of the tracer is not discriminated from that of the tracee and that the labelled and unlabelled molecule follow the same metabolic pathway [4, 5]. Under steady state conditions – i.e. constant contractions of tracee and tracer as well as unchanged pool size – of continuous isotope infusion, the basic assumption is given by

$$F/R_a = [Tracer]/[Tracee] \ [4, 5]$$

where F is the infusion rate of the labelled compound (tracer) and R_a the rate of appearance of the endogenous metabolite (tracee), respectively (Fig. 4).

Gas chromatography/mass spectrometry in the selective ion monitoring mode is used to detect the relative concentrations, and it is clear from the equation that the measurement of absolute concentrations is not required but only the fraction between [tracer] and [tracee], i.e. the isotope enrichment. Choosing an appropriate tracer then allows to monitor organ specific metabolic pathways. Table 1 shows the most commonly used isotopes with their natural abundance and body content as well as normal and experimental uptake [4, 5].

Two different isotope techniques can be used for the monitoring of the splanchnic region. First, the infusion of 6,6-D_2-glucose, i.e. deuterium-labelled glucose, allows to determine endogenous glucose production rate. Since the labelling of the C6-atom does not recirculate [4, 6], the R_a of this tracer is directly related to the endogenous gluconeogenesis. In addition, the determination of glucose production rate with this method is a rather organ-specific marker of hepatic metabolic performances. Although during epinephrine infusion renal glucose release may account for up to 40% of total endogenous glucose formation [29] in healthy volunteers, it is generally conjected that extrahepatic synthesis of glucose contributes for only 5–10% to overall gluconeogenesis [30], in particular

Fig. 4. Basic principle for the use of stable isotopes in a single compartment model. Under steady state conditions, the tracer is infused into the serum pool with the infusion rate F, and the ratio of F and the rate of appearance R_a of the tracee is equal to the concentration quotient of tracer and tracee. (Adapted from [4, 5])

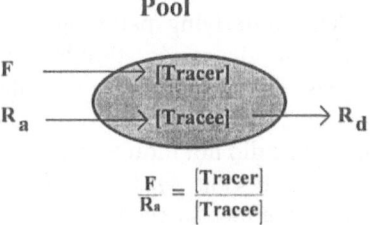

Table 1. Natural abundance, natural content and uptake under normal as well as experimental conditions of commonly used stable isotopes. (Adapted from [4])

Isotope	Natural enrichment, %	Body content, mg/kg	Body content, mg/70 kg	Normal uptake, mg/kg	Uptake during study, mg/kg
^2H	0.015	15	1050	6.9	0.05
^{13}C	1.107	1980	138600	99.9	0.11
^{15}N	0.366	111	7700	0.15	0.12
^{18}O	0.204	130	9100	133.40	0.15

in patients with multiple organ failure when acute renal failure is present. Since in addition hepatic glucose production accounts for about 50% of hepatic O_2 uptake [31], it can be assumed to be also related to hepatic perfusion and O_2 delivery. Second, the fate of enterally administered leucine can be used to evaluate the splanchnic region [4, 6]. Orally given, leucine is absorbed in the small bowel and partially metabolized in the liver, i.e. it undergoes a first pass effect. Since intravenously administered leucine does not follow this pathway, the first pass effect as a fraction of total leucine turnover can be measured as a combined marker of intestinal function, portal blood flow as well as hepatic metabolic capacity [4, 6].

Stable Isotope Approaches for the Monitoring of Hepato-Splanchnic Metabolism

Several studies have investigated the effects of pharmacologic or other therapeutic interventions on the metabolic response of the liver as assessed by hepatic glucose production. In healthy volunteers infusing either epinephrine [32] or norepinephrine [33] in doses comparable to those routinely used in the ICU setting (0.1 and 0.14 μg/kg/min, respectively), significantly increased endogenous glucose formations. While epinephrine nearly doubled the glucose release, the effect was less pronounced during norepinephrine administration. This response is apparently linked to the increased intracellular cAMP concentrations: in the perfused rat, liver administration of enoximone together with epinephrine had a synergistic effect on hepatic glucose release [34]. In contrast to the effects of these endogenous catecholamines, the synthetic adrenergic agonists, dobutamine (6 μg/kg/min) and dopexamine (2.25 μg/kg/min), had hardly any effect on the metabolic response in volunteers [33]. This difference is probably due to their less pronounced β_2-adrenergic activity resulting in only scarce increases of intracellular cAMP levels [35], in particular when low doses are infused [33, 35].

The underlying pathology, however, may substantially alter the metabolic effect of adrenergic stimulation. We compared the course of hepatic glucose release after epinephrine stimulation in normal healthy volunteers with that of patients with alcoholic liver cirrhosis [36]: in contrast to normal volunteers, epinephrine did not induce any change in hepatic glucose production in the cirrhotic patients (Fig. 5). Compromised hepatic perfusion did not account for this striking effect since there was no difference in the simultaneously measured

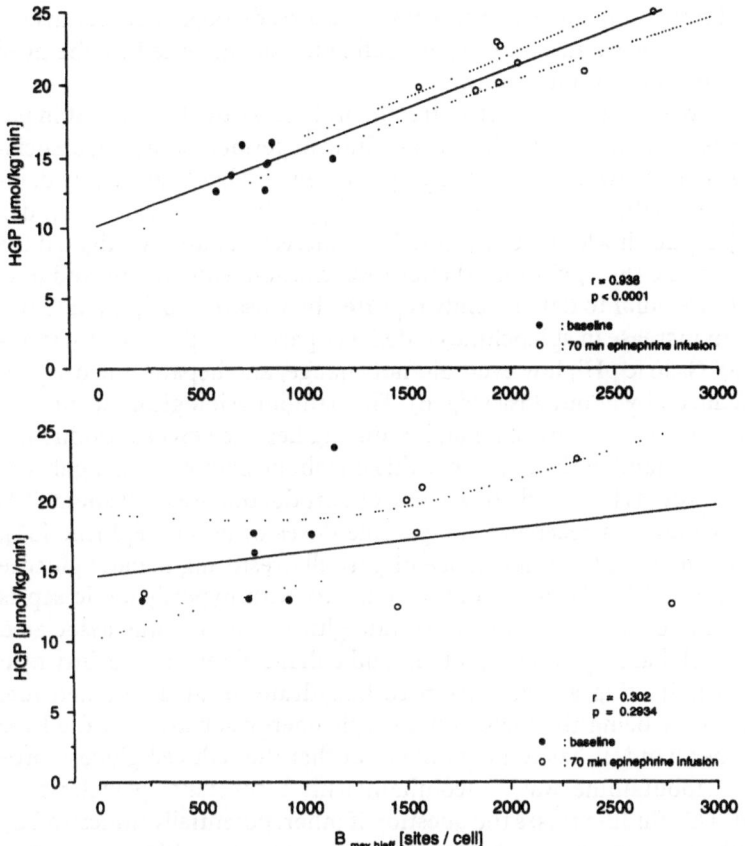

Fig. 5. Hepatic glucose production as a function of the density of high affinity β-adrenoreceptor binding sites in normal volunteers (*upper panel*) and patients with liver cirrhosis (*lower panel*) before (*solid symbols*) and during epinephrine infusion (*open symbols*). While there was a linear positive correlation in the normal volunteers, no significant relation could be found in the cirrhotic patients. The comparable increase of the number of adrenoreceptor sites suggests that epinephrine infusion was not able to stimulate glucose production due to a postreceptor defect. (Adapted from [36])

glycerol clearance which is almost complete at low serum levels during one single transhepatic passage [37]. In addition to the metabolic response, the density of β₂-adrenergic receptor sites on lymphocytes was determined (Fig. 5). While there was a linear positive correlation between the number of receptor sites in the volunteers, no significant relation was found in the cirrhotic patients suggesting that a post-receptor defect is responsible for the lacking increase in hepatic glucose release.

Obviously, the hormonal status may also influence the course of hepatic glucose production during therapeutic interventions. In 7 mechanically ventilated patients with hemodynamically stable sepsis, infusing prostacyclin did not cause any change in glucose production [38]. In these patients, however, who received total parenteral nutrition, glucose production was already depressed because of the absolute insulin resistance and hyperinsulinemia documented by the need for exogenous insuline administration.

The metabolic response to vasoactive treatment is of particular interest in patients with sepsis or septic shock where splanchnic hypermetabolism in association with a mismatch between local O_2 supply and demand has been clearly demonstrated [26, 39, 40]. In 12 patients with hyperdynamic (cardiac index >4 L/min/m^2) septic shock due to necrotizing pancreatitis, we investigated the effects of dobutamine (5–7 µg/kg/min) after resuscitation with volume and norepinephrine [41]. Similar to data recently reported by Uusaro et al. [42], dobutamine induced an increase in splanchnic O_2 delivery parallel to the global systemic effect (Fig. 6). Gastric pHi, however, did not change, and hepatic glucose production was reduced by about 25% (Fig. 6). The pathophysiological meaning of this finding is equivocal: on the one hand, reducing hepatic glucose production decreases the O_2 demand of the liver since this metabolic pathway is a highly energy consuming process [31], and, in fact, glucose production was still about 50% higher than in volunteers receiving comparable doses of norepinephrine [33]. We could show the potential importance of partially restoring hepatic glucose production to normal levels in a group of patients with hyperdynamic sepsis receiving enoximone [43]: the drop in hepatic glucose release was associated with a decreased global respiratory quotient and enhanced serum free fatty acid levels (Table 2) indicating a switch from carbohydrate to fat dominated fuel utilization, the latter being the major physiologic energy substrate of the liver [44]. On the other hand, it has to be pointed out that the reduced glucose production during dobutamine was concomitant with a constant splanchnic O_2 uptake (Fig. 6). This finding raises the question if other, potentially undesired O_2 consuming pathways assumed further importance, a concern which was underscored by the pHi levels which did not respond to the dobutamine treatment either.

The effects of incremental PEEP on hepatic venous O_2 saturation and glucose production further underscore the impact of the patient's pathology on the interaction of hemodynamic and metabolic responses. In 15 patients with hyperdynamic septic shock, we measured hepatic venous O_2 saturation as well as glucose production during ventilation with PEEP levels of 5, 10 and 15 cmH$_2$O [45] after conventional resuscitation goals had been achieved. Increasing PEEP induced the well-known fall in cardiac output concomitant with a decreased hepatic venous O_2 saturation suggesting impaired hepatic blood flow and O_2 delivery. This hemodynamic effect was paralleled by reduced hepatic glucose production (Fig. 7), the mean values being comparable to those of healthy volunteers in the

Fig. 6. Effects of dobutamine (5–7 µg/kg/min) in 12 patients with hyperdynamic (CI >4 L/ min/m^2) septic shock due to necrotizing pancreatitis on splanchnic O_2 kinetics (**A**, *upper panel*), gastric pHi (**A**, *lower panel*) as well as hepatic glucose production (**B**). While dobutamine significantly incrased splanchnic O_2 delivery (**A**, *solid line, closed squares*) proportional to systemic O_2 delivery, splanchnic O_2 uptake and pHi remained unchanged. Hepatic glucose production decreased significantly, but remained significantly lower than in healthy normal volunteers. (Adapted from [41])

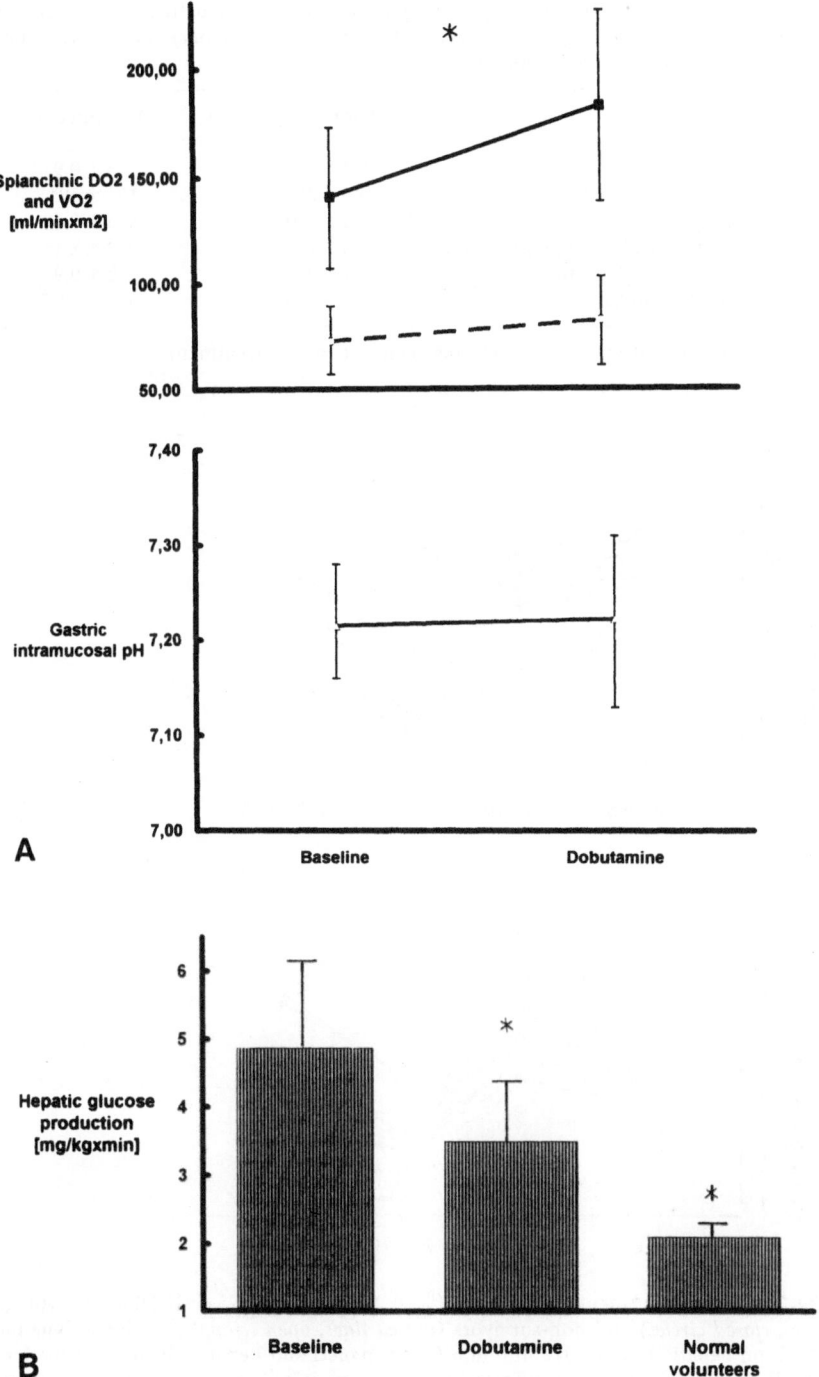

Table 2. Cardiac index, oxygen uptake, respiratory quotient, hepatic glucose production, lactate turnover and serum free fatty acid levels before and after 2 h of enoximone treatment in patients with abdominal sepsis. (Adapted from [43])

	Before enoximone	120 min enoximone
Cardiac index, L/min/m²	5.4 ± 1.0	5.3 ± 0.9
Oxygen uptake, mL/min/m²	148 ± 26	181 ± 30*
Respiratory quotient	0.93 ± 0.10	0.85 ± 0.12*
Hepatic glucose production, mg/kg/min	5.8 ± 2.4	4.2 ± 2.1*
Lactate turnover, mg/kg/min	4.2 ± 0.8	4.2 ± 0.9
Free fatty acids, μmol/L	282 ± 113	580 ± 221*

All values mean ± SD; n = 6; * $p < 0.05$ between control and treatment

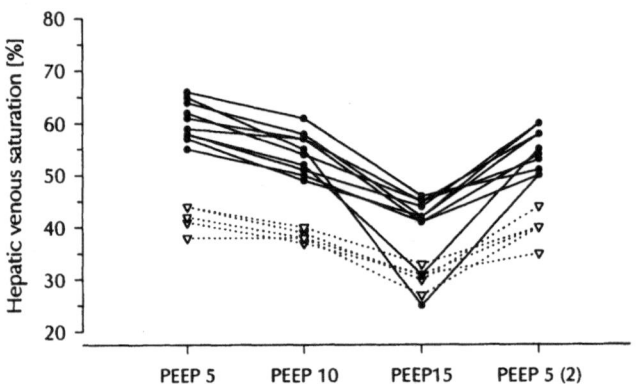

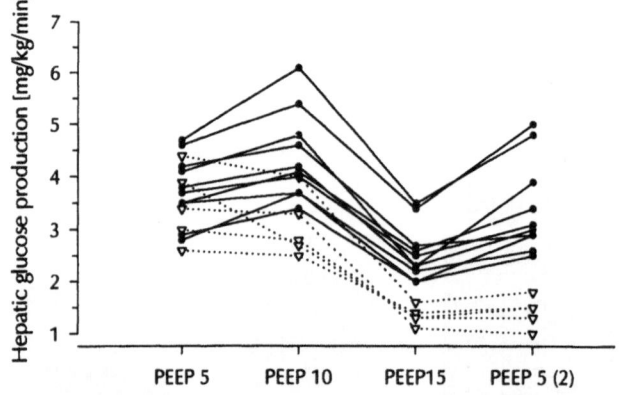

Fig. 7. Effect of incremental PEEP levels (5, 10, 15 and a second 5 cmH₂O) in survivors (*straight lines, closed circles*) and non-survivors (*dotted lines, open triangles*) of hyperdynamic septic shock on hepatic venous O₂ saturation (*upper panel*) and hepatic glucose production (*lower panel*). Note that in the non-survivors, hepatic venous O₂ saturation was significantly lower than in the survivors, and that hepatic glucose production did not return to baseline levels in this group when hepatic venous O₂ saturation was restored with the removal of PEEP. (Adapted from [45])

survivors, and markedly subnormal in the non-survivors. Returning PEEP to the baseline level resulted in restored global hemodynamics as well as hepatic venous O_2 saturation suggesting recovery of hepatic perfusion and O_2 delivery. Strikingly, glucose production only returned to the control values in the survivors while it remained markedly depressed in the non-survivors (Fig. 7). In contrast to the survivors, the non-survivors had exhibited significantly lower hepatic venous O_2 saturation levels far below the normal range already in the control period. It is tempting therefore to speculate that the PEEP-induced fall in cardiac output caused a drop in regional O_2 delivery below a critical threshold which resulted in a concomitant depression of hepatic metabolic performance.

When the pathophysiological significance of a single metabolic response is difficult to evaluate the simultaneous determination of another metabolic pathway may help, such as demonstrated in mechanically ventilated patients with abdominal sepsis [46]. In this study, measuring glucose production was combined with estimating the leucine first pass effect (see above). Volume loading and subsequent addition of dopamine resulted in reduced hepatic glucose production which, however, did not attain normal levels (Fig. 8). The fact that the therapeutic interventions allowed to almost completely restore the leucine first pass effect, a parameter depending on intestinal perfusion as well as liver blood flow and metabolic capacity, suggests that in these patients the reduced glucose release reflected a probably beneficial effect on splanchnic O_2 balance.

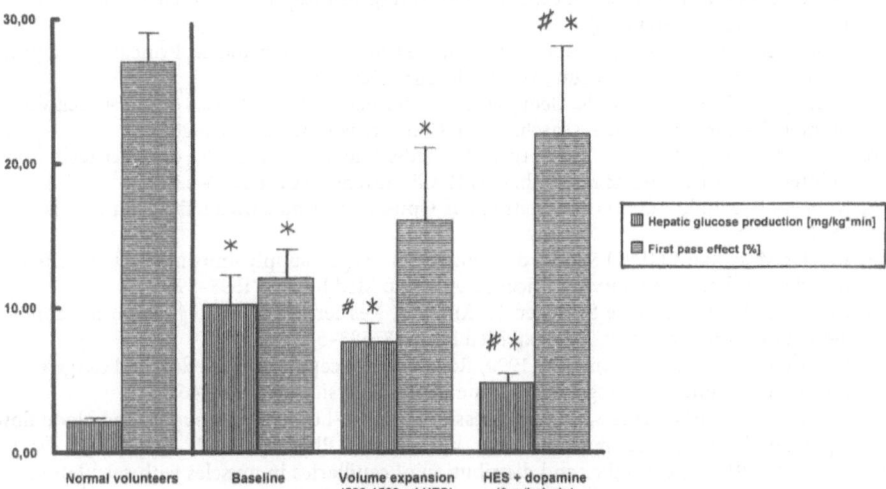

Fig. 8. The influence of volume expansion with hydroxyethyl starch (HES, 500–1500 mL) until a pulmonary artery occlusion pressure of 15 mmHg was achieved and additional dopamine (6 µg/kg/min) on hepatic glucose production and the first pass effect of enterally administered leucine in the liver in mechanically ventilated patients with abdominal sepsis ($n = 8$, mean ± SD). It has to be noted that despite hemodynamic improvement, hepatic metabolic function remained depressed associated with a persistent more than twofold increase in glucose production rate when compared to values in healthy volunteers. # $p < 0.05$ versus baseline, * $p < 0.05$ versus normal range. (Adapted from [46])

Conclusion

In this chapter, we reviewed the potential role of remission spectrophotometry using EMPHO for the assessment of capillary hemoglobin oxygenation and stable isotope approaches for the evaluation of metabolic effects in the splanchnic region. In animal experiments, EMPHO measurements closely correlated with other parameters of splanchnic microcirculatory blood flow and O_2 kinetics. Since there are only limited clinical data available, further studies are warranted to estimate the role of EMPHO for patient management. Experience with stable isotope approaches is far more important, and the results clearly show that the metabolic response to pharmacologic or other therapeutic interventions cannot always be inferred from regional hemodynamic and O_2 kinetic data. Depending on the underlying pathology, the information obtained from these metabolic measurements might even lead to reconsidering the currently valid interpretation of routinely available measurements.

References

1. Takala J (1995) Assessment of splanchnic tissue perfusion. Clin Intensive Care 6:80–82
2. Frank KH, Kessler M, Appelbaum K, Dümmler W (1989) The Erlangen micro-lightguide spectrophotometer EMPHO I. Phys Med Biol 34:1883–1900
3. Kuchenreuther S, Adler J, Eichelbrönner O, Georgieff M (1996) The Erlanger micro-lightguide photometer: A new concept for monitoring intracapillary oxygen supply of tissue. J Clin Monitoring (In press)
4. Wolfe RR (1992) Radioactive and stable isotope tracers in biomedicine. Principles and practice of kinetic analysis. 2nd edn., Wiley-Liss Inc., New York
5. Ensinger H, Vogt J, Träger K, Georgieff M, Radermacher P (1995) Use of tracer techniques in intensive care medicine research. Part I. Clin Intensive Care 6:283–285
6. Ensinger H, Vogt J, Träger K, Georgieff M, Radermacher P (1996) Use of tracer techniques in intensive care medicine research. Part II. Clin Intensive Care 7:30–33
7. Kubelka P, Munk F (1931) Ein Beitrag zur Optik der Farbanstriche. Z Techn Physik 11a:76–77
8. Kessler M, Höper J (1992) Spatial distribution of oxygen supply units in heart and skeletal muscle and their regulatory significance. Adv Exp Med Biol 317:593–598
9. Harrison DK, Birkenhake S, Hagen N, Knauf S, Kessler M (1989) Regulation of capillary blood flow: A new concept. Adv Exp Med Biol 248:583–588
10. Harrison DK, Kessler M, Knauf S (1990) Regulation of capillary blood flow and oxygen supply in skeletal muscle in dogs during hypoxemia. J Physiol 420:431–446
11. Harrison DK, Birkenhake S, Knauf S, Kessler M (1990) Local oxygen supply and blood flow regulation in contracting muscle in dogs and rabbits. J Physiol 422:227–243
12. Krogh A (1919) The number and distribution of capillaries in muscles with calculations of the oxygen pressure necessary for supplying the tissue. J Physiol 52:409–415
13. Krogh A (1919) The supply of oxygen to the tissues and the regulation of the capillary circulation. J Physiol 52:457–477
14. Kessler M, Klövekorn WP, Höper J, et al (1984) Local oxygen supply and regional wall motion of the dog's heart during critical stenosis of the LAD. Adv Exp Med Biol 169:331–340
15. Chance B, Oshino N, Sugano T, Mayevski A (1973) Basic principles of tissue oxygen determination from mitochondrial signals. Adv Exp Med Biol 37:277–292
16. Kessler M, Höper J, Harrison DK, et al (1984) Tissue oxygen supply under normal and pathological conditions. Adv Exp Med Biol 169:69–80

17. Sato N, Kamada T, Schichiri M, Kawano S, Abe H, Hagihara B (1979) Measurement of hemoperfusion and oxygen sufficiency in gastric mucosa *in vivo*. Gastroenterology 76: 814–819
18. Leung FW, Morishita T, Livingston EH, Reedy T, Guth PH (1987) Reflectance spectrophotometry for the assessment of gastroduodenal mucosal perfusion. Am J Physiol 252: G797–G804
19. Casadevall M, Panés J, Piqué JM, Bosch J, Terés J, Rodés J (1992) Limitations of laser-Doppler velocimetry and reflectance spectrophotometry in estimating gastric mucosal blood flow. Am J Physiol 263:G810–G815
20. Hasibeder W, Germann R, Sparr H, et al (1994) Vasomotion induces regular major oscillations in jejunal mucosal tissue oxygenation. Am J Physiol 266:G978–G986
21. Germann R, Haisjackl M, Hasibeder W, et al (1994) Dopamine and mucosal oxygenation in the porcine jejunum. J Appl Physiol 77:2845–2852
22. Eichelbrönner O, Kuchenreuther S, Nemeth P, Adler J, Radermacher P, Georgieff M (1995) Intracapillary HbO_2 and Hb of gastric mucosa during sepsis monitored by use of the EMPHO and compared with the pHi. Clin Intensive Care 6 (Suppl):94 (Abst)
23. Sato N, Hayashi N, Kawano S, Kamada T, Abe H (1983) Hepatic hemodynamics in patients with chronic hepatitis or cirrhosis as assessed by organ-reflectance spectrophotometry. Gastroentrology 84:611–616
24. Specht M, Morciniec P, Kuhly P, et al (1995) Assessment of local hemoglobin oxygenation in gastric and duodenal mucosa: First measurements with the EMPHO II spectrophotometer. Clin Intensive Care 6 (Suppl):95 (Abst)
25. Specht M, Morciniec P, Kuhly P, et al (1995) Influence of PEEP on hemoglobin oxygenation and blood flow velocimetry in gastric and duodenal mucosa. Intensive Care Med 21:S199 (Abst)
26. Temmesfeld-Wollbrück B (1995) Spectrophotometric assessment of gastric mucosal perfusion. Clin Intensive Care 6:37–38
27. Hawker F (1994) SIRS: Is it a liver disease? Int J Intensive Care 1:113
28. Wilmore DW, Goodwin CW, Aulick LH, Powanda MC, Mason AD, Pruitt BA (1980) Effect of injury and infection on visceral metabolism and circulation. Ann Surg 192:491–504
29. Sturmvoll M, Chintalapudi U, Priello G, Welle S, Gutierrez O, Gerich J (1995) Uptake and release of glucose by the human kidney. Postabsorptive rates and responses to epinephrine. J Clin Invest 96:2528–2533
30. Löffler G (1979) Intermediärstoffwechsel II: Kohlenhydrate. In: Löffler G, Petrides PE, Weiss L, Harper HA (eds) Physiologische Chemie, 2nd edn. Springer Verlag, New York, pp 315–357
31. Jungas RL, Halperin ML, Brosnan JT (1992) Quantitative analysis of amino acid oxidation and related gluconeogenesis in humans. Physiol Rev 72:419–448
32. Ensinger H, Träger K, Geisser W, et al (1994) Glucose and urea production and leucine, ketoisocaproate and alanine fluxes at supraphysiological plasma adrenaline concentrations in volunteers. Intensive Care Med 20:113–118
33. Geisser W, Träger K, Vogt J, et al (1996) Glucose production during infusion of different catecholamines in healthy volunteers. Intensive Care Med 22 (Suppl):S77 (Abst)
34. Weidenbach H, Beckh K, Schricker T, Georgieff M, Adler G (1995) Enhancement of hepatic glucose release and bile flow by the phosphodiesterase-III-inhibitor enoximone in the perfused rat liver. Life Sciences 56:172–176
35. MacGregor DA, Prielipp RC, Butterworth JF, James RL, Boyster RL (1996) Relative efficacy and potency of β-adrenoreceptor agonists for generating cAMP in human lymphocytes. Chest 109:194–200
36. Schricker T, Albuszies G, Weidenbach H, et al (1996) Effect of epinephrine on glucose metabolism in patients with alcoholic liver cirrhosis. J Hepatology (In press)
37. Sestoft L, Fleron P (1975) Kinetics of glycerol uptake by the perfused rat liver. Biochem Biophys Acta 375:462–471
38. Scheeren T, Susanto F, Reinauer H, Tarnow J, Radermacher P (1994) Prostacyclin improves glucose utilization in patients with sepsis. J Crit Care 9:175–184

39. Gump FE, Price JE, Kinney GM (1970) Whole body and splanchnic blood flow and oxygen consumption measurements in patients with intraperitoneal infections. Ann Surg 171: 321–328
40. Ruokonen E, Takala J, Kari A, Saxén H, Mertsola J, Hansen EJ (1993) Regional blood blood flow and oxygen transport in septic shock. Crit Care Med 21:1296–1303
41. Reinelt H, Fischer G, Wiedeck H, et al (1996) Effects of increased regional blood flow on splanchnic metabolism. Intensive Care Med 22 (Suppl):S75 (Abst)
42. Uusaro A, Ruokonen E, Takala J (1995) Estimation of splanchnic blood flow by the Fick principle in man and problems in the use of indocyanine green. Cardiovasc Res 30:106–112
43. Schricker T, Radermacher P, Träger K, Kugler B, Georgieff M (1996) Metabolic and hemodynamic response to the phosphodiesterase-III-inhibitor enoximone in septic patients. Clin Intensive Care (In press)
44. Newsholm EA, Leech AR (1983) Catabolism of lipids. In: Newsholm EA, Leech AR (eds) Biochemistry for the Medical Sciences, John Wiley & Sons, New York, pp 246–299
45. Träger K, Radermacher P, Georgieff M (1996) PEEP and hepatic metabolic performance in septic shock. Intensive Care Med 22 (Suppl):S127 (Abst)
46. Bagley JS, Wan JMF, Georgieff M, Forse RA, Blackburn G (1991) Cellular nutrition in support of early multiple organ failure. Chest 100:182S–188S

Growth Factors and the Intestine

P. Fürst and J. L. Rombeau

Introduction

One of the most exciting achievements of the medical research community has been the characterization of a diverse family of signal molecules, the growth factors (GF), which are involved in the control of cell growth and differentiation, and may play a crucial role in numerous diseased conditions. The origin of this research lies in the studies of S. Cohen, R. Levi-Montalchini, D. Metcalf and others who first used complex biological assays to characterize epidermal and nerve GF and the colony stimulating factors (CSF), respectively. Indeed, these works stimulated many groups to establish methods for elucidation of both their biological role and mechanism of molecular action through specific receptors. Particularly important to the development of the field has been the ability to employ characterized single peptide species. The availability of pure factors and modern molecular and cellular techniques has firmly established the central role of these signal molecules in many aspects of biology. The realization that the factors trigger through specific receptors, the generation of second messengers and hence intracellular enzyme cascades generated new insight into the mechanisms which may be operating in diseases and during critical illness. In addition, these studies have stimulated the introduction of novel methods for manipulating GF-induced signal cascades which could be important in many pathological conditions.

In recent years, the role of GF in intestinal growth and function has received considerable interest. This chapter describes current knowledge of structure and function of selected relevant GF with particular emphasis on their potential therapeutic utilities.

General Classification

Classification of selected GF based on biological function is summarized in Figs. 1–4 [1].

In group 1, short chain 4-α helical GF are to be considered in immunohemopoietic regulation. Granulocyte macrophage CSF (GM-CSF) using β-common chain receptor is participating in innate immunity. GM-CSF and stem cell factor (SCF) are involved in producing immunohemopoietic cells from the bone mar-

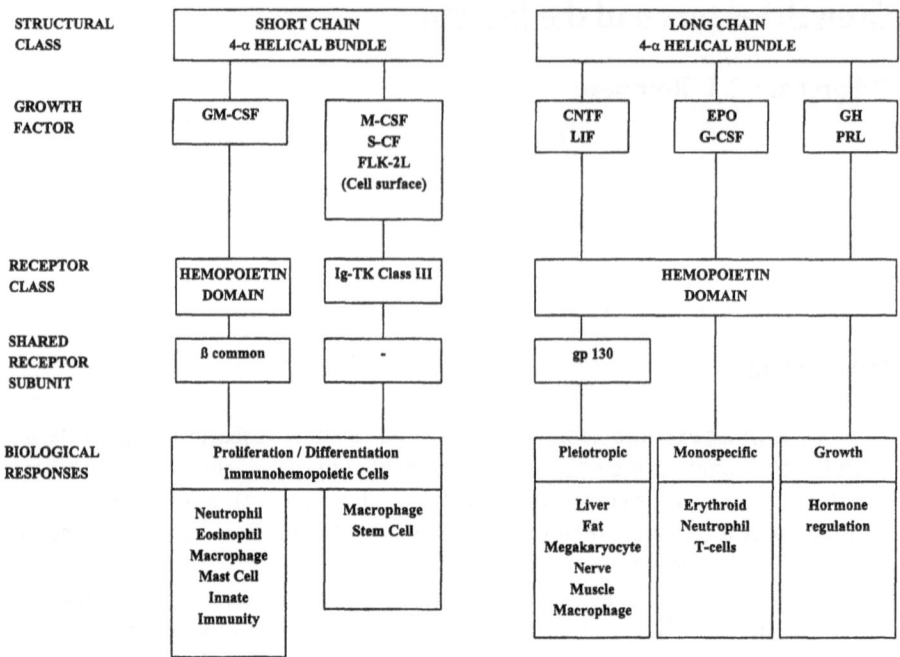

Fig. 1. Subclassification of group 4-α helical growth factor.
CSF: colony stimulating factor; G: granulocyte; M: macrophage SCF: stem cell factor; FLK-2L: fetal liver kinase-2 ligand; LIF: leukemia inhibitory factor; EPO: erythropoietin; CNTF: ciliary neutrotrophic factor; GH: growth hormone; PRL: prolactin. (Modified from [1])

row. Long chain 4-α GF, erythropoietin (EPO) and G-CSF are mostly specific generating erythroid and neutrophilic cells, and ciliary neutrotrophic factor (CNTF) is one of the most pleiotropic factors [2]. Growth hormone (GH) and prolactin (PRL) exhibit a classical endocrine role in whole body metabolism (Fig. 1).

Group 2 GF are involved primarily in growth and differentiation of a variety of epithelial, endothelial and neural tissues [3]. Many of these factors appear to play an essential role during tissue modelling in development. The ligands for the cell surface antigens CD40L, CD27L and FASL belongs to the β-jelly roll structural class and are involved in immune regulatory events, and especially the acute phase response to injury and infection (Fig. 2).

The group 3 GF (Fig. 3) mediate various biological responses. The epidermal GF (EGF) class of GF is involved in the proliferation of epithelial cells and in wound healing, while insulin-like GF are promoting proliferation and differentiation of mesenchymal cells and metabolic responses in tissue cells [4].

The group 4 mosaic GF (Fig. 4) have important biological activities. The hepatocyte GF (HGF) has an unique structure and is involved as a mitogen for hepatocytes, endothelial and intestinal epithelial cells [5].

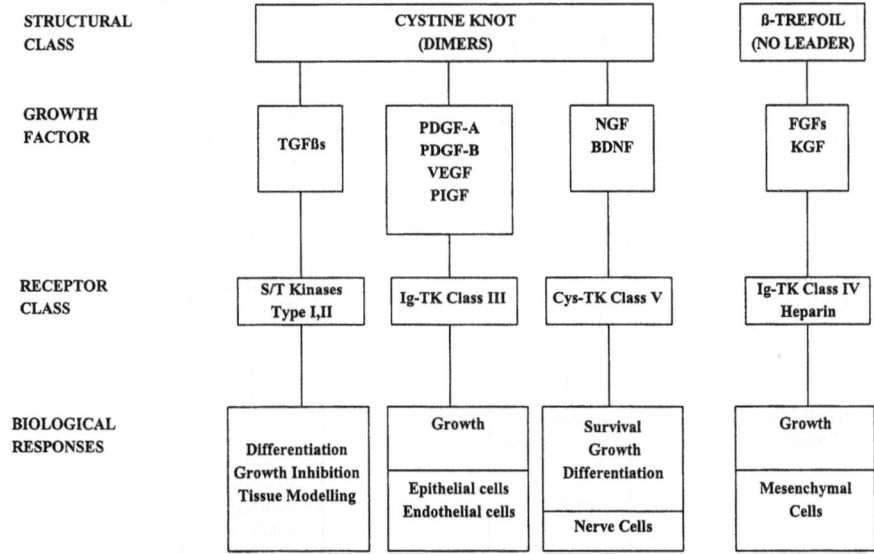

Fig. 2. Subclassification of group 2-β sheet rich growth factors.
TGF: transforming growth factor; PDGF: platelet derived growth factor; VEGF: vascular endothelial cell growth factor; PIGF: placenta growth factor; NGF: nerve growth factor; KGF: kerato-
nocyte growth factor; FGF: fibroblast growth factor; S/T: serine/threonine; TK: tyrosine kinase;
Cys: cysteine rich. (Modified from [1])

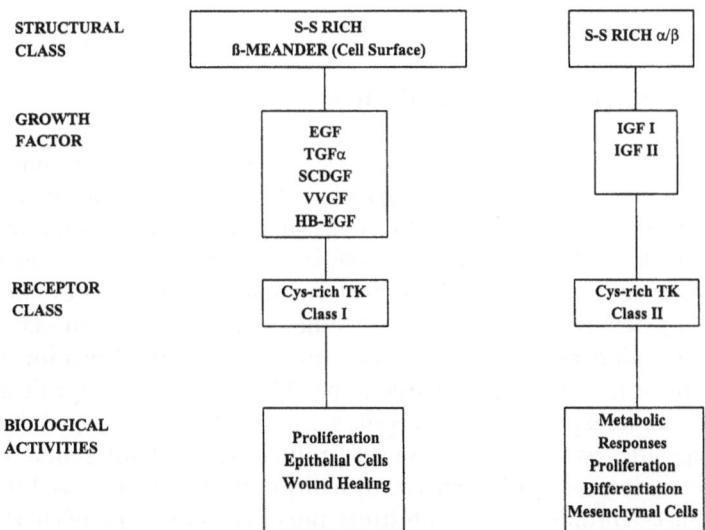

Fig. 3. Subclassification of group 3 small α/β-growth factors.
EGF: epidermal growth factor; TGF: transforming growth factor; SCDGF: Schwann-cell-derived
growth factor; VVGF: vaccinia virus-derived growth factor; HB-EGF: heparinbinding EGF; IGF:
insulin-like growth factor; TK: tyrosine kinase. (Modified from [1])

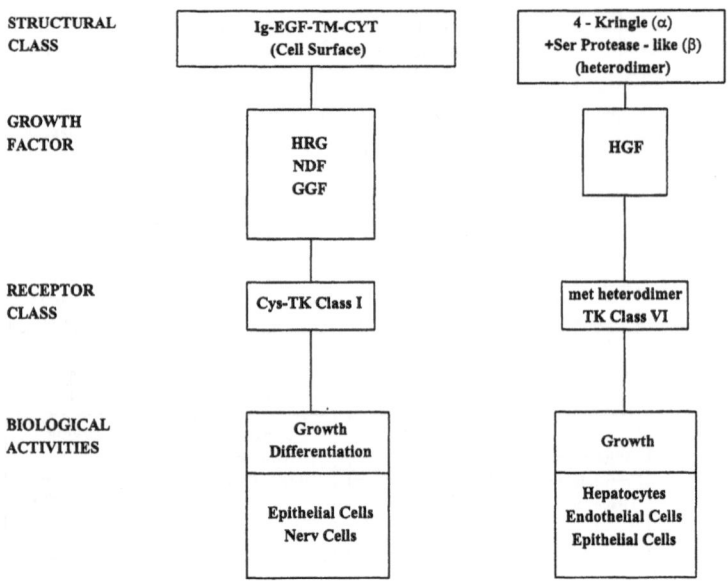

Fig. 4. Subclassification of group 4 mosaic growth factors.
HRG: heregulin; NDF: new differentiation factor; GGF: glial growth factor; HGF: hepatocyte growth factor; Cys: cysteine-rich domain; TK: tyrosine kinase; Ig: immunoglobuline-like; EGF: epidermal growth factor like; TM: transmembrane domain; CYT: cytoplasmic domain. (Modified from [1])

Growth Factors and the Intestine

A number of GF listed in figures 1–4 reveal regulatory functions in the small intestine and colon. Established methods of studying their effects in the gut include stimulation of endogenous GF production, administration of exogenous GF, and inhibition of GF synthesis [6]. New approaches using molecular biologic techniques have improved our understanding in evaluating the relationship between GF and the gut. Studies of gene expression may reveal changes in GF and/or receptor synthesis in intestinal growth; direct information about GF effects in the gut is proposed to be obtained from transgenic animals that over- or underexpress GF or receptor genes [7]. Indeed, many of the effects are tissue specific, yet their impact on cell proliferation and differentiation appears to be a common mechanism shared by many of the GF (Figs. 1–4). Important GF affecting cell proliferation in intestinal mucosa include hepatocyte HGF, GH, prolactin (PRL), EGF, neurotensin (NT), insulin-like GF (IGFs), fibroblast GF (FGFs), transforming GF (TGFα and TGFβ) and endothelins (ETs). Principal GF that influence intestinal cell proliferation and differentiation are summarized in Table 1.

Hepatocyte Growth Factor (HGF)

Alternative names are scatter factor (SF), human lung fibroblast-derived mitogen, hepatopoietin A and hepatotropin. HGF is αβ-hetero-dimeric glycoprotein secreted by mesodermal cells. HGF stimulates mitogenesis and cell motility. HGF is a multi-functional factor for several epithelial cells. It stimulates growth of endothelial cells, keratinocytes and melanocytes [5], and it dissociates layers of epithelial cells (scattering effect), increasing their motility and invasiveness [8].

HGF is produced by non-parenchymal liver, kidney, lung and by intestinal cells. Cells in these tissues express the high level of HGF receptor in humans. The receptor is expressed at a particularly high level in epithelial cells of the gastrointestinal (GI) tract [9, 10].

HGF has been purified to homogeneity [11], the gene of human HGF has been cloned [12] and the locus was mapped [13]. Although this highly interesting GF may possess therapeutical potential, it is not yet available for clinical trials.

The Growth Hormone (GH)/Prolactin (PRL) Family

These pituary hormones define an expanding family of approximately 22 GF that also encompasses the placental lactogenes (PLs), proliferins and somatolactin. GH is alternatively referred to as somatotropin. Human GH, PRL and PL can be efficiently expressed in *E. coli*, and purified recombinant extracellular binding domains of receptors are available for direct binding assay [14]. Alternatively, the proliferation of myeloid cell lines transfected with full-lengths receptors affords a cell-based assay for bioactivity [14, 15]. Unlike most other mammalian GHs, primate GHs have broad specificity and bind tightly to both the GH (somatogenic) and PRL (lactogenic) receptors. GH release is primarily controlled by the opposing actions of the hypothalamic hormones GHRH and somatostatin, and importantly, is pulsatile and mainly nocturnal [16].

The trophic effects of GH on intestinal mucosa are well known. However, there is still some uncertainty as to whether these effects are a direct consequence of GH or secondary to improved nutrition, hyperphagia, or nutrient-stimulated release of secondary hormones such as gastrin and somatostatin [17]. In an early study, GH demonstrated a mitogenic effect on crypt cells of the duodenum in hypophysectomized rats [18]. Subsequent studies showed that GH induced GI tract hypertrophy in hypophysectomized rats as well as histogenesis in fetal rat intestinal transplants [19].

The growth-promoting effects of GH in the small intestine and colon have traditionally been considered to be mediated by IGF-I [20], and it is known that binding to GH receptors stimulates IGF gene transcription [21]. One study, however, indicates that discrete epithelial cell subpopulations of the intestinal mucosa are directly responsive to GH [22]. The crypt base columnar, villous columnar, goblet, and enteroendocrine cells of the small intestine, and the crypt base and surface columnar cells of the colon all possess GH receptors of hetero-

Table 1. Summary and description of principle growth factors that influence intestinal cell proliferation and differentiation

Growth factor	Receptor/Location	Intestinal cell action	Comments
HGF	HGF receptor • Small intestine and colon	Mucosal growth Stimulates cell motility and dissociation of epithelial sheets	Expression of receptor highly increased in tumors

GH	GH receptor
	• Small intestine
	  – Crypt base columnar cells
	  – Villous columnar cells
	  – Goblet cells
	  – Enteroendocrine cells
	• Colon
	  – Crypt base cells
	  – Surface columnar cells
		Mucosal growth
		Increases cell longevity
		Increases cell proliferation (?)
			Probably mediated by IGF-I

PRL	PRL receptor • Small intestine and colon	Mucosal growth? Release regulated by VIP	Mediated by GH Overexpression associated with intestinal tumors
EGF*	EGF/TGFα receptors • Small intestine and colon • Apical and basolateral surfaces of cell membranes • Intrinsic protein-tyrosine kinase activity	Mucosal growth Increases crypt cell production Enhances cell maturation in fetal intestine Regulates water, sodium, chloride and glucose transport	Mediated by TGFα Parenteral effects > enteral effects

NT	NT receptors
	• Small intestine and colon
		Increases mucosal growth
		Small intestine (mostly jejunum)
		  Cell proliferation
		Colon
		  Increases cell proliferation in young
		  Causes cell hypertorphy in adult
		  Increases postresection adaptive hyperplasia
			NT mRNA found in small intestine (mostly distal) and colon
			Posttranscriptional mechanism regulates NT production in intestinal mucosa

Table 1. Cont.

Growth factor	Receptor/Location	Intestinal cell action	Comments

IGF-I, IGF-II	IGF-I, II receptors
	• Small intestine
	  – Crypt base cells
	  – Villous columnar cells
	• Colon
	  – Crypt base cells
	  – Apical columnar cells
	• Binding activity
	  – Colon > small intestine
	• Receptor density
	  – Crypt > apex
		Mucosal growth
		Crypt cell proliferation
		Increases DNA and protein synthesis
		Increases postresection adaptive hyperplasia
			IGFBPs modulate
			  IGF receptor interaction
			IGF-I ten times more potent than
			  IGF-II

FGFs	FGF receptors	Promote intestinal cell growth Enhance mucosal cell differentiation	Mostly found in heparin bound form (HSPGs)

TGFα	EGF/TGFα receptors present
	throughout small intestine and
	colon
		Increases mucosal growth
		  Increases cell proliferation
		  Increases cell migration
		  Enhances cell differentiation
		  Epithelial cell restitution
		  (wound healing)
			Similar in structure and activity
			  to EGF

TGFβ	specific TGFβ receptor (?) throughout small intestine and colon	Inhibits cell proliferation Cell migration Induces cell differentiation/maturation Enhances cell restitution (wound healing)	Production and function apex > crypt base
ETs	ETₐ and ET_b receptors?	Stimulation of smooth muscle cell proliferation	ET receptors are linked to calcium channels

* cf. TGFα

geneous distribution [22]. The localization of these specific GH receptors supports the importance of GH in the proliferation of intestinal epithelial cells [23]. Thus, GH may act independently, via second messengers such as IGF-I, or synergistically with IGF-I as a growth promoter in the small intestine and colon. Among the activities that are probably also direct is the initiation of adipocyte differentiation in which c-fos and c-jun transcription is rapidly induced [16].

A model of chronic GH excess, transgenic mice with bovine GH gene linked to mouse metallothionein I promoter demonstrates increased growth of small-bowel mucosa [24]. Chronic GH excess increases jejunal villus height, small-bowel weight, mucosal mass, and DNA protein content accompanied by an increase in intestinal IGF-I mRNA expression in mouse small intestine. Furthermore, this effect in transgenic mice appears not to be secondary to increased rate of enterocyte proliferation. This finding suggests GH may have a prolonging effect on the life span of intestinal mucosal cells [24].

PRL also has a multitude of effects on metabolism, development and behavior. PRL receptor expression is widespread (liver, adipose tissue, intestine, brain, heart and skeletal muscle [16, 25]) and is regulated by factors like GH and PRL as well as steroids. Release of PRL from pituitary lactotrops is stimulated in humans by factors such as thyrotrophin-releasing hormone (TRH) and vasoactive intestinal peptide (VIP). In burned patients, VIP may be involved in the multiple metabolic and hormonal responses. Following burn injury plasma concentrations of VIP decrease, presumably reflecting enhanced utilization or complex hormonal regulation. Enteral nutrition is associated with an elevation of the polypeptide concentration [26].

Epidermal Growth Factor (EGF)

EGF is a low molecular weight (Mr = 6045) polypeptide. There are 5 distinct mammalian gene products that can be identified as EGF-like molecules; EGF, TGFα, amphiregulin, heparin binding EGF (Hb-EGF), and betacellulin [27]. The mature forms of EGF and TGFα are of 53 and 50 residues, respectively. They are stable to heat and acidic pH. Mature EGF can be isolated and is available as a recombinant protein (including human EGF and TGFα) from numerous commercial sources.

EGF is a well-known mitogen that stimulates cell proliferation *in vitro* and *in vivo,* and its administration results in hyperproliferation of various epithelial tissues [27]. This has led to the idea that EGF may be the "maintenance" factor for the continuous renewal of epithelial cell populations. In addition to mitogenic responses, the administration of EGF produces several non-mitogenic responses such as the inhibition of gastric acid secretion [27]. The trophic effects of EGF occur in many types of epithelial cells, especially in those of the intestinal mucosa [28, 29]. Although its underlying mechanisms are still unknown, recombinant human EGF (urogastrone) effectively stimulates intestinal cell production in adult rats and humans [30]. Some of these EGF-induced effects may be mediated by the analog TGFα [31]. Since EGF and TGFα share the same intestinal cell-surface receptors (EGF/TGFα receptor), many effects of EGF may also apply to TGFα [32]. Nevertheless, EGF is important in cell proliferation and maturation of pre- and postnatal intestine [33]. In suckling mice, repeated injections of EGF stimulates intestinal DNA synthesis and production of certain absorptive enzymes [34]. Furthermore, EGF promotes maturation of small intestine and differentiation of brush border membranes in fetal mice [35].

While a single dose of EGF does not affect cell proliferation, repeated daily injections or parenteral nutrition (TPN) with EGF greatly enhances this process in small intestine and colon [36]. The effect of EGF differs when administered enterally or parenterally [36, 37]. In one study, EGF given enterally did not stimulate cell proliferation in rat colon [38], whereas intravenous recombinant EGF reversed marked intestinal hypoplasia characteristically found in TPN-fed rats. TPN with EGF restores CCPR in small intestine to levels found in orally fed rats and increases labelling (tritiated thymidine) per crypt in the colon more than twice that of enterally fed rats [39]. Subcutanous infusion of EGF following massive small bowel resection (6.25 µg/kg/h) results in increased animal weight, mucosal thickness, and most importantly, small bowel length. These effects may be of great benefit to the host. It will be interesting to see whether the striking increase in bowel length can be demonstrated in human EGF studies [40].

In another study, following massive proximal resection, adaptation of intestinal digestive and absorptive function does not parallel ileal mucosal hyperplasia. Administration of EGF (oral 40 µg/kg/day) to resected animals (rabbits) enhances glucose absorption. Consequently, EGF stimulates maltase specific activity and may have therapeutic potential in management of short gut syndrome [41].

EGF receptors are present throughout the intestine and have been located on both basolateral and brush-border membranes [42]. Such receptors with intrinsic protein-tyrosine kinase activity phosphorylate several endogenous proteins [43]. While their role in signaling cell proliferation and mucosal growth remains unknown, EGF receptors may regulate water, sodium, chloride, and glucose transport in the gut. *In vivo* transport studies reveal that EGF-receptor interactions increase chloride, glucose, sodium, and water absorption in rabbit jejunum [44]. Thus, EGF upregulates electrolyte and nutrient absorption in the small bowel, which may partially explain its function in both normal and stressed intestine.

Neurotensin (NT)

Neurotensin is a tridecapeptide found in mucosal endocrine cells of the jejunum and ileum [45]. It has a trophic effect in many tissues in the GI tract, including small intestine and colon [46, 47]. Long-term NT administration stimulates colonic mucosal growth in both young and adult rats [46]. Although NT increases colonocyte proliferation in young rats, it appears to only increase colonocyte size (hypertrophy) in adult rats. Subcutaneous injections of NT reverse small-bowel mucosal hypoplasia associated with liquid elemental diets in aged rats. Neurotensin apparently stimulates cell proliferation in rat small intestine that is most pronounced in the jejunum [48].

Neurotensin may also be important in the intestinal regeneration after small-bowel resection [49]. A recent study suggests NT augments adaptive hyperplasia in intestinal mucosa after small-bowel resection. Within 7 to 8 days after resection, maximal mucosal hyperplasia usually occurs in the residual small intestine. After 7 days of administration, NT increased DNA, RNA, and protein content in residual small intestinal mucosa after distal or proximal enteroectomy. Thus, NT has the capability to promote cell proliferation usually stimulated solely by small-bowel resection [50].

Recent Northern blot analysis and hybridization of rat encoding gene for NT and neuromedin-N has been utilized to map the intestinal distribution of NT mRNA and to study the regulation of NT expression during periods of fasting and refeeding in rats [51]. Neurotensin mRNA transcripts are distributed throughout rat small intestine and proximal colon with the greatest amount found in the distal small bowel. Furthermore, rats fasted for 72 h have profoundly reduced NT intestinal tissue concentrations, while such animals re-fed for 24 h returned NT concentrations to normal levels. Interestingly, the amount of NT mRNA and its transcription are not affected by periods of fasting and feeding. Such results strongly suggest that a yet undefined posttranscriptional mechanism regulates NT production in intestinal mucosa [51].

Insulin-like Growth Factors (IGFs)

IGF-I and IGF-II are GF with structures similar to insulin but which are primarily involved in normal growth and development of vertebrates. The major source of circulating (endocrine) IGFs is the liver, though most extrahepatic tissues synthesize IGFs where they operate as paracrine/autocrine regulators of the differentiated function of these tissues including epithelium of the intestinal tract. IGFs are alternatively named somatomedins. In developing fetal tissues, IGF is expressed primarily by mesenchymal derived cells, which suggests that it plays an important role in tissue development [52].

IGF-I and II are polypeptides that play an important role in mucosal growth by modulating intestinal crypt cell proliferation. IGF-I induces increased DNA and protein synthesis in intestinal crypt cells *in vitro* and enhances intestinal mucosal adaptation after gut resection [53–55]. It interacts with its receptors throughout the small intestine and colon and is considered a primary mediator of postnatal trophic effects of GH [56]. Similar to IGF-I, IGF-II stimulates DNA and protein synthesis in IEC-6 cells. In concentration response experiments, IGF-I is about ten times more potent than IGF-II in stimulating DNA and protein syntheses in IEC-6 cells [57]. An important role for IGF-I in colonic adaptation after intestinal resection is indicated by enhanced colonic mucosal growth and water absorption after IGF-I treatment. Upregulation of colonic IGF-I mRNA as well as alteration of IGFBP-3 and IGFBP-4 mRNA expression suggests that the IGF-I action pathway may mediate, at least in part, the colonic adaptative response. This would mean that exogenous IGF-I administration or manipulation of intestinal IGF-I action may provide therapeutic benefit in patients suffering from short bowel syndrome [58].

Currently, a constant intraluminal infusion of IGF-I by jejunostomy has been suggested [59, 60]. Intraluminal delivery of IGF-I appears to be an efficacious and potentially safer route than systemic therapy to deliver the growth-promoting effects of IGF-I directly to adapting intestinal mucosa. Intraluminally delivered IGF-I is not detectable in the systemic circulation and, therefore, may avoid the potential side effects of systemic delivery. While short-term, focal effects of IGF-I delivered to the bowel mucosa have been reported previously [59], administration of intraluminal IGF-I in this post-resection jejunostomy model demonstrates a safe route of delivery to long segments of adapting bowel which may have direct clinical applications for patients recovering from massive bowel resection [60].

Once considered to be primarily synthesized in the liver, IGFs are now known to be produced locally within many organs, including the gut [53]. Studies with *in situ* hybridization and Nothern blot techniques have revealed mRNA for IGF-I and IGF-II in fetal human and rat intestine [61]. Intestinal synthesis of IGF as well as many of the binding proteins suggests that these growth factors function predominantly through either autocrine or paracrine mechanisms as well [56, 57, 62, 63].

Despite intestinal synthesis of several types of IGF-binding proteins (IGFBPs) [64], their roles have not been clearly determined. Several *in vitro* studies suggest that endogenous production of IGFBPs may facilitate or inhibit IGF action. However, most studies demonstrate an inhibitory role for IGFBPs that prevents IGFs from interacting with intestinal cell-surface IGF receptors [65]. If these findings are correct, decreased IGF potency *in vivo* may correlate with IGFBPs binding. In a recent animal study *in vivo*, decreased ileal synthesis of IGFBP-3 enhanced IGF-I bioability to stimulate ileal cell proliferation and adaptation after massive small-bowel resection [66]. Other research, however, indicates that the mitogenic effect of IGF-I is actually dependent on its ability to bind IGFBPs [67]. Thus, the mitogenic effects of IGFs are most likely the result of complex interactions between IGFBPs and IGF cell receptors. Interestingly, IGF-I alone, in contrast to TGFβ and PDGF, had no effect on wound-breaking strength. However, the combination of IGF-I and IGFBP-1 significantly increased wound-breaking strength, probably due to post-translation modification of the binding protein (dephosphorylation). Thus, IGF-I is a potent stimulant of incisional wound healing but it must be combined with one of its specific binding protein [68].

Receptors for IGF-I and IGF-II have higher expressions in proliferative crypt cells when compared to the apical cells of the rat small intestine and colon, although these receptors are present on a variety of cells in the intestinal epithelium [56]. Additionally, heterogeneity among receptors exists between the small intestine and colon as well as among the various layers within each organ. Interestingly, binding activity to IGF receptors is higher in the colon than in the rest of the GI tract in the rat [56]. Receptor density in the intestinal epithelium is much greater in the crypts than in the villi, which suggests that IGF receptors modulate crypt cell proliferation and decrease in expression with intestinal cell differentiation [69].

It is notable that each of IGF-I and EGF uses a distinct tyrosine kinase receptor but the receptors share some common signal transduction pathways. An interesting idea is whether EGF and IGF-I interact to regulate intestinal epithelial cell growth. EGF and IGF-I alone each stimulated DNA synthesis in IEC-6 cells, but the combined effects of the two GF were synergistic. Indeed, the IEC-6 cells express high levels of type I IGF receptor mRNA, while IGF-I *per se* decreases expression of this receptor mRNA, and EGF attenuates this effect. Both GF reduce IGFBP2 mRNA expression. EGF, but not IGF-I, potently and rapidly induce c-fos and c-jun mRNAs and induce total AP-1 transcriptional activity. IGF-I, but not EGF, induce c-jun phosphorylation and transactivation. These distinct effects of the two GF on the intracellular signal transduction mechanisms leading to transcriptional activation of AP-I may contribute to their synergistic effects on DNA synthesis [70].

Combination of IGF-I and glutamine exerts also differential effects on IGFBPs. Following bowel resection, increased intestinal growth was associated with increased levels of IGFBP-4 with administration of IGF-I, but not with glutamine treatment [71].

Administration of IGF-I improves intestinal structure and glucose absorption in the rat small bowel allograft. Both IGF-I and glutamine reduce bacterial translocation to mesenteric lymph nodes. The combination of IGF-I and glutamine increases water absorption [72].

IGF receptors are polarized on the apical membranes of proximal colon mucosa with apical colonocytes possessing only type I IGF receptors [73]. Although abundant IGF-I and IGF-II receptors have been identified in the human colon, their role in mucosal growth and adaptation in both small intestine and colon is not fully understood [74, 75].

Fibroblast Growth Factors (FGFs)

FGFs are a family of 15–32 kDA single chain polypeptides having a role in a variety of biological processes such as cell growth, differentiation, tissue repair and transformation [76, 77]. At present the FGF family consists of 9 members.

FGFs are potent mitogens for a wide variety of cells. FGF have trophic effects on endothelial and epithelial cells of the intestinal mucosa. FGF stimulates cultured endothelial cells to mirror a basement membrane matrix, a process dependent upon the proteolytic enzymes collagenase and plasminogen activator. Many of the FGFs in tissues are apparently present in heparin bound forms [78], binding heparin sulphate proteoglycans (HSPGs) on the cell surface and in the extracellular matrix. Tissue FGFs in the HSPG-matrix-bound form promote intestinal cell growth [79]. The FGF receptors are expressed in a large variety of cells, and ligand binding may induce differentiation responses in wide a range of biological processes such as tissue development, tissue repair and survival and differentiation [79, 80].

Transfected FGF constructs are capable of cellular transformation through autocrine or paracrine mechanisms. Exogenous administration of FGF has been found to promote angiogenesis, intestinal epithelial growth and also progression of various tumors [76]. In addition FGFs are involved in the differentiation of a variety of cells including those of intestinal mucosa [81].

Transforming Growth Factors (TGFs)

TGFβ was originally discovered as a secreted factor that induced malignant transformation *in vitro*. It is now recognized as a prototype member of a growing superfamily of secreted, disulfide-linked homodimeric polypeptides. These factors affect a variety of biological processes in both transformed and normal cells including regulation of cellular proliferation and differentiation [82, 83]. TGFα is expressed throughout the GI tract with the highest amounts found in the colon [84]. Similar to EGF in structure and activity, TGFα stimulates intestinal cell proliferation and may promote cell migration and modulate intestinal membrane transport [85, 86]. It promotes migration of many cell types, including intestinal epithelial cells. In the normal human adult, TGFα is localized in small intestinal villi and restricted to the upper third of colonic crypts [87]. This pattern of distribution within the differentiated regions of the intestinal epithelium suggests TGFα, along with proliferative effects, may play an equally important role in cell differentiation. Such mediated migration may not only be important in cell differentiation from crypt to luminal surface, but also in rapid restitution of the gut barrier after injury to the intestinal epithelium [88].

As mentioned, TGFα and EGF share the same intestinal cell-surface receptor (EGF/TGFα receptor) on intestinal epithelial cells. Because EGF is limited within the intestinal tract, TGFα is probably the natural ligand for this receptor. Indeed, coexpression of TGFα and EGF/TGFα receptor transcripts from morphologically normal human colonic epithelium has been reported [89]. Nevertheless, how these TGFα stimulated receptors signal or promote specific physiologic effects in the gut via an autocrine or paracrine mechanism remains to be determined.

In contrast to TGFα, TGFβ appears to inhibit cell proliferation *in vitro* and *in vivo* [90]. TGFβ has the ability to induce differentiation and maturation by activating cells to develop into a non-proliferative state [91]. In HT29 colon carcinoma sublines, TGF-β1 blocks or restricts cells in early G1 phase of the cell cycle where immature colonocytes begin to differentiate [92]. Although initially thought to be greatest in crypt cells and least in columnar villous cells [93], recent studies have demonstrated that TGFβ activity and mRNA content are greatest in columnar villous cells and least in the crypt cells [91, 94]. In embryonic mice, isoform-specific antibodies intensively stain TGF-β1 in differentiated cells localized in villi and crypt surfaces of small intestine and colon, respectively [95].

As with TGFα, TGFβ may mediate rapid restitution of the gut barrier after injury to the intestinal epithelium. Although addition of this peptide inhibits cell proliferation in IEC-6 monolayers after "injury" with a razor blade, TGFβ nevertheless enhances restitution by quickening cell migration into the artificially induced wounds [96]. Thus, TGFβ may accelerate healing of intestinal epithelial cells *in vivo* by inducing rapid cell migration into wounds. Injection of TGFβ *in vivo* induces hypercellular lesions probably due to a chemoattractant activity on fibroblasts and monocytes which undergo subsequent activation, rather than a direct proliferative effect [97].

TGFβ, a multifunctional growth factor, binds specifically and with high affinity to a wide variety of cell types [98, 99]. The most widely distributed high affinity TGFβ receptors present on the cell surface are the types I and II receptors. The type I receptor forms together with the type II receptor a heteromeric signaling receptor complex that seems essential for mediating the antiproliferative effects of TGFβ.

Endothelins

Endothelins belong to a family of peptides with 21 amino acids. Endothelin-1 is a product of endothelial cells, in addition, the human genome processes the genes for endothelin-2 and endothelin-3. The production of endothelins is increased during critical illness (hypoxia) or receptor-operating agonists like catecholamines, platelet-derived products, angiotensin II, arginine vasopressin and interleukin-1. Endothelin production is inhibited by endothelin-derived nitric oxide via the formation of guanosine monophosphate as well as by a putative smooth muscle cell-derived inhibitory factor [100–102].

The biological role of endothelin is yet uncertain, but clearly the peptides have potent biological properties such as vasoconstruction, vasodilation, and in the intestinal tract, proliferation of different cell lines [100–102].

Conclusion

It seems clear that a large number of growth factors remain to be characterized, and it is to be expected that the understanding of their receptor signal transduction mechanisms will allow the design of specific antagonists. It remains to be seen whether the selectivity of these antagonists will be useful for therapeutic manipulation because many distinct differentiated cell types may respond to the same factor with fundamentally different consequences. This crosstalk probably reflects the modulation of a cell's response, in developmental time and location, by a panel of synergistically acting factors. The unravelling of these complex responses is an enormously challenging task. The whole growth factor field is at a very exciting stage because we will see in the next few years answers to questions of basic research which have therapeutic implications. Indeed, newly acquired experience gained by efforts of scientists is rapidly accepted and absorbed by mankind. Panta rei: nothing is static, everything changes. Surprising and exciting medical progress of yesterday belongs today to the common daily medical practice.

References

1. Nicola NA (1994) An introduction to the cytokines. In: Nicola NA (ed) Cytokines and their receptors. Oxford University Press, Oxford, New York, Tokyo, pp 1-7
2. Boulay J, Paul WE (1993) Hemapoietin sub-family classification based on size, gene organization and sequence homology. Current Biology 3:573-581
3. Bazan JF (1991) Neuropoietic cytokines in the hematopoetic fold. Neuron 7:197-208
4. Sprang SR, Bazan JF (1993) Cytokine structural taxonomy and mechanisms of receptor engagement. Curr Opin Structural Biol 3:815-827
5. Bussolino F, DiRenzo MF, Ziche M, et al (1992) Hepatocyte growth factor is a potent angiogenic factor which stimulates endothelial cell motility and growth. J Cell Biol 119:629-641
6. Vanderhoof JA (1993) Regulatory peptides and intestinal growth. Gastroenterology 104:1205-1208
7. Lund PK, Ulshen MH, Rountree DB, et al (1990) Molecular biology of gastrointestinal peptides and growth factors: Relevance to intestinal adaptation. Digestion 46 (Suppl):66-73
8. Weidner KM, Behrens J, Vandekerckhove J, et al (1990) Scatter factor: Molecular characteristics and effect on the invasiveness of epithelial cells. J Cell Biol 111:2097-2108
9. DiRenzo MF, Narsimhan RP, Olivero M, et al (1991) Expression of the Met/HGF receptor in normal and neoplastic human tissues. Oncogene 6:1997-2003
10. Prat M, Narsimhan RP, Crepaldi T (1991) The receptor encoded by the human c-MET oncogene is expressed in hepatocytes, epithelial cells and solid tumours. Int J Cancer 49:323-328
11. Gherardi E, Stoker M (1991) Hepatocyte growth factor - scatter factor: Mitogen, motogen, and met. Cancer Cells 3:227-232
12. Seki T, Hagiya M, Shimonishi M, et al (1991) Organization of the human hepatocyte growth factor-encoding gene. Gene 102:213-219
13. Saccone S, Narsimhan RP, Gaudino G, et al (1992) Regional mapping of the human hepatocyte growth factor (HGF)-scatter factor gene to chromosome 7q21.1 Genomics 13:912-914
14. Wells JA, Cunningham BC, Fuh G, et al (1993) The molecular basis for growth hormone-receptor interactions. Recent Prog Hormone Res 48:253-275
15. Fuh G, Colosi P, Wood WI, et al (1993) Mechanism-based design of prolactin receptor antagonists. J Biol Chem 268:5376-5381
16. Kelly PA, Ali S, Rozakis M, et al (1993) The growth hormone/prolactin receptor family. Recent Prog Hormone Res 48:123-164
17. Konturek SJ (1990) Role of growth factors in gastroduodenal protection and healing of peptic ulcers. Gastroenterol Clin North Am 19:41-65
18. Leblond CP, Carriere R (1955) The effect of growth hormone and thyroxine on the mitotic rate of the intestinal mucosa of the rat. Endocrinology 56:265-270
19. Cooke PS, Yonemura CU, Russel SM, et al (1986) Growth and differentiation of fetal rat intestine transplants: Dependence on insulin and growth hormone. Biol Neonate 49:211-215
20. Read LC, Lemmey AB, Howarth GS, et al (1991) The gastrointestinal tract is one of the most responsive target tissues for IGF-I and its potent analogs. In: Spencer EM (ed) Modern Concepts of Insulin-like Growth Factors, Amsterdam, Elsevier, pp 225-234
21. Behringer RR, Lewin TM, Quaife CJ, et al (1990) Expression of insulin-like growth factor I stimulates normal somatic growth in growth hormone-deficient transgenic mice. Endocrinology 127:1033-1040

390   P. Fürst and J.L. Rombeau

22. Lobie PE, Breipohl W, Waters MJ (1990) Growth hormone receptor expression in the rat gastrointestinal tract. Endocrinology 126:299–306
23. Hart MH, Phares CK, Erdman SH, et al (1987) Augmentation of post-resection mucosal hyperplasia by pleroceroid growth factor. Dig Dis Sci 32:1275–1278
24. Ulshen MH, Dowling RH, Fuller CD, et al (1993) Enhanced growth of small bowel in transgenic mice overexpressing bovine growth hormone. Gastroenterology 104:973–980
25. Matthews LS (1991) Molecular biology of growth hormone receptors. Trends Endocrinol Metab 2:176–180
26. Vaubourdolle M, Salvucci M, Cynober L (1986) Plasma concentrations of vasoactive intestinal polypeptide in severely burned patients: Influence of enteral nutrition. Clin Nutr 5:217–220
27. Carpenter G, Wahl MI (1990) In: Sporn MB, Roberts AB (eds) Peptide growth factors and their receptors. Springer, Berlin, pp 69–171
28. Al Nafussi AI, Wright NA (1982) The effect of epidermal growth factor (EGF) on cell proliferation of the gastrointestinal mucosa in rodents. Virchows Arch Cell Pathol 40:63–69
29. Conteas CN, Majumdar APN (1987) The effects of gastrin, epidermal growth factor, and somatostatin on DNA synthesis in a small intestinal crypt cell line (IEC-6). Proc Soc Exp Biol Med 184:307–311
30. Sullivan PB, Brueton MJ, Tabara Z, et al (1991) Epidermal growth factor in necrotising enteritis. Lancet 338:53–56
31. Derynck R (1988) Transforming growth factor α. Cell 43:593–595
32. Downward J, Yarden Y, Mayes E, et al (1984) Close similarity of epidermal growth factor receptor and V-er^6 B oncogene protein sequences. Nature 307:521–527
33. Weaver LH, Walker WA (1988) Epidermal growth factor and the developing human gut. Gastroenterology 94:845–847
34. Malo C, Menard D (1982) Influence of epidermal growth factor on the development of suckling mouse intestinal mucosa. Gastroenterology 83:28–35
35. Beaulieu JF, Calvert R (1981) The effect of epidermal growth factor on the differentiation of the rough endoplasmic reticulum in fetal mouse small intestine in organ culture. J Histochem Cytochem 29:765–770
36. Goodlad R, Wilson TJ, London W, et al (1987) Intravenous but not intragastric urogastrone EGF is trophic to the intestine of parenterally fed rats. Gut 28:573–582
37. Ulshen MH, Lyn-Cook L, Roasch R (1986) Effects of intraluminal epidermal growth factor on mucosal proliferation in the small intestine of adult rats. Gastroenterology 91:1134–1140
38. Foster HM, Whitehead RH (1990) Intravenous but not intracolonic epidermal growth factor maintains colonocyte proliferation in defunctioned rat colorectum. Gastroenterology 99:1710–1714
39. Goodlad RA, Lee CY, Wright NA (1992) Cell proliferation in the small intestine and colon of intravenously fed rats: Effects of urogastrone-epidermal growth factor. Cell Prolif 25:393–404
40. Chaef MS, Arya G, Ziegler MM, Warner BW (1994) Epidermal growth factor enhances intestinal adaptation after massive small bowel resection. J Pediatric Surg 29:1035–1039
41. O'Loughlin E, Winter M, Shun A, Hardin A, Gall GD (1994) Structural and functional adaptation following jejunal resection in rabbits. Effect of epidermal growth factor. Gastroenterology 107:87–93
42. Thompson J (1988) Specific receptors for epidermal growth factor in rat intestinal microvillus membranes. Am J Physiol 254:G429–G435
43. Carpenter G (1987) Receptors for epidermal growth factor and other polypeptide mitogens. Ann Rev Biochem 56:881–914
44. Opleta-Madsen K, Hardin J, Gall DG (1991) Epidermal growth factor upregulates intestinal electrolyte and nutrient transport. Am J Physiol 260:G807–G814
45. Helmstaedter V, Feurle GE, Forssmann WG (1977) Ultrastructural identification of a new cell type the N-cell as the source of neurotensin in the gut mucosa. Cell Tissue Res 184:445–452

46. Wood JG, Hoang HD, Bussjaeger LJ, et al (1988) Neurotensin stimulates growth of small intestine in rats. Am J Physiol 255:G812–G817
47. Izukura M, Parekh D, Evers BM, et al (1990) Neurotensin stimulates colon growth in rats. Gastroenterology 98:A416 (Abst)
48. Evers BM, Izukura M, Townsend CM Jr, et al (1992) Neurotensin prevents intestinal mucosal hypoplasia in rats fed an elemental diet. Dig Dis Sci 37:425–431
49. Evers BM, Izukura M, Chung DH, et al (1991) Molecular mechanisms of intestinal adaptation after resection. Surg Forum 42:130–132
50. Izukura M, Evers BM, Parekh D, et al (1992) Neurotensin augments intestinal regeneration after small bowel resection in rats. Ann Surg 215:520–527
51. Evers BM, Beauchamp RD, Ishizuka J, et al (1991) Post-transcriptional regulation of neurotensin in the gut. Surgery 110:247–252
52. Bondy CA, Werner H, Roberts CT Jr, et al (1990) Cellular pattern of insulin-like growth factor-I (IGF-I) and type I IGF receptor gene expression in early organogenesis: Comparison with IGF-II gene expression. Mol Endocrinol 4:1386–1398
53. Daughaday WH, Rotwein P (1989) Insulin-like growth factor I and II. Peptide, messenger ribonucleic acid and gene structures, serum and tissue concentration. Endocrinol Rev 10:68–91
54. Lemmey AB, Martin AA, Read LC, et al (1991) IGF-I and the truncated analogue des-(1-3) IGF-I enhance growth in rats after gut resection. Am J Physiol 260:E213–E219
55. Vanderhoof JA, McCusker RH, Clark R, et al (1992) Truncated and native insulin-like growth factor I enhance mucosal adaptation after jejunoileal resection. Gastroenterology 102:1949–1956
56. Laburthe M, Rouyer-Fessard C, Gammeltoft S (1988) Receptors for insulin-like growth factors I and II in rat gastrointestinal epithelium. Am J Physiol 254:G457–G462
57. Park JHY, McCusker RH, Vanderhoof JA, et al (1992) Secretion of insulin-like growth factor II (IGF-II) and IGF-binding protein-2 by intestinal epithelial (IEC-6) cells: Implications for autocrine growth regulation. Endocrinology 131:1359–1368
58. Mantell MP, Ziegler TR, Adamson WT, Roth JA, et al (1995) Resection-induced colonic adaptation is augmented by IGF-I and associated with upregulation of colonic IFG mRNA. Am J Physiol 269:G974–G980
59. Olanrewaju H, Patel L, Seidel ER (1992) Trophic action of local intra-ileal infusion of insulin-like growth factor I: Polyamine dependence. Am J Physiol 263:E282–E286
60. Adamson WT, Lew JI, Smith RJ, Rombeau JL (1995) Intraluminal delivery of IGF-I augments post-resection intestinal adaptation without systemic absorption. Surgical Forum 46:184–187
61. Han VKM, d'Ercole AJ, Lund PK (1987) Cellular localization of somatomedin/insulin-like growth factor mRNAs in the human fetus. Science 236:193–197
62. Humbel RE (1990) Insulin-like growth factors I and II. Eur J Biochem 190:445–462
63. Park JHY, Vanderhoof JA, Blackwood D, et al (1990) Characterization of type I and II insulin-like growth factor receptors in an intestinal epithelial cell line. Endocrinology 126:2998–3005
64. Orlowski CC, Brown AL, Ooi GT, et al (1990) Tissue, developmental and metabolic regulation of messenger ribonucleic acid encoding a rat insulin-like growth factor-binding protein. Endocrinology 126:644–652
65. Gopinath R, Watson PE, Etherton TD (1989) An acid-stable insulin-like growth factor (IGF-)binding protein from pig serum inhibits binding of IGF-I and IGF-II to vascular endothelial cells. J Endocrinol 120:231–236
66. Albiston AL, Taylor RG, Herington AC, et al (1992) Divergent ileal IGF-I and IGFBP-3 gene expression after small bowel resection: A novel mechanism to amplify IGF action? Mol Cell Endocrinol 83:R17–R20
67. Blum WF, Jenne EW, Reppin F, et al (1989) Insulin-like growth factor I (IGF-I) binding protein complex is a better mitogen than free IGF-I. Endocrinology 125:766–772
68. Jyung RW, Mustoe TA, Busby WH, Clemmons DR (1994) Increased wound-breaking strength induced by IGF-I in combination with IGFBP-1. Surgery 115:233–239

69. Termanini B, Nardi RV, Finam TM, et al (1990) Insulin-like growth factor I receptors in rabbit gastrointestinal tract. Characterization and autoradiographic localization. Gastroenterlogy 99:51–60
70. Simmons JG, Hoyt, EC, Westwick HK, Brenner DA, et al (1995) Insulin-like growth factor-I and epidermal growth factor interact to regulate growth and gene expression in IEC-6 intestinal epithelial cells. Molecular Endocrinology 9:1157–1165
71. Ziegler TR, Mantell MP, Robeau JL, Smith RL (1994) Effects of glutamine and IGF-I pathway after partial small bowel resection. J Parent Enteral Nutr 18:205
72. Zhang W, Bain A, Robeau JL (1995) Insulin like growth factor-I (IGF-I) and glutamine improve structure and function in the small bowel allograft. J Surg Res (In press)
73. Pilion DJ, Haskell JF, Atchison JA, et al (1989) Receptors for IGF-I, but not for IGF-II, on proximal colon epithelial cell apical membranes. Am J Physiol 257:E27–E34
74. Rouyer-Fessard C, Gammeltoft S, Laburthe M (1990) Expression of two types of receptor for insulin-like growth factor in human colonic epithelium. Gastroenterology 98:703–707
75. Grey V, Rouyer-Fessard C, Gammeltoft S, et al (1991) Insulin-like growth factor II/mannose-6-phosphate receptors are transiently increased in the rat distal intestinal epithelium after resection. Mol Cell Endocrinol 75:221–227
76. Basilico C, Moscatelli D (1992) The FGF family of growth factor and oncogenes. Adv Cancer Res 59:115–165
77. Partanen J, Vainikka S, Alitalo K (1993) Structural and functional specificity of FGF receptors. Biol Sci 340:297–303
78. Yayon A, Klagsbrun M, Esko JD, et al (1991) Cell surface, heparin-like molecules are required for binding of basic fibroblast growth factor to its high affinity receptor. Cell 64:841–848
79. Salmvirta M, Heino J, Jalkanen M (1992) Basic fibroblast growth factor-syndecan complex at cell surface or immobilized to matrix promotes cell growth. J Biol Chem 267:17606–17610
80. Peters KG, Ornitz D, Werner S, et al (1993) Unique expression pattern of the FGF receptor 3 gene during mouse organogenesis. Rev Biol 155:423–430
81. Wanaka A, Milbrandt J, Johnson EM Jr (1991) Expression of FGF receptor gene in rat development. Development 111:455–468
82. Derynck R (1996) The biological complexity of transforming growth factor-β. In: Thompson A (ed) The cytokine handbook. Academic Press (In press)
83. Massagué J (1990) The transforming growth factor-β family. Annu Rev Cell Biol 6:597–641
84. Cartlidge SA, Elder JB (1989) Transforming growth factor α and epidermal growth factor levels in normal human gastrointestinal mucosa. Br J Cancer 60:657–660
85. Suemori S, Ciacci C, Podolsky DK (1991) Regulation of transforming growth factor expression in rat intestinal epithelial cell lines. J Clin Invest 87:2216–2221
86. Roberts AB, Sporn MB (1990) The transforming growth factor-βs. In: Sporn ME, Roberts AB (eds) Peptide growth factor and their receptors. Springer, Heidelberg, pp 419–472
87. Thomas DM, Nasim MM, Gullick WJ, et al (1992) Immunoreactivity of transforming growth factor in the normal adult gastrointestinal tract. Gut 33:628–631
88. Moore R, Carlson S, Madara JL (1989) Rapid barrier restitution in an *in vitro* model of intestinal epithelial injury. Lab Invest 60:237–244
89. Markowitz SD, Molkentin K, Gerbic C, et al (1990) Growth stimulation by coexpression of transforming growth factor and epidermal growth factor-receptor in normal and adenomatous human colon epithelium. J Clin Invest 86:356–362
90. Roberts AB, Anzano MA, Sporn MB, et al (1985) Type β transforming growth factor: A bifunctional regulator of cellular growth. Proc Natl Acad Sci USA 82:119–123
91. Barnard JA, Beauchamp RD, Coffey RJ, et al (1989) Regulation of intestinal epithelial cell growth by transforming growth factor type β. Proc Natl Acad Sci USA 86:1578–1582
92. Hafez MM, Hsu S, Yan Z, et al (1992) Two roles for transforming growth factor β1 in colon enterocytic cell differentiation. Cell Growth Differ 3:753–762
93. Koyama SY, Podolsky DK (1989) Differential expression of transforming growth factor α and β in rat intestinal epithelial cells. J Clin Invest 83:1768–1773

94. Barnard JA, Beauchamp RD, Coffey RJ, et al (1989a) Transforming growth factors and intestinal epithelium. More questions than answers. Gastroenterology 97:1587–1588
95. Pelton RW, Saxena B, Jones M, et al (1992) Immunolocalization of TGF-β1, TGF-β2 and TGF-β3 in the mouse embryo: Expression patterns suggest multiple roles during embryonic development. J Cell Biol 115:1091–1105
96. Mahida YR, Ciacci C, Podolsky DK (1992) Peptide growth factors: Role in epithelial-lamina propria cell interactions. Ann NY Acad Sci 664:148–156
97. Moses HL, Yang EY, Pietenpol JA (1990) TGF-β stimulation and inhibition of cell proliferation: New mechanistic insights. Cell 63:245–247
98. Segarini P (1991) Clinical application of TGFβ. In: Ciba Foundation Symposium, Wiley, Chichester, pp 29–50
99. Lin HY, Lodish HF (1993) Receptors for the TGF-β superfamily: Multiple polypeptides and serine/threonine kinases. Trends Cell Biol 3:14–19
100. Lüscher TF, Oemar BS, Boulanger CM, et al (1993) Molecular and cellular biology of endothelin and its receptors. Part I. J Hypertension 11:7–11
101. Lüscher TF, Oemar BS, Boulanger CM, et al (1993) Molecular and cellular biology of endothelin and its receptors. Part II. J Hypertension 11:121–126
102. Yanagisawa M, Masaki T (1989) Biochemistry and molecular biology of the endothelins. Tr Pharmacol Sci 10:374–378

Subject Index

Springer-Verlag
and the Environment

$\mathbf{W}$e at Springer-Verlag firmly believe that an international science publisher has a special obligation to the environment, and our corporate policies consistently reflect this conviction.

$\mathbf{W}$e also expect our business partners – paper mills, printers, packaging manufacturers, etc. – to commit themselves to using environmentally friendly materials and production processes.

$\mathbf{T}$he paper in this book is made from low- or no-chlorine pulp and is acid free, in conformance with international standards for paper permanency.